John Dalton's Colour Vision Legacy

John Dalton's Colour Vision Legacy

Selected proceedings of the international conference

EDITED BY

CHRISTINE DICKINSON, IAN MURRAY

AND

DAVID CARDEN

Department of Optometry and Vision Sciences,
UMIST, Manchester, UK

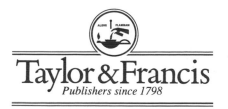

Taylor & Francis
Publishers since 1798

UK   Taylor & Francis Ltd, 1 Gunpowder Square, London EC4A 3DE
USA   Taylor & Francis Inc., 1900 Frost Road, Suite 101, Bristol, PA 19007

British Library Cataloguing in Publication Data

A catalogue record for this book is available from the British Library.
ISBN 0-7484-0310-8 (cased)

Library of Congress Cataloging Publication data are available

Cover design by Ian Youngs

Typeset in Times 10/12pt by Poole Typesetting (Wessex) Ltd

Printed in Great Britian by T. J. International Ltd

Contents

SECTION 5 Development and Colour Vision Defects

SECTION 6 Techniques in Colour Visual Testing

SECTION 9 **Models of Colour Vision**

SECTION 10 **Colour Applications**

Preface

Readers of this book cannot help but reflect on the depth of knowledge and range of techniques represented by the discipline loosely referred to as colour science. This volume marks a particularly appealing example. Firstly, John Dalton, a classical empiricist and philosopher in the traditions of his time, makes some observations about his colour vision which at the time may have been startling for those with normal colour vision but, despite their compelling detail, rather banal for those who had come to live with a colour vision abnormality.

Enter, 200 years later, a technique ideally suited to settle the issue of whether Dalton's peculiarity of colour perception was due to loss of either long or medium wavelength receptors. It is hard to imagine a technique apparently further removed from colour science than polymerase chain reaction (PCR). Imagine Dalton's response if he were told that from a tiny fragment of his 200 year old retina it would be possible to amplify the strand of DNA which carried the code for his unusual colour vision. When one adds the historical accidents it is tempting to speculate on divine intervention; Ransome, who removed Dalton's eyes after his death left one of them intact not realising that this would allow a tiny undisturbed sample of retina to be obtained; the eyes survived the ravages of the Second World War being removed from Dalton Hall in Manchester to the premises of the Manchester Literary and Philosophical Society (which was bombed) and subsequently to the Manchester Museum of Science and Industry. Against all odds, the story which began in Manchester in 1794 reached its culmination exactly 200 years later.

Yet there are other examples, many in the chapters which follow, of how colour science seems to have attracted the attention of numerous branches of science. Many diverse techniques have been used to establish that the majority of non-primate mammals have quite poor colour discrimination, being mainly dichromatic. Techniques based on molecular genetics have shown that the New World monkeys appear to have a kind of genetically-based half-way house between dichromacy and full trichromacy. Due to polymorphism many of these species have the potential of expressing three distinct cone types.

The importance of colour discrimination in primates is almost a biological luxury compared with the requirements of some of the lower vertebrates such as bees and some shallow water fishes. Here colour vision reaches true tetrachromacy with many of these species having equally spaced receptor sensitivity ranging from the near ultra violet to the infra red. Intracellular electrophysiological techniques have shown that bees possess interneurons with a similar function to that of human retinal ganglion cells, showing colour opponency. Furthermore, although the receptors of vertebrates and invertebrates are totally different, the post-receptoral processes are remarkably similar, with chromatic adaptation and colour constancy phenomena appearing in many species. Behavioural experiments on goldfish match the electrophysiology; they have revealed not only some striking morphological changes linked to changes in adaptation, but also the remarkable effects of the drug ethambutol on post-receptoral colour opponent cells. In large doses, ethambutol cancels colour opponency; perhaps even more remarkable is the observation that it has similar effects in humans.

Despite the staggering range of techniques and disciplines applied to colour vision in the last two hundred years and the apparent acceleration in progress over the last two decades, some might be forced to the conclusion that two hundred years is a short time in colour science; there are still many gaps in our understanding. Not least of these is the complexity of the neurophysiological processing of colour information and the formidable problems surrounding so-called colour constancy. Understanding how the stability of the perceived colour of a surface is achieved, regardless of the ambient illumination is attractive to neurophysiologists, psychologists and mathematicians alike. Here is a problem exceptional in its complexity. The effects are perceptually robust and there is an area in the monkey brain which has the necessary neural processing power and sampling characteristics to take account of ambient illumination. Despite this evidence to the contrary, many authors continue to insist that retinal processing accounts for constancy effects. In 200 years' time colour scientists may marvel at the progress made in the 20th century; they may also reflect on the naivety which made us try to identify a single anatomical site for a process as complex as colour constancy.

ACKNOWLEDGEMENTS

A meeting such as The John Dalton Conference cannot be successful without the efforts of a small group of committed people. We are particularly grateful to Janus Kulikowski who inspired us with the idea for the conference but was prepared to take a back seat role. We would also like to thank all those who worked so competently both during the conference and for the many months beforehand, such as Jacqui Grant, all the staff of The Visual Sciences Laboratory in the Department of Optometry and Visual Sciences at UMIST, and the Manchester Library Theatre, in particular Chris Honer. Thanks are also due to the Applied Vision Association who gave us a vote of confidence by agreeing to underwrite the project. The following kindly agreed to referee the chapters which for the most part were submitted on time and in the correct format: Professor Janus Kulikowski, Dr Malik Nacer, Professor David Foster, Professor Keith Ruddock, Professor Neil Charman, Professor Jack Moreland, Ms Sarah Hosking and Dr Vince Walsh. Finally and perhaps most importantly we would like to thank all those who attended the conference and contributed chapters. Without them we would not have been able to mark this singular moment in the history of colour science with this volume.

Contributors

S.L. ALVAREZ
College of Optometry, Ohio State University, 338W 10th Avenue, Columbus, Ohio 43210, USA

D. V. de ALWIS
Sussex Eye Hospital, Eastern Road, Brighton, East Sussex, UK

M. BACH
Universität-Augenklinik, University of Freiburg Killianstrasse 5, 79106 Freiburg, Germany

W. BACKHAUS
Institut für Neurobiologie, Freie Universität Berlin, Thielallee 63, 14195 Berlin, Germany

B.G. BATCHELOR
Department of Computing Mathematics, University of Wales Cardiff, PO Box 916, Senghennydd Road, Cardiff CF2 4YN, Wales, UK

L. BEDARIDA
Istituto Policattedra di Discipline Biologiche, Università di Pisa, Pisa, Italy

V. BIASI
Department of Psychology, 1st University of Rome, Via dei Marsi 78, 00185 Rome, Italy

J. BIRCH
Applied Vision Research Centre Department of Optometry and Visual Science, The City University, Northampton Square, London EC1V OHB, UK

B. BLUM
Department of Physiology and Pharmacology, Sackler School of Medicine, Tel Aviv University, Ramat Aviv, Tel Aviv 69978, Israel

M. BONAIUTO
Department of Developmental and Social Psychology, 1st University of Rome, Via dei Marsi 78, 00185 Rome, Italy

P. BONAIUTO
Department of Psychology, 1st University of Rome, Via Caio Mario 8, 00192 Rome, Italy

J.K. BOWMAKER
Department of Visual Science, Institute of Ophthalmology, University of London, Bath Street, London EC1V 9EL, UK

J. VAN BRAKEL
Institute of Philosophy, University of Leuven, Kardinaal Mercierplein 2, 3000 Leuven, Belgium

P.J. BRENT
Biophysics Section, Physics Department, Imperial College, Prince Consort Rd, London SW7 2BZ, UK

C. BURDEN
Applied Vision Research Centre, Department of Optometry and Visual Science, The City University, London EC1V OHB, UK

D.C. BURR
Istituto di Neurofisiologia del CNR, Via San Zeno 51, 56100 Pisa, Italy

A. BUSBY
Upbury Manor School, Gillingham, Kent, UK

J. B. CALDERONE
Department of Psychology, University of California, Santa Barbara, CA 93106, USA

M. A. CARBON
160 Waring Way, Merritt Island FL 32952–6213, USA

D. CARDEN
Visual Sciences Laboratory, Department of Optometry and Vision Sciences, UMIST, PO Box 88, Sackville Street, Manchester M60 1QD, UK

A.G. CASSWELL
Sussex Eye Hospital, Eastern Road, Brighton, East Sussex, UK

W.N. CHARMAN
Department of Optometry and Vision Sciences, UMIST, PO Box 88, Sackville Street, Manchester M60 1QD, UK

A.S. CAMPERIO CIANI
Department of General Psychology, University of Padua, via Venezia 8, 35139, Padua, Italy

B.L. COLE
Department of Optometry, University of Melbourne, Carlton, Victoria 3053, Australia

K. CONNOLLY
University of Prince Edward Island, Charlottetown, Prince Edward Island, CIA 4P3, Canada

F. DEAN
Sussex Eye Hospital, Eastern Road, Brighton, East Sussex, UK

G. DEREFELDT
National Defence Research Establishment, Department of Human Studies, Division of Human Factors, FOA 53, PO Box 1165, S-58111 Linköping, Sweden

S.S. DHURI
Department of Chemical Technology, University of Bombay, Matunga, Bombay 400019, India

C. DICKINSON
Department of Optometry and Vision Sciences, UMIST, PO Box 88, Sackville Street, Manchester M60 1QD, UK

K.S. DULAI
Department of Molecular Genetics, Institute of Ophthalmology, University of London, Bath Street, London EC1V 9EL, UK

M.J. EARLEY
College of Optometry, Ohio State University, 338W 10th Avenue, Columbus, OH 43210, USA

S.N. ENDRICHOVSKY
Helmholtz Scientific Research Institute of Eye Disease, Sadovaja-Chernogrjasskaja 14/19, Moscow, Russia

B.J.W. EVANS
Institute of Optometry, 56–62 Newington Causeway, London, SE1 6DS, UK

M.D. FAIRCHILD
Munsell Colour Science Laboratory, Center for Imaging Science, Rochester Institute of Technology, 54 Lomb Memorial Drive, Rochester, NY 14623–5604, USA

G.D. FINLAYSON
Department of Computer Science, University of York, York, YO1 5DD, UK

R. FLAVELL
The Management School, Imperial College, London SW7 2PG, UK

D.H. FOSTER
Department of Vision Sciences, Aston University, Birmingham B4 7ET, UK

B.V. FUNT
School of Computing Science, Simon Fraser University, Vancouver, British Columbia V5A 1S6, Canada

J. GERLING
Universität-Augenklinik, University of Freiburg, Killianstrasse 5, 79106 Freiburg, Germany

A.M. GIANNINI
Department of Psychology, 1st University of Rome, Via dei Marsi 78, 00185, Rome, Italy

R.T. GILDAY
School of Engineering, University of Sussex, Brighton, East Sussex BN1 9QT, UK

P. GRASSIVARO GALLO
Via S. Pietro 128/b, 35139, Padova, Italy

V.C. GUPTE
Milton Roy, Bombay, India

C.J. HAWKYARD
Department of Textiles, UMIST, PO Box 88, Sackville Street, Manchester M60 1QD, UK

J.K. HOVIS
School of Optometry, University of Waterloo, Waterloo, Ontario N2L 3G1, Canada

D.M. HUNT
Department of Molecular Genetics, Institute of Ophthalmology, University of London, Bath Street, London EC1V 9EL, UK

M. IKEDA
School of Architecture, Faculty of Engineering, Kyoto University, Yoshida-Honmachi, Sakyo-Ku, Kyoto 606-01, Japan

M. ISHIWATA
Department of Image Science, Chiba University, 1-33 Yayoicho, Inage-ku, Chiba 263, Japan

T. ITO
School of Science and Engineering, Waseda University, 3-4-1 Ohkubo, Shinjuku, Tokyo 169, Japan

G.H. JACOBS
Department of Psychology, University of California, Santa Barbara, CA 93106, USA

K.L. JACOBS
110 Main Street, Bloomingdale, Ontario N0B 1K0, Canada

R. JEANES
MRC Applied Psychology Unit, 15 Chaucer Road, Cambridge CB2 2EF, UK

G. JORDAN
Department of Experimental Psychology, University of Cambridge, Dawning Street, Cambridge CB2 3EB, UK

H. JORDAN
School of Psychology, University of Wales, Bangor, Gwynedd, LL57 2DG, UK

P.E. KING-SMITH
College of Optometry, Ohio State University, 338 W 10th Avenue, Columbus, OH 43210, USA

P.J. KNOWLES
Sussex Eye Hospital, Eastern Road, Brighton, East Sussex, UK

C. KON
Eye Department, St George's Hospital, Tooting, London, UK

J.M. KRAFT
Department of Psychology, University of Colorado at Boulder, Campus Box 345, Colorado 80309-0345, USA

J. KRAUSKOPF
Center for Neural Science, New York University, 6 Washington Place, Room 809, New York 10003, USA

J.J. KULIKOWSKI
Visual Sciences Laboratory, Department of Optometry and Vision Sciences, UMIST, PO Box 88, Sackville Street, Manchester M60 1QD, UK

I. KURIKI
Imaging Science and Engineering Laboratory, Tokyo Institute of Technology, 4259 Nagatsuta, Midori-ku, Yokohama 227, Japan

N. LAUINGER
Institut für Optosensorik IOS, Kalsmunt-Westhang 9, 35578 Wetzlar, Germany

P. LAYCOCK
Mathematics Department, UMIST, PO Box 88, Sackville Street, Manchester M60 1QD, UK

S.J. LEAT
School of Optometry, University of Waterloo, Waterloo, Ontario N2L 3 G1, Canada

B.B. LEE
Department of Neurobiology, Max Planck Institut for Biophysical Chemistry, Am Fassberg, 37077 Göttingen, Germany

K.J. LINNELL
School of Psychology, Birmingham University, Edgbaston, Birmingham, B15 2TT, UK

A.D. LOGVINENKO
School of Psychology, Queen's University, Belfast, BT9 5BP, UK

J.J. McCANN
Vision Research Laboratory, Polaroid Corporation, 750 Main Street, Cambridge, MA 02178, USA

J.H. MacDONALD
Biophysics Section, Physics Department, Imperial College, London SW7 2BZ, UK

W. McILHAGGA
McGill Vision Research Centre, 687 Pine Ave West, H4–14, Montreal, Quebec H3A 1A1, Canada

D.J. McKEEFRY
Department of Anatomy, University College London, Gower Street, London, WC1E 6BT, UK

D.I.A. MacLEOD
Department of Psychology, University of California, San Diego, 9500 Gilman Drive, La Jolla, CA 92093-0109, USA

J.D. MADDOCKS
Department of Optometry, University of Melbourne, Carlton, Victoria 3053, Australia

T. MEIGEN
Universitäts Augenklinik, University of Freiburg, Killianstr. 5, 79106 Freiburg, Germany

K.F. MIDDLETON
Biophysics Section, Physics Department, Imperial College, London SW7 2BZ, UK

B. MODÉER
National Defence Research Establishment, Department of Human Sciences, Division of Human Factors, FOA 53, PO Box 1165, S 58111 Linköping, Sweden

Y. MOHRI
Department of Image Science, Chiba University, 1-33 Yayoicho, Inage-ku, Chiba 263, Japan

J.D. MOLLON
Department of Experimental Psychology, University of Cambridge, Downing Street, Cambridge CB2 3EB, UK

K. MOMOSE
Department of Electrical and Electronic Engineering, Kanagawa Institute of Technology, 1030 Shimo-ogino, Atsugi, Kanagawa 243–02, Japan

I.R. MOORHEAD
W4 Division, Defence Research Agency, Fort Halstead, Sevenoaks, Kent TN14 7BP, UK

C. MORA-FERRER
Institut für Zoologie III, J. Gutenberg-Universität, 55099 Mainz, Germany

J.D. MORELAND
Communication and Neuroscience Department, University of Keele, Keele, Staffordshire ST5 5BG, UK

A.B. MORLAND
Biophysics Section, Physics Department, Imperial College, London SW7 2BZ, UK

M.C. MORRONE
Istituto di Neurofisiologia del CNR, Via San Zeno 51, 56100, Pisa, Italy

K.T. MULLEN
McGill Vision Research Centre, Department of Ophthamology, McGill University, 687 Pine Avenue West H4-14, Montréal, Québec, Canada

I.J. MURRAY
Visual Sciences Laboratory, Department of Optometry and Vision Sciences, UMIST, PO Box 88, Sackville Street, Manchester, M60 1QD, UK

A.M. NACER
Visual Sciences Laboratory, Department of Optometry and Vision Sciences, UMIST, PO Box 88, Sackville Street, Manchester, M60 1QD, UK

Y. NAKANO
Department of Information Machines and Interfaces, Hiroshima City University, 151-5 Numata-cho, Ozuka, Asa-minami-ku, Hiroshima 731-31, Japan

S. NAKAUCHI
Department of Information and Computer Sciences, Toyohashi University of Technology, 1–1 Hibarigoaka Tempaku, Toyohashi 441, Japan

S.M.C. NASCIMENTO
Department of Physics, University of Minho, 4710 Braga Codex, Portugal

L.I. NESTERUK
Helmholtz Scientific Research Institute of Eye Disease, Sadovaja-Chernogrjasskaja 14/19, Moscow, Russia

C. NEUMEYER
Institute für Zoologie III, J. Gutenberg Universität, Saarstrasse 21, 55099 Mainz, Germany

T. NILSSON
Psychology Department, University of Prince Edward Island, Charlottetown, PEI C1A 4P3, Canada

E. O'DONOGHUE
Manchester Royal Eye Hospital, Oxford Road, Manchester M13 9WH, UK

A. OGAWA
School of Science and Engineering, Waseda University, 3-4-1 Ohkubo, Shinjuku, Tokyo 169, Japan

J.A. OGILVIE
Biophysics Section, Physics Department, Imperial College, Prince Consort Road, London SW7 2BZ, UK

D. OSORIO
School of Biological Sciences, Sussex University, Falmer, Brighton BN1 9QG, UK

A. ORAZEM
Physiologisches Institut II der Universität Düsseldorf, Moorenstrasse 5, D-40225 Düsseldorf, Germany

N.R.A. PARRY
Department of Ophthalmology, Manchester Royal Eye Hospital, Oxford Road, Manchester, M13 9WH, UK

U. PERSSON
National Defence Research Establishment, Department of Human Sciences, Division of Human Factors, FOA 53, PO Box 1165, S 58111 Linköping, Sweden

V. PETRAUSKAS
Sensory Research Group, Vilnius University, Ciurlionio 110–805, Vilnius 2015, Lithuania, CIS

A. PETROV
Russian Research Center, Kurchatov Institute, Kurchatov Sq 1, Moscow 123182, Russia

G.E. PIERCE
College of Optometry, Ohio State University, 338W 10th Avenue Columbus, OH 43210, USA

J.P. REFFIN
School of Engineering, University of Sussex, Brighton, East Sussex, BN1 9QT, UK

L.G. RIPLEY
School of Engineering, University of Sussex, Brighton, East Sussex, BN1 9QT, UK

A.G. ROBSON
12 Hadassah Street, Siddal, Halifax HX3 9AP, UK

L. ROMANA
ISEF of Bologna, Padua Section, Padua, Italy

M.M. ROMANO
Department of Psychology, 1st University of Rome, Via dei Marsi 78, 00185 Rome, Italy

L. ROUTLEDGE
Visual Sciences Laboratory, Department of Optometry and Vision Sciences, UMIST, PO Box 88, Sackville Street, Manchester M60 1QD, UK

J. ROSS
Department of Psychology, The University of Western Australia, Perth, Australia

K.H. RUDDOCK
Department of Physics (Biophysics Section), Imperial College, Prince Consort Road, London SW7 2BZ, UK

B.A.C. SAUNDERS
Department of Anthropology, University of Utrecht, PO Box 80-140, 3508 TC Utrecht, The Netherlands

B.E. SCHEFRIN
Department of Psychology, University of Colorado, Boulder, CO 80309-0345, USA

H. SCHEIBNER
Physiologisches Institut II der Universität Düsseldorf, Moorenstrasse 5, 40225 Düsseldorf, Germany

S. SCHMID
Universität-Augenklinik, University of Freiburg, Killianstrasse 5, D-79106 Freiburg, Germany

A.M. SHAMSHINOVA
Helmholtz Scientific Research Institute of Eye Disease, Sadovaja-Chernogrjasskaja 14/19, Moscow, Russia

SHARANJEET-KAUR
Department of Optometry and Vision Sciences, UMIST, PO Box 88, Sackville Street, Manchester M60 1QD, UK

K. SHINOMORI
Department of Psychology, University of Colorado at Boulder, Muenzinger Psychology Building, Campus Box 345, Boulder, Colorado 80309-0345, USA

S. SHIOIRI
Department of Image Science, Chiba University, 1-33 Yayoicho, Inage-ku, Chiba 263, Japan

S.R. SHUKLA
Department of Chemical Technology, University of Bombay, Nathalal Parik Marg, Matunga, Bombay 400019, India

J. SMALLEY
Human Performance and Operational Feedback Section, Nuclear Electric, Barnwood GL4 7RS, UK

H. SPEKREIJSE
The Laboratory of Medical Physics and Informatics, University of Amsterdam, PO Box 12141, AC Amsterdam-Z0, The Netherlands

Z. STANKEVICIUS
Department of Physics, Vilnius University, Vilnius, Lithuania, CIS

J.F. STEIN
University Laboratory of Physiology, Oxford University, Parks Road, Oxford, OX1 3PT, UK

J.M. STEWARD
Department of Optometry, University of Melbourne, Carlton, Victoria 3053, Australia

T. SUGIYAMA
Imaging Science and Engineering Laboratory, Tokyo Institute of Technology, Nagatsuta, Midori-ku, Yokohama 227, Japan

T. SWARTLING
National Defence Research Establishment, Department of Human Sciences, Division of Human Factors, FOA 53, PO Box 1165, S-58111 Linköping, Sweden

V. TANNER
Sussex Eye Hospital, Eastern Road, Brighton, East Sussex, UK

D.Y. TELLER
Guthrie Hall NI 25, University of Washington, Department of Psychology, Seattle, WA 98195, USA

S.J. TREGEAR
Glasgow Caledonian University, City Campus, Cowcaddens Road, Glasgow, G4OBA, UK

M.F. TRITSCH
Institut für Zoologie III (Biophysik), Johannes Gutenberg Universität Mainz, 55099 Mainz, Germany

T. TROSCIANKO
Department of Psychology, University of Bristol, 8 Woodland Road, Bristol BS8 ITN, UK

K. UCHIKAWA
Department of Intelligence Science, Tokyo Institute of Technology, Graduate School, 4259 Nagatsuta, Midori-ku, Yokohama 227, Japan

A. UCHIYAMA
School of Science and Engineering, Waseda University, 3-4-1 Ohkubo, Shinjuku, Tokyo 169, Japan

H. UJIKE
Human Informatics Department, National Institute of Bioscience and Human Technology, 1-1 Higashi, Tsukuba 305, Japan

I. UMBERS
Human Performance and Operational Feedback Section, Nuclear Electric, Barnwood GL4 7RS, UK

S. USUI
Department of Information and Computer Sciences, Toyohashi University of Technology, 1-1

Hibarigaoka Tempaka, Toyohashi: 441, Japan

H.H. VAITKEVICIUS
Sensory Research Group, Vilnius University, Ciurlionio 110-805, Vilnius, Lithuania, CIS

R. VAN ARSDEL
USAEHA/HSHB M0-V (Vision Conservation), APG-EA, MD 21010, USA

D. VAN LAAR
Department of Psychology, University of Portsmouth, King Charles Street, Portsmouth PO1 2ER, UK

S.V. VICKERS
Sussex Eye Hospital, Eastern Road, Brighton, East Sussex, UK

F. VIVIANI
Department of General Psychology, Universita Degli Studi di Padova, Piazza Capitaniato 3, 35139 Padova, Italy

J.S. WERNER
Department of Psychology, University of Colorado, Boulder, CO 80309-0345, USA

P.F. WHELAN
School of Engineering, Dublin City University, Dublin, Ireland

H.D. WHITEFOOT
Department of Optometry and Vision Sciences, UMIST, PO Box 88, Sackville Street, Manchester M60 1QD, UK

J.J. WIETSMA
The Laboratory of Medical Physics and Informatics, University of Amsterdam, PO Box 12141, AC Amsterdam-ZO, The Netherlands

A.J. WILKINS
MRC Applied Psychology Unit, 15 Chaucer Road, Cambridge CB2 2EF, UK

J.R.WRIGHT
Biophysics Section, Physics Department, Imperial College, Prince Consort Road, London SW7 2BZ, UK

A.A. YACOVLEV
Helmholtz Scientific Research Institute of Eye Disease, Sadovaja-Chernogrjasskaja 14/19, Moscow, Russia

H. YAGUCHI
Department of Image Science, Chiba University, 1–33 Yayoicho, Inage-ku, Chiba 263, Japan

K. YOKOI
Imaging Science and Engineering Laboratory, Tokyo Institute of Technology, 4259 Nagatsuta, Midori-ku, Yokohama 227, Japan

T. YOSHIZAWA
MATTO Lab for Human Information Systems, Kanazawa Institute of Technology, 3–1 Yatsukaho, Matto, Ishikawa 924, Japan

Conference Participants

W. BACKHAUS
Institute für Neurobiologie, Freie Universität Berlin, Thielallee 63, 14195 Berlin, Germany

B.G. BATCHELOR
Department of Computing Mathematics, University of Wales Cardiff, PO Box 916, Senghennydd Road, Cardiff CF2 4YN, Wales, UK

S.S. BERGSTROM
Department of Applied Psychology, University of Umea, Umea, S-90187, Sweden

J. BIRCH
Applied Vision Research Centre, Department of Optometry and Visual Science, The City University, Northampton Square, London EC1V 0HB, UK

B. BLUM
Department of Physiology and Pharmacology, Sackler School of Medicine, Tel Aviv University, Ramat Aviv, Tel Aviv 69978, Israel

P. BONAIUTO
Department of Psychology, 1st University of Rome, Via Caio Mario 8, 00192 Rome, Italy

J.K. BOWMAKER
Department of Visual Science, Institute of Ophthalmology, University of London, Bath Street, London EC1V 9EL, UK

J. VAN BRAKEL
Institute of Philosophy, University of Leuven, Kardinaal Mercierplein 2, 3000 Leuven, Belgium

P.J. BRENT
Biophysics Section, Physics Department, Imperial College, Prince Consort Road, London SW7 2BZ, UK

J. BRISTOW
Biophysics Section, Physics Department, Imperial College, Prince Consort Road, London SW7 2BZ, UK

J.A. BROWN
The Mount, Cliffe Terrace, Baildon, West Yorkshire BD17 5LA, UK

D.C. BURR
Instituto di Neurofisiologia del CNR, Via San Zeno 51, 56100 Pisa, Italy

M.A. CARBON
160, Waring Way, Merritt Island, FL 32952–6213, USA

D. CARDEN
Visual Sciences Laboratory, Department of Optometry and Vision Sciences, UMIST, PO Box 88, Sackville Street, Manchester M60 1QD, UK

W.N. CHARMAN
Department of Optometry and Vision Sciences, UMIST, PO Box 88, Sackville Street, Manchester M60 1QD, UK

B.L. COLE
Head, Department of Optometry, University of Melbourne, Carlton, Victoria 3053, Australia

S. DAIN
School of Optometry, University of New South Wales, Sydney 2052, Australia

G. DEREFELDT
National Defence Research Establishment, Department of Human Studies, Division of Human Factors, FOA 53, PO Box 1165, S-58111 Linköping, Sweden

C. DICKINSON
Department of Optometry and Vision Sciences, UMIST, PO Box 88, Sackville Street, Manchester, M60 1QD, UK

N. DRASDO
Clinical Neurophysiology Unit, Department of Vision Sciences, Aston University, Birmingham B4 7ET, UK

B.J.W. EVANS
Institute of Optometry, 56–62 Newington Causeway, London SE1 6DS, UK

M.D. FAIRCHILD
Munsell Colour Science Laboratory, Center for Imaging Science, Rochester Institute of Technology, 54 Lomb Memorial Drive, Rochester, NY 14623-5604, USA

G.D. FINLAYSON
Department of Computer Science, University of York, York, YO1 5DD, UK

D.H. FOSTER
Department of Vision Sciences, Aston University, Birmingham B4 7ET, UK

A.M. GIANNINI
Department of Psychology, 1st University of Rome, Via dei Marsi 78, 00185 Rome, Italy

R.T. GILDAY
School of Engineering, University of Sussex, Brighton, East Sussex BN1 9QT, UK

S.L. GUTH
School of Optometry, Indiana University, Bloomington, Indiana 47405, USA

T. HASEGAWA
University of the Sacred Heart, Department of Psychology, 4-3-1 Hiroo, Shibuya-ku, Tokyo 150, Japan

C.J. HAWKYARD
Department of Textiles, UMIST, PO Box 88, Sackville Street, Manchester M60 1QD, UK

J.K. HOVIS
School of Optometry, University of Waterloo, Waterloo, Ontario N2L 3G1, Canada

P.A. HOWARTH
Department of Human Sciences, Loughborough University of Technology, Loughborough, Leicestershire LE11 3TU, UK

E.G. HUBERT
Combined Studies Office, Faculty of Science and Engineering, Manchester Metropolitan University, Manchester M1 5GD, UK

D.M. HUNT
Department of Molecular Genetics, Institute of Ophthalmology, University of London, Bath Street, London EC1V 9EL, UK

T. JAASKELAINEN
Vaisala Laboratory, University of Joensuu, PO Box 111, FIN-80101 Joensuu, Finland

G.H. JACOBS
Department of Psychology, University of California, Santa Barbara, CA 93106, USA

K.L. JACOBS
110 Main Street, Bloomingdale, Ontario N0B 1K0, Canada

H. JORDAN
School of Psychology, University of Wales, Bangor, Gwynedd, LL57 2DG, UK

P.E. KING-SMITH
College of Optometry, Ohio State University, 338 W 10th Ave Columbus, OH 43210, USA

J.M. KRAFT
Department of Psychology, University of Colorado at Boulder, Campus Box 345, Colorado 80309-0345, USA

J. KRAUSKOPF
Center for Neural Science, New York University, 6 Washington Place, Room 809, New York 10003, USA

J.J. KULIKOWSKI
Visual Sciences Laboratory, Department of Optometry and Vision Sciences, UMIST, PO Box 88, Sackville Street, Manchester M60 1QD, UK

I. KURIKI
Imaging Science and Engineering Laboratory, Tokyo Institute of Technology, 4259 Nagatsuta, Midori-ku, Yokohama 227, Japan

A. KURTENBACH
Universitäts-Augenklinik, Schleichstrasse 12, Tubingen 72076, Germany

N. LAUINGER
Institut für Optosensorik IOS, Kalsmunt-Westhang 9, 35578 Wetzlar, Germany

B.B. LEE
Department of Neurobiology, Max Planck Institut for Biophysical Chemistry, Am Fassberg, 37077 Göttingen, Germany

B. LING
56 Johnston Parade, South Coogee, NSW 2034, Australia

K.J. LINNELL
School of Psychology, Birmingham University, Edgbaston, Birmingham, B15 2TT, UK

A.D. LOGVINENKO
School of Psychology, Queen's University, Belfast BT9 5BP, UK

J.J. McCANN
Vision Research Laboratory, Polaroid Corporation, 750 Main Street, Cambridge, MA 02178, USA

W. McILHAGGA
McGill Vision Research Centre, 687 Pine Ave West, H4–14, Montreal, Quebec H3A 1A1, Canada

T. MEIGEN
Universitäts Augenklinik, University of Freiburg, Killianstr. 5, D-79106 Freiburg, Germany

B. MERTSCHING
Department of Computer Science, University of Hamburg, Vogt-Kolln-Str 30, D-22527 Hamburg, Germany

J.D. MOLLON
Department of Experimental Psychology, University of Cambridge, Downing Street, Cambridge CB2 3EB, UK

K. MOMOSE
Department of Electrical and Electronic Engineering, Kanagawa Institute of Technology, 1030 Shimo-ogino, Atsugi, Kanagawa, 243–02, Japan

I.R. MOORHEAD
W4 Division, Defence Research Agency, Fort Halstead, Sevenoaks, Kent TN14 7BP, UK

J.D. MORELAND
Communication and Neuroscience Department, University of Keele, Keele, Staffordshire ST5 5BG, UK

A.B. MORLAND
Biophysics Section, Physics Department, Imperial College, London SW7 2BZ, UK

M.C. MORRONE
Istituto di Neurofisiologia del CNR, Via San Zeno 51, 56100 Pisa, Italy

I.J. MURRAY
Visual Sciences Laboratory, Department of Optometry and Vision Sciences, UMIST, PO Box 88, Sackville Street, Manchester M60 1QD, UK

A.M. NACER
Visual Sciences Laboratory, Department of Optometry and Vision Sciences, UMIST, PO Box 88, Sackville Street, Manchester M60 1QD, UK

Y. NAKANO
Department of Information Machines and Interfaces, Hiroshima City University, 151-5 Numata-cho, Ozuka, Asa-minami-ku, Hiroshima 731-31, Japan

S. NAKAUCHI
Department of Information and Computer Sciences, Toyohashi University of Technology, 1-1 Hibarigaoka Tempaku, Toyohashi 441, Japan

S.M.C. NASCIMENTO
Department of Physics, University of Minho, 4710 Braga Codex, Portugal

C. NEUMEYER
Institute für Zoologie III, J. Gutenberg Universität, Saarstrasse 21, 55099 Mainz, Germany

T. NILSSON
Psychology Department, University of Prince Edward Island, Charlottetown, Prince Edward Island C1A 4P3, Canada

J.A. OGILVIE
Biophysics Section, Physics Department, Imperial College, Prince Consort Road, London SW7 2BZ, UK

D. OSORIO
School of Biological Sciences, Sussex University, Falmer, Brighton BN1 9QG, UK

O. PACKER
Center for Visual Science, University of Rochester, Rochester, NY 14627, USA

J. PARKKINEN
Department of Information Technology, Lappeenranta University of Technology, PO Box 20, FIN-53851 Lappeenranta, Finland

N.R.A. PARRY
Vision Science Centre, Manchester Royal Eye Hospital, Oxford Road, Manchester, M13 9WH, UK

V. PETRAUSKAS
Sensory Research Group, Vilnius University, Ciurlionio 110–805, Vilnius 2015, Lithuania, CIS

A.P. PETROV
Russian Research Center, Kurchatov Institute, Kurchatov Sq 1, Moscow 123182, Russia

L.G. RIPLEY
School of Engineering, University of Sussex, Brighton, East Sussex BN1 9QT, UK

A.G. ROBSON
12 Hadassah Street, Siddal, Halifax HX3 9AP, UK

K.H. RUDDOCK
Department of Physics (Biophysics Section), Imperial College, Prince Consort Road, London SW7 2BZ, UK

M.H.A. RUSSELL
17 Ivy Green Rd, Chorlton-cum-Hardy, Manchester M21 1FS, UK

M. SATO
Department of Intelligence Science, Tokyo Institute of Technology, 4259 Nagatsuta, Midori-ku, Yokohama 227, Japan

H. SCHEIBNER
Physiologisches Institut II der Universität Dusseldorf, Moorenstrasse 5, D-40225 Dusseldorf, Germany

A.M. SHAMSHINOVA
Helmholtz Scientific Research Institute of Eye Disease, Sadovaja-Chernogrjasskaja 14/19, Moscow, Russia

K. SHINOMORI
Department of Psychology, University of Colorado at Boulder, Muenzinger Psychology Building, Campus Box 345, Boulder, Colorado 80309-0345, USA

S.R. SHUKLA
Department of Chemical Technology, University of Bombay, Nathalal Parikh Mary, Matunga, Bombay 400019, India

P. SILFSTEN
Department of Information Technology, Lappeenranta University of Technology, PO Box 20, FIN-53851, Lappeenranta, Finland

K.J. SMITH
38 Ladybridge Avenue, Worsley, Manchester M28 3BP, UK

J.A.B. SPALDING
5 Curzon Road, Weybridge, Surrey KT13 8UW, UK

J.F. STEIN
University Laboratory of Physiology, Oxford University, Parks Road, Oxford OX1 3PT, UK

S. SUMI
Psychology Laboratory, Keio University, Hiyoshi, Kohoku-ku, Yokohama 223, Japan

C.M. SUTTLE
Department of Vision Sciences, Aston University, Aston Triangle, Birmingham B4 7ET, UK

D.Y. TELLER
Guthrie Hall NI 25, University of Washington, Department of Psychology, Seattle, WA 98195, USA

S. TORII
University of the Sacred Heart, 4-3-1 Shibuya, Hiroo, Tokyo 150, Japan

T. TORII
Department of Psychology, Japan Women's University, 1-1-1 Nishiikuta, Tamaku, Kawasaki, Kanagawa, Japan

S.J. TREGEAR
Glasgow Caledonian University, City Campus, Cowcaddens Road, Glasgow G4 0BA, UK

M.F. TRITSCH
Institut für Zoologie III (Biophysik), Johannes Gutenberg Universität Mainz, 55099 Mainz, Germany

K. UCHIKAWA
Department of Intelligence Science, Tokyo Institute of Technology, Graduate School, 4259 Nagatsuta, Midori-ku, Yokohama 227, Japan

H. UJIKE
Human Informatics Department, National Institute of Bioscience and Human Technology, 1–1 Higashi, Tsukuba 305, Japan

H.H. VAITKEVICIUS
Sensory Research Group, Vilnius University, Ciurlionio 110-805, Vilnius, Lithuania, CIS

D. VAN LAAR
Department of Psychology, University of Portsmouth, King Charles Street, Portsmouth PO1 2ER, UK

F. VIVIANI
Department of General Psychology, Università degli Studi di Padova, Piazza Capitanato 3, 35139 Padova, Italy

C.M. DE WEERT
NICI, University of Nymegen, PO Box 9104, 6500 HE Nymegen, The Netherlands

A.J. WILKINS
MRC Applied Psychology Unit, 15 Chaucer Road, Cambridge CB2 2EF, UK

B. WINN
Department of Optometry, University of Bradford, West Yorkshire BD7 1DP, UK

J.R. WRIGHT
Biophysics Section, Physics Department, Imperial College, Prince Consort Road, London SW7 2BZ, UK

W.D. WRIGHT
25 Craig Mount, Radlett, Hertfordshire WD7 7LW, UK

H. YAGUCHI
Department of Image Science, Chiba University, 1-33 Yayoicho, Inage-ku, Chiba 263, Japan

T. YAJIMA
Department of Intelligence Science, Tokyo Institute of Technology, 4259 Nagatsuta, Midori-ku, Yokohama 227, Japan

T. YOSHIZAWA
MATTO Lab for Human Information Systems, Kanazawa Institute of Technology, 3-1 Yatsukaho, Matto, Ishikawa 924, Japan

Section 1 – Dalton's Colour Vision

Dalton – Letter

J. Dalton

The flower was pink but it appeared to me almost an exact sky-blue by day; in candlelight however it was astonishingly changed, not having then any blue in it but being what I called red – a colour which forms a striking contrast to blue.

When John Dalton made this observation, and was then surprised to find that only his brother shared the same perception, he was finally convinced of the unusual nature of his own colour vision. As a result of a series of meticulous observations he believed it was 'almost beyond doubt that one of the humours of my eye . . . is a coloured medium'. In fact he left instructions for a post mortem examination of his eyes, but no trace was found of the blue colouration he had predicted. Thirty-six years earlier in 1808, Young had already suggested that congenital colour vision defects arose from the photoreceptors, but Dalton refused to believe it. Despite this, congenital colour vision deficiency is still known as 'Daltonism' in recognition of the fact that Dalton's paper to the Manchester Literary and Philosophical Society on 31 October 1794 was the first description of the condition, and offered a stimulus to many investigators. It was to celebrate the 200th anniversary of this lecture that the John Dalton Conference was held in Manchester in 1994.

John Dalton was born in Eaglesfield in the English Lake District in early September 1766. He was the son of a farmer engaged in the weaving trade and was educated in the village school, but by the age of 11 years he had started his own school in the village. In 1781, at the age of 15, he joined his brother teaching in a school in Kendal, and first met John Gough, the man who taught him the orderly scientific method of careful observation and meticulous recording. His first interest was in meteorology, and he kept a daily journal of his findings until the day before he died. In 1793, he was appointed as teacher of mathematics at New College, Manchester. This school had been set up by religious dissenters to whom the doors of the universities were closed – as in fact they were to Dalton, who was himself a Quaker. On 3 October 1794, Dalton was elected as a member of the 'Lit and Phil', and one month later was reading that first paper 'Extraordinary facts relating to the vision of colours with observations'.

In 1800, he left New College and began private tutoring and public lecturing – one notable pupil was James Prescott Joule. In 1808 he published the atomic theory for which he is chiefly remembered:

every particle of water is like every other particle of water; every particle of hydrogen is like every other particle of hydrogen ... Chemical analysis and synthesis go no farther than to the separation of particles one from another, and to their reunion. No new creation or destruction of matter is within the reach of chemical agency ...

In 1817, he became President of the Lit and Phil, and remained in office until his death, working from a room in the Society's house that had been set aside as a study and laboratory.

Manchester was slow to honour its first internationally-recognised scientist during his lifetime, but he was given a large public funeral preceded by a lying in state attended by over 40 000 Mancunians. Manchester Town Hall contains his statue and portrait, and there is a city centre street named after him.

1.1.1 EXTRACT FROM MANCHESTER MEMOIRS

(*Memoirs and Proceedings of the Manchester Literary and Philosophical Society*, 1924, **68**(9), 113–117, *reproduced by kind permission of the Manchester Literary and Philosophical Society*)

The Society has a most interesting letter of Dalton's, written in February 1794, soon after his arrival in Manchester. It is addressed 'Elihu Robinson, Eaglesfield, near Cockermouth' and is printed below with a few notes.

Manchester, 2d mo. 20th 1794.

Dear Cousin,

Amidst an increasing variety of pursuits. – amidst the abstruse and multifarious speculations resulting from my profession, together with frequent engagements to new friends and acquaintances, shall I find a vacant hour to inform thee where I am, & what I am doing? Yes: certainly one hour out of sixteen some day may be spared for the purpose. I need not inform thee that Manchester was [sic] a large and flourishing place. – Our Academy is a large & elegant building in the most elegant retired Street of the place; it consists of a front & two wings; the first floor of the front is the hall where most of the business is done; over it is a Library with about 3,000 volumes; over this are two rooms, one of which is mine; it is about 8 yards by 6, and above 3 high, has two windows & a fire place, is handsomely papered, light, airy & retired; whether it is that philosophers like to approach as near to the stars as they can, or that they choose to soar above the vulgar into a purer region of the atmosphere, I know not; but my apartment is full 10 yards above the surface of the earth. One of the wings is occupied by Dr Barne's family, he is one of the tutors, & superintendent of the seminary; the other is occupied by a family who manage the boarding, and 17 In-students, with 2 tutors, each individual having a separate room, &c. Our out-students from the town and neighbourhood, at present amount to 9, which is as great a number as has been since the institution: they are of all religious professions; one friend's son from the town has entered since I came: The tutors are all Dissenters. Terms for In-students, 40 Guineas per session (10 months): Out-students, 12 Guineas. Two tutors and the In-students all dine, &c, together in a room on purpose; we breakfast on tea at $8\frac{1}{2}$, dine at $1\frac{1}{2}$, drink tea at 5, and sup at $8\frac{1}{2}$; we fare as well as it is possible for anyone to do. At a small extra Expence we can have any friend to dine, etc., with us in our respective Rooms. My official department of tutor only requires my attendance upon the Students 21 hours in the week: but I find it often expedient to prepare my Lectures previously.

There is in this town a large library,[1] furnished with the best books in every art, science and language, which is open to all, gratis; when thou art apprized of this & such like circumstances, when thou considerest me in my private apartment, undisturbed, having a good fire, & a philosophical apparatus around me, thou wilt be able to form an opinion whether I spend my time in slothful inactivity of body & mind. – The watch word for my retiring to rest, is 'past – 12 o'clock – cloudy morning.'

Now that I have mentioned clouds it leads me to observe that I continue my meteorological journal, have two rain-gages [sic] about a mile off, at a friend's house; one gage is in the garden, & the other upon the flat roof of his house, 10 yards higher than the former. I find that the lower gage catches 12 parts of rain for the upper 11. From my correspondence with my brother it appears they have had about twice the rain we have.

I hope my friends there are not altogether disappointed with my Essays[2] – please make the following correction, & intimate it occasionally to such as have them. Page 37 total rain at Kendal 1790 should be 62.363, and for 1791, 66.200.

Among my late experiments, have had some on the artificial production of cold, but have not been able to freeze quicksilver. I find that two parts of snow & one of common salt, mixed & stirred, produce a cold regularly of $-7°$, or $7°$ below 0. I have sunk the thermometer below 0 in a common wine glass, half-filled with the mixture.

Here is a very considerable body of friends here; near 200 attend our first day meetings. I have received particular civilities from most of them, & am often at a loss where to drink tea on a first day afternoon, being pressed on some many hands. – On first day lately I took a walk, in company with another, to Stockport; there are but few friends there, but the most elegant little meeting house that can be conceived; the Walls and ceiling perfectly white; the wainscot, seats, gallery, &c., all white as possible; the gallery rail turned off at each end in fine serpentine form; a white chandelier; the floor as smooth as a mahogany table, & covered with a light red sand, the house is well-lighted, & in as neat order as possible; it stands upon a hill; in short, in a fine sunny day it is too brilliant an object to be attended, by a stranger at least, with the composure required.

I am at present engaged in a very curious investigation: – I discovered last summer with certainty, that colours appear different to me to what they do to others: The flowers of most of the Cranesbills appear to me in the day, almost exactly *sky blue*, whilst others call them *deep pink*; but happening once to look at one in the night by candle light I found it of a colour as different as possible from day light; it seemed then very near yellow, but with a tincture of red; whilst no body else said it differed from the daylight appearance, my brother excepted, who seems to see as I do. I never till now set about an examination into the matter; I have collected specimens of ribbands, &c, of various colours, and the result, as far as I have yet gone, is nearly as follows. The primary colours, *orange, yellow & blue* appear to me much the same in the night as they do in the day, & I always distinguish them and call them by their proper names, as well as several Drabs and other mixed colours; some *reds*, for instance vermillion, appear the same or alike day & night; but others, & more especially the different shades of *pink*, confound me most completely in the day, they all appearing *light blue*: all the dyed *greens* seem to have little or no green about them; they appear inclining to *red* or to *brown* in the day, & almost *blue* in the night; the *pinks* and *light blues* which appear almost off the same piece in the day, are as opposite as black and white in the night, or by candle light. A piece of silk ribband, which some call a *very deep pink* & others *crimson*, appears to me in the day to be a *very dark drab*, & exactly like another which they call a *mud* colour; in the night however the former seems *red or crimson*, & the latter unchanged. – I was

the other day at a friend's house, who is a dyer; there was present himself and Wife, a
Physician, and a young woman. His wife brought me a piece of cloth, – I said I was there
in a coat just of the colour a few weeks before, which I called a reddish snuff colour; they
told me they had never seen me in any such coat, for that cloth was one of the finest *grass
greens* they had seen. I saw nothing like grass about it. They tell me my Table cloth is
green, but I say not, and further that I never saw a green table cloth in my life, but one,
and everybody else said it had lost its *green* colour. In short my observations have
afforded a fund of diversion to all, & something more to philosophers for they have been
puzzled beyond measure, as well as myself, to account for the Circumstances. – I mean
to communicate my observations to the world through the channel of some philosophical Society. The young women tell me they will never suffer me to go on to the
gallery with a *green* coat; & I tell them I have no objection to their going on with me in
a *crimson* (that is) dark drab gown.

It seems that another of your maids is become mistress; – a good omen for the next,
whoever she may be. – Methinks there may be a question started from some side of the
fire, when this is read, 'I wonder whether John is going to marry yet, or not?'. May
answer that my head is too full of triangles, chymical processes, & electrical experiments, &c. to think much of marriage. I must not however omit to mention that I was
completely Sir Roger de Coverleyed a few weeks ago.

The occasion was this: being desired to call upon a widow, a friend, who thought of
entering her son at the academy, I went, & was struck with the sight of the most perfect
figure that ever human eyes beheld, – in a plain, but neat dress, her person, her features
were engaging beyond all description – upon enquiry after I found that she was
universally allowed to be the handsomest woman in Manchester. – Being invited by her
to tea a few days after, along with a worthy man here, a public friend, I should have in
any other circumstances been highly pleased with an elegant Tea equipage, American
apples of the most delicious flavour, & choice wines, but in the present, these were only
secondary objects. Deeming myself however full proof against *mere beauty*, & knowing
that its concomitants are often ignorance & vanity, I was not under much apprehension;
but when she began to descant upon the excellence of an exact acquaintance with
English grammar & the art of Letter writing – to compare the merits of Johnson's and
Sheridan's dictionaries, – to converse upon the use of 'dephlogisticated marine acid in
bleaching' – upon the effects of opium on the animal system, &c., &c., I was no longer
able to hold out, but surrendered at discretion. During my *captivity*, which lasted about
a week, I lost my appetite, and had other symptoms of bondage about me, as incoherent
discourse, &c., but have now happily regained my freedom.

Having now wrote till I have tired my hand, & probably thy eyes in reading, I shall
conclude with my Love to Cousin Ruth and thyself and to all enquiring Friends,

JOHN DALTON

1.1.2   NOTES

1. Chetham's Library.
2. 'Meteorological Observations and Essays', published 1793.

Extraordinary Facts Relating to the Vision of Colours: With Observations By Mr John Dalton

Read 31 October 1794

First published in *Memoirs of the Manchester Literary and Philosophical Society*, Volume 5, p. 28–45, 1798; reproduced with the kind permission of the Manchester Literary and Philosophical Society.

It has been observed, that our ideas of colours, sounds, tastes, &c. excited by the same object may be very different in themselves, without our being aware of it; and that we may nevertheless converse intelligibly concerning such objects, as if we were certain the impressions made by them on our minds were exactly similar. All, indeed, that is required for this purpose, is, that the same object should uniformly make the same impression on each mind; and that objects which appear different to one should be equally so to others. It will, however, scarcely be supposed, that any two objects, which are every day before us, should appear hardly distinguishable to one person, and very different to another, without the circumstance immediately suggesting a difference in their faculties of vision; yet such is the fact, not only with regard to myself, but to many others also, as will appear in the following account.

I was always of the opinion, though I might not often mention it, that several colours were injudiciously named. The term *pink*, in reference to the flower of that name, seemed proper enough; but when the term *red* was substituted for pink, I thought it highly improper; it should have been *blue*, in my apprehension, as pink and blue appear to me very nearly allied; whilst pink and red have scarcely any relation.

In the course of my application to the sciences, that of optics necessarily claimed attention; and I became pretty well acquainted with the theory of light and colours before I was apprized of any peculiarity in my vision. I had not, however, attended much to the practical discrimination of colours, owing, in some degree, to what I conceived to be a perplexity in their nomenclature. Since the year 1790, the occasional study of botany obliged me to attend more to colours than before. With respect to colours that were *white*, *yellow*, or *green*, I readily assented to the appropriate term. *Blue*, *purple*, *pink*, and *crimson* appeared rather less distinguishable; being, according to my idea, all referable to *blue*. I have often seriously asked a person whether a flower was blue or pink, but was generally considered to be in jest. Notwithstanding this, I was never convinced of a peculiarity in my vision, till I accidentally observed the colour of the flower of the *Geranium zonale* by candle-light in the Autumn of 1792. The flower was pink, but it appeared to me almost an exact sky-blue by day; in candle-light, however, it was astonishingly changed, not having then any blue in it, but being what I called red, a colour which forms a striking contrast to blue. Not then doubting but that the change of colour would be equal to all, I requested some of my friends to observe the phenomenon; when I was surprised to find they all agreed, that the colour was not materially different from what it was by day-light, except my brother who saw it in the same light as myself. This observation clearly proved, that my vision was not like that of other persons; – and, at the same time, that the difference between day-light and candle-light, on some colours, was indefinitely more perceptible to me than to others. It was nearly two years after that time, when I entered upon an investigation of the subject, having procured the assistance of a friend, who, to his acquaintance with the theory of colours, joins a practical knowledge of their names and constitutions. I shall now proceed to state the facts ascertained under the three following heads:

I.   An account of my own vision.
II.   An account of others whose vision has been found similar to mine.
III. Observations on the probable cause of our anomalous vision.

I. Of my own vision

It may be proper to observe, that I am short-sighted. Concave glasses of about five inches focus suit me best. I can see distinctly at a proper distance; and am seldom hurt by too much or too little light; nor yet with long application.

My observations began with the solar *spectrum*, or coloured image of the sun, exhibited in a dark room by means of a glass prism. I found that persons in general distinguish six kinds of colour in the solar image; namely, *red, orange, yellow, green, blue* and *purple*. Newton, indeed, divides the purple into *indigo* and *violet*; but the difference between him and others is merely nominal. To me it is quite otherwise: – I see only *two* or at most *three* distinctions. These I should call *yellow* and *blue*; or *yellow, blue* and *purple*. My yellow comprehends the *red, orange, yellow* and *green* of others; and my *blue* and *purple* coincide with theirs. That part of the image which others call red, appears to me little more than a shade, or defect of light; after that the orange, yellow and green seem *one* colour, which descends pretty uniformly from an intense to a rare yellow, making what I should call different shades of yellow. The difference between the green part and the blue part is very striking to my eye: they seem to be strongly contrasted. That between the blue and purple is much less so. The purple appears to be blue much darkened and condensed. In viewing the flame of a candle by night through the prism, the appearances are pretty much the same, except that the red extremity of the image appears more vivid than that of the solar image.

I now proceed to state the results of my observations on the colours of bodies in general, whether natural or artificial, both by day-light and candle-light. I mostly used ribbands for the artificial colours.

Red
(By day-light.)

Under this head I include *crimson, scarlet, red* and *pink*. All crimsons appear to me to consist chiefly of dark blue; but many of them seem to have a strong tinge of dark brown. I have seen specimens of *crimson, claret*, and *mud*, which were very nearly alike. Crimson has a *grave* appearance, being the reverse of every shewy and splendid colour. Woollen yarn dyed crimson or dark blue is the same to me. *Pink* seems to be composed of nine parts of light blue, and one of red, or some colour which has no other effect than to make the light blue appear dull and faded a little. Pink and light blue therefore compared together, are to be distinguished no otherwise than as a splendid colour from one that has lost a little of its splendour. Besides the pinks, roses, &c. of the gardens, the following British *flora* appear to me blue; namely, *Statice Armeria, Trifolium pratense, Lychnis Floscuculi, Lychnis dioica*, and many of the *Gerania*. The colour of a florid complexion appears to me that of a dull, opake, blackish blue, upon a white ground. A solution of sulphate of iron in the tincture of galls (that is, dilute black ink) upon white paper, gives a colour much resembling that of a florid complexion. It has no resemblance of the colour of blood. *Red* and *scarlet* form a genus with me totally different from pink. My idea of red I obtain from *vermilion, minium, sealing wax, wafers, a soldier's uniform*, &c. These seem to have no blue whatever in them. Scarlet has a more splendid appearance than red. Blood appears to me red; but it differs much from the articles mentioned above. It is much more dull, and to me is not unlike that colour called *bottle-green*. Stockings spotted with blood or with dirt would scarcely be distinguishable.

Red
(By candle-light.)

Red and scarlet appear much more vivid than by day. Crimson loses its blue and becomes yellowish red. Pink is by far the most changed; indeed it forms an excellent contrast to what it is by day. No blue now appears; yellow has taken its place. Pink by candle-light seems to be three parts yellow and one red, or a reddish yellow. The blue, however, is less mixed by day than the yellow by night. Red, and particularly scarlet, is a superb colour by candle-light; but by day some reds are the least shewy imaginable: I should call them dark drabs.

Orange & yellow
(By day-light and candle-light.)

I do not find that I differ materially from other persons in regard to these colours. I have sometimes seen persons hesitate whether a thing was white or yellow by candle-light, when to me there was no doubt at all.

Green
(By day-light.)

I take my standard idea from grass. This appears to me very little different from red. The face of a laurel-leaf (*Prunus Lauro-cerasus*) is a good match to a stick of red sealing-wax; and the back of the leaf answers to the lighter red of wafers. Hence it will be immediately concluded, that I see either red or green, or both, different from other people. The fact is, I believe that they both appear different to me from what they do to others. Green and orange have much affinity also. Apple green is the most pleasing kind to me; and any other that has a tinge of yellow appears to advantage. I can distinguish the different vegetable greens one from another as well as most people; and those which are nearly alike or very unlike to others are so to me. A decoction of bohea tea, a solution of liver of sulphur, ale, &c. &c. which others call brown, appear to me green. Green woollen cloth, such as is used to cover tables, appears to me a dull, dark, brownish red colour. A mixture of two parts mud and one red would come near it. It resembles a red soil just turned up by the plough. When this kind of cloth loses its colour, as other people say, and turns yellow, then it appears to me a pleasant green. Very light green paper, silk, &c. is white to me.

Green
(By candle-light.)

I agree with others, that it is difficult to distinguish greens from blues by candle-light; but, with me, the greens only are altered and made to approach the blues. It is the real greens only that are altered in my eye; and not such as I confound with them by day-light, as the brown liquids abovementioned, which are not at all tinged with blue by candle-light, but are the same as by day, except that they are paler.

Blue
(By day-light and candle-light.)

I apprehend this colour appears very nearly the same to me as to other people, both by day-light and candle-light.

Purple
(By day-light and candle-light.)

This seems to me a slight modification of blue. I seldom fail to distinguish purple from blue; but should hardly suspect purple to be a compound of blue and red. The difference between day-light and candle-light is not material.

Miscellaneous observations

Colours appear to me much the same by moon-light as they do by candle-light.[1]

Colours viewed by lightning appear the same as by day-light; but whether exactly so, I have not ascertained.

Colours seen by electric light appear to me the same as by day-light. That is, pink appears blue, &c.

Colours viewed through a transparent sky-blue liquid, by candle-light, appear to me as well as to others the same as by day-light.

Most of the colours called drabs appear to me the same by day-light and candle-light.

A light drab woollen cloth seems to me to resemble a light green by day. These colours are, however, easily distinguished by candle-light, as the latter becomes tinged with blue, which the former does not. I have frequently seen colours of the drab kind, said to be nearly alike, which appeared to me very different.

My idea of *brown* I obtain from a piece of white paper heated almost to ignition. This colour by day-light seems to have a great affinity to green, as may be imagined from what I have said of greens. Browns seem to me very diversified; some I should call red: – dark brown woollen cloth I should call black.

The light of the rising or setting sun has no particular effect; neither has a strong or weak light. Pink appears rather duller, all other circumstances alike, in a cloudy day.

All common combustible substances exhibit colours to me in the same light; namely, *tallow, oil, wax, pit-coal.*

My vision has always been as it is now.

II. An account of others whose vision has been found similar to mine

It has been already observed that my brother perceived the change in the colour of the geranium such as myself. Since that time having made a great number of observations on colours, by comparing their similarities, &c. by day-light and candle-light, in conjunction with him, I find that we see as nearly alike as any other persons do. He is shorter sighted than myself.

As soon as these facts were ascertained, I conceived the design of laying our case of vision before the public, apprehending it to be a singular one. I remembered, indeed, to have read in the Philosophical Transactions for 1777, an account of *Mr. Harris* of Maryport in Cumberland,[2] who, it was said, 'could not distinguish colours' but his case appeared to be different from ours. Considering, however, that one anomaly in vision may tend to illustrate another, I reperused the account; when it appeared extremely probable that if his vision had been fully investigated, and a relation of it given in the first person, he would have agreed with me. There were four brothers in the same predicament, one of whom is now living. Having an acquaintance in Maryport, I solicited him to propose a few queries to the survivor, which he readily did (in conjunction with another brother, whose vision has nothing peculiar), and from the answers transmitted to me, I could no longer doubt of the similarity of our cases. To render it still more circumstantial, I sent about twenty specimens of different coloured ribbands, with directions to make observations upon them by day-light and candle-light: the result was exactly conformable to my expectation.

It then appeared to me probable, that a considerable number of individuals might be found whose vision differed from that of the generality, but at the same time agreed with my own. Accordingly I have since taken every opportunity to explain the circumstances amongst my acquaintance, and have found several in the same predicament. Only one or two I have heard of who differ from the generality and from us also. It is remarkable that, out of twenty-five pupils I once had, to whom I explained this subject, two were found to agree with me; and, on another similar occasion, one. Like myself, they could see no material difference betwixt pink and light blue by day, but a striking contrast by candle-light. And, on a fuller investigation, I could not perceive they differed from me materially in other colours. They, like all the rest of us, were not aware of their actually seeing colours different from other people; but imagined there was great perplexity in the *names* ascribed to particular colours. I think I have been informed already of nearly twenty persons whose vision is like mine. The family at Maryport consisted of six sons and one daughter; four of the sons were in the predicament in question. Our family consisted of three sons and one daughter who arrived at maturity; of whom two sons are circumstanced as I have described. The others are mostly individuals in families, some of which are numerous. I do not find that the parents or children in any of the instances have been so, unless in one case. Nor have I been able to discover any physical cause whatever for it. Our vision, except as to colours, is as clear and distinct as that of other persons. Only two or three are short sighted. It is remarkable that I have not heard of one female subject to this peculiarity.

From a great variety of observations made with many of the abovementioned persons, it does not appear to me that we differ more from one another than persons in general do. We certainly agree in the principal facts which characterize our vision, and which I have attempted to point out below. It is but justice to observe here, that several of the resemblances and comparisons mentioned in the preceding part of this paper were first suggested to me by one or other of the parties, and found to accord with my own ideas.

Characteristic facts of our vision

1. In the solar spectrum three colours appear; yellow, blue and purple. The two former make a contrast; the two latter seem to differ more in degree than in kind.
2. *Pink* appears, by day-light, to be sky-blue a little faded; by candle-light it assumes an orange or yellowish appearance, which forms a strong contrast to blue.
3. *Crimson* appears a muddy blue by day; and crimson woollen yarn is much the same as dark blue.
4. *Red* and *scarlet* have a more vivid and flaming appearance by candle-light than by day-light.
5. There is not much difference in colour between a stick of red sealing wax and grass, by day.
6. Dark green woollen cloth seems a muddy red, much darker than grass, and of a very different colour.
7. The colour of a florid complexion is dusky blue.
8. Coats, gowns, &c. appear to us frequently to be badly matched with linings, when others say they are not. On the other hand, we should match crimsons with claret or mud; pinks with light blues; browns with reds; and drabs with greens.
9. In all points where we differ from other persons, the difference is much less by candle-light than by day-light.

III. Observations tending to point out the cause of our anomalous vision

The first time I was enabled to form a plausible idea of the cause of our vision, was after observing that a sky-blue transparent liquid modified the light of a candle so as to make it similar to day-light; and, of course, restored to pink its proper colour by day, namely, light blue. This was an important observation. At the same time that it exhibited the effect of a transparent coloured medium in the modification of colours, it seemed to indicate the analogy of solar light to that resulting from combustion; and that the former is modified by the transparent blue atmosphere, as the latter is by the transparent blue liquid. Now the effect of a transparent coloured medium, as Mr. Delaval has proved, is to transmit more, and consequently imbibe fewer of the rays of its own colour, than of those of other colours. Reflecting upon these facts, I was led to conjecture that one of the humours of my eye must be a transparent, but *coloured*, medium so constituted as to absorb *red* and *green* rays principally, because I obtain no proper ideas of these in the solar spectrum; and to transmit blue and other colours more perfectly. What seemed to make against this opinion however was, that I thought red bodies, such as vermilion, should appear black to me, which was contrary to fact. How this difficulty was obviated will be understood from what follows.

Newton has sufficiently ascertained, that opake bodies are of a particular colour from their reflecting the rays of light of that colour more copiously than those of the other colours; the unreflected rays being absorbed by the bodies. Adopting this fact we are insensibly led to conclude, that the more rays of any one colour a body reflects, and the fewer of every other colour, the more perfect will be the colour. This conclusion, however, is certainly erroneous. Splendid coloured bodies reflect light of every colour copiously; but that of their own most so. Accordingly we find, that bodies of all colours, when placed in homogeneal light of any colour, appear of that particular colour. Hence a body that is red may appear of any other colour to an eye that does not transmit red, according as those other colours are more copiously reflected from the body, or transmitted through the humours of the eye.

It appears therefore almost beyond a doubt, that one of the humours of my eye, and of the eyes of my fellows, is a *coloured* medium, probably some modification of blue. I suppose it must be the vitreous humour; otherwise I apprehend it might be discovered by inspection, which has not been done. It is the province of physiologists to explain in what manner the humours of the eye may be coloured, and to them I shall leave it; and proceed to shew that the hypothesis will explain the facts stated in the conclusion of the second part.

1. This needs no further illustration.
2. *Pink* is known to be a mixture of red and blue; that is, these two colours are reflected in excess. Our eyes only transmit the blue excess, which causes it to appear blue; a few red rays pervading the eye may serve to give the colour that faded appearance. In candle-light, red and orange, or some other of the higher colours, are known to abound more proportionably than in day-light. The orange light reflected may therefore exceed the blue, and the compound colour consist of red and orange. Now, the red being most copiously reflected, the colour will be recognized by a common eye under this small modification; but the red not appearing to us, we see chiefly the orange excess: it is consequently to us not a modification but a new colour.
3. By a similar method of reasoning, *crimson* being compounded of red and dark blue, must assume the appearances I have described.
4. Bodies that are red and scarlet probably reflect orange and yellow in greatest plenty, next after red. The orange and yellow, mixed with a few red rays, will give us our idea of red, which is heightened by candle-light, because the orange is then more abundant.
5. Grass-green is probably compounded of green, yellow, and orange, with more or less blue. Our idea of it will then be obtained principally from the yellow and orange mixed with a few green rays. It appears, therefore, that red and green to us will be nearly alike. I do not, however, understand why the greens should assume a bluish appearance to us and to every body else, by candle-light, when it should seem that candle-light is deficient in blue.
6. The green rays not being perceived by us, the remaining rays may, for aught that is known, compound a muddy red.
7. The observations on the phaenomena of pink and crimson, will explain this fact.
8. Suppose a body to reflect red rays as the number 8, orange rays as the number 6, and blue as 5; and another body red 8, orange 6, and blue 6: then it is evident that a common eye, attending principally to the red, would see little difference in those colours; but we, who form our ideas of the colours from the orange and blue, should perceive the latter to be bluer than the former.
9. From the whole of this paper it is evident, that our eyes admit blue rays in greater proportion than those of other people; therefore when any kind of light is less abundant in blue, as is the case with candle-light compared to day-light, our eyes serve in some degree to temper that light, so as to reduce it nearly to the common standard. This seems to be the reason why colours appear to us by candle-light, almost as they do to others by day-light.

I shall conclude this paper by observing, that it appears to me extremely probable, that the sun's light and candle-light, or that which we commonly obtain from combustion, are originally constituted alike; and that the earth's atmosphere is properly a *blue fluid*, and modifies the sun's light so as to occasion the commonly perceived difference.

1.2.1 NOTES

1. Mr Boyle observed colours by moon-light to differ from those by day-light. *Priestley on Vision*, p. 145.
2. A translation of this account, to which is annexed the extraordinary case of M. Colardeau, is inserted in Rozier, *Observations sur la Physique, &c.*, p. 87.

Dalton's Colour Blindness: An Essay in Molecular Biography

John D. Mollon, Kanwaljit S. Dulai and David M. Hunt

1.3.1 HISTORICAL BACKGROUND

John Dalton was already in his 20s when he first suspected that his colour perceptions were abnormal. Shortly after he had moved from Kendal to Manchester in the spring of 1793, he wrote in a letter to Elihu Robinson:

> The flowers of most of the Cranesbills appear to me in the day, almost exactly *sky blue*, whilst others call them *deep pink*; but happening once to look at one in the night by candle light I found it of a colour as different as possible from day light; it seemed then very near yellow, but with a tincture of red. (Source: Lonsdale, 1874)

His brother experienced the same dramatic failure of colour constancy, but most saw no change.

In his first paper to the Manchester Literary and Philosophical Society, on 31 October 1794, Dalton systematically analysed his colour deficiency (Dalton, 1798). There the inconstant Cranesbill is identified as *Geranium zonale*; and from contemporary descriptions (Martyn, 1799) we can be fairly certain that Dalton was referring to the plant now named *Pelargonium zonale*, a native of South Africa cultivated in England as early as 1710 (van der Walt, 1977) (Figure 1.3.1, see colour section). In general, he found that he confounded crimsons with blues and scarlets with greens. '*Red* and *scarlet* form a genus with me totally different from pink.' The vermilion colour of sealing wax was a good match to the outer face of the leaf of the laurel (*Prunus laurocerasus*). And in a phrase that was often to be repeated, he described the red end of the solar spectrum as 'little more than a shade or defect of light'.

By enquiries Dalton came to know of nearly 20 persons similarly affected, including two in one of his classes of 25. Significantly he remarked: 'I have not heard of one female subject to this peculiarity'. In explanation of his defect, he proposed that his eye must contain a blue filter, selectively absorbing long wavelengths. As no coloration was visible by external inspection, he suggested that it was his vitreous that was tinted.

Owing perhaps to his later fame as a chemist, the term 'daltonism' was adopted as the term for colour blindness in languages as diverse as Spanish and Russian. The source of this eponym was probably Prevost of Geneva, who used the term *daltonien* in print as early as

1827. British commentators objected to the association of a visual defect with the name of their distinguished countryman (Whewhell, 1841), but Dalton himself was unperturbed. Holding to the end of his life that his eye must contain a blue filter, he gave instructions that his eyes should be examined upon his death. He died on 27 July 1844, and the following day his medical attendant, Joseph Ransome, conducted a post-mortem (Henry, 1854). Ransome dissected one eye, and found the aqueous to be 'perfectly pellucid', as was the vitreous, while the lens was slightly amber-coloured 'as usual in persons of advanced age'. The second eye Ransome very shrewdly left largely intact, removing the posterior pole by a vertical section and examining scarlet and green through it, as though through a lens. Colours remained distinct when observed in this way and thus Dalton's own hypothesis was refuted. But the remains of one eye survived, stored dry between watch glasses, first in the possession of Dalton Hall (Brockbank, 1944) and then of the Manchester Literary and Philosophical Society. We report in this chapter the results of an analysis of DNA from this preserved tissue. For permission to take samples, we are grateful to the Society, and to the Manchester Museum of Science and Industry, who currently have care of the eye (Figure 1.3.2, see colour section).

Ransome's observations showed conclusively that Dalton's own hypothesis was mistaken. The most prominent alternative explanation of colour blindness in 1844 supposed that its origin was cerebral. A Mr Bally, a phrenologist and former assistant to Spurzheim, was present at the post-mortem. Although not sympathetic to phrenology, Joseph Ransome felt bound to record that Bally 'pointed out a remarkable prominence on the frontal portion of the orbital plates (which represents the phrenological site of the "*organ of colour*"), and the imperfect or deficient development of the convolution of the anterior lobes, which rested upon them'.

However, an explanation of a modern kind was already available in the literature when Dalton gave his paper to the Manchester Literary and Philosophical Society. In 1777 a London glass-seller and entrepreneur, George Palmer, had proposed that the retina contained three classes of fibre, corresponding to three physical kinds of light (Mollon, 1993; Palmer, 1777; Walls, 1956). Prompted perhaps by the early descriptions of colour blindness that appeared in the literature of the late 1770s (Huddart, 1777; Lort, 1778), Palmer subsequently proposed that colour blindness arose from either the inactivity or the constitutive over-activity of either one or two of the three kinds of retinal 'molecule' (Voigt, 1781). An explanation of this kind was applied to Dalton's case by Thomas Young, who was the first to grasp that the physical variable underlying hue was a continuous one whereas our own visual system imposed a trichromatic limitation on normal colour perception. Listing Dalton's 1794 paper in the bibliography of his *Lectures on Natural Philosophy and the Mechanical Arts*, Young (1807) remarks in a note:

> ... He (Dalton) thinks it probable that the vitreous humour is of a deep blue tinge: but this has never been observed by anatomists, and it is much more simple to suppose the absence or paralysis of those fibres of the retina, which are calculated to perceive red; this supposition explains all phenomena, except that greens appear to become bluish when viewed by candlelight: but in this circumstance there is perhaps no great singularity.

1.3.2 MOLECULAR BASIS OF COLOUR VISION

We now know that Young's three-receptor hypothesis is an essentially correct account of the first stage of normal colour vision. Trichromatic vision is achieved by combining the signals from three cone types: short-wave (SW) cones with peak sensitivity (λ_{max}) near 430 nm, middle-wave (MW) cones with λ_{max} near 530 nm, and long-wave cones (LW) with λ_{max} near 560 nm (Dartnall *et al.*, 1983; Schnapf *et al.*, 1987). The spectral sensitivities of the cones depend on photopigment molecules embedded in the multiply-infolded membranes of the outer segments. Each type of photopigment consists of a protein moiety bound to a chromophore, retinal, a derivative of vitamin A_1. The protein has a heptahelical structure of seven transmembrane α-helices that are linked by intracellular and extracellular loops to form a palisade that encloses the chromophore (Applebury and Hargrave, 1986; Hargrave, 1982). Small variations in the amino acid sequence of the helical regions determine the λ_{max} values of the different pigments. The protein moiety (opsin) of the SW pigment is coded by a gene on the short arm of chromosome 7 (Fitzgibbon *et al.*, 1994; Nathans *et al.*, 1986b) whereas the MW and LW opsins are coded by adjacent genes on the X chromosome (Vollrath *et al.*, 1988).

Spectroradiometric measurements have shown that the two forms of dichromatic vision, protanopia and deuteranopia (Figure 1.3.3), are commonly associated with the absence of either the LW or the MW cone pigment respectively (Mollon *et al.*, 1984; Rushton, 1971), and molecular biology has revealed that the corresponding gene on the X-chromosome is either altered or absent (Deeb *et al.*, 1992; Nathans *et al.*, 1986a,b). In modern terms, Young's hypothesis is that Dalton was a protanope and this interpretation has been shared by most authoritative commentators (e.g. Abney, 1913; Helmholtz, 1896; Wright, 1967).

1.3.3   THE USE OF THE POLYMERASE CHAIN REACTION FOR THE AMPLIFICATION OF ANCIENT DNA

The ability to analyse DNA from preserved or dried tissue depends entirely on a relatively new technique called the polymerase chain reaction (PCR). This technique, developed by Mullis *et al.* (1986), enables tiny quantities of DNA to be amplified up to workable levels for cloning and sequencing. Two short single-stranded molecules of DNA (oligonucleotides) of about 20 bases in length and complementary to the DNA sequence on either side of the region to be amplified are used to prime the synthesis of a new strand (Figure 1.3.4). Synthesis is carried out by a heat-stable DNA polymerase, *Taq* polymerase, isolated from the thermophilic bacterium *Thermus aquaticus*; this heat-stability is critical to PCR because amplification is achieved by cycling through a sequence consisting of (1) annealing of primers at around 60°C, (2) synthesis of DNA at 72°C and (3) strand separation at 94°C. After each cycle, there is a doubling of template sequence; after 30–35 cycles, the target sequence will have undergone an amplification of about 10^6.

This method has been successfully used to amplify the tiny quantities of DNA that can be isolated from ancient soft and bony tissues. The first successful application of this method was carried out by Pääbo *et al.* (1988) who amplified short fragments of mitochondrial DNA from a 7000-year-old brain in a skeleton buried in a peat bog at a site in Windover, Florida, USA, and, more recently, nuclear genes have been amplified from the same human source (Lawlor *et al.*, 1991).

1.3.4   AMPLIFICATION AND CLONING OF VISUAL PIGMENT GENE FRAGMENTS FROM JOHN DALTON'S DNA

A major problem in the analysis of DNA amplified from ancient tissue is that the high sensitivity of PCR means that contamination with only a few molecules of foreign DNA

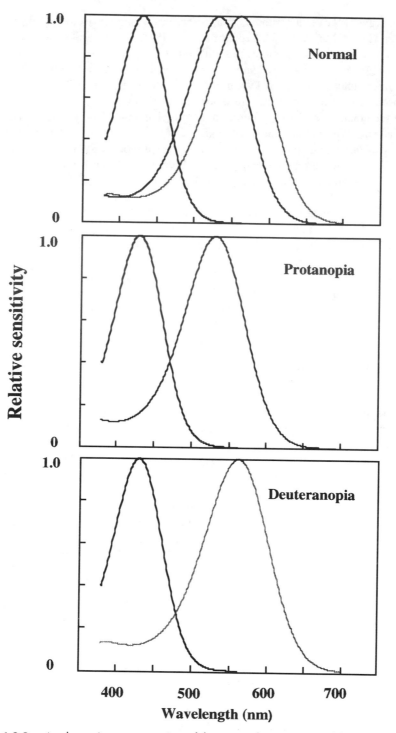

Figure 1.3.3. A schematic representation of the spectral sensitivities of the three types of cone in the normal retina (top panel). The middle panel represents protanopia, where the LW photopigment is missing, and the lowermost panel represents deuteranopia, where the MW photopigment is missing.

can lead to a spurious result with all amplified products derived from the contaminating source (Hagelberg *et al.*, 1991; Hagelberg, 1994). To minimise the risk of contamination from previous examinations, we took samples from a region in the interior of Dalton's eye, which is unlikely to have been handled. This region was tentatively identified as peripheral retina. Several small samples were removed with a sterile scalpel blade and placed immediately into sterile 1.5 ml eppendorf tubes. At all times, sterile surgical gloves were worn. New pipettors and reagents were used in all subsequent procedures and all experiments were set up in a room previously unused for work on visual pigments. Each PCR used a different sample of eye tissue yet gave the same overall result.

Each tissue sample was divided into fragments of about 1 mm³. Initial attempts to isolate DNA by a standard phenol/chloroform extraction method after proteinase K digestion proved ineffective. An alternative method that uses GeneReleaser™ (BioVentures, Inc) was adopted. GeneReleaser serves two purposes, it avoids the need to purify DNA and it sequesters products that might inhibit polymerase activity. The resulting extracts were used as a source of template DNA for amplification of opsin gene fragments by PCR as detailed in Figure 1.3.5. Details of the primer pairs used are given in Table 1.3.1, including annealing temperatures for the second round PCRs. Amplified products were separated by electrophoresis in a 1.2 per cent low-melting-point agarose gel using 0.5 × TAE buffer and visualised after staining with ethidium bromide. Blank tubes lacking DNA were carried through both first- and second-round PCRs. No amplified fragments were seen in these tubes. The primer pairs were tested on a normal male observer, an anomalous male

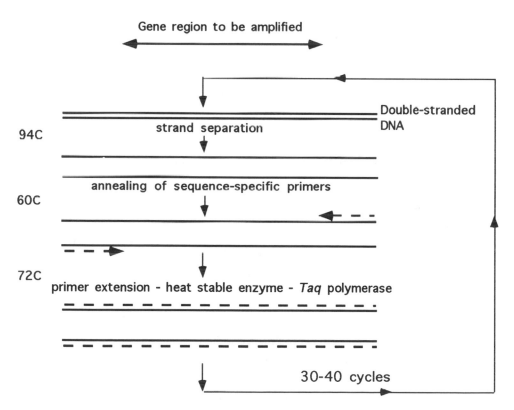

Figure 1.3.4. The polymerase chain reaction (PCR). Parameters for the amplification from John Dalton's DNA are given in Figure 1.3.5.

Table 1.3.1 Primer pairs used for the polymerase chain reaction amplification of opsin gene fragments. Numbers in parentheses refer to the 5′ and 3′ ends of amplified coding regions

Primer pairs	Amplified region	Temperature of annealing
R4+/R5−, G4+/G5−, R4+/G5−, G4+/R5−	Exon 4, intron 4, exon 5 (721-868)	62ºC
E3+/E3−	Exon 3 (480-596)	56ºC
E4+/E4−	Exon 4 (650–761)	56ºC
E5+/E5−	Exon 5 (830–983)	58ºC
I4+/I5−	Intron 4, exon 5, intron 5	68ºC

trichromat and a male deuteranope; in these cases, a single PCR was carried out with the DNAs from these subjects using the parameters of the second-round PCR for Dalton, except that 1 μl of template DNA (isolated by conventional methods from blood samples) was added in place of the first-round mix. The sequence and gene specificity of all primers used are given in Table 1.3.2.

Bands of the correct size were excised and placed in 1.5 ml eppendorf tubes containing 50 μl sterile water. DNA was eluted overnight, followed by a brief heating to 68°C for 5 min. Amplified fragments were TA cloned (Invitrogen) into pCRII and cycle-sequenced

---

1. Tissue fragments (about 1 mm³) were added to 20 μl of GeneReleaser™ (BioVentures, Inc) in 0.2 ml eppendorf tubes.

2. The tube was heated as follows: 65°C for 30 sec, 8°C for 30 sec, 97°C for 180 sec, 8°C for 60 sec, 65°C for 180 sec, 97°C for 60 sec, 65°C for 60 sec, 80°C for 1 hour.

3. The PCR mix was added either immediately or after storage at 4°C overnight. This mix contained 200 μM each of dATP, dCTP, dGTP and dTTP, 0.5 units of *Taq* polymerase, 9 mM MgCl$_2$, 30 μM of each primer and 2 μl Perfect Match (Stratagene) in a final volume of 50 μl.

4. A first-round PCR was carried by heating at 94°C for 180 sec, before 35 cycles of 94°C for 20 sec, 62°C for 30 sec, 72°C for 120 sec, and a final step of 72°C for 600 sec. No products from this first-round PCR could be seen.

5. A second-round PCR was then carried out by adding 1 μl of the first-round mix to 49 μl of PCR mix prepared as before but pre-heated to 94°C.

Figure 1.3.5. Protocol for preparation and amplification of template DNA from preserved eye tissue.

Table 1.3.2 Specificity and sequence of primer oligonucleotides

Primers	Specificity	Sequence (5'–3')
R4+	LW opsin exon 4	GCTGCATCATCCCACTCGC
G4+	MW opsin exon 4	GCTGCATCACCCCACTCAG
R5–	LW opsin exon 5	GACGCAGTACGCAAAGATC
G5–	MW opsin exon 5	GAAGCAGAATGCCAGGACC
E3+	MW/LW opsin exon 3	TCACAGGTCTCTGGTCTCTGG
E3–	MW/LW opsin exon 3	CTCCAACCAAAGATGGGCGG
E4+	MW/LW opsin exon 4	CACGGCCTGAAGACTTCATGC
E4–	MW/LW opsin exon 4	CGCTCGGATGGCCAGCCACAC
E5+	MW/LW opsin exon 5	GAATTCCACCCAGAAGGCAGAG
E5–	MW/LW opsin exon 5	GTCGACGGGGTTGTAGATAGTGGC
I4+	MW/LW opsin intron 4	ACGTGGAATTCCCTCTCCTCCTCCCCACAAC
I5–	MW/LW opsin intron 5	ACGTGAAGCTTCAGGTGGGGCCATCACTGCA

with *Taq* polymerase, dye-tagged dideoxy nucleotides and either the T7 or Sp6 sequencing primers. The products of the reaction were visualised in an Applied Biosystems Model 373 DNA Sequencer System.

1.3.5 MOLECULAR GENETICS OF JOHN DALTON'S DICHROMACY

The MW and LW opsin genes, juxtaposed on the X chromosome (Vollrath *et al.*, 1988), show an almost identical gene structure of six coding regions (exons) interrupted by five non-coding regions (introns); the only difference is that intron one is usually shorter in the MW gene (Lund Jorgensen *et al.*, 1990; Nathans *et al.*, 1986a). Both genes specify opsin proteins of 364 amino acids in length. The MW and LW opsins (Figure 1.3.6) differ for only 15 amino acids (Nathans *et al.*, 1986a) and substitutions at a number of these sites (Table 1.3.3) are known to contribute to the spectral shift in the wavelength of maximal absorbance (λ_{max}) between the two pigments (Asenjo *et al.*, 1994; Merbs and Nathans, 1992, 1993), although changes at only three of these sites are responsible for most of the spectral displacement (Ibbotson *et al.*, 1992; Merbs and Nathans, 1992, 1993; Neitz *et al.*, 1991; Williams *et al.*, 1992). These key substitutions are at amino acids 180 (serine/alanine), 277 (tyrosine/phenylalanine) and 285 (threonine/alanine); in each case, the gain of an hydroxyl-bearing amino acid (serine, threonine, tyrosine) results in a red shift in λ_{max} (Table 1.3.3). Substitution at site 180 (alanine or serine), however, is polymorphic (Neitz and Jacobs, 1990; Winderickx *et al.*, 1992, 1993) with two forms of each opsin gene present in the population. An otherwise LW pigment with serine-180 gives a pigment with λ_{max} of 563 nm whereas alanine-180 gives 556 nm; the corresponding MW pigments give λ_{max} values of 534 and 532 nm (Asenjo *et al.*, 1994).

As the only amino acid substitutions that clearly differentiate MW and LW pigments are at sites 277 and 285, both coded by exon 5, we used codon differences in this exon, together with gene-specific differences in exon 4, to determine whether a MW and/or a LW opsin gene is present in Dalton's DNA. Two primer pairs were used (Deeb *et al.*, 1992): one pair (R4+, R5–) is specific for LW exons 4 and 5 and the other (G4+, G5–) is specific for MW exons 4 and 5 (Figure 1.3.7a). In other combinations (R4+, G5– and G4+, R5–), these primers will also generate fragments from any hybrid gene that contains a MW exon 4 and LW exon 5 or *vice versa*. The results in Figure 1.3.8a show that only primer pair R4+, R5– generated a fragment of the correct size (about 1.7 kb) from Dalton's DNA, indicating that a LW but no MW opsin gene is present. Southern blotting and probing of the PCR products with an exon 5 probe confirmed that only this set of primers amplified an opsin gene fragment (Figure 1.3.8b). The specificity of these primers was confirmed with a number of test DNA samples; as expected, the DNA from a normal observer yielded fragments of the

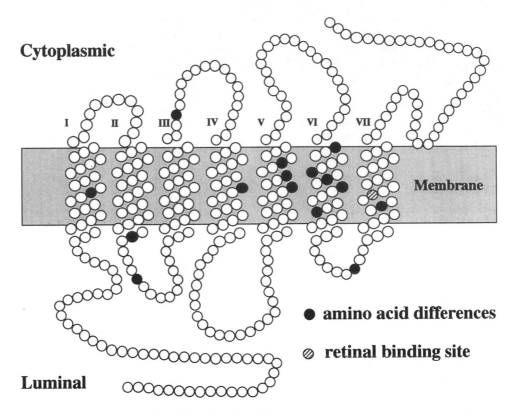

Figure 1.3.6. Two-dimensional model of MW/LW cone opsin. The position and length of each transmembrane region is based on the model of Baldwin (1993).

Table 1.3.3 Hybrid pigments derived from a LW pigment with key amino acids separately substituted

Amino acids						λ_{max} (nm)	Change in
180	**230**	**233**	**277**	**285**	**309**		λ_{max} (nm)
ser	ile	ala	tyr	thr	tyr	563*	
ala	ile	ala	tyr	thr	tyr	556	−7
ser	thr	ala	tyr	thr	tyr	561	−2
ser	ile	ser	tyr	thr	tyr	560	−3
ser	ile	ala	phe	thr	tyr	553	−10
ser	ile	ala	tyr	ala	tyr	547	−16
ser	ile	ala	tyr	thr	phe	561	−2

Data is from Asenjo *et al.* (1994). Each pigment was generated by site-directed mutagenesis and expressed in mammalian COS cells.

*   Maximal λ_{max} for LW pigment.

correct size with the R4+, R5– and G4+, G5– combinations, a known anomalous trichromat produced, in addition to the two present in the normal observer, a third fragment with the R4+, G5– combination, indicating the presence of a hybrid gene, whereas only the R4+, R5– primer pair amplified a fragment from the DNA of a known deuteranope (Figure 1.3.8c).

In order to confirm that the fragment amplified by the R4+, R5– primer pair from Dalton's DNA was indeed derived from an opsin gene, the fragment was cloned and partial DNA sequences were obtained from 10 separate clones. The sequence details of this fragment are shown in Figure 1.3.9a and confirm that the fragment was amplified from an opsin gene. Moreover, on the basis of sequence differences between the MW and LW genes at nucleotides 740 and 747 in exon 4, we can infer that this gene coded for a LW visual pigment.

To check further whether only a single LW opsin gene was present in John Dalton's DNA, we used four additional primer pairs (Table 1.3.2) that do not differentiate between MW and LW genes (Dulai *et al.*, 1994; Ibbotson *et al.*, 1992; Nathans *et al.*, 1993). Three of these pairs amplify within exons 3, 4 and 5 respectively and the fourth amplifies between

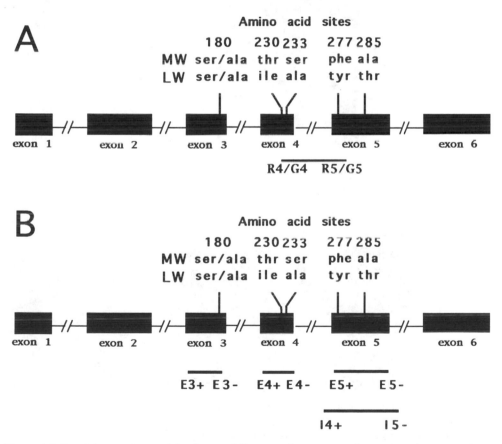

Figure 1.3.7. Primer pairs used for the amplification of opsin gene fragments. The LW and MW opsin genes are both composed of six exons. The position of key amino acid substitutions in relation to the amplified regions are shown. (A) Gene-specific primers; (B) Non-specific primers.

introns 4 and 5, that is across exon 5 (Figure 1.3.7b). For each primer pair, a number of clones were sequenced (Table 1.3.4) and in each case, only a single sequence was identified (Figure 1.3.9a); for exons 4 and 5, all the clones were identical to the sequence of the LW opsin gene as previously reported (Nathans *et al.*, 1986a), whereas all the exon 3 clones were identical to the second most common variant of this highly polymorphic region of the LW opsin gene (Winderickx *et al.*, 1993) with G at nucleotide 538 coding for alanine-180. A total of 27 different clones containing amplified fragments generated with this range of non-specific primers (Table 1.3.4) are thus consistent in identifying a single LW gene in Dalton's DNA.

From our data therefore, we are able to confirm that John Dalton was indeed a dichromat but, contrary to previous interpretations, he was a *deuteranope with a single LW opsin gene coding for a LW visual pigment*. The presence of alanine at position 180, together with

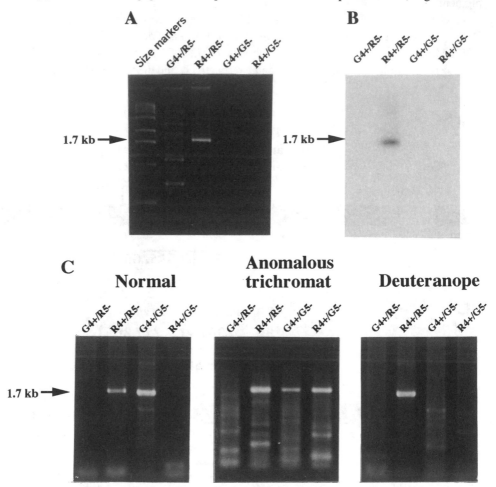

Figure 1.3.8. Amplification products obtained from different combinations of the gene-specific R4 + /G4 + and R5 + /G5- primers. The position of the 1.7 kb fragment is shown. (A) Amplified products from Dalton's DNA. The size marker bands are 0.506, 1.018, 1.636, 2.036, and 3.054 kb. (B) Southern blot of gel A, hybridised with a ^{32}P-labelled exon 5 probe amplified from normal genomic DNA with the non-specific I4 + /I5- primers. (C) Amplification products from a normal male observer, an anomalous male trichromat and a male deuteranope.

A

```
MW    C ATC ATC GTG CTC TGC TAC CTC CAA GTG TGG CTG GCC ATC CGA GCG - 785
LW    T ... ... A.. ... ... ... ... ... ... ... ... ... ... ... ...
Dalton T ... ... A.. ... ... ... ... ... ... ... ... ... ... ... ...
```

B

Exon 3

	Amino acid	
	153	180
LW1	leu	ser
LW2	leu	ala
Dalton	leu	ala

Exon 4

	Amino acid		
	230	233	236
MW	thr	ser	val
LW	ile	ala	met
Dalton	ile	ala	met

Exon 5

	Amino acid						
	274	275	277	279	285	298	309
MW	val	leu	phe	phe	ala	pro	phe
LW	ile	phe	tyr	val	thr	ala	tyr
Dalton	ile	phe	tyr	val	thr	ala	tyr

C

Amino acid											
153	180	230	233	236	274	275	277	279	285	298	309
leu	ala	ile	ala	met	ile	phe	tyr	val	thr	ala	tyr

Figure 1.3.9.   Sequence of fragments amplified from Dalton's DNA. (A) Nucleotide sequence of exon 4 amplified with the LW-specific R4+/R5- primer pair. (B) Deduced amino acid sequence of fragments amplified with non-specific primer pairs. (C) Deduced amino acid sequence of John Dalton's LW pigment.

Table 1.3.4 Summary of sequence analysis of cloned PCR fragments generated with non-specific MW and LW opsin gene primers

Amplified region	Number of clones analysed	MW	LW
Exon 3	5	0	5*
Exon 4	5	0	5
Exon 5	15	0	15
Intron 4, exon 5, intron 5	2	0	2

The four pairs of PCR primers used do not differentiate between the LW and MW opsin genes (Dulai *et al.*, 1994; Nathans *et al.*, 1993). Sequences are classified on the basis of homology to the sequences of the MW and LW genes reported by Nathans *et al.* (1986a).
*Exon 3 is highly polymorphic; the sequence present in John Dalton's DNA is identical to the second most common LW variant (Winderickx *et al.*, 1993).

tyrosine-277 and threonine-285 (Figure 1.3.9b), would produce a pigment with the shorter λ_{max} of 556 nm, compared to a λ_{max} of 563 nm for the serine-180 pigment.

How confident can we be that contamination has been avoided and that the sequenced opsin gene was indeed derived from John Dalton's DNA? As described above, we took every possible precaution to avoid contact with other sources of DNA. Our result depends on the absence, rather than the presence, of a gene – a gene whose adjacent LW fellow we have successfully amplified. Only contamination by the DNA from another deuteranope would have given the same result. As far as we are aware, no workers in our laboratory at the time of this study have any defect in colour vision and certainly none are dichromats. The deuteranope that we used for test purposes was not known to us until after all the PCR experiments on John Dalton's tissue had been carried out. For these reasons, therefore, we are confident that our result is not an artefact.

1.3.6   ASSESSMENT OF DALTON'S PHENOTYPE

Long tradition holds that John Dalton was a protanope (Abney, 1913; Helmholtz, 1896; Young, 1807; Wright, 1967). Two honourable exceptions to this tradition are Keyser (1943) and Walls (1956), who both suggest that Dalton was a deuteranope. Sadly, neither gives reasons. Can our molecular result be reconciled with the historical evidence for his phenotype? Protanopes and deuteranopes can be distinguished by their spectral sensitivity and by their colour matches. We consider these two aspects of Dalton's phenotype in turn.

The classical sign of protanopia is the foreshortening of the red end of the spectrum. In fact, the physicists Sir John Herschel and Sir David Brewster each questioned Dalton directly and both reported that he did not see the spectrum as foreshortened at long wavelengths. Thus, Brewster in his *Letters on Natural Magic* writes:

> In all those cases which have been carefully studied, at least in three of them in which I have had the advantage of making personal observations, namely, those of Mr. Troughton, Mr. Dalton, and Mr. Liston, the eye is capable of seeing the whole of the prismatic spectrum, the red space appearing to be yellow.
>
> (Brewster, 1842)

while Herschel, in a letter dated 20 May 1833, writes directly to Dalton:

> It is clear to me that you and all others so affected perceive *as light* every ray, which others do. The retina *is excited* by every ray which reaches it. . . . The question, then, is reduced to one of pure sensation. It seems to me, that we have three primary sensations when you have only two.

We refer or can refer in imagination, all colours to three, red, yellow, blue. All other colours we think we perceive to be mixtures of these... Now to eyes of your kind it seems to me that all your tints are referable to two, which I shall call A and B; the equilibrium of A and B producing *your* white ... (Henry, 1854).

And finally we may record a footnote by Richard Taylor, the scientific publisher: 'Dr Dalton has never stated that the spectrum he saw was *shorter* than the spectrum seen by others' (Wartmann, 1846). It remains, however, to explain Dalton's own remark that red appears as 'little more than a shade or defect of light' (Dalton, 1798). In fact, even for a deuteranope, the red part of a spectrum will look dim compared to the juxtaposed yellow and orange regions. The yellow, orange and red regions may have the same hue for the deuteranope,[1] but the red region must have reduced luminosity, since the LW pigment peaks in the yellow-green (see Figure 1.3.2, in the colour section) and its sensitivity falls rapidly at long wavelengths. For the deuteranope the red end of the spectrum does not offer the *Farbenglut*, the extra vividness of saturated colours which derives from the LW-MW opponent signal and which enhances the brightness of long wavelengths for the normal observer (Kohlrausch, 1923).

John Dalton found that sealing wax and the outer face of a laurel leaf (*Prunus laurocerasus*) were a good match in colour. We have accordingly measured the reflectance of samples of eighteenth-century sealing wax and laurel leaves using a Photo Research PR650 spectroradiometer and a Macbeth daylight lamp. The measured chromaticities of these samples are plotted in the CIE diagram of Figure 1.3.10: they fall on a confusion line that is at least as compatible with deuteranopia as with protanopia. Dalton identified a number of British flowers that appeared pink to the normal eye but 'blue' to him. We have measured the chromaticities of several of these flora. All of them, even the eye-catching crimson of the male red campion, *Lychnis diocia* (Figure 1.3.1, see colour section), lie on the 'blue' side of a line passing through the deutan confusion point and the chromaticity of northern daylight, a line that represents the set of chromaticities which appear neutral to a deuteranope. These measurements do not unequivocally require a diagnosis of deuteranope – they would be equally compatible with protanopia – but they do dispose of a misconception that has bedeviled earlier interpretations of Dalton, the misconception that it could only be the lack of a 'red-sensitive' receptor that caused his failure to see the redness in pink flowers.

1.3.6 COLOUR CONSTANCY IN DICHROMATS

We end our consideration of Dalton's colour perceptions by returning to the failure of colour constancy that initiated his self-analysis. He had observed that the flowers of *Pelargonium zonale* looked 'near sky blue' to him by daylight and yet yellowish or reddish by candlelight. The two colours were explicitly of opposite quality for Dalton, lying on different sides of neutral.

Constancy failures of this type can be predicted, in principle, without direct testing of a dichromatic subject. They can be derived purely from a knowledge of where the subject's confusion point lies in a chromaticity diagram. We need adopt only the assumption – common to virtually all theories of colour constancy – that the subject sees as neutral any surface that reflects equally all the component wavelengths of the illuminant. Surfaces that we call white or grey exhibit a non-selective spectral reflectance of this kind. We can then derive the dichromat's hue shift from purely physical measurements. We must measure (1) the radiance spectrum of the two illuminants (here daylight and candlelight) and (2) the spectral flux that reaches the eye from the test surface under the two illuminants.

Figure 1.3.11 illustrates such measurements for the pink flowers of one specimen of *Pelargonium zonale*. When the illuminant is daylight, *P. zonale* plots to the left of the line that represents the set of colours that must appear neutral to a dichromat. In other words, the flower must exhibit a hue on the 'cold' or bluish side of neutral. Candlelight is very deficient in short wavelengths and all natural surfaces are shifted rightwards in the chromaticity diagram, but the critical result for this specimen of *P. zonale* is that the flower now lies on the right of the deuteranope's neutral line: its hue must be counted among the 'warm' or yellowish colours.

Thus, since Dalton was a deuteranope, his failure of colour constancy is fully predictable from these physical measurements.[2] Interestingly (at least for this sample of *P. zonale* and

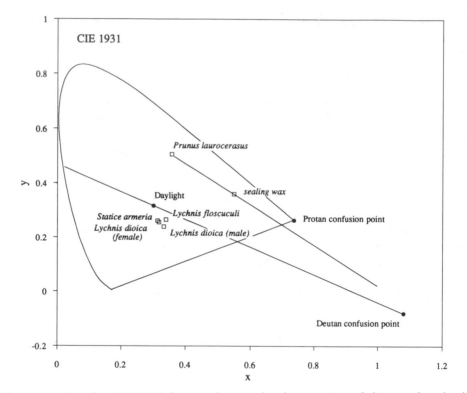

Figure 1.3.10.   The CIE (1931) diagram showing the chromaticities of objects referred to by Dalton. In this diagram, subsets of colours that are confusable by a protanope lie on lines that converge at $x = 0.747$, $y = 0.253$ (the 'protan confusion point'). The corresponding deutan confusion point is less well specified, in part because of properties of the diagram and in part because of genetic heterogeneity of the LW pigment; we plot the value given by Wyszecki and Stiles (1982). Sealing wax and the face of a laurel leaf give a confusion line that is at least as compatible with deuteranopia as with protanopia. We also show several British flora that appeared blue to Dalton: thrift (*Statice armeria*, now *Armeria maritima*), ragged robin (*Lychnis floscuculi*), and the red campion (*Lychnis dioica*). Male and female red campions differ in saturation and are plotted separately. Although all these flowers appear pink to the normal eye, they plot to the left of the deuteranopic confusion line that passes through the chromaticity of our standard daylight source; so they would be expected to look bluish both to a protanope and a deuteranope.

for the candlelight we used) a protanope would explicitly not experience a shift from one hue to its opposite as the illuminant was changed. The change in illuminant does not translate *P. zonale* to the 'yellow' side of the protanope's neutral line. Dalton's failure of constancy, which has so often been taken to indicate protanopia, in fact favours a diagnosis of deuteranopia.

In summary, contemporary reports of Dalton's spectral sensitivity favour a diagnosis of deuteranopia, and his colour matches are consistent with deuteranopia. Our analysis of the chromaticities of *P. zonale* also favours deuteranopia. Thus our molecular finding, that

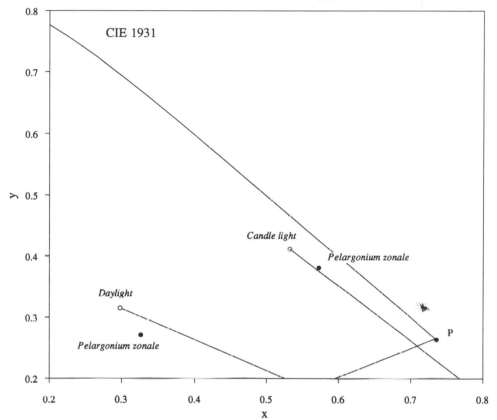

Figure 1.3.11. A magnified region of the CIE (1931) diagram showing the chromaticities of a specimen of *Pelargonium zonale* in daylight (Macbeth easel light) and in candle light. The pelargonium was grown from stock collected in South Africa by Celia James. A spectroradiometer was used to make measurements of individual petals and of a white reference plaque in the two illuminants. The measurements of the plaque give the chromaticities of the illuminants. In daylight illumination, *P. zonale* lies to the left of the deutan confusion line that passes through the chromaticity of the illuminant: for a deuteranope, it must therefore lie on the 'bluish' side of neutral. Candle light compresses the whole gamut of colours into a small region of the chromaticity diagram. *P. zonale* now lies to the right of a deutan confusion line that passes through the illuminant: it must thus be translated to the opposite – 'warm' – side of neutral. On the other hand, the pelargonium would straddle a line that passed through candle light and the *protan* copunctal point (P). Thus, from spectroradiometric measurements of actual objects and from established estimates of confusion lines, one can predict a failure of constancy in deuteranopes. One can also show that a shift between daylight and candle light is less likely to cause a protanope to judge that *P. zonale* has changed from one hue to its opposite.

Dalton retains the LW and lacks the MW gene, is fully compatible with the historical evidence for his phenotype.

1.3.7   POSTSCRIPT: MOLECULAR BIOGRAPHY

The present study may represent the first instance where a hereditary defect has been identified in an historical figure and where both phenotype and genotype are known in detail. It is unlikely to be the last such case and we should like to propose the term 'molecular biography' for this new discipline. The famous and the infamous have often left fragments of themselves behind, if only locks of hair; and as more is understood of the genetic basis of human variation and disease, it should become possible to answer unsolved historical questions about the illnesses and the mental aberrations of figures from the past.

However, several conditions must be met before an exercise in molecular biography is feasible: (1) tissue must exist from which uncontaminated DNA can be recovered; (2) the provenance of the tissue must be relatively certain; (3) the ethical permission of the donor or the donor's descendants must be given (since genetic analysis of relatively recent figures may reveal attributes of the living); (4) phenotypic evidence must exist that suggests a specific genetic disorder or anomaly in the historical subject; and, perhaps most importantly, (5) the sequence must be known for the gene or genes that determine the condition in question. In the present case, the conditions were very much in our favour: the eye tissue was in a dry state that facilitates survival of DNA; there are written references to the removal of the tissue and its subsequent ownership; Dalton explicitly left his eyes for the study of daltonism; he also provided a detailed account of his phenotype; and the psychophysical and molecular bases of dichromacy are rather well understood. Only a few other historical figures will provide so attractive a subject for molecular biography.

1.3.8   ACKNOWLEDGEMENTS

This work was supported by the Wellcome Trust and the Medical Research Council. We thank the Manchester Literary and Philosophical Society for permission to take samples from Dalton's eye; the Manchester Museum of Science & Industry for giving us access to the material; the Director of the Botanic Garden and the Keeper of Manuscripts, Cambridge University, for access to colorimetric samples; H. Key, E. Spong and C. James for specimens of *Pelargonium zonale*, and D. Hull and E. N. Willmer for botanical advice. An account of this work has also been published in *Science*, 1995, **267**, 984–988.

1.3.9   NOTES

1. Insofar as we cannot share another's sensations, we cannot know for certain what this sensation might be. If we suppose it similar to the normal's yellow, then there is the interesting possibility that dark versions of the hue would look different in quality to the dichromat, in the sense that a normal sees brown as different in quality from yellow. The critical point for the present purpose is that the red part of the spectrum would, for Dalton, *match* a darkened yellow.
2. We have in fact shown a specimen of *P. zonale* to the modern deuteranope whose DNA we analysed as a test for the gene-specific primer pairs. In northern daylight he described the flowers as blue, comparing them to a part of the sky that exhibited a slightly desaturating haze. Shown the flower a few minutes later in candlelight, he described the colour as red.

1.3.10   REFERENCES

ABNEY, W. (1913) *Researches in Colour Vision and the Trichromatic Theory*, London: Longmans, Green & Co.

APPLEBURY, M. L. & HARGRAVE, P. A. (1986) Molecular biology of the visual pigments, *Vision Research*, **26**, 1881–1895.

ASENJO, A. B., RIM, J. & OPRIAN, D. D. (1994) Molecular determinants of human red/green color discrimination, *Neuron*, **12**, 1131–1138.

BALDWIN, J. (1993) The probable arrangement of the helices in G protein-coupled receptors, *European Molecular Biology Organisation Journal*, **12**, 1693–1703.

BREWSTER, D. (1842) *Letters on Natural Magic, addressed to Sir Walter Scott, Bart.*, London: J. Murray.

BROCKBANK, E. M. (1944) *John Dalton*, Manchester: Manchester University Press.

DALTON, J. (1798) Extraordinary facts relating to the vision of colours, *Memoirs of the Manchester Literary and Philosophical Society*, **5**, 28.

DARTNALL, H. J. A., BOWMAKER, J. K. & MOLLON, J. D. (1983) Human visual pigments: microspectrophotometric results from the eyes of seven persons, *Proceedings of the Royal Society*, **B220**, 115–130.

DEEB, S. S., LINDSEY, D. T., HIBIYA, Y., SANOCKI, E., WINDERICKX, J., TELLER, D. Y. & MOTULSKY, A. G. (1992) Genotype-phenotype relationships in human red/green color-vision defects: molecular and psychophysical studies, *American Journal of Human Genetics*, **51**, 687–700.

DULAI, K. S., BOWMAKER, J. K., MOLLON, J. D. & HUNT, D. M. (1994) Sequence divergence, polymorphism and evolution of the middle-wave and long-wave visual pigment genes of Great Apes and Old World monkeys, *Vision Research*, **34**, 2483–2491.

FITZGIBBON, J., APPUKUTTAN B., GAYTHER, S., WELLS, D., DELHANTY, J. & HUNT, D. M. (1994) Localisation of the human blue cone pigment gene to chromosome band 7q31.3-32, *Human Genetics*, **93**, 79–80.

HAGELBERG, E. (1994) Dried samples: hard tissues. In: Herrmann B. & Hummel S. (Eds), *Ancient DNA*, New York: Springer-Verlag.

HAGELBERG, E., GRAY, I. C. & JEFFREYS, A. J. (1991) Identification of the skeletal remains of a murder victim by DNA analysis, *Nature*, **352**, 427–429.

HARGRAVE, P. A. (1982) Rhodopsin chemistry, structure and topography, *Progress in Retinal Research*, **1**, 1–51.

VON HELMHOLTZ, H. (1896) *Handbuch der Physiologischen Optik*, Hamburg: Vos.

HENRY, W. C. (1854) *Memoirs of the Life and Scientific Researches of John Dalton*, London: Cavendish Society.

HUDDART, J. (1777) An account of persons who could not distinguish colours, *Philosophical Transactions of the Royal Society*, **67**, 260–265.

IBBOTSON, R. E., HUNT, D. M., BOWMAKER, J. K. & MOLLON, J. D. (1992) Sequence divergence and copy number of the middle- and long-wave photopigment genes in Old World monkeys, *Proceeding of the Royal Society*, **B247**, 145–154.

KEYSER, G. W. (1943) *Über Wertung angeborener Fehler des Farbensehens*, Oslo: Broggers.

KOHLRAUSCH, A. (1923) Theoretisches und Praktisches zur heterochromen Photometrie, *Pflügers Archiv ges. Physiol. Menschen Tiere*, **200**, 216–219.

LAWLOR, D. A., DICKEL, C. D., HAUSWIRTH, W. W. & PARHAM, P. (1991) Ancient HLA genes from 7,500-year-old archaeological remains, *Nature*, **349**, 785–788.

LONSDALE, H. (1874) *The Worthies of Cumberland, Volume 5, John Dalton*, London: Routledge.

LORT, M. (1778) An account of a remarkable imperfection of sight, *Philosophical Transactions of the Royal Society*, **68**, 611.

LUND JORGENSEN, A., DEEB, S. S. & MOTULSKY, A. G. (1990) Molecular genetics of X chromosome-linked color vision among populations of African and Japanese ancestry: high frequency of a shortened red pigment gene among Afro-Americans, *Proceedings of the National Academy of Science, USA*, **87**, 6512– 6516.

MARTYN, T. (1799) *Thirty-eight Plates with Explanations: Intended to Illustrate Linnaeus's System of Vegetables*, London: J. White.

MERBS, S. L. & NATHANS, J. (1992) Absorption spectra of human cone pigments, *Nature*, **356**, 433–435.

MERBS, S. L. & NATHANS, J. (1993) Role of hydroxyl-bearing amino acids in differentially tuning the absorption spectra of the human red and green cone pigments, *Photochemistry and Photobiology*, **58**, 706–710.

MOLLON, J. D. (1993) George Palmer. In: Nicholls, C. S. (Ed.) *The Dictionary of National Biography*, Oxford: Oxford University Press, pp. 509–510.

MOLLON, J. D., BOWMAKER, J. K., DARTNALL, H. J. A. & BIRD, A. C. (1984) Microspectrophotometric and psychophysical results for the same deuteranopic observer. In: Verriest, G. (Ed.) *Colour Vision Deficiencies VII*, The Hague: Dr. W. Junk, pp. 303– 310.

MULLIS, K., FALOONA, F., SCHARF, S., SAIKI, R., HORN, G. & ERLICH, H. (1986) Specific enzymatic amplification of DNA in vitro: the polymerase chain reaction, *Cold Spring Harbor Symposium of Quantitative Biology*, **51**, 263–273.

NATHANS, J., MAUMENEE, I. H., ZRENNER, E., SADOWSKI, B., SHARPE, L. T., LEWIS, R. A., HANSEN, E., ROSENBERG, T., SCHWARTZ, M., HECKENLIVELY, J. R. *et al.* (1993) Genetic heterogeneity among blue-cone monochromats, *American Journal of Human Genetics*, **53**, 987–1000.

NATHANS, J., THOMAS, D. & HOGNESS, D. S. (1986a) Molecular genetics of human color vision: The genes encoding blue, green, and red pigments, *Science*, **232**, 193–202.

NATHANS, J., PIANTANIDA, T. P., EDDY, R. L., SHOWS, T. B. & HOGNESS D. S. (1986b) Molecular genetics of inherited variation in human colour vision, *Science*, **232**, 203–210.

NEITZ, J. & JACOBS, G. H. (1990) Polymorphism in normal human color vision and its mechanism, *Vision Research*, **30**, 621–636.

NEITZ, M., NEITZ, J. & JACOBS, G.H. (1991) Spectral tuning of pigments underlying red-green color vision, *Science*, **252**, 971–974.

PÄÄBO, S., GIFFORD, J. A. & WILSON, A. C. (1988) Mitochondrial DNA sequences from a 7000-year-old brain, *Nucleic Acids Research*, **16**, 9775–9787.

PALMER, G. (1777) *Theory of Colours and Vision*, London: S. Leacroft.

RUSHTON, W. A. H. (1971) Color vision: An approach through the cone pigments, *Investigative Ophthalmology*, **10**, 311–322.

SCHNAPF, J. L., KRAFT, T. W. & BAYLOR, D. A. (1987) Spectral sensitivities of human cone photoreceptors, *Nature*, **325**, 439–441.

VAN DER WALT, J. J. A. (1977) *Pelargoniums of Southern Africa*, Cape Town: Purnell.

VOIGT, J. H. (1781) Des Herrn Giros von Gentilly Muthmassungen über die Gesichtsfehler bey Untersuchung der Farben, *Magazin für das Neueste aus der Physik und Naturgeschichte (Gotha)*, **1**, 57–61.

VOLLRATH, D., NATHANS, J. & DAVIES, R. W. (1988) Tandem array of human visual pigment genes at Xq28, *Science*, **240**, 1669–1672.

WALLS, G. L. (1956) The G. Palmer story, *Journal of the History of Medicine*, **11**, 66–96.

WARTMANN, E. (1846) Memoir on daltonism (or colour blindness), *Taylor's Scientific Memoirs*, **4**, 156–187.

WHEWHELL, W. (1841) Eleventh Meeting of the British Association for the Advancement of Science, *Athenaeum*, **722**, 669.

WILLIAMS, A. J., HUNT, D. M., BOWMAKER, J. K. & MOLLON, J. D. (1992) The polymorphic photopigments of the marmoset: spectral tuning and genetic basis, *European Molecular Biology Organisation Journal*, **11**, 2039–2045.

WINDERICKX, J., LINDSEY, D. T., SANOCKI, E., TELLER, D. Y., MOTULSKY, A. G. & DEEB, S. S. (1992) Polymorphism in red photopigment underlies variation in colour matching, *Nature*, **356**, 431–433.

WINDERICKX, J., BATTISTI, L., HIBIYA, Y., MOTULSKY, A. G. & DEEB, S. S. (1993) Haplotype diversity in the human red and green opsin genes: evidence for frequent sequence exchange in exon 3, *Human Molecular Genetics*, **2**, 1413–1421.

WRIGHT, W. D. (1967) *The Rays are not Coloured*, London: Hilger.
WYSZECKI, G. & STILES, W. S. (1982) *Color Science*, New York: Wiley.
YOUNG, T. (1807) *A Course of Lectures on Natural Philosophy and the Mechanical Arts*, London: J. Johnson.

Section 2 – Pigments and Genetics

Primate Visual Pigments: Their Spectral Distribution and Evolution

J.K. Bowmaker, D.M. Hunt and J.D. Mollon

Although we may sometimes consider our own colour vision to be superior to that of other animals, the culmination of the evolution of colour vision is not necessarily to be found within primates nor even within mammals, but is most probably represented amongst the diurnal birds, reptiles and shallow-living teleost fish. In these 'lower' vertebrate groups, vision extends over a spectral range greater than that of most mammals, ranging from the near ultraviolet (about 320 nm) through to the far red (about 750–800 nm), and colour vision is subserved by at least four spectrally distinct cone populations regularly spaced within this extended visible spectrum (for a review, see Bowmaker, 1991). Indeed, many of these species are probably truly tetrachromatic (Neumeyer, 1992; Palacios and Varela, 1992). In contrast, most non-primate mammals would appear to be dichromats, with a colour vision system based on only two classes of cone, one that is maximally sensitive in the green/yellow spectral region (530–565 nm) and the second, forming a rather sparse population of short-wave-sensitive (SWS) cones, maximally sensitive in the violet/blue region (420–460 nm). In some nocturnal mammals these SWS cones are displaced into the near ultraviolet (for a review of mammalian colour vision, see Jacobs, 1993).

Amongst the mammals, it is only within the primates that trichromacy has evolved, but even here, monkeys from the New World remain basically dichromatic. Nevertheless, New World monkeys have achieved a limited degree of trichromacy through a remarkable polymorphism of their visual pigments. Within the two major groups, the *Callitrichidae* and the diurnal *Cebidae*, three cone visual pigments maximally sensitive in the red/green spectral region are available to each species (Jacobs and Neitz, 1987; Jacobs *et al.*, 1987; Mollon *et al.*, 1984; Tovée *et al.*, 1992; Travis *et al.*, 1988). However, all males are dichromats with only a single longer-wave pigment in addition to a typically mammalian SWS cone, whereas some two thirds of females are behaviourally trichromatic and possess two spectrally distinct classes of cone maximally sensitive in the red/green (Figure 2.1.1). The polymorphism is a consequence of three allelic variants of a single gene coding for the cone opsin, each producing a visual pigment with a slightly different wavelength of maximum absorbance (λ_{max}) (Mollon *et al.*, 1984; Neitz *et al.*, 1991; Williams *et al.*, 1992). As the gene is located on the X chromosome, all males can have only one copy and express only one of the three pigments, whereas females, who are heterozygous for the gene locus, are able to express two spectrally distinct cone pigments. As a result of X chromosome inactivation, only one of the alleles will be expressed in any given cone and the animal's nervous system is flexible enough to be able to extract the available wavelength information (Tovée *et al.*, 1992).

Within any one species of platyrrhine, therefore, there are six forms of colour vision: three forms of dichromacy exhibited by all the males and the homozygous females, and three forms of trichromacy possessed by the two-thirds of females that are heterozygous for

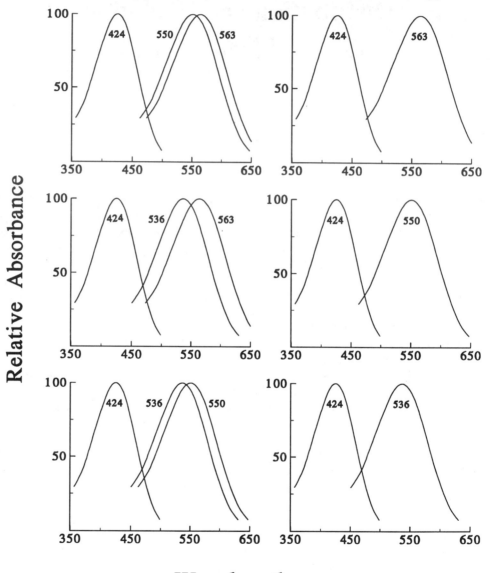

Wavelength, nm

Figure 2.1.1. Polymorphism of visual pigments in a New World monkey. Absorbance spectra of the visual pigment complements of the six forms of colour vision in the squirrel monkey. The three right hand panels show the three forms of dichromacy exhibited by males and those females homozygous for the LWS/MWS opsin gene. The three left hand panels illustrate the three forms of trichromacy exhibited by the two thirds of females heterozygous for the gene locus. Data taken from Mollon *et al.* (1984).

this opsin gene locus. The polymorphism is presumably maintained because of hetero-zygous advantage: the only way to have the benefit of at least some members of the species possessing trichromacy is to maintain the polymorphism of the opsin gene (Mollon *et al.*, 1984; Tovée *et al.*, 1992). The set of three pigments expressed as a consequence of the polymorphism differs between the two major groups of platyrrhines: in the *Callitrichidae*, the marmosets and tamarins have pigments with λ_{max} at about 543, 556 and 563 nm (Jacobs *et al.*, 1987; Travis *et al.*, 1988), whereas in the *Cebidae*, the squirrel monkey and capuchin monkey have pigments with λ_{max} at about 536, 550 and 563 nm (Figure 2.1.1) (Jacobs and Neitz, 1987; Mollon *et al.*, 1984; Shyue *et al.*, 1995).

Only in Old World primates, including humans, is full trichromacy achieved. In these species, the single ancestral genetic locus for the longer-wave pigment has become duplicated so that even in males, the single X chromosome can give the benefit of two spectrally distinct cone populations. The striking polymorphism exhibited by platyrrhines is not found and the available data suggests that all catarrhines, including the Great Apes and humans, normally possess cone pigments with λ_{max} restricted to two spectral locations close to 535 and 563 nm (Bowmaker *et al.*, 1978; Bowmaker *et al.*, 1991; Dulai *et al.*, 1994; Hárosi, 1987; Ibbotson *et al.*, 1992). Nevertheless, polymorphisms of a different kind do occur in Old World monkeys and humans, where sequence variations appear to be relatively common (Deeb *et al.*, 1994, 1995; Dulai *et al.*, 1994; Ibbotson *et al.*, 1992; Nathans *et al.*, 1986a; Neitz and Neitz, 1995; Winderickx *et al.*, 1993) and where, at least in humans, hybrid genes account for much of the colour deficiency that is found in about eight per cent of male Caucasians and about 0.5 per cent of females (e.g. Hunt *et al.*, 1995b; Merbs and Nathans, 1992b; Nathans *et al.*, 1986b; Neitz *et al.*, 1995; Winderickx *et al.*, 1992).

As all these visual pigments are composed of a G-protein-linked opsin molecule enclosing the chromophore retinal, the spectral differences between the various cone pigments must depend on differences in the structure of opsin (Knowles and Dartnall, 1977). To displace an absorbance maximum to longer wavelengths, for instance, requires that there is a smaller energy difference between the ground and excited states of the molecule: the protein-chromophore interaction must increase delocalisation in the π electron shell of the chromophore. This could be through substitutions of differently charged amino acids or amino acids with different polar properties. The opsin molecules of the primate long-wave-sensitive (LWS) and middle-wave-sensitive (MWS) cone pigments are composed of 364 amino acids (Nathans *et al.*, 1986a), but it is only those amino acids that lie on the inner surfaces of the membrane helices and in close proximity to retinal that probably have the principal role in spectral tuning. A model for the three-dimensional arrangement of the seven helices, based on comparisons of the amino acid sequences of a large number of G-protein receptors and the two-dimensional crystal structure of rhodopsin (Schertler *et al.*, 1993), has recently been proposed (Baldwin, 1993). In this model, each α-helix is composed of 26 residues, although only the central 18 or so residues are thought to be embedded in the membrane (Figure 2.1.2). The spectral shifts in λ_{max} between the various primate LWS/MWS cone pigments have been shown to depend primarily on amino acid substitution at just three sites in these trans-membrane regions and, in each case, it is the gain or loss of a hydroxyl-bearing amino acid that is important (Asenjo *et al.*, 1994; Merbs and Nathans, 1992a; Nathans *et al.*, 1986a; Neitz *et al.*, 1991; Williams *et al.*, 1992).

The three sites are 164 in helix IV (serine/alanine) and 261 (tyrosine/phenylalanine) and 269 (threonine/alanine) in helix VI (Figure 2.1.2). (These site numbers correspond with bovine rhodopsin and would be 180, 277 and 285 respectively in the LWS/MWS cone opsins). The shortest-wave pigments with λ_{max} at about 536 nm have the non-hydroxyl bearing amino acids at all three sites, whereas the longest-wave pigments with λ_{max} close to 563 nm have the hydroxyl-bearing amino acid at the three sites. The pigments with intermediate λ_{max} have combinations of both non-hydroxyl and hydroxyl-bearing amino acids. Thus, in the *Callitrichidae*, the 543-nm pigment has one hydroxyl replacement from the 536-nm pigment, tyrosine at 261, whereas the 557-nm pigment has one non-hydroxyl replacement from the 563-nm pigment, alanine at 164. The 550-nm pigment of the *Cebidae* also has a single hydroxyl replacement from the 536-nm pigment, but in this case it is threonine at 269. This simple 'additive' concept ignores the role of any other amino acid differences between the pigments and it is now apparent that a number of other sites can have a small influence in determining the λ_{max}, causing spectral displacements of perhaps 1 or 2 nm (Asenjo *et al.*, 1994).

In contrast, much less is known about spectral differences and spectral tuning of the SWS cone pigments. Perhaps because they are not often associated with colour deficiencies, SWS cones have been rather ignored, at least in terms of their exact spectral location. This is not so surprising, because determining their λ_{max} is not as simple as it is for the LWS/MWS cones. First, they are rare, comprising only about five per cent of the total cone

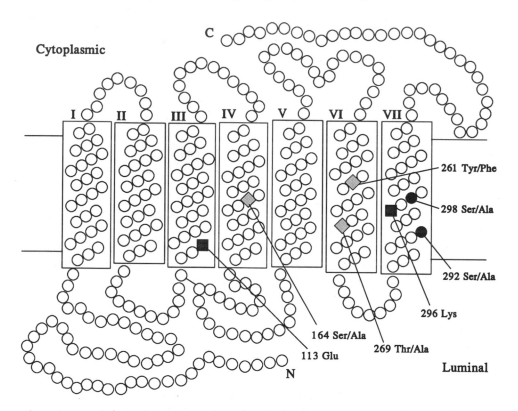

Figure 2.1.2.   Schematic representation of opsin showing the seven α-helical membrane segments (Baldwin, 1993; Nathans *et al.*, 1986a). Sites 164, 261 and 269 in helices IV and VI are involved in the spectral tuning of primate LWS/MWS cone pigments. Sites 292 and 298 in helix VII are proposed as tuning sites for primate SWS cones. Retinal is attached to opsin at lysine 296 in helix VII and glutamate 113 in helix III acts as a counter ion to the protonated Schiff's base linkage of retinal.

population, so that direct measurements by microspectrophotometry or electrophysio-logical techniques are more difficult, and, second, psychophysical and electrorctinographic measurements of short-wave sensitivity have to take into account pre-receptoral screening, especially by the lens. Nevertheless, although the SWS cone pigments of New and Old World primates show maximal absorbances in a narrow range of the violet region of the spectrum, small inter-species differences do occur.

We have looked at the SWS cones from eight species of Old World monkey and the λ_{max} values all lie close to 430 nm (Bowmaker *et al.*, 1991). In only two species have we measured sufficient numbers of SWS cones to fix the λ_{max} with some precision: in the moustached guenon (*Cercopithecus cephus*) the λ_{max} was 432 nm and in the talapoin (*Miopithecus talapoin*) 431 nm (Figure 2.1.3) (Bowmaker *et al.*, 1991; Hunt *et al.*, 1995a). Similar values have also been determined for macaques by microspectrophotometry (Hárosi, 1987; Mansfield *et al.*, 1984) and by determinations of spectral sensitivity using suction electrode techniques (Baylor *et al.*, 1987). In humans, however, the SWS cones have their maximum absorbance shifted to slightly shorter wavelengths with λ_{max} at 420 nm (Bowmaker, 1991; Dartnall *et al.*, 1983) (Figure 2.1.3). Amongst the New World monkeys differences in the λ_{max} of SWS cones also occur. In the marmoset the mean λ_{max} is 424 nm

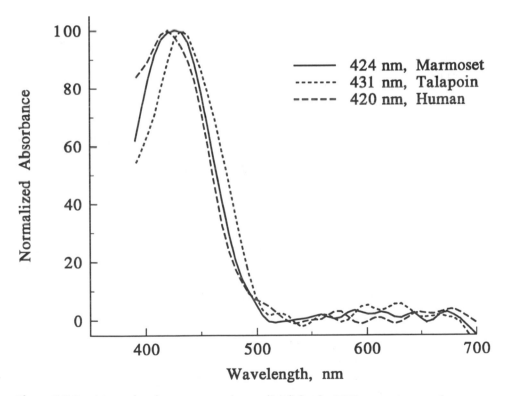

Figure 2.1.3. Mean absorbance spectra (normalized) for the SWS cone pigments from marmoset, talapoin and human as recorded by microspectrophotometry. The spectra are means from 13 marmoset, 7 talapoin and 8 human SWS cones. The data have been smoothed using a non-parametric smoothing algorithm that uses locally weighted least-squares linear regressions to obtain smoothed values for each absorbance value at each given wavelength value.

(Tovée *et al.*, 1992; Travis *et al.*, 1988), lying between the λ_{max} of talapoin and human SWS cones (Figure 2.1.3). Earlier data from squirrel monkeys show that in this species, SWS cones have a λ_{max} similar to that of Old World monkeys and close to 430 nm (Bowmaker *et al.*, 1985; Mollon *et al.*, 1984).

The spectral differences, about 11 nm between human and talapoin monkey and about 7 nm between marmosets and talapoin, are of a similar order to the differences within the platyrrhine MWS/LWS cone pigments. Are amino acids bearing hydroxyl groups important here in spectral tuning and are the same set of amino acids that determine spectral tuning in the LWS and MWS pigments again involved? We have sequenced the SWS cone opsin genes from a marmoset, talapoin and human and have used the deduced amino acid sequences to identify candidate sites for the inter-species spectral shifts. The sequence of the human gene is identical to that published by Nathans *et al.* (1986a) and the SWS cone opsin proteins show considerable inter-species homology in amino acid sequence (Hunt *et al.*, 1995a).

In terms of spectral tuning between the SWS pigments from the different species, the only site in the human and talapoin SWS pigments that shows a loss or gain of an hydroxyl-bearing amino acid in an α-helical trans-membrane region is at position 292 of helix VII (Figures 2.1.2 and 2.1.4). This residue faces the centre of the chromophore binding pocket and is close to the lysine residue that forms the Schiff's base linkage with the chromophore. We propose that substitution of serine for alanine at this site in the SWS cone opsin is responsible for the spectral shift from 431 nm in talapoin monkey to 420 nm in human. It is interesting that substitution by site-directed mutagenesis of alanine by aspartate at this site in bovine rhodopsin has been shown to result in a similar blue shift of about 10 nm (Nakayama and Khorana, 1991).

As the marmoset is identical to talapoin at site 292, an additional amino acid substitution must be responsible for the 7 nm blue shift that places the spectral peak of the marmoset pigment at 424 nm, approximately mid-way between the human and talapoin pigments. The marmoset pigment differs from talapoin and human in an hydroxyl-bearing amino acid at the following amino acid positions/helical sites: 46/9 and 56/19 in helix I, 155/5 and 159/9 in helix IV, 217/16 in helix V, and 298/13 in helix VII (Figure 2.1.4) (Hunt *et al.*, 1995a). However, from alignment with the conserved sites in each helix, all except position 298 are on lipid-facing aspects of the helices (Figure 2.1.4). We propose, therefore, that substitution of serine for alanine at site 298 accounts for the blue spectral shift from 431 nm in talapoin to 424 nm in marmoset.

We cannot, of course, rule out the possibility that other differences in amino acids between the three opsins at additional sites contribute to the observed spectral differences. It would seem probable, though, that such contributions, if any, are small in relation to the shifts of 6–11 nm resulting from the alanine/serine differences at sites 292 and 298. At the three hydroxyl/non-hydroxyl sites in the LWS/MWS primate cone pigments, the presence of a hydroxyl-bearing amino acid leads to a red shift, but in the SWS pigments, serine at either site 292 or 298 leads to a blue shift. This opposite spectral displacement may be either a consequence of the overall spectral location of the different pigment groups, about 420–430 nm as opposed to 530–560 nm or, more probably, a consequence of the different positions of the amino acids in opsin in relation to retinal. Amino acids in helices IV and VI probably interact with the β-ionone ring of retinal, whereas those in helix VII are closely associated with the Schiff's base linkage of retinal to lysine at site 296.

What is it in the environment of primates that has dictated the peak sensitivities of the different cone classes? The major difference between the New and Old World monkeys is in the polymorphism of cone pigments in the New World contrasted with the more conserved spectral locations of the MWS/LWS pigments in the Old World. As discussed previously, the polymorphism in the platyrrhincs is probably maintained by the advantages of trichromacy that it endows on two-thirds of the females. Presumably, the duplication of the ancestral MWS/LWS gene that occurred in catarrhines has failed to occur in platyr-rhines. A biological explanation is still required for the spectral differences between the two sets of pigments in the cebids and the callitrichids. One possibility is that the differences relate to variations in diet and to the relative quantity of fruit that each group prefers: the *Callitrichidae* are more specialised for eating gums and saps (Tovée *et al.*, 1992). In Old World monkeys, the λ_{max} of the LWS and MWS cones are usually separated by about 30 nm. Again, their λ_{max} may be dictated by diet: many catarrhines are frugivorous and select primarily yellow fruits (Gautier-Hion *et al.*, 1985). Mollon (1991) has suggested that the spectral location of the two cone classes is ideally suited for discriminating such yellow fruits against the 'dappled' background of foliage.

A biological explanation for the small differences in the λ_{max} of the SWS cone pigments is not so apparent. Why should the human SWS cone be maximally sensitive at a shorter wavelength than that of Old World monkeys? One major factor may be the transparency of the lens to short wavelengths. Most vertebrate lenses absorb violet and near ultraviolet light to a greater or lesser extent and there is a clear correlation between lens transparency and ultraviolet sensitivity (Bowmaker, 1991; Goldsmith, 1991). In humans, the lens shows

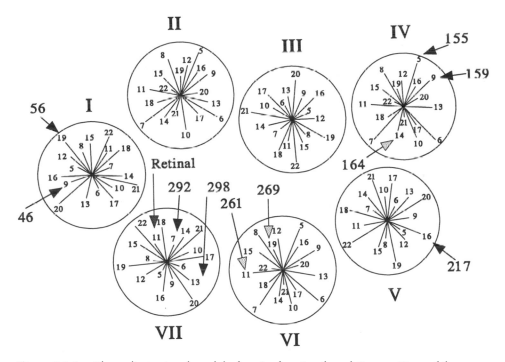

Figure 2.1.4. Three dimensional model of opsin showing the relative positions of the seven α-helical trans-membrane regions (Baldwin, 1993). Each circle represents an α-helix and each radiating line within the circle represents an amino acid. The position of each line indicates the location of each amino acid around the circumference of the helix and the length of each line indicates the depth of the amino acid within the helix. Sites 164, 261 and 269 are primarily responsible for spectral differences between primate LWS/MWS cone pigments; sites 292 and 298 are proposed as tuning sites for primate SWS cone pigments. The chromophore, 11-*cis* retinal, is attached to a lysine in helix VII.

increasing absorbance into the violet (Wyszecki and Stiles, 1982), though this varies between individuals and increases with age, whereas data for Old World monkeys suggests that, at least in macaques, the lens is yellower than in humans, with a density at 400 nm nearly twice that of humans (Kennedy and Milkman, 1956; Cooper and Robson, 1969). There is then a simple correlation of lens absorbance with the λ_{max} of SWS cones in catarrhines, with the shorter λ_{max} associated with the more transparent lens.

Open environments contain relatively more short-wave light and are therefore 'whiter' than the yellow/green of forest shade (Endler, 1993), and it may be that the evolution of humans from an arboreal ancestor to an open savannah biped makes increased short-wave sensitivity an advantage. It would be interesting to know the λ_{max} of SWS cones in the great apes: the lens absorbance of baboons appears to be closer to human than to macaque (Cooper and Robson, 1969). Similar considerations cannot be applied to New World monkeys because squirrel monkeys and marmosets are both arboreal. Squirrel monkeys have lenses with absorbance similar to macaques (Cooper and Robson, 1969), but marmosets, with a shorter λ_{max} SWS cone pigment, have even yellower lenses (Tovée et al., 1992).

2.1.1   REFERENCES

ASENJO, A.B., RIM, J. & OPRIAN, D.D. (1994) Molecular determinants of human red/green color discrimination, *Neuron*, **12**, 1131–1138.

BALDWIN, J.M. (1993) The probable arrangement of the helices in G protein-coupled receptors, *European Molecular Biology Organisation Journal*, **12**, 1693–1703.

BAYLOR, D.A., NUNN, B.J. & SCHNAPF, J.L. (1987) Spectral sensitivity of cones of the monkey *Macaca fascicularis*, *Journal of Physiology*, **390**, 145–160.

BOWMAKER, J.K. (1991) Evolution of visual pigments and photoreceptors. In: Gregory, R.L. & Cronly-Dillon, J.R. (Eds.) *Evolution of the Eye and Visual System*, Vol.2, London: Macmillan, pp. 63–81.

BOWMAKER, J.K., DARTNALL, H.J.A., LYTHGOE, J.N. & MOLLON, J.D. (1978) The visual pigments of rods and cones in the Rhesus monkey *Macaca mulatta*, *Journal of Physiology*, **274**, 329–348.

BOWMAKER, J.K., JACOBS, G.H., SPIEGELHALTER, D.J. & MOLLON, J.D. (1985) Two types of trichromatic squirrel monkey share a pigment in the red-green spectral region, *Vision Research*, **25**, 1937–1946.

BOWMAKER, J.K., ASTELL, S., HUNT, D.M. & MOLLON, J.D. (1991) Photosensitive and photostable pigments in the retinae of Old World monkeys, *Journal of Experimental Biology*, **156**, 1–19.

COOPER, G.F. & ROBSON, J.G. (1969) The yellow colour of the lens of man and other primates, *Journal of Physiology*, **203**, 411–417.

DARTNALL, H.J.A., BOWMAKER, J.K. & MOLLON, J.D. (1983) Human visual pigments: microspectrophotometric results from the eyes of seven persons, *Proceedings of the Royal Society of London*, **B 220**, 115–130.

DEEB, S.S., JORGENSEN, A.L., BATTISTI, L., IWASAKI, L. AND MOTULSKY, A.G. (1994) Sequence divergence of the red and green visual pigments in great apes and humans, *Proceedings of the National Academy of Sciences*, **91**, 7262–7266.

DEEB, S.S., ALVAREZ, A., MALKKI, M. and MOTULSKY, A.G. (1995) Molecular-patterns and sequence polymorphisms in the red and green visual pigment genes of Japanese men, *Human Genetics*, **95**, 501–506.

DULAI, K.S., BOWMAKER, J.K., MOLLON, J.D. & HUNT, D.M. (1994) Sequence divergence, polymorphism and evolution of the middle-wave and long-wave visual pigments of Great Apes and Old World monkeys, *Vision Research*, **34**, 2483–2491.

ENDLER, J.A. (1993) The color of light in forests and its implications, *Ecological Monographs*, **63**, 1–27.

GAUTIER-HION, A., DUPLANTIER, J.-M., QURIS, R., FEER, F., SOURD, C., DECOUX, J.-P., DUBOST, G., EMMONS, L., ERARD, C., HECKETSWEILER, P., MOUNGAZI, A., ROUSSILHON, C. & THIOLLAY, J.-M. (1985) Fruit characteristics as a basis of fruit choice and seed dispersal in a tropical forest community, *Oecologia*, **65**, 324–337.

GOLDSMITH, T.H. (1991) The evolution of visual pigments and colour vision. In: Gouras, P. (Ed.) *The Perception of Colour*, Vol. 6, London: Macmillan, pp. 62–89.

HÁROSI, F.I. (1987) Cynomologus and Rhesus monkey visual pigments, *Journal of General Physiology*, **89**, 717– 743.

HUNT, D.M., COWING, J.A., BOWMAKER, J.K., PATEL, R., APPUKUTTAN, B. & MOLLON, J.D. (1995a) Sequence and evolution of the blue cone pigment gene in Old and New World primates, *Genomics*, **27**, 535–538.

IBBOTSON, R.E., HUNT, D.M., BOWMAKER, J.K. & MOLLON, J.D. (1992) Sequence divergence and copy number of the middle- and long-wave photopigment genes in Old World monkeys, *Proceedings of the Royal Society of London*, **B 247**, 145–154.

JACOBS, G.H. (1993) The distribution and nature of colour vision among the mammals, *Biological Reviews*, **68**, 413– 471.

JACOBS, G.H. AND NEITZ, J. (1987) Inheritance of color vision in a New World monkey (*Saimiri sciureus*), *Proceedings of the National Academy of Sciences*, **84**, 2545–2549.

JACOBS, G.H., NEITZ, J. & CROGNALE, M.A. (1987) Color vision polymorphism and its photopigment basis in a callitrichid monkey (*Saguinus fusicollis*), *Vision Research*, **27**, 2089–2100.

KENNEDY, D. & MILKMAN, R.D. (1956) Selective light absorption by the lenses of lower vertebrates, and its influence on spectral sensitivity, *Biological Bulletin*, **111**, 375–386.

KNOWLES, A. & DARTNALL, H.J.A. (1977) The photobiology of vision. In: Davson, H. (Ed.) *The Eye*, Vol.2B, 2nd edn, New York: Academic Press, pp. 1–689.

MANSFIELD, R.J.W., LEVINE, J.S., LIPETZ, L.E., COLLINS, B.A., RAYMOND, G. & MacNICHOL, E.F. (1984) Blue-sensitive cones in the primate retina: microspectrophotometry of the visual pigment, *Experimental Brain Research*, **56**, 389–394.

MERBS, S.L. & NATHANS, J. (1992a) Absorption spectra of the human cone pigments, *Nature*, **356**, 433–435.

MERBS, S.L. & NATHANS, J. (1992b) Absorption spectra of the hybrid pigments responsible for anomalous color vision, *Science*, **258**, 464–466.

MOLLON, J.D. (1991) The uses and evolutionary origins of primate colour vision. In: Gregory, R.L. & Cronly-Dillon, J.R. (Eds.) *Evolution of the Eye and Visual System*, Vol.2, London: Macmillan, pp. 306–319.

MOLLON, J.D., BOWMAKER, J.K. & JACOBS, G.H. (1984) Variations of colour vision in a New World Primate can be explained by polymorphism of retinal photopigments, *Proceedings of the Royal Society of London*, **B 222**, 373–399.

NAKAYAMA, T.A. & KHORANA, H.G. (1991) Mapping of the amino acids in membrane-embedded helices that interact with the retinal chromophore in bovine rhodopsin, *Journal of Biological Chemistry*, **266**, 4269–4275.

NATHANS, J., THOMAS, D. & HOGNESS, D.S. (1986a) Molecular genetics of human color vision: the genes encoding blue, green and red pigments, *Science*, **232**, 193–203.

NATHANS, J., PIANTANIDA, T.P., EDDY, R.L., SHOWS, T.B. & HOGNESS, D.S. (1986b) Molecular genetics of inherited variations in human color vision, *Science*, **232**, 203–210.

NEITZ, M. and NEITZ, J. (1995) Numbers and ratios of visual pigment genes for normal red-green color vision, *Science*, **267**, 1013–1016.

NEITZ, M., NEITZ, J. & JACOBS, G.H. (1991) Spectral tuning of pigments underlying red-green color vision, *Science*, **252**, 971–974.

NEITZ, M., NEITZ, J. and JACOBS, G.H. (1995) Genetic basis of photopigment variations in human dichromats, *Vision Res.*, **35**, 2095–2103.

NEUMEYER, C. (1992) Tetrachromatic color vision in goldfish: evidence from color mixture experiments, *Journal of Comparative Physiology*, **A 171**, 639–649.

PALACOIS, A.G. & VARELA, F.J. (1992) Color mixing in the pigeon (*Columba livia*) II: a psychophysical determination in the middle, short and near-uv wavelength range, *Vision Research*, **32**, 1947–1953.

SCHERTLER, G.X., VILLA, C. & HENDERSON, R. (1993) Projection structure of rhodopsin, *Nature*, **362**, 770–772.

SHYUE, S.K., HEWETTEMMETT, D., SPERLING, H.G., HUNT, D.M., BOWMAKER, J.K., MOLLON, J.D. & LI, W.H. (1995) Adaptive evolution of color vision genes in higher primates, *Science*, **269**, 1265–1267.

TOVÉE, M.J., MOLLON, J.D. & BOWMAKER, J.K. (1992) The relationship between cone pigments and behavioural sensitivity in a New World monkey (*Callithrix jacchus jacchus*), *Vision Research*, **32**, 867–878.

TRAVIS, D.S., BOWMAKER, J.K. & MOLLON, J.D. (1988) Polymorphism of visual pigments in a callitrichid monkey, *Vision Research*, **28**, 481–490.

WILLIAMS, A.J., HUNT, D.M., BOWMAKER, J.K. & MOLLON, J.D. (1992) The polymorphic photopigments of the marmoset: spectral tuning and genetic basis, *European Molecular Biology Organisation Journal*, **11**, 2039–2045.

WINDERICKX, J., LINDSEY, D.T., SANOCKI, E., TELLER, D.Y., MOTULSKY, A.G. & DEEB, S.S. (1992) Polymorphism in red photopigment underlies variation in colour matching, *Nature*, **356**, 431–433.

WINDERICKX, J., BATTISTI, L. HIBIYA, Y., MOTULSKY, A.G. and DEEB, S.S. (1993) Haplotype diversity in the human red and green opsin genes: evidence for frequent sequence exchange in exon 3, *Human Molecular Genetics*, **2**, 1413–1421.

WYSZECKI, G. & STILES, W.S. (1982) *Color Science*, 2nd edn, New York: John Wiley & Sons.

Evaluation of the Genetic Contribution to Individual Variations in the Spectral Sensitivity of Deuteranopes

Gerald H. Jacobs and Jack B. Calderone

2.2.1 INTRODUCTION

Studies of the spectral sensitivity of dichromatic humans have historically been central both to colour theory and to attempts to infer mechanisms for defective colour vision. Although there have been a considerable number of attempts to measure the spectral sensitivity of deuteranopes, and thereby define the spectral properties of the photopigments underlying dichromacy, most of these studies have been largely unconcerned with the issue of individual variability. Table 2.2.1 summarises some results from a number of studies that have included information about spectral variability in deuteranopes. Listed in the table are indications of the ranges of measured peak sensitivity (λ_{max}) for the sample and, where available, a statistic describing variability. Estimates are included both for several psycho-physical determinations and for two studies that used objective measurement techniques. The most thorough of these investigations are likely to have been those of Alpern and colleagues who inferred λ_{max} values for a large sample of deuteranopes from the anomalo-scope brightness matches made between a yellow primary light and various red/green test light mixtures (Alpern, 1987; Alpern and Wake, 1977; Alpern and Pugh, 1977). In a detailed examination of a subset of these subjects, Alpern and Pugh (1977) conducted experiments to show that the spectral variation among their subjects could not be attributed solely to individual variations in the screening properties of the ocular media, to individual differences in the optical properties of the cones, or to individual differences in pigment optical density. Rather, they concluded that there must be inherent individual variations in the spectra of the deuteranope L-cone pigment. Note that the magnitude of individual variation documented for deuteranopes by Alpern *et al.* is similar to that found in two other recent studies (Table 2.2.1).

The nature of individual variations in spectral sensitivity has recently taken on new interest with the discovery that the genes specifying M- and L-cone opsins are polymorphic (Nathans *et al.*, 1986). A subset of these polymorphisms are known to be important for the spectral tuning of the photopigment. Of these, the gene polymorphism of interest here is one that results in an amino-acid substitution (serine/alanine) at position 180 in the cone opsin. This substitution is associated with a small but significant shift in the λ_{max} value of the photopigment. As estimated by comparisons of the spectra of pigments resulting from

Table 2.2.1. Published estimates of variations in the λ_{max} of the L-cones of deuteranopes

Technique	λ_{max}		Reference	
	Range	SD	n	
Psychophysics	28	-	18*	Wald and Brown, 1965
Psychophysics	6.35	1.6	38	Alpern and Wake, 1977
Psychophysics	7.4	2.4	8	Alpern and Pugh, 1977
Psychophysics	5–6	-	9	Sanocki et al., 1993
MSP	16	4.4	10**	Mollon et al., 1984
ERG	5	1.4	11	Jacobs and Neitz, 1991

* Includes both deuteranomalous and deuteranopic subjects
** Number of individual cone spectra measured; in all other cases it represents the number of individuals tested.
Range and SD values are specified in nm. ERG, electroretinogram; MSP, microspectrophotometry.

action of the two alternative versions of the gene, the shift in peak value of the pigment is in the range of 4–7 nm (Asenjo et al., 1994; Neitz et al., 1991; Merbs and Nathans, 1993; Neitz et al., 1995). Recently, Sanocki et al. (1993) reported that deuteranopes believed to have the two polymorphic variants of the L-cone pigment gene showed correlated variations in the λ_{max} values of their pigments. The λ_{max} values for the pigments of these deuteranopes were estimated from anomaloscope brightness matches. So estimated, the average λ_{max} differences for two groups of deuteranopes (consisting of five and four subjects respectively) was 4.3 nm. We have now examined spectra obtained from deuteranopes to see if evidence for this polymorphic variation can be detected in a larger sample of subjects whose spectral sensitivities had been measured with an objective technique.

2.2.2 METHODS

The subjects were 23 young (18–25 years of age), male deuteranopes. They were initially screened for deutan defects by their performance on standard plate tests (Ishihara and AO-HRR). The diagnosis of dichromacy was made by their subsequent failure to set a unique Rayleigh match in a test involving the use of a Maxwellian-view optical system. The test field was a 3°–10° centred annulus and the Rayleigh equation was 589 nm = 546 nm + 670 nm with the primary and comparison lights presented in temporal alternation (Neitz and Jacobs, 1990).

Spectral sensitivity was measured with electroretinogram (ERG) flicker photometry (Neitz and Jacobs, 1984). The pupil of the test eye was dilated and ERGs were differentially recorded using a DTL electrode. With the aid of a dental bite, a large stimulus field (57°) was presented in Maxwellian-view. ERGs were recorded from trains of light pulses that originated from two sources. One beam (achromatic, 3.54 log td) served as the reference light of the photometer. The test beam provided monochromatic lights in steps of 10 nm from 450 to 660 nm. At each test wavelength the intensity of the light was varied until it was equal in effectiveness to the reference light. Equations were made twice for each test light. The total pulse rate of the photometer was 62.5 Hz.

The spectral sensitivity values for each deuteranope were corrected for lens absorption (Wyszecki and Stiles, 1982) and these data arrays were best fit with standard visual pigment absorption curves (Dawis, 1981) that were shifted in steps of 1 nm along a log wave-number axis. The data of concern here are the peak values of these best-fitting functions.

2.2.3   INDIVIDUAL VARIATIONS IN ERG SPECTRA OBTAINED FROM DEUTERANOPES

We have reported previously that highly reliable measurements can be made with ERG flicker photometry. For instance, the variability seen with this technique is considerably lower than that obtained with heterochromatic flicker photometry, a standard psycho-physical technique used to measure spectral sensitivity (Jacobs and Neitz, 1993). The spectra obtained with ERG flicker photometry can be well characterised by photopigment absorption curves. Figure 2.2.1 shows two examples of the spectra that were obtained from deuteranopic subjects. Included there are results from the individual subject whose data were best fitted by this procedure, and results from the individual whose data yielded the single poorest fit to the absorption curves. Note that even the poorest data set obtained for any of the 23 subjects allows a reasonably compelling estimate of peak sensitivity.

Figure 2.2.2 shows the distribution of λ_{max} values obtained for the sample of deuter-anopes. The total range of peak values, 7 nm, is virtually identical to that obtained from the psychophysical measurements by Alpern *et al.* summarized in Table 2.2.1, and the measure of variability of these λ_{max} values (SD = 2.08 nm) is not dissimilar to that of the previous reports.

A considerable list of factors can be compiled that might contribute to the variation in the λ_{max} values of Figure 2.2.2. These would include individual variations in preretinal filtering,

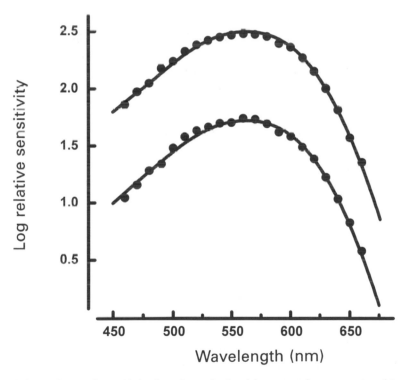

Figure 2.2.1.   Spectral sensitivity functions obtained from two deuteranopic subjects with ERG flicker photometry. The solid circles are individual sensitivity measurements; the solid lines are the best-fitting photopigment absorption functions. The two data sets represent, respectively, the subjects whose data yielded the best (top) and poorest (bottom) fits to photopigment curves from among 23 subjects similarly tested. For both subjects the estimated λ_{max} value was 560 nm.

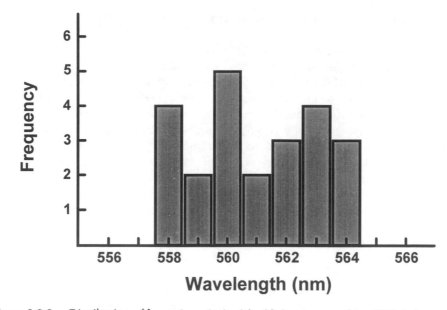

Figure 2.2.2. Distribution of λ_{max} values obtained for 23 deuteranopes from ERG flicker photometric measurements.

individual variations in photopigment density, and the error inherent in the measurement technique itself, as well as any individual variations in the spectra of the deuteranopic photopigment (Alpern and Pugh, 1977). One standard approach to such a data set would be to make assumptions about the effects of each of these factors and then to examine the nature of residual variation after each of these, in turn, has been compensated or argued to be insignificant. We have elected to use an alternative approach, one which may allow a separation of the genetic factors underlying spectral variation from the several other sources. It involves a comparison of the distribution of λ_{max} values from these deuteranopes to a distribution of λ_{max} values obtained from a sample of nonhuman primates. The assumption is that the latter show no individual variation in the genetic mechanisms for spectral tuning, although they are likely to be subject to all of the other sources of variation. Comparison of these two data sets thus might be thought to allow a determination of whether any of the variation in the deuteranope data may be traced to genetically-controlled variations in spectral tuning.

2.2.4   COMPARISONS OF DEUTERANOPE AND MONKEY L-CONE SPECTRA

It is now well established that a significant number of species of platyrrhine monkey have a striking L/M cone photopigment polymorphism (reviewed in Jacobs, 1993). For present purposes, the important fact is that this polymorphism yields many individuals who have only a single class of L/M photopigment. Data obtained both from classical genetic analysis and from molecular approaches provides strong support for the view that these individuals have only a single X-chromosome photopigment gene and that gene is invariant among individuals sharing a given photopigment phenotype (Hunt *et al.*, 1993; Jacobs and Neitz, 1987; Jacobs *et al.*, 1993). Although the particular L/M photopigments vary among these playtrrhine monkeys, each species so far studied has been found to contain individuals whose single L/M photopigment has a λ_{max} value very similar to that for the human deuteranopes, i.e. about 560 nm.

Figure 2.2.3 shows the distribution of λ_{max} values obtained from a total of 39 platyrrhine monkeys. This collection includes representatives from five genera (*Ateles*, *Callicebus*, *Cebus*, *Saimiri* and *Saguinous*). These results were obtained in ERG recording experiments that were, for all practical purposes, identical to those employed to measure the spectra for deuteranopes. Probably most important, the monkeys were tested using the same lights and other stimulus configurations that were used for the human subjects. The data analysis was also the same. The only manipulation unique to the monkey data set is that prior to combining the results from the different species, the collections of λ_{max} values for each species were slid along the wavelength scale so that all had a common mean λ_{max} value. This amounted to an adjustment of 0, 1 or 2 nm for the various species. The adjustment keeps intact any of the within-species variation that might reasonably be thought traceable to some of the non-genetic factors noted above. The λ_{max} distribution for this sample of monkeys does not deviate significantly ($\chi^2 = 6.13$; df = 5; ns) from a normal distribution (solid line in Figure 2.2.3) having a SD value of 1.36 nm.

As noted above, there is considerable evidence for two polymorphic versions of the human L-cone opsin gene that produce pigments of different spectra. Action of either one of them might be expected to yield a distribution of λ_{max} values similar to the monkey data of Figure 2.2.3 (hereafter referred to as the 'single-gene distribution'). If both versions of the L-cone gene were expressed in our sample of deuteranopes, the λ_{max} distribution should be better accounted for by the combination of two distributions like that of Figure 2.2.3, rather than by only one such distribution. To see if this was so, we compared the fits to the deuteranope data obtained for the case of the operation of a single gene and for alternative

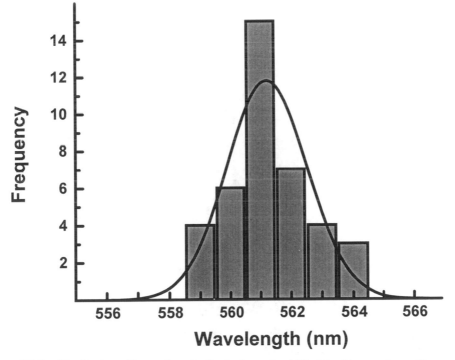

Figure 2.2.3. Distribution of λ_{max} values for the L-pigments of 39 platyrrhine monkeys. The smooth curve is the best-fitting normal distribution.

scenarios where there were two genes in the sample that generate pigments variably separated in their λ_{max} values. To accomplish this, we used a computer program that uses maximum likelihood to determine whether one distribution or two provides a better fit to the data. The parameters explored by the program are the spectral displacement between the two distributions and the proportions of cases falling in the two distributions. The distribution of deuteranope λ_{max} values deviate significantly from the single gene distribution ($\chi^2 = 56.7$; df = 6; $p < .005$); they were best accounted for by two single-gene distributions that had a λ_{max} separation of 3.5 nm ($\chi^2 = 3.15$; df = 6; ns). These two distributions are shown in Figure 2.2.4. This analysis sorts roughly equal numbers of deuteranopes (12 and 11 subjects respectively) into the two groups.

Some support for the validity of the idea embodied in the results of Figure 2.2.4 comes from an attempt to similarly fit data from human protanopes with the distribution from the monkey λ_{max} values. Evidence suggests that the polymorphism affecting position 180 is of higher frequency in the deuteranope L-cone pigment genes than it is in protanope M-cone pigment genes (Neitz *et al.*, 1995; Sanocki *et al.*, 1993). If this is so, one would expect to encounter genetically-based variations in spectral sensitivity much more frequently in deuteranopes than in protanopes. We fit a distribution of λ_{max} values obtained for 14 protanopes using the single-gene distribution of Figure 2.2.3. Unlike the results for deuteranopes, the protanope distribution was fit very closely by the monkey λ_{max} distribution and, in particular, the single-gene distribution fit these data better than did any two such distributions at various λ_{max} separations.

As there are undoubtedly other factors that influence the nature of the distribution of values for our deuteranopic sample, some of which were mentioned above, it is not appropriate to assume that the separation suggested by the analysis (3–4 nm) gives an accurate estimate of the actual spectral separation of alternative versions of the L-cone

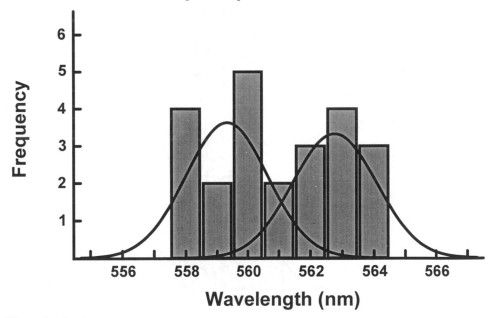

Figure 2.2.4. Results of an analysis showing the best-fit of distributions appropriate for λ_{max} values obtained from platyrrhine monkeys (from Figure 2.2.3) to the distribution of λ_{max} values for the human deuteranopes. The two distributions shown by the continuous lines have peaks separated by about 4 nm. See text for further discussion.

photopigment. Nevertheless, this value is not far from the earlier estimates of the spectral step associated with polymorphic variation at position 180 (Asenjo *et al.*, 1994; Merbs and Nathans, 1993; Neitz *et al.*, 1991; Neitz et al., 1995). At the minimum this analysis indicates that some fraction of the individual variation traditionally detected in the spectral sensitivity of deuteranopes is traceable to gene-controlled photopigment variation. Our experiment thus supports the conclusion that Alpern (1987) earlier reached from an analysis of psychophysical data. However, the discrete nature of the gene-controlled variation now believed to characterise deuteranope λ_{max} variations differs from his conception of a continuous variation in the λ_{max} values. These results also add weight to the general conclusion that the cone pigment gene polymorphisms, now widely reported in molecular studies, have measurable impacts on human visual physiology and visual behaviour.

2.2.5   ACKNOWLEDGEMENTS

The research summarised here was supported by a grant from the National Eye Institute (EY02052).

2.2.6   REFERENCES

ALPERN, M. (1987) Variation in the visual pigments of human dichromats and human trichromats. In: Committee on Vision, National Research Council (Ed.) *Frontiers of Visual Science*, Washington: National Academy Press, pp. 169–193.

ALPERN, M. & PUGH, JR., E. N. (1977) Variation in the action spectrum of erythrolabe among deuteranopes, *Journal of Physiology*, **266**, 613–646.

ALPERN, M. & WAKE, T. (1977) Cone pigments in human deutan colour vision defects, *Journal of Physiology*, **266**, 595–612.

ASENJO, A. B., RIM, J. & OPRIAN, D. D. (1994) Molecular determinants of human red/green colour discrimination, *Neuron*, **12**, 1131–1138.

DAWIS, S. M. (1981) Polynomial expressions of pigment nomograms, *Vision Research*, **21**, 1427–1430.

HUNT, D. M., WILLIAMS, A. J., BOWMAKER, J. K. & MOLLON, J. D. (1993) Structure and evolution of the polymorphic photopigment gene of the marmoset, *Vision Research*, **33**, 147–154.

JACOBS, G. H. (1993) The distribution and nature of color vision among the mammals, *Biological Reviews*, **68**, 413–471.

JACOBS, G. H. & NEITZ, J. (1987) Inheritance of color vision in a New World monkey (*Saimiri sciureus*), *Proceedings of the National Academy of Sciences USA*, **84**, 2545–2549.

JACOBS, G. H. & NEITZ, J. (1991) Deuteranope spectral sensitivity measured with ERG flicker photometry, *Documenta Ophthalmologica Proceedings Series*, **10**, 405–411.

JACOBS, G. H. & NEITZ, J. (1993) Electrophysiological estimates of individual variation in the L/M cone ratio. In: Drum, B. (Ed.) *Colour Vision Deficiencies XI*, Dordrecht: Kluwer, pp. 107–112.

JACOBS, G. H., NEITZ, J. & NEITZ, M. (1993) Genetic basis of polymorphism in the colour vision of platyrrhine monkeys, *Vision Research*, **33**, 269–274.

MERBS, S. L. & NATHANS, J. (1993) Role of hydroxyl-bearing amino acids in differentially tuning the absorption spectra of the human red and green cone pigments, *Photochemistry and Photobiology*, **58**, 706–710.

MOLLON, J. D., BOWMAKER, J. K., DARTNALL, H. J. A. & BIRD, A. C. (1984) Microspectrophotometric and psychophysical results for the same deuteranopic observer, *Documenta Ophthalmologica Proceedings Series*, **7**, 303–310.

NATHANS, J., THOMAS, D. & HOGNESS, D. S. (1986) Molecular genetics of human colour vision: The genes encoding blue, green, and red pigments, *Science*, **232**, 193–202.

NEITZ, J. & JACOBS, G. H. (1984) Electroretinogram measurements of cone spectral sensitivity in dichromatic monkeys, *Journal of the Optical Society of America*, **A 1**, 1175–1180.

NEITZ, J. & JACOBS, G. H. (1990) Polymorphism in normal human colour vision and its mechanism, *Vision Research*, **30**, 621–636.

NEITZ, M., NEITZ, J. & JACOBS, G. H. (1991) Spectral tuning of pigments underlying red-green colour vision, *Science*, **252**, 971–974.

NEITZ, M., NEITZ, J. & JACOBS, G. H. (1995) Genetic basis of photopigment variations in human dichromats, *Vision Research*, **35**, 2095–2103.

SANOCKI, E., LINDSEY, D. T., WINDERICKX, J., TELLER, D. Y., DEEB, S. S. & MOTULSKY, A. G. (1993) Serine/alanine amino acid polymorphism of the L and M cone pigments: Effects on Rayleigh matches among deuteranopes, protanopes and colour normal observers, *Vision Research*, **33**, 2139–2152.

WALD, G. & BROWN, P. K. (1965) Human colour vision and colour blindness, *Cold Spring Harbor Symposium on Quantitative Biology*, **30**, 345–359.

WYSZECKI, G. & STILES, W. S. (1982) *Colour Science*, New York: Wiley.

Induced Colour Blindness in Goldfish

Christa Neumeyer, Carlos Mora-Ferrer, Jan Jaap Wietsma and Henk Spekreijse

2.3.1 INTRODUCTION

The goldfish is ideal for studying colour vision. Having been domesticated for at least one thousand years (Hervcy and Ilems, 1968), it can easily be tamed and used for behavioural experiments. Especially suitable are training experiments that give insight into all the different aspects of colour vision. Earlier measurements of spectral sensitivity and wavelength discrimination led to the conclusion that colour vision in goldfish is trichromatic (see, for review, Jacobs, 1981), which was in line with the finding of three cone types maximally sensitive at about 450 nm, 535 nm and 620 nm (Marks, 1965; Tomita, 1965). The assumed similarity to human colour vision and the specific advantages of the fish retina stimulated extensive electrophysiological investigations that showed so-called colour opponent neurons and double opponent neurons for the first time (for review, see Djamgoz and Yamada, 1990). The findings indicated that the neural basis of colour vision in goldfish is comparable to that in primates (i.c. Old World monkeys), and so it was assumed that the goldfish could be regarded as a model system for understanding human colour vision. To test whether this notion was indeed justified, we first reinvestigated spectral sensitivity and wavelength discrimination with a two-choice behavioural training technique (Neumeyer, 1984, 1986). These measurements, together with additive colour mixture experiments, showed that colour vision in goldfish is even more complicated than human colour vision: it is tetrachromatic, with an ultraviolet cone as the fourth photoreceptor type (Neumeyer, 1985, 1992).

In other respects, however, colour vision in goldfish seems to be very similar to human colour vision, indicating comparable principles in the processing of colour specific information: as in human colour vision, for example, simultaneous colour contrast, and colour constancy could be shown (Dörr and Neumeyer, 1993, 1994; Ingle, 1985). One of the most striking similarities, however, is the effect of the drug ethambutol. This tuberculostatic pharmaceutical may cause a deficiency in red/green discrimination after prolonged application in high doses (for example: 200–400 g in total, over eight months) in human patients (Zrenner and Krüger, 1981). Exactly the same effect could be observed in goldfish when cthambutol was given in the food for 2–3 weeks (Spekreijse *et al.*, 1991). Very similar changes in wavelength discrimination and in spectral sensitivity could also be measured when the overall room illumination was reduced to about 1 lux, which brings the visual system of the goldfish into a mesopic state of adaptation (Neumeyer and Arnold, 1989). As known from neuroanatomical and electrophysiological investigations, the change in the state of adaptation is accompanied by striking morphological and physiological transitions (Weiler and Wagner, 1984). For this plasticity of the retina, dopamine probably plays a decisive role (see, for review, Negishi *et al.*, 1990). To prove this possibility, we tested dopamine antagonists, and found the same loss of red-green discrimination as after ethambutol treatment or under a room illumination of 1 lux.

In the following we will describe the different cases in which red/green colour blindness was induced in more detail.

2.3.2 ETHAMBUTOL

The inability to discriminate between red and green after prolonged application of ethambutol in humans was shown to be based not on defects on the receptor level, as in inherited deuter- or protanopia, but on alterations in the neural interactions between the different cone mechanisms (Zrenner and Krüger, 1981). In fish (carp), van Dijk and Spekreijse (1983) investigated the action spectra of ganglion cells in the isolated retina, and found a change in the response characteristics of colour opponent cells. That ethambutol indeed has an effect on colour vision was shown in training experiments with goldfish given ethambutol (500–1000 mg kg^{-1} body weight day^{-1}) in the form of food pellets for 2–3 weeks. Wavelength discrimination was tested in a two-choice discrimination task, with the training wavelength shown on one test-field, and a comparison wavelength on the second test-field (Spekreijse *et al.*, 1991). Three training wavelengths were used, located in the ranges of best discrimination ability at 400 nm, 500 nm and 610 nm. When trained on 404 nm or 509 nm, no change in the choice behaviour was observed in comparison to a control fish. However, with training wavelength 608 nm, choice frequency hardly exceeded 60 per cent when comparison wavelengths between 535 nm and 700 nm were tested. This indicated that wavelength discrimination was completely eliminated in the mid and long wavelength part of the spectrum. The effect of ethambutol was entirely reversible, and red/green discrimination recovered 3–4 weeks after the end of the treatment.

The reason for this lack of red-green colour discrimination was assumed to be a reduced contribution of the long wavelength cone type to colour vision. This was concluded from the finding that in ethambutol-treated goldfish spectral sensitivity in the range of the long-wavelength maximum at 660 nm was reduced by about 1 log unit (Spekreijse *et al.*, 1991, Figure 4). This sensitivity reduction, however, was not due to a sensitivity loss in the long wavelength cone type itself, but must have been based on a changed neural interaction between the mid and long wavelength cone mechanisms. This was concluded from the finding that no difference between ethambutol-treated and untreated fish was observed: first, in ERG measurements, and, second, in measurements of spectral sensitivity in which the fish obviously discriminated on the basis of brightness, but not on the basis of hue (Neumeyer *et al.*, 1991; Spekreijse *et al.*, 1991, Figure 3). Thus, ethambutol affects only the contribution of the long wavelength cone type to colour vision, but not its contribution to brightness perception.

2.3.3 MESOPIC STATE OF ADAPTATION

Measuring wavelength discrimination under an overall white room illumination of 1 lux (instead of 20 lux), we found to our great surprise that colour vision in the goldfish was tri- and not tetrachromatic, using the ultraviolet, the blue and the green cone types only. Discrimination between the mid- and the long-wavelength range was impossible. This was again accompanied by a decrease of sensitivity in the long-wavelength range (Neumeyer and Arnold, 1989). As in the case of ethambutol, the missing contribution of the long-wavelength cone type to colour vision is not based on the receptor mechanism, but must be due to changed neural interactions (Neumeyer et al., 1991).

2.3.4 DOPAMINE-ANTAGONISTS

At the transition from the light adapted to the dark adapted state, the horizontal cells in the goldfish retina show an interesting plasticity: amongst others, the biphasic H2-horizontal cells become monophasic, and the spinules at the horizontal cell dendrites disappear (Weiler and Wagner, 1984). Furthermore, the concentration of dopamine in the retina was found to be higher in the light than in the dark adapted retina (Kolbinger et al., 1990).

If dopamine is essential for bringing the retina into the light adapted state, and if red-green discrimination is possible only when the retina is light adapted, dopamine antagonists should also induce a red-green colour vision deficiency. Thus, following a suggestion by Reto Weiler, we first tested the non-specific dopamine-antagonist haloperidol injected into the vitreous of trained goldfish. About one hour after injection into the dark adapted eyes, wavelength discrimination was measured under a white room illumination of 20 lux (light adapted state). The results were similar to the findings under ethambutol or under 1 lux room illumination: wavelength discrimination was almost entirely eliminated between about 560 nm and 630 nm, but was about normal in the violet and blue-green spectral ranges (400–450 nm, and 450–520 nm) (Mora-Ferrer and Neumeyer, 1994). A corresponding result was obtained when we tested the specific D1-receptor antagonist SCH 23390 with the same method. Figure 2.3.1 shows the results for three individual goldfish that are representative for the 3–4 animals tested for each condition. When trained on 404 nm, or 495 nm (low and middle part of Figure 2.3.1), injection of SCH 23390 did not have much effect: the relative choice frequency on the training wavelength was only slightly reduced. However, when trained on 599 nm, discrimination ability was lost or impaired when wavelengths 570 nm or 640 nm were shown for comparison.

A further indication of the importance of D1-dopamine receptors for red-green discrimination was obtained in an experiment in which 6-OH dopamine, a drug known to destroy selectively dopaminergic cells (Negishi et al., 1990), was injected into the vitreous of both eyes. In the range between 461 nm and 540 nm, discrimination ability was normal in three fishes trained on 495 nm. However, as shown in Figure 2.3.2, discrimination ability was greatly reduced in the mid- to long-wavelength range 1–3 days after injection. When, however, the specific D1-receptor dopamine *agonist* SKF 38393 was injected into the eyes of the same fish (nine days after injection of 6-OH dopamine) a complete recovery of red-green discrimination was found, which lasted for about one hour.

2.3.5   BICUCULLINE

Injecting the GABA$_A$ receptor antagonist bicuculline into one eye of trained goldfish using the second eye for control measuments, we found the same specific wavelength discrimina-

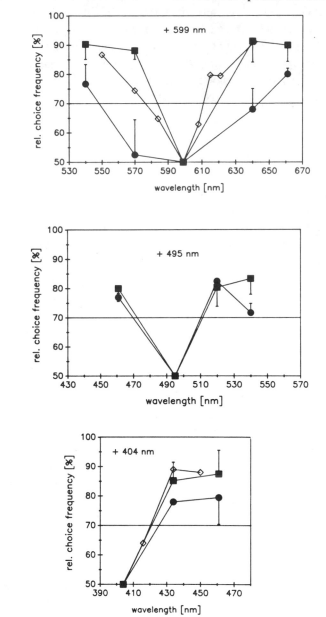

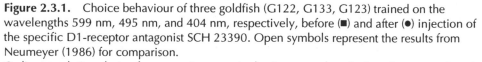

Figure 2.3.1.   Choice behaviour of three goldfish (G122, G133, G123) trained on the wavelengths 599 nm, 495 nm, and 404 nm, respectively, before (■) and after (●) injection of the specific D1-receptor antagonist SCH 23390. Open symbols represent the results from Neumeyer (1986) for comparison.

Ordinate: relative choice frequency in percent; abscissa: wavelength given for comparison in the two-choice discrimination task.

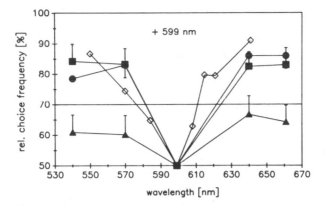

Figure 2.3.2. Choice behaviour of a goldfish (G130) treated with 6-OH-dopamine, and subseding injection of the specific D1-receptor agonist SFK 38393. (■) wavelength discrimination before applying the dopaminergic agents; training wavelength was 599 nm. (▲) choice behaviour 1–8 days after injection of 6-OH-dopamine. (●) choice behaviour one hour after injection of SFK 38393, on day 9 after injection of 6-OH-dopamine. Open symbols represent the results from Neumeyer (1986) for comparison.

tion loss, and a similar reduction of sensitivity in the long wavelength part of the spectrum as in the cases described above (Wietsma and Spekreijse, 1991).

2.3.6 DISCUSSION

The loss of red-green discrimination ability found after intraocular injection of specific drugs indicates that the defect must be of retinal origin. A localisation of the affected site in the retina would answer the question of which retinal neuron types are essential for red-green discrimination. It is a general notion that all cell types with so-called colour opponent and double opponent response characteristics are involved in colour coding. However, what does this mean more specifically? For example, which role is played by the biphasic or triphasic horizontal cells, or bipolar and ganglion cells showing red-green opponency in colour vision, and do they play a role at all?

The effect of bicuculline, a GABA_A-receptor antagonist, indicates that inhibitory interactions are involved. On the level of horizontal cells in roach and carp retina, it was shown that the GABA antagonists picrotoxin and bicuculline selectively eliminated the depolarising component of the biphasic H2-responses (Djamgoz and Ruddock, 1979; Murakami et al., 1982). On the ganglion cell level, bicuculline showed an effect on some cells; for example, it suppressed the 'on' response of a red 'on'/green 'off' cell (Wietsma, 1994). The inhibitory influence of GABA on colour coding can be located in the outer as well as in the inner plexiform layer, as horizontal and amacrine cells are GABAergic (for review see Lasater, 1990, and Kamermans and Spekreijse, 1995).

The effect of ethambutol, which can be studied so easily in behavioural experiments, is unfortunately still unknown on the cellular level. When it is given orally, a more central effect cannot be entirely excluded. In the isolated retina, ethambutol eliminated the opponent character of red-green ganglion cells (van Dijk and Spekreijse, 1983; Wietsma, 1994). In biphasic horizontal cells it caused an increased hyperpolarisation of the resting potential, and a reduction of the depolarising response amplitude (Spekreijse et al., 1991). A re-measurement (Wietsma, 1994) showed, however, that the effects were transient and disappeared with a prolonged (about 10 minutes) application. Furthermore, in goldfish fed with ethambutol for several weeks we had expected to find a reduced number of biphasic horizontal cells. However, the distribution of mono-, bi-, and triphasic horizontal cells was the same as in untreated fish, and also the spinules of the horizontal cell dendrites in cone pedicles were normal (Wietsma, 1994). This led us to the conclusion that the effect of ethambutol is most probably restricted to the inner plexiform layer of the retina.

The morphological and physiological changes in photoreceptors, pigment epithelial cells, horizontal and ganglion cells at different states of adaptation are well investigated (see, for review, Wagner, 1990). Dopamine, which is released from interplexiform cells in teleost retina, seems to be involved in light adaptation (Kohler *et al.*, 1990; Kolbinger *et al.*, 1990). When the non-specific dopamine antagonist haloperidol was injected into the vitreous of a dark adapted fish, the biphasic horizontal cells in the subsequently light adapted isolated retina showed less spinules and a reduced depolarising component of the response in comparison with control retinae (Djamgoz *et al.*, 1989). Similar results were obtained by using specific dopamine antagonists (Kirsch *et al.*, 1991). The same substances and solvents in comparable concentrations were used in the behavioural experiments, and caused selectively red-green colour blindness as described above. Therefore, it is tempting to assume that horizontal cells are decisive for colour discrimination. A first try to localise D1-receptors in the goldfish retina using SCH 23390 combined with a fluorescent dye gave a pronounced staining in the outer plexiform layer (Behrens, 1994; Wagner and Behrens, 1993). However, electrophysiological investigations very recently showed dopamine dependent responses in bipolar cell terminals that might be mediated by D1-dopamine receptors (Heidelberger and Matthews, 1994). Thus, to be entirely certain where D1-receptors are localised in the retina, immunocytochemical investigations are required.

An interesting question is why a directly or indirectly disturbed influence of GABA selectively affects red/green discrimination, and not colour vision in total. So far, it is not known whether colour opponent horizontal, bipolar and ganglion cells with short wavelength cone input are also affected by the drugs used in this study. It cannot be excluded that here the pharmacology is different, using for example mainly glycine as an inhibitory transmitter, or involving other GABA receptors. However, it is also possible that in the retina the signals of only two cone types (mid- and long-wavelength) are already combined providing the basis for red-green discrimination, whereas the information of the short wavelength and UV mechanisms are compared with the other mechanisms at more central levels.

The behavioural findings that after treatment with ethambutol and under the mesopic state of adaptation the contribution of the long-wavelength cone type was affected only in colour vision and visual acuity, but not in brightness, flicker and motion perception (Neumeyer and Schaerer, 1992; Schaerer and Neumeyer, 1993) are also important. They indicate the existence of two different pathways of long-wavelength cone contribution in the retina: a direct one (L-cones, bipolar cells, ganglion cells) involved in brightness and motion perception, and an indirect one involving horizontal and/or amacrine cells for colour vision. Thus, two types of long-wavelength-cone driven ganglion cells should exist. By making use of the different response behaviour at the transition from the dark to a light adapted state, we tried to identify these two ganglion cell types by electrophysiological recordings. A few cells were indeed found that could belong to the 'colour' class (Neumeyer *et al.*, 1991). Thus, this study, in which behavioural experiments were combined with neuropharmacological methods, provides us with a tool to test whether specific neurons play a role in colour vision.

2.3.7 ACKNOWLEDGEMENTS

We are very grateful to Neil Beckhaus for correcting the English manuscript. The study was supported by Deutsche Forschungsgemeinschaft (Ne 215 7–9) and Human Frontier Science Program (H. Spekreijse).

2.3.8 REFERENCES

BEHRENS, U.D. (1994) Dopamin-D1-Rezeptor vermittelte Prozesse bei der Lichtadaptation in der Fischnetzhaut. Thesis, Universität Tübingen.

DJAMGOZ, M.B.A. & RUDDOCK, K.H. (1979) Effects of picrotoxin and strychnine on fish retinal S-potentials: evidence for inhibitory control of depolarizing responses, *Neuroscience Letters*, **12**, 329–334.

DJAMGOZ, M.B.A. & YAMADA M. (1990) Electrophysiological characteristics of retinal neurons: synaptic interactions and functional outputs. In: Douglas, R.H. & Djamgoz, M.B.A. (Eds) *The Visual System of Fish*, London: Chapman & Hall.

DJAMGOZ, M.B.A., KIRSCH, M. & WAGNER, H.-J. (1989) Haloperidol suppresses light-induced spinule formation and biphasic responses of horizontal cells in fish (roach) retina, *Neuroscience Letters*, **107**, 200–204.

DÖRR, S. & NEUMEYER, C. (1993) Simultaneous color contrast in goldfish, *Investigative Ophthalmology and Visual Science*, **34**, 747.

DÖRR, S. & NEUMEYER, C. (1994) Color constancy in goldfish – aspects of a quantitative study. In: Elsner, N. & Breer, H. (Eds) *Proceedings of the 22nd Göttingen Neurobiology Conference 1994*, Vol. II, Stuttgart: Thieme, p. 483.

HEIDELBERGER, R. & MATTHEWS, G. (1994) Dopamine enhances Ca^{2+} responses in synaptic terminals of retinal bipolar neurons, *NeuroReport*, **5**, 729–732.

HERVEY, G.F. & HEMS, J. (1968) *The Goldfish*, London, Faber.

INGLE, D.J. (1985) The goldfish as a retinex animal, *Science*, **227**, 651–653.

JACOBS, G.H. (1981) *Comparative Color Vision*, New York: Academic Press, pp. 106ff.

KAMERMANS, M. & SPEKREIJSE, H. (1995) Spectral behavior of cone-driven horizontal cells in teleost retina, *Progress in Retinal and Eye Research*, **14**, 313–360.

KIRSCH, W., WAGNER, H.-J. & DJAMGOZ, M.B.A. (1991) Dopamine and plasticity of horizontal cell function in the teleost retina: regulation of a spectral mechanism through D1-receptors, *Vision Research*, **31**, 401–412.

KOHLER, K., KOLBINGER, W., KURZ-ISLER, G. & WEILER, R. (1990) Endogeneous dopamine and cyclic events in the fish retina II: Correlation of retinomotor movement, spinule formation and connexon density of gap junctions with dopamine activity during light/dark cycles, *Visual Neuroscience*, **5**, 417–428.

KOLBINGER, W., KOHLER, K., OETTING, H. & WEILER, R. (1990) Endogeneous dopamine and cyclic events in the fish retina, I: HPLC assay of total content, release, and metabolic turnover during different light/dark cycles, *Visual Neuroscience*, **5**, 143–149.

LASATER, E.M. (1990) Neurotransmitters and neuromodulators of the fish retina. In: Douglas, R.H. & Djamgoz, M.B.A. (Eds) *The Visual System of Fish*, London: Chapman & Hall.

MARKS, W.B. (1965) Visual pigments of single goldfish cones, *Journal of Physiology*, **178**, 14–32.

MORA-FERRER, C. & NEUMEYER, C. (1994) Dopamine antagonists impair 'red-green' discrimination in goldfish after intravitreal injection. In: Drum, B. (Ed.) *Colour Vision Deficiencies XII*, Dordrecht: Kluwer.

MURAKAMI, M., SHIMODA, Y., NAKATANI, K., MIYACHI, E. & WATANABE, S. (1982) GABA-mediated negative feedback and color opponency in carp retina, *Japanese Journal of Physiology*, **32**, 927–935.

NEGISHI, K.T., TERANISHI, T. & KATO, S. (1990) The dopamine system of the teleost fish retina, *Progress in Retinal Research*, **9**, 1–48.

NEUMEYER, C. (1984) On spectral sensitivity in the goldfish: evidence for neural interactions between different 'cone mechanisms', *Vision Research*, **24**, 1123–1131.

NEUMEYER, C. (1985) An ultra-violet receptor as a fourth receptor type in goldfish color vision, *Naturwissenschaften*, **72**, 162–163.

NEUMEYER, C. (1986) Wavelength discrimination in the goldfish, *Journal of Comparative Physiology*, **158**, 203–213.

NEUMEYER, C. (1992) Tetrachromatic color vision in goldfish: evidence from color mixture experiments, *Journal of Comparative Physiology A*, **171**, 639–649.

NEUMEYER, C. & ARNOLD, K. (1989) Tetrachromatic color vision in the goldfish becomes trichromatic under white adaptation light of moderate intensity, *Vision Research*, **29**, 1719–1727.

NEUMEYER C. & SCHAERER, S. (1992) Two separate pathways in the processing of L-cone type information in goldfish: color and acuity vs. brightness and flicker, *Investigative Ophthalmology and Visual Science*, **33**, 703.

NEUMEYER, C., WIETSMA, J.J. & SPEKREIJSE, H. (1991) Separate processing of 'color' and 'brightness' in goldfish, *Vision Research*, **31**, 537–549.

SCHAERER, S. & NEUMEYER C. (1993) Parallel processing of motion and color in goldfish, *Investigative Ophthalmology and Visual Science*, **34**, 1033.

SPEKREIJSE, H., WIETSMA, J.J. & NEUMEYER, C. (1991) Induced color blindness in goldfish: a behavioral and electrophysiological study, *Vision Research*, **31**, 551–562.

TOMITA, T. (1965) Electrophysiological study of the mechanisms subserving color coding in fish retina, *Cold Spring Harbor Symposium on Quantitative Biology*, **30**, 559–566.

VAN DIJK, B.W. & SPEKREIJSE, H. (1983) Ethambutol changes the color coding of carp retinal ganglion cells reversibly, *Investigative Ophthalmology and Visual Science*, **24**, 128–133.

WAGNER, H.-J. (1990) Retinal structure of fishes. In: Douglas, R.H. & Djamgoz, M.B.A. (Eds) *The Visual System of Fish*, London: Chapman & Hall.

WAGNER, H.-J. & BEHRENS, U.D. (1993) Microanatomy of the dopaminergic system in the rainbow trout retina, *Vision Research*, **33**, 1345–1358.

WEILER, R. & WAGNER, H.-J. (1984) Light-dependent change of cone-horizontal cell interactions in carp retina, *Brain Research*, **298**, 1–9.

WIETSMA, J.J. (1994) Induced color blindness. A behavioral and electrophysiological study on pharmacologically induced color vision disturbances in goldfish, Thesis, University of Amsterdam.

WIETSMA, J.J. & SPEKREIJSE, H. (1991) Bicuculline produces reversible red-green color blindness in goldfish, as revealed by monocular behavioral testing, *Vision Research*, **31**, 2101–2107.

ZRENNER, E. & KRÜGER, C.J. (1981) Ethambutol mainly affects the function of red/green opponent neurons, *Documenta Ophthalmologica Proceedings Series*, **27**, 13–25.

Section 3 – Pathways and Channels

Parallel Pathways in Primate Retina

Barry B. Lee

3.1.1 INTRODUCTION

It is now widely accepted that the parvocellular and magnocellular pathways of the primate visual system carry parallel streams of visual information, and represent a functional division of major significance. Recent anatomical studies have suggested that the ganglion cell types of these systems are not only physiologically distinct but represent different anatomical cell types with very specific connectivity within the primate retina. At a behavioural level, the presence of luminance and chromatic channels within the human visual system was first proposed on the basis of psychophysical observation (e.g. Kelly and van Norren, 1977; King-Smith and Carden, 1976). It is generally accepted that cell types and systems bear some kind of relation to these psychophysical channels. How close is this relationship? The recent developments in primate retinal anatomy and physiology are reviewed below and the physiological and psychophysical evidence for a link between cell classes and psychophysical channels is discussed.

Of the two cell systems passing information through the lateral geniculate nucleus to the cortex, the parvocellular pathway contains at least six identifiable cell classes, all of which display cone and colour opponency; cells of the parvocellular pathway without opponency are extremely rare (e.g. Derrington *et al.*, 1984). Red-green opponent cells receive antagonistic input from middle- (M) and long-wavelength (L) sensitive cones, and appear to be divisible into four types: red on-centre, green on-centre, red off-centre and green off-centre. Two types of cells with short-wavelength (S) cone input are present, the S-cone providing either excitatory or inhibitory input opposed by some combination of the M- and L-cones. The magnocellular pathway contains on- and off-centre cells with M-and L-cone input to both centre and surround.

The terms magnocellular and parvocellular refer of course to the lamination of cells within the lateral geniculate nucleus. In the retina, the parasol ganglion cells of Polyak (1941) project to the magnocellular layers and his midget ganglion cells to the parvocellular layers (Perry *et al.*, 1984). Both parasol and midget ganglion cells contain sub-types with dendritic trees ramifying in the inner and outer sub-laminae of the inner plexiform layer (IPL) (Watanabe and Rodieck, 1989). Cells of these pathways are often called M- and P-cells respectively, but will here be termed MC- and PC-cells to avoid confusion with the M-cone.

65

3.1.2 ANATOMICAL PATHWAYS THROUGH THE RETINA

Recent evidence has revealed a high degree of anatomical specificity in the retinal pathways associated with the parvocellular and magnocellular systems, beginning at the bipolar cell level. Diffuse bipolar cells are associated with the parasol or MC-cells and midget bipolar cells with M,L-cone opponent PC-cells, while at least one further bipolar cell type is associated with the S-cone pathways (see Wässle and Boycott, 1991 for review). It has recently been shown that midget bipolar cells continue to provide input to midget ganglion cells until far out into the retinal periphery (Wässle *et al.*, 1994). At these eccentricities midget ganglion cells receive input from several midget bipolars and their dendritic morphology suggests cone specificity (Dacey, 1993b), and thus colour opponency.

It has recently become possible to record and stain primate retinal ganglion cells *in vitro* (Dacey and Lee, 1994b) and this has permitted anatomical identification of physiological types, as summarised in Table 3.1.1 which also includes an approximate estimate of the percentage of ganglion cells belonging to each class. It is well established that ganglion cells with dendritic trees ramifying in the inner, vitreal half of the IPL usually have an on-centre field structure, and those with trees branching in the outer, scleral half, an off-centre field structure (e.g. Famiglietti and Kolb, 1976). As expected, on-centre MC-cells were found to correspond to the inner parasols, and off-centre MC-cells to outer parasols (Dacey and Lee, 1994b). A specific ganglion cell, the small bistratified, has been identified as the blue-on + S-(ML) physiological type (Dacey and Lee, 1994a). This cell type has one layer of dendrites ramifying in the outer layer of the IPL and another close to the cell body in a layer where the S-cone bipolar terminates (Dacey, 1993a). Another cell type with a large dendritic tree ramifying in the inner half of the IPL near the S-cone bipolar terminals and a small cell body has been tentatively identified as the physiological cell type with

Table 3.1.1   Anatomical identity of physiological ganglion cell types

Pathway	Physiological cell type	Anatomical cell type	Bipolar input	Proportion
Magnocellular	On-centre MC-cell	Inner parasol	Invaginating diffuse bipolar	5%
	Off-centre MC-cell	Outer parasol	Flat diffuse bipolar	5%
Parvocellular	Blue on, + S-(ML) PC-Cell	Small bistratified	S-cone bipolar	10%
	Blue off, Yellow on -S + (ML) PC-Cell	Large-field inner cell?	Unknown	10%
	Green and red on-centre cells	Inner midget	Invaginating midget bipolars	30%
	Green and red off-centre cells	Outer midget	Flat midget bipolars	30%
Unknown	Various transient, non-opponent cells	Other cell types	Unknown	10%

inhibitory S-cone input (Dacey and Lee, unpublished observations). The small cell body size of this cell type (about the size of a midget) may account for the low encounter rate during retinal recording, but until more anatomical data are available any estimate as to its numerosity is only approximate.

Midget ganglion cells so far recorded have displayed M,L-cone opponency (Dacey and Lee, 1994b). However, Table 3.1.1 makes apparent a unique feature of red-green PC-cells. Inner midgets apparently consist of two cell groups, red and green on-centre cells. Anatomical evidence suggests that there is only one mosaic of this cell type tiling the retina (Dacey, 1993b). Likewise, outer midgets are made up of red and green off-centre cells. Except for the receptors themselves, mosaics of retinal neurones previously described (e.g. Wässle et al., 1981) have always been physiologically homogeneous and two different cell types sharing the same mosaic is a most unusual feature. A further unusual feature of the midget mosaics is that the dendritic trees of neighbouring cells show no overlap (Dacey, 1993b). Again, retinal neurones of very diverse types usually show an overlap of dendritic trees with neighbouring members of their mosaic, often to give a coverage factor of 3–4 (Wässle and Boycott, 1991). No overlap implies a coverage factor of one or less. The functional significance of these unique features of the red-green PC-cell mosaics is obscure.

There exist several other ganglion cell types that may be recorded in the *in vitro* preparation, although these cells make up only a few per cent of the total count. It is currently uncertain which, if any, of these types project to the lateral geniculate nucleus and which to midbrain loci. However, all cell types encountered until now have shown transient, non-opponent responses to visual stimulation (Dacey and Lee, unpublished observations). It had been suggested that a separate red-green opponent cell class corresponded to the Type II cell of Wiesel and Hubel (1966) and might be responsible for red-green colour vision (Rodieck, 1991). However, quantitative physiological measurements have failed to reveal a clear Type I/Type II dichotomy (Derrington et al., 1984) but rather suggest a continuum in which surround size is often not much bigger than the centre (Reid and Shapley, 1992). The anatomical candidate for Type II, the small bistratified, is now known to be the blue-on cell so that a further red-green opponent pathway appears unlikely.

These recent studies of retinal circuitry in the primate suggest considerable specificity in retinal connectivity, with physiological cell classes mapping on to clearly identifiable ganglion cell types. It may be the case that cone and colour opponency is restricted to a few clearly defined cell types. In any event, parallel pathways in the primate retina now have a firm anatomical basis.

3.1.3   CELL CLASSES, PSYCHOPHYSICAL CHANNELS AND TEMPORAL MODULATION

The most convincing psychophysical evidence for multiple channels within the visual system has been derived from experiments involving temporal modulation (Kelly and van Norren, 1977). A convincing link between psychophysical channels and physiological cell types has been developed by employing psychophysical protocols to explore the properties of ganglion cells. A good example of this approach has been the study of phase shifts in heterochromatic flicker photometry (HFP). In HFP, two lights are modulated in counterphase (180 degrees) and their relative intensities adjusted until the percept of flicker is minimised. At moderate temporal frequencies (5–10 Hz) with red and green lights, residual flicker can be further reduced if a small phase shift away from 180 degrees is introduced (de Lange, 1958). Alternatively, modulation thresholds may be measured as a function of the relative phase of the lights (Lindsey *et al.*, 1986; Swanson *et al.*, 1987). A sketch of the waveforms involved is shown in Figure 3.1.1A. Modulation depth is adjusted to threshold at a variety of relative phases of the red and green lights which have the same luminance and modulation depth. An example of data so obtained is shown in Figure 3.1.1B, in which an observer's modulation thresholds at 6.5 Hz are plotted as a function of relative phase of the lights. A four degree foveal target was used, with 1000 tds retinal illuminance, and the thresholds (a mean of three) were obtained by a method of adjustment. The threshold curve follows a U-shaped course. Thresholds are maximum not at counterphase (± 180 degrees) but at about 140 degrees. This corresponds to the phase of minimum flicker in the conventional task. Other evidence suggests that MC-cells form the physiological substrate for HFP (Lee *et al.*, 1988). The presence of phase shifts similar to those observed psychophysically in the response of MC-cells has provided strong corrobora-

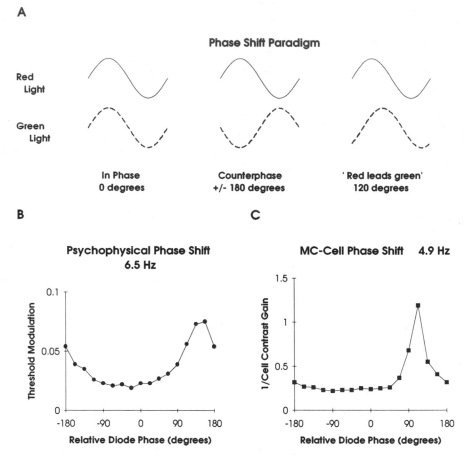

Figure 3.1.1A. Structure of the phase varying stimulus. **B.** Psychophysical thresholds as a function of relative phase of red and green lights. **C.** 1/contrast gain plotted against relative diode phase for an on-centre MC-cell. A 20 per cent modulation depth was used and the amplitude of the first harmonic derived from Fourier analysis. Contrast gain is then given by imp/s/per cent modulation. Cell receptive field was parafoveal in location, otherwise stimulus conditions were similar to the psychophysical tests. Data replotted from Kremers *et al.*, (1994), reproduced by permission.

tion for this link (Smith *et al.*, 1992). In Figure 3.1.1C the reciprocal of contrast gain of an MC-cell as a function of relative phase of the lights is plotted. A U-shaped function is again found with a similar axis of symmetry to the psychophysical data. Phase of minimum sensitivity as a function of temporal frequency is very similar in both physiological and psychophysical data (Figure 15, Smith *et al.*, 1992).

For detection of luminance and chromatic modulation, there is also substantial evidence for different psychophysical detection mechanisms having different cell types as their physiological substrates (Kremers *et al.*, 1992; Lee *et al.*, 1990). Separable psychophysical detection mechanisms may be usefully revealed by plotting thresholds in cone contrast co-ordinates (Cole *et al.*, 1993; Stromeyer *et al.*, 1985) and when cell responsivities are also plotted in such co-ordinates parallel behaviour is observed (Lee *et al.*, 1993a).

Cumulative evidence thus suggests that discrete mechanisms for psychophysical detection of luminance and chromatic change map closely onto different cell classes within the afferent visual pathway.

3.1.4 CELL CLASSES, PSYCHOPHYSICAL CHANNELS AND SPATIAL VISION

The role of different ganglion cell populations in spatial vision is less easy to define. Spectral sensitivity when measured with acuity targets resembles the luminosity function (e.g. Pokorny *et al.*, 1968), and it is often assumed that an achromatic or luminance mechanism may underlie high spatial frequency vision. As PC-cells are more numerous than MC-cells and may have smaller receptive fields (but see below), there have been several attempts to show that outputs of the colour opponent PC-cells can be combined to form such an achromatic mechanism (e.g. Ingling, 1991; Lennie and D'Zmura, 1988). However, such mechanisms although theoretically attractive, have not been shown to be physiologically realistic; a number of assumptions are hidden within them (Lee, 1993). Although it is commonly stated that MC-cells have large receptive fields and thus can only be responsible for vision at low spatial frequencies (e.g. Schiller *et al.*, 1990), a number of studies have demonstrated that their receptive fields are small enough to permit them to respond to several tens of cycles per degree in the fovea (Blakemore and Vital-Durand, 1986; Crook *et al.*, 1988; Derrington and Lennie, 1984), probably approaching the visual resolution of the behaving macaque (Cavonius and Robbins, 1973). If, as the anatomical evidence suggests, centres of red-green PC-cells receive input from only a single cone, this should permit them to respond to many tens of cycles/degree even in the parafovea. This is not the case, and MC- and PC-cells seem to respond up to similar spatial frequencies at any given eccentricity (Blakemore and Vital-Durand, 1986; Crook *et al.*, 1988).

One serious problem for support of achromatic spatial vision by PC-cells is their low responsivity to achromatic contrast (Kaplan and Shapley, 1986; Lee *et al.*, 1989), for human vision maintains a high degree of spatial accuracy down to 10 per cent contrast and below (Wehrhahn and Westheimer, 1990). Although it can be argued that PC-cells could band together to improve the sensitivity of the PC-pathway as a whole (Watson, 1992), it is not clear whether the necessary spatial summation might be incompatible with a high-resolution spatial signal. In recent studies measuring retinal signals associated with the hyperacuities, it has been possible to show that only the matrix of MC-cells can deliver an adequate signal to support human performance, especially at low contrast (Lee *et al.*, 1993b; Lee *et al.*, 1994).

Although an achromatic spatial vision channel based on the PC-pathway may be physiologically unrealistic, there are problems with reliance on the MC-pathway for an achromatic spatial signal. MC-cell density is below the two-dimensional Nyquist limit required for psychophysical performance (e.g. Wässle and Boycott, 1991). It might be argued that the two-dimensional Nyquist limit only applies to reconstruction of patterns in which the Nyquist frequency is simultaneously approached in both of two orthogonal directions, and the grating patterns usually employed to measure visual resolution are only one dimensional. Thus, a strict sampling limit may not apply to a system that assumes that lines and edges are extended in space. The orientation selective mechanisms of the visual cortex would be just such a system. Nevertheless, the resolution of these issues remains controversial.

3.1.5   CONCLUSIONS

The concept of parallel channels within the human visual system dealing with chromatic and luminance information was first postulated from psychophysical evidence. Physiological identification of different opponent and non-opponent cell types provided a possible substrate for these channels. Although this link has been controversial, the evidence in its favour is now quite strong, especially for temporal processing. Recent data, demonstrating that different physiological cell types can be distinguished anatomically, have provided further support for the concept of parallel channels passing through the retina.

At this point one might well ask whether the demonstration of parallel pathways at such a peripheral level is relevant for central processing of afferent signals. Other psychophysical data, such as masking experiments (Gegenfurtner and Kiper, 1992), indicate that, centrally, chromatic mechanisms may emerge that have been substantially modified in comparison with the outputs of retinal channels. Nevertheless, insofar as specific psychophysical effects can be revealed to have a physiological substrate at the ganglion cell level (as in Figure 3.1.1), parallel afferent pathways carrying different types of information would appear to be a useful concept when interpreting psychophysical data. With more complex visual tasks than simple detection paradigms, such as the perception of movement, contributions from magnocellular and parvocellular pathways may be more difficult to disentangle, although it seems likely that knowledge of the afferent signals through these pathways is a useful requisite for interpreting cortical responses and modelling cortical processing (Gegenfurtner et al., 1994).

3.1.6   ACKNOWLEDGEMENTS

I would like to thank Dennis Dacey for permission to quote from unpublished work, and the numerous colleagues who have assisted with the experiments cited in the text.

3.1.7   REFERENCES

BLAKEMORE, C. & VITAL-DURAND, F. (1986) Organisation and post-natal development of the monkey's lateral geniculate nucleus, *Journal of Physiology*, **380**, 453–492.

CAVONIUS, C.R. & ROBBINS, D.O. (1973) Relationship between luminance and visual acuity of the rhesus monkey, *Journal of Physiology*, **232**, 501–511.

COLE, G.R., HINE, T. & MCILHAGGA, W. (1993) Detection mechanisms in L-, M- and S-cone contrast space, *Journal of the Optical Society of America*, A **10**, 38–51.

CROOK, J.M., LANGE-MALECKI, B., LEE, B.B. & VALBERG, A. (1988) Visual resolution of macaque retinal ganglion cells, *Journal of Physiology*, **396**, 205–224.

DACEY, D.M. (1993a) Morphology of a small field bistratified ganglion cell type in the macaque and human retina: is it the blue-ON cell?, *Visual Neuroscience*, **10**, 1081–1098.

DACEY, D.M. (1993b) The mosaic of midget ganglion cells in the human retina, *Journal of Neuroscience*, **13**, 5334–5335.

DACEY, D.M. & LEE, B.B. (1994a) The blue-ON opponent pathway in primate retina originates from a distinct bistratified ganglion cell type, *Nature*, **367**, 731–735.

DACEY, D.M. & LEE, B.B. (1994b) Physiology of identified ganglion cell types in an in vitro preparation of macaque retina, *Investigative Ophthalmology and Visual Science*, **35**, 2001.

DE LANGE, H. (1958) Research into the dynamic nature of the human fovea-cortex systems with intermittent and modulated light, *Journal of the Optical Society of America*, **48**, 779–789.

DERRINGTON, A.M. & LENNIE, P. (1984) Spatial and temporal contrast sensitivities of neurones in lateral geniculate nucleus of macaque, *Journal of Physiology*, **357**, 219–240.

DERRINGTON, A.M., KRAUSKOPF, J. & LENNIE, P. (1984) Chromatic mechanisms in lateral geniculate nucleus of macaque, *Journal of Physiology*, **357**, 241–265.

FAMIGLIETTI, E.V. & KOLB, H. (1976) Structural basis for ON- and OFF-center responses in retinal ganglion cells, *Science*, **194**, 193–195.

GEGENFURTNER, K.R. & KIPER, D.C. (1992) Contrast detection in luminance and chromatic noise, *Journal of the Optical Society of America*, A **9**, 1880–1888.

GEGENFURTNER, K.R., KIPER, D.C., BEUSMANS, J.M.H., CARANDINI, M., ZAIDI, Q. & MOVSHON, J.A. (1994) Chromatic properties of neurons in macaque MT, *Visual Neuroscience*, **11**, 455–466.

INGLING, C.R. (1991) Psychophysical correlates of parvo channel function. In: Valberg, A. & Lee, B.B. (Eds) *From Pigments to Perception; Advances in Understanding Visual Processes*, New York and London: Plenum Press, pp. 413–424.

KAPLAN, E. & SHAPLEY, R.M. (1986) The primate retina contains two types of ganglion cells with high and low contrast sensitivity, *Proceedings of the National Academy of Sciences U.S.A.*, **83**, 2755–2757.

KELLY, D.H. & VAN NORREN, D. (1977) Two-band model of heterochromatic flicker, *Journal of the Optical Society of America*, **67**, 1081–1091.

KING-SMITH, P.E. & CARDEN, D. (1976) Luminance and opponent-color contributions to visual detection and adaptation and to temporal and spatial integration, *Journal of the Optical Society of America*, **66**, 709–717.

KREMERS, J., LEE, B.B. & KAISER, P.K. (1992) Sensitivity of macaque retinal ganglion cells and human observers to combined luminance and chromatic modulation, *Journal of the Optical Society of America*, A **9**, 1477–1485.

KREMERS, J., YEH, T. & LEE, B.B. (1994) The response of macaque ganglion cells and human observers to heterochromatically modulated lights: the effect of stimulus size, *Vision Research*, **34**, 217–221.

LEE, B.B. (1993) Macaque ganglion cells and spatial vision, *Progress in Brain Research*, **95**, 33–43.

LEE, B.B., MARTIN, P.R. & VALBERG, A. (1988) The physiological basis of heterochromatic flicker photometry demonstrated in the ganglion cells of the macaque retina, *Journal of Physiology*, **404**, 323–347.

LEE, B.B., MARTIN, P.R. & VALBERG, A. (1989) Sensitivity of macaque retinal ganglion cells to chromatic and luminance flicker, *Journal of Physiology*, **414**, 223–243.

LEE, B.B., POKORNY, J., SMITH, V.C., MARTIN, P.R. & VALBERG, A. (1990) Luminance and chromatic modulation sensitivity of macaque ganglion cells and human observers, *Journal of the Optical Society of America*, A **7**, 2223–2236.

LEE, B.B., MARTIN, P.R., VALBERG, A. & KREMERS, J. (1993a) Physiological mechanisms underlying psychophysical sensitivity to combined luminance and chromatic modulation, *Journal of the Optical Society of America*, A **10**, 1403–1412.

Lee, B.B., Wehrhahn, C., Westheimer, G. & Kremers, J. (1993b) Macaque ganglion cell responses to stimuli that elicit hyperacuity in man: Detection of small displacements, *Journal of Neuroscience*, **13**, 1001–1009.

Lee, B.B., Wehrhahn, C., Westheimer, G. & Kremers, J. (1994) The spatial precision of macaque ganglion cell responses and vernier acuity, *Investigative Ophthalmology and Visual Science*, **35** (Suppl.), 2064.

Lennie, P. & D'Zmura, M.D. (1988) Mechanisms of color vision, *CRC Critical Reviews in Neurobiology*, **3**, 333–400.

Lindsey, D.T., Pokorny, J. & Smith, V.C. (1986) Phase-dependent sensitivity to heterochromatic flicker, *Journal of the Optical Society of America*, A **3**, 921–927.

Perry, V.H., Oehler, R. & Cowey, A. (1984) Retinal ganglion cells that project to the dorsal lateral geniculate nucleus in the macaque monkey, *Neuroscience*, **12**, 1110–1123.

Pokorny, J., Graham, C.H. & Lanson, R.N. (1968) Effect of wavelength on foveal grating acuity, *Journal of the Optical Society of America*, **58**, 1410–1414.

Polyak, S.L. (1941) *The Retina*, Chicago: University of Chicago Press.

Reid, R.C. & Shapley, R.M. (1992) Spatial structure of cone inputs to receptive fields in primate lateral geniculate nucleus, *Nature*, **356**, 716–718.

Rodieck, R.W. (1991) Which cells code for color? In: Valberg, A. & Lee, B.B. (Eds) *From Pigments to Perception*, New York and London: Plenum, pp. 83–94.

Schiller, P.H., Logothetis, N.K. & Charles, E.R. (1990) Function of the colour-opponent and broad-band channels of the visual system., *Nature*, **343**, 68–70.

Smith, V.C., Lee, B.B., Pokorny, J., Martin, P.R. & Valberg, A. (1992) Responses of macaque ganglion cells to the relative phase of heterochromatically modulated lights, *Journal of Physiology*, **458**, 191–221.

Stromeyer, C.F., III, Cole, G.R. & Kronauer, R.E. (1985) Second-site adaptation in the red-green chromatic pathways, *Vision Research*, **25**, 219–237.

Swanson, W.H., Pokorny, J. & Smith, V.C. (1987) Effects of temporal frequency on phase-dependent sensitivity to heterochromatic flicker, *Journal of the Optical Society of America*, A **4**, 2266–2273.

Wässle, H. & Boycott, B.B., (1991) Functional architecture of the mammalian retina, *Physiological Reviews*, **71**, 447–480.

Wässle, H., Boycott, B.B. & Illing, R.-B. (1981) Morphology and mosaic of on- and off-beta-cells of the cat retina and some functional considerations, *Proceedings of the Royal Society*, B **212**, 177–195.

Wässle, H., Grünert, U., Martin, P.R. & Boycott, B.B. (1994) Immunocytochemical characterisation and spatial distribution of midget bipolar cells in the macaque monkey retina, *Vision Research*, **34**, 561–579.

Watanabe, M. & Rodieck, R.W. (1989) Parasol and midget ganglion cells of the primate retina, *Journal of Comparative Neurology*, **289**, 434–454.

Watson, A.B. (1992) Transfer of contrast sensitivity in linear visual networks, *Visual Neuroscience*, **8**, 65–76.

Wehrhahn, C. & Westheimer, G. (1990) How vernier acuity depends on contrast, *Experimental Brain Research*, **80**, 618–620.

Wiesel, T. & Hubel, D.H. (1966) Spatial and chromatic interactions in the lateral geniculate body of the rhesus monkey, *Journal of Neurophysiology*, **29**, 1115–1156.

Chromatic Adaptation After-effects on Luminance and Chromatic Channels

Ichiro Kuriki and Donald I.A. MacLeod

3.2.1 INTRODUCTION

During exposure to a chromatic illuminant, the human visual system adapts to the illuminant. As a result of adaptation, the visual system shifts its sensitivity, and this makes the colour appearance of the adapting light more whitish than before. This phenomenon is quite common and it may seem to last several seconds after the disappearance of the adapting light. However, there has been little investigation of this long-lasting after-effect of chromatic adaptation (Fairchild and Lennie, 1992; Jameson *et al.*, 1979).

We have investigated the dynamics of chromatic adaptation, by measuring the magnitude and time course of the after-effect following various durations of chromatic adaptation. In addition, we tried to investigate what stage of the visual processing system is responsible for this slow chromatic adaptation: the receptors or the later stages. Pre-exposure to coloured light not only changes colour appearance; it can also change the spectral sensitivity of the visual system, and these two phenomena should be correlated if receptoral sensitivity changes underlie them both.

3.2.2 METHOD

Our experiment compared the effects of chromatic adaptation on the luminance and chromatic channels, by using either equal-luminance or unique-yellow settings during the after-effect. If the results for both tasks are the same, this would suggest that the after-effect occurs at a stage before the separation of the luminance and chromatic channels, such as the photoreceptors. We can assess the difference between the effect in the luminance and chromatic channels by measuring the difference between equal-luminance and unique-yellow settings for the same adapting conditions. The experiments were made on TEKTRONIX 690SR CRT screen, controlled by an IBM/PC computer with a Number Nine graphic board.

3.2.2.1 Procedure

The observer first made either equal luminance or unique-yellow settings without chromatic adaptation, in a dark room. Red and green pre-adapting conditions followed this control condition.

3.2.2.2 Stimulus sequence

There were five different lengths of pre-adapting period: 4 s, 12 s, 20 s, 40 s and 60 s. The length of adapting period and the type of test stimulus were fixed within a session. The test cycle started with the chosen duration of adaptation to a red or green uniform adapting stimulus (Figure 3.2.1).

The adapting stimulus was a full screen of the maximum intensity of red phosphor or a full screen of green phosphor of the same luminance. The luminance was about 40 cdm^{-2}, and the angular subtense was 8 degrees vertical by 10 degrees horizontal. Five seconds of test stimulus (10 cdm^{-2}) immediately followed this pre-adapting stimulus. In the main experiment a uniform grey screen followed the test stimulus to let the visual system recover from pre-adaptation. This lasted for twice the duration of the pre-adaptation stimulus. The entire cycle was repeated as necessary.

To characterise the dynamics of the adaptive changes, we used a technique we term 'parametric adjustment': the observer varied both the initial test stimulus and its rate of change over time, so as to produce a setting (either an equal luminance setting, or a unique yellow setting) that appeared valid both at the onset and at the offset of the test period. The x- and y-axes of a trackball respectively determined the test stimulus value at the onset of the test stimulus and at its offset five seconds later, and the cycle was repeated until the observer reached a satisfactory setting. The test stimulus changed linearly between the onset and offset values, and this linear gradient generally appeared satisfactory throughout the duration of the test stimulus.

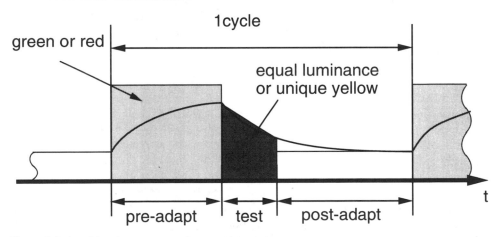

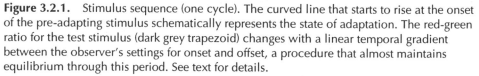

Figure 3.2.1. Stimulus sequence (one cycle). The curved line that starts to rise at the onset of the pre-adapting stimulus schematically represents the state of adaptation. The red-green ratio for the test stimulus (dark grey trapezoid) changes with a linear temporal gradient between the observer's settings for onset and offset, a procedure that almost maintains equilibrium through this period. See text for details.

3.2.2.3 Test stimuli

We used three kinds of test stimuli: unique-yellow, minimum motion and flicker balance settings. For the unique-yellow setting, the observer was asked to change the ratio between red and green phosphor intensity, so that the colour patch appear neither reddish nor greenish.

The minimum motion and flicker balance settings were presented to measure the change in equal luminance settings. For the minimum motion settings, the observer was asked to null motion perception using the procedure of Anstis and Cavanagh (Anstis and Cavanagh, 1983).

The flicker balance procedure is a new refinement of heterochromatic flicker photometry (Figure 3.2.2).

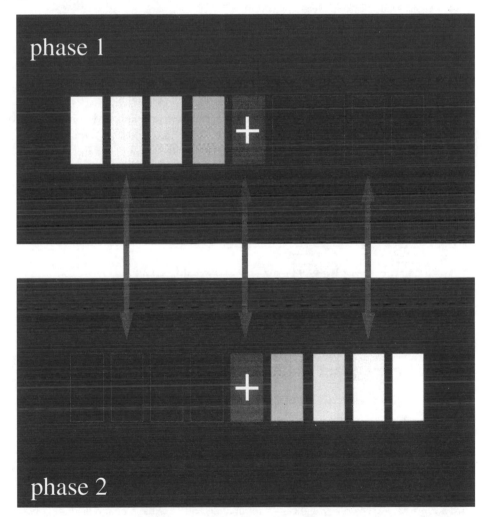

Figure 3.2.2.   Flicker balance technique. Arrays of test lights (phase 1) and standard lights (phase 2) are presented in rapid alternation phases at a frequency. Intensity of the patches are changed progressively, so that the patches except the equi-luminant pair are flickering. The observer's adjustments increase or decrease all test intensities by the same factor, by allowing the equiluminant point to be steered to the centre of the display.

The stimulus consists of an array of flicker patches, that progressively change the ratio between test and standard light intensities across the screen. Adjustments by the observer varied the intensity of all the test patches by the same factor. If the test intensity was set too high, a flicker null appeared at one side of the array. If it was too low, the null appeared at the opposite side of the array. The observer's task was to steer the flicker null into the centre of the screen, and the flicker amplitude then appeared equal on the two sides of the stimulus. This allowed the observer to make a quick and accurate equal luminance setting, which is essentially equivalent to ordinary HFP (Kuriki and MacLeod, in preparation). The observer made at least five settings for each condition.

3.2.2.4 Analysis: Relative M-cone weight

We express the results in terms of the weight for M-cone output into either luminance or chromatic channels, relative to that for the L-cones. Figure 3.2.3 shows our simple model for the luminance and chromatic channels, taken from Ahn and MacLeod (Ahn and MacLeod, 1993).

If the adaptation occurs at the photoreceptor, the changes of relative M-cone weight for different adapting conditions will be the same for both unique-yellow and equal-luminance settings. On the other hand, if the adaptation processes that differentially suppress L or M

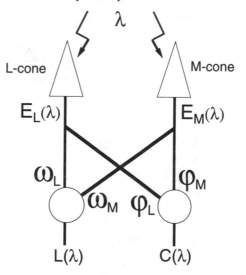

Relative M-cone weight :

$$\omega = \omega_M / \omega_L \text{ (luminance channel)}$$
$$\varphi = \varphi_M / \varphi_L \text{ (chromatic channel)}$$

Figure 3.2.3. L- and M-cone weights into luminance and chromatic channels. $E_M(\lambda)$ and $E_L(\lambda)$ stand for the excitation of M- and L-cones to the incident light λ, respectively. ω_M and ω_L are the weights applied for $E_M(\lambda)$ and $E_L(\lambda)$ at the input to the luminance channel, which generates an output $L(\lambda) = \omega_L E_L(\lambda) + \omega_M E_M(\lambda)$. φ_M and φ_L are the weights for $E_M(\lambda)$ and $E_L(\lambda)$ at the input to the chromatic channel, which generates an output $C(\lambda) = \varphi_L E_L(\lambda) - \varphi_M E_M(\lambda)$. See Ahn and MacLeod (1993) for detail.

cone signals are different for the L and M cone inputs routed to the chromatic and achromatic post-receptoral channels, then the relative M-cone weight may behave differently in the unique-yellow and equal luminance settings. In this model, the characterisation of all adaptation effects by an M-cone weight, rather than (for instance) a bias, means that all such effects are attributed to changes of sensitivity, either in the receptors themselves or in the 'links' between the receptors and the channels. Changes of sensitivity within the channels do not affect the M-cone weight once the L and M cone inputs have been combined for that channel.

3.2.3   RESULTS

3.2.3.1 Unique-yellow setting

Figure 3.2.4 shows the results for unique-yellow settings for observers IK and RS. The two panels show the two different observers, and the different symbols show the different adapting conditions; filled circles for green adaptation, open circles for red adaptation. The horizontal axis shows the total time elapsed from the *onset* of adapting stimulus. Each line segment is for a single adapting condition and represents the first five seconds of recovery immediately following the offset of the adapting stimulus. Thus the symbols at the left and right end of each line show the settings for the onset and offset of the test stimulus, respectively. The vertical axis shows log relative M-cone weight, introduced in the previous section. If the chosen setting were the pure red or pure green phosphor (that is, if the preadapting stimuli themselves came to appear yellow), the symbol would fall on the top or bottom horizontal line. The dotted horizontal line shows the unique-yellow setting in the control condition.

For both observers, the symbols at the left end of each line show that the effect of adaptation grows slowly, and takes several tens of seconds to build up to a maximum. The magnitude of the difference between red and green adapting conditions is about 0.25 to 0.3 log unit at most in each observer; this corresponds to the factor of two or to 10–15 jnd steps. The effect of adaptation was not large enough, however, to change the appearance of red or green phosphor into neither reddish nor greenish, even with 60s of pre-adaptation. The symbols at the right end of each line show that the effect of adaptation began to fade during the five seconds after the adapting stimulus had disappeared. Yet at the end of the five second period of measured recovery, a substantial fraction of the initial adaptive shift in unique yellow still remained.

Figure 3.2.5 gives a more extended picture of recovery, following 20 s of pre-adaptation. In this experiment we asked the observer to make the unique-yellow setting for various lengths of test period, using the parametric adjustment procedure with a linear gradient of red/green ratio in each case.

For observer IK, the time to recover from chromatic adaptation was twice as long as it took for preceding adaptation; 40 s, in this case. The settings for both conditions for observer IK return to the control baseline at 60 s, while the results for observer RS reached a plateau at around 40 s to 50 s. The observer RS reported some residual difference in the appearance of the texture of the test patch at 60 s, and the same phenomenon was reported also by observer IK. We suspect that this may be responsible for the large offset in the results for the observer RS.

3.2.3.2 Minimum motion setting

Figure 3.2.6 shows the result for the minimum motion setting. The meanings of the axes and symbols are the same as in the Figure 3.2.5. The results for observer IK show almost no difference between red and green pre-adapting experiments, although at 40 s and 60 s, there may be a small difference.

The results for observer RS show a fairly large standard deviation for each setting and it is very difficult to see any systematic difference between the two adapting conditions. However, where reliable differences appear, the red adapting condition produces a *smaller* log relative M-cone weight. This is the opposite from the effect seen in the unique-yellow setting. Therefore, the change in log relative M-cone weight for unique-yellow and minimum motion settings are clearly not the same.

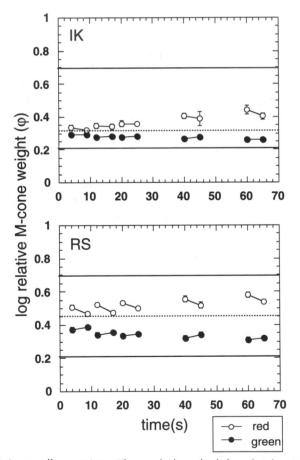

Figure 3.2.4.   Unique-yellow settings. The symbols at the left and right end of the each line segment shows the settings chosen by parametric adjustment for the onset and offset of the test period respectively. The error bars show 95 per cent confidence intervals.

3.2.3.3 Flicker balance setting

Figure 3.2.7 shows the results for the flicker balance setting. The meanings of the symbols are the same as in Figure 3.2.6. For observer IK, the difference between the red and green adapting conditions is small, as in the results for minimum motion setting. For observer RS, the standard deviations for the shorter adapting time conditions are smaller, and the results are almost the same as for the minimum motion setting.

3.2.4   INTENSE ADAPTING FIELD EXPERIMENTS

These results show that the effect of chromatic adaptation on spectral sensitivity is generally smaller than the effect on colour appearance; but for the longer duration adaptations, it is possible that the two effects become comparable in magnitude. To test this point, we made additional experiments using intense adapting lights, in an effort to increase the magnitude of the adaptive changes. The adapting lights were provided by a Maxwellian view system superimposed on the CRT screen by means of a beam splitter. The adapting

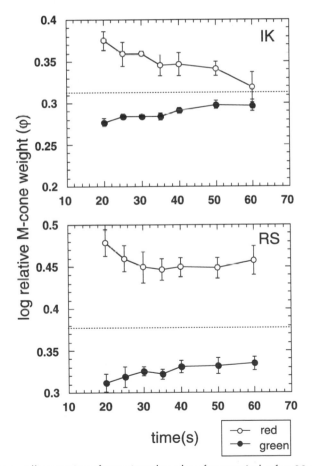

Figure 3.2.5. Unique-yellow settings for various lengths of test period, after 20 s of pre-adaptation. The error bars show 95 per cent confidence intervals.

light was generated using a KODAK #92 wratten filter and a 500-nm interference filter for the red and green adapting stimuli. The adapting field intensity was about 1000 td.

3.2.5   RESULTS

Figure 3.2.8 shows the results for unique-yellow and minimum motion settings for observer IK. The difference between red and green adaptation for the unique-yellow setting is larger than in the CRT-adaptation experiment, and its magnitude in relative M-cone weight is about 0.4 log unit. On the other hand, the difference between the two adapting conditions is now smaller in minimum motion settings, where the magnitude in relative M-cone weight is less than 0.1 log unit. This result clearly shows that the effects of chromatic adaptation on the luminance and chromatic channels are different from each other.

In runs using test stimuli of different intensity (not shown), the unique-yellow setting and

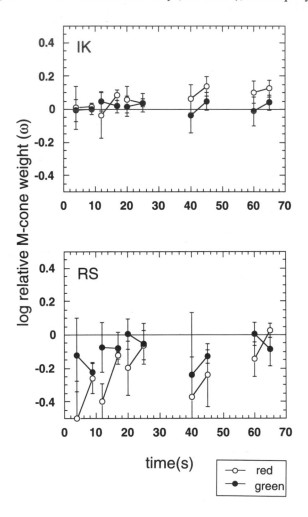

Figure 3.2.6.   Minimum motion settings. The error bars show 95 per cent confidence intervals.

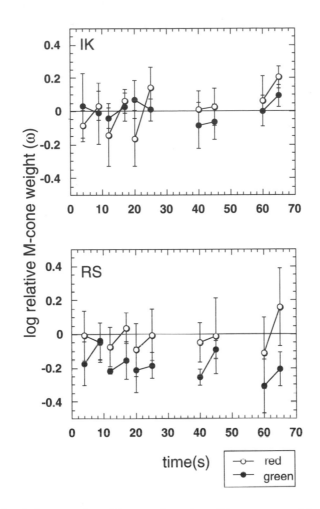

Figure 3.2.7. Flicker balance settings. The error bars show 95 per cent confidence intervals.

M-cone weight were not substantially dependent on test intensity. This supports the assumption inherent to the model, that the effects of adaptation under these conditions are analogous to a change of weight or gain rather than a bias.

3.2.6   SUMMARY AND CONCLUSION

In summary, our results show that: (1) the chromatic adaptation after-effect grows slowly over several tens of seconds; (2) recovery from chromatic adaptation takes about as long as it took for pre-adaptation; and (3) preceding chromatic adaptation affects unique-yellow settings relatively strongly but has little or no effect on equal-luminance settings.

It follows that the chromatic adaptation process responsible for these adaptation after-effects occurs not at the photo-receptor, or at stages where the signals from different types of photoreceptor remain segregated, but at the later stages of the visual system.

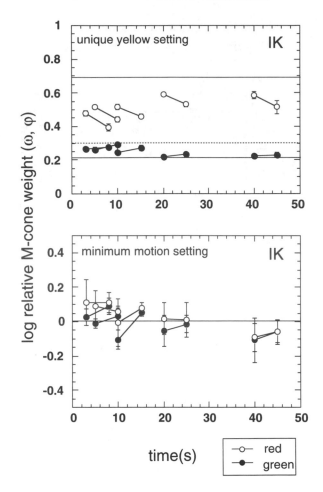

Figure 3.2.8. Unique-yellow and minimum motion settings for observer IK with a high-intensity adapting field. Top panel shows the results for unique-yellow settings; and the bottom panel shows the results for minimum-motion settings. The persisting effect of pre-adaptation is stronger for unique-yellow settings but weaker or non-existent for the minimum-motion settings.

3.2.7 REFERENCES

AHN, S. & MacLEOD, D.I.A. (1993) Link-specific adaptation in the luminance and chromatic channels, *Vision Research*, **33**, 2271–2286.

ANSTIS, S. & CAVANAGH, P. (1983) A minimum motion technique for judging equiluminance. In: Mollon, J.D. & Sharpe, L. D. (Eds), *Colour Vision Physiology and Psychophysics*, London: Academic Press, pp. 155–166.

FAIRCHILD, M. D. & LENNIE, P. (1992) Chromatic adaptation to natural and incandescent illuminants, *Vision Research*, **32**, 2077–2085.

JAMESON, D., HURVICH, L. M. & VARNER, F. D. (1979) Receptoral and postreceptoral visual processes in recovery from chromatic adaptation, *Proceedings of the National Academy of Sciences*, **76**, 3034–3038.

KURIKI, I. & MacLEOD, D.I.A., Flicker balance technique for heterochromatic photometry, in preparation.

Selectivity Limits of Spectral Sensitivity Functions for Chromatic and Achromatic Mechanisms

A. Nacer, I.J. Murray, Sharanjeet-Kaur and J.J. Kulikowski

3.3.1 INTRODUCTION

Two basic post-receptoral spectral sensitivity functions (SSFs) can be obtained by presenting a 1° test spot on a white (1000 td) background; 1 Hz presentations are detected by the chromatic-opponent system with its characteristic three peaks, whereas 25 Hz stimulates the achromatic system reflecting the luminosity (V_λ) function (King-Smith, 1975; King-Smith and Carden, 1976). Various intermediate shapes of SSFs are obtained when temporal frequency varies between 1 and 25 Hz. Three additional functions can be obtained using coloured backgrounds (Stiles's (1939) method modified by M. Marre, 1973) that can isolate the so-called cone mechanisms.

At low spatial and temporal frequencies of the test spot and photopic luminance levels, detection is said to depend on the luminance contrast between the test and the background fields (see Shapley and Enroth-Cugell, 1984). Thus, the luminance threshold (ΔL) increases in direct proportion to background luminance (L) according to Weber's law (i.e. sensitivity decreases in inverse proportion, showing a slope of -1 on a log-log scale).

This is not the case for higher temporal frequencies (> 30 Hz) when the Weber fraction ($\Delta L/L$) is found to be very small (nearly zero), indicating a 'non-contrast' detection of luminance change, which is pure flicker detection (King-Smith and Kulikowski, 1975).

The aim of this study is to re-evaluate the temporal characteristics of these SSFs, use various methods to isolate constituent mechanisms and discuss them in the context of other recent results obtained in psychophysics and electrophysiology.

3.3.2 OBJECTIVE

The objectives of the present study were (1) to show that there are not two but at least three different mechanisms underlying spectral sensitivity responses over a wide range of temporal frequencies, and (2) to show that pure flicker mechanisms, unambiguously associated with the V_λ function, are revealed only at presentation rates of 33 Hz and higher.

3.3.3   METHODS

A 3-channel Maxwellian view optical system was used for all experiments. The first and second channels were derived from the same light source (a Philips 50 W tungsten lamp) and provided both the small and large backgrounds (1.1° and 10° respectively). The third channel was used to present the test flash which was a 1.1° spot having a square-wave luminance distribution. The test light (Philips 50 W) was derived from a single-prism monochromator with exit slit of 1 mm and a half bandwidth of 4 nm. Narrow-band Balzer filters were used to calibrate the monochromator by measuring the maximum light transmission in the blue, green and red regions of the spectrum. A precision neutral density wedge (0–6 log units) mounted on a stepper motor, was used to control test brightness. The wedge settings were read by a BBC microcomputer. The computer was programmed to calculate relative sensitivity values based on calibrations of the wedge and bulbs made over a 6 log unit range using a photomultiplier (Thorn EMI). The radiant flux in quanta sec^{-1} deg^{-2} of the stimulus was also calculated and converted to relative sensitivity. The backgrounds were calibrated by measuring the luminance on a perfect diffuser positioned 10 cm behind the final image (which is at the plane of the pupil in a Maxwellian view system), according to the method described by Westheimer (1966). The stimulus was viewed through a 3 mm artificial pupil. Four small spots were positioned symmetrically around the stimulus to aid fixation.

Test duration was checked by the same photomultiplier used for radiance calibrations together with an oscilloscope and the error was within 0.50 ms for shortest durations and lower for longer durations.

Using the method of adjustment, the subjects (AN, 29 and SK, 28) were asked to set test brightness to detection threshold at low frequencies of the test stimulus, and to set flicker detection threshold when temporal frequencies were high (i.e. > 5–6 Hz). The experiments were controlled by computer and average threshold sensitivity was accepted as the mean of three determinations. A light adaptation of one minute preceded each experiment when a white background was used. This adaptation time was two minutes when coloured filters were used to isolate blue cones.

3.3.4   RESULTS

3.3.4.1 1 Hz versus 25 Hz SS functions

Typical spectral (1 Hz) and flicker (25 Hz) sensitivity functions are shown in Figure 3.3.1. In normal subjects, the 1 Hz curve reveals three peaks (450 nm, 530 nm and 610 nm) and two troughs (500 nm and 575 nm), indicating post-receptoral processing of colour-opponent mechanisms (Sperling and Harwerth, 1971).

The 25 Hz curve however, shows only one broad peak near 550 nm and resembles the CIE (1978) V_λ function. It was argued (King-Smith and Carden, 1976) that this curve was the response of the non-opponent or the achromatic mechanism.

Figure 3.3.2 shows a smooth transition between the chromatic-opponent and achromatic non-opponent characteristics with increasing temporal frequency for a background luminance of 2000 td. For normal subjects, flicker-based spectral sensitivity is similar to the shape of the luminosity function at 25 Hz and retains this shape for higher temporal frequencies. However, the crucial test for the operation of a pure luminance detection system is that flicker detection is independent of background luminance. The shape of the 25 Hz function, although similar to the luminosity V_λ curve, cannot be regarded as

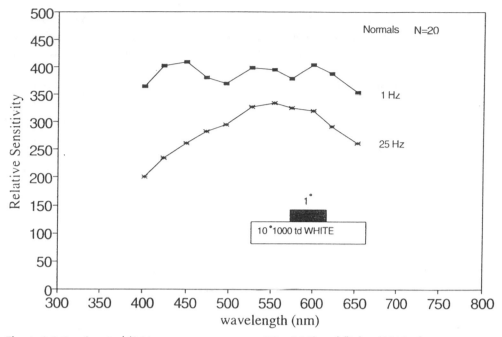

Figure 3.3.1. Spectral (1 Hz, upper curve, mean SD = 0.15) and flicker (25 Hz, lower curve, mean SD = 0.12) sensitivity functions for 1° test spots on large 10° 1000 td white background. Data are the mean of 35 normal eyes. Adapted from Russell (1991).

conclusive on its own. Note that although the curve is similar in shape to V_λ at 12.5 and 17.5 Hz, the peak is shifted away from 555 nm as indicated by the small vertical lines on each curve. At 25 Hz and above, the peak corresponds to that of the V_λ curve at 555 nm.

3.3.4.2 Flicker sensitivity

Figure 3.3.3 shows the relationship between background luminance and sensitivity to a 1° target on a large white background for four spectral lights (474, 527, 574 and 601 nm) over a range of temporal frequencies, from 1 Hz to 35.6 Hz. Sensitivity is almost linearly related to background luminance up to 25 Hz; $\Delta L/L$ approx 1. Above 35 Hz, Weber fraction $\Delta L/L$ is nil indicating that sensitivity is independent of background luminance. Detection for these high frequencies is solely determined by pure flicker, which is not the case for the 25 Hz frequency when $\Delta L/L$ is around 0.9.

3.3.4.3 Temporal characteristics

Figure 3.3.4 illustrates temporal frequency characteristics for four different stimulus conditions. In Figure 3.3.4a, a white pedestal (see inset) is projected on the large white background and made spatially coincident with the test spot, $\lambda = 450$ nm. Sensitivity for a range of temporal frequencies reveals a single function (most likely the blue-yellow opponent mechanism), with maximum sensitivity at low temporal frequencies. This is what would be expected if, as suggested by Foster and Snelgar (1983), the pedestal reduced the sensitivity of achromatic mechanisms – leaving only the chromatic channel to respond to the stimulus. Figure 3.3.4b shows that a single mechanism is also obtained with a 1000 td yellow coincident field without the white background. Here the yellow background suppresses the red and green cone-mechanisms. The result is an isolated blue-cone response. It is evident that maximum responses are obtained at low frequencies (< 1 Hz) with both the white and yellow backgrounds.

The 'blue' mechanism (test spot 450 nm) is easiest to isolate by using an additional pedestal co-extensive in size with the test spot. When the pedestal is yellow the blue-cone mechanism is obtained, whereas the white pedestal and white background reveal the operation of the blue-yellow opponent function; in both cases pedestals minimise achromatic intrusions. The temporal frequency (low-pass) characteristics in these two cases are very similar, as though it was a unitary mechanism, related to colour opponent function, rather than to the receptoral properties.

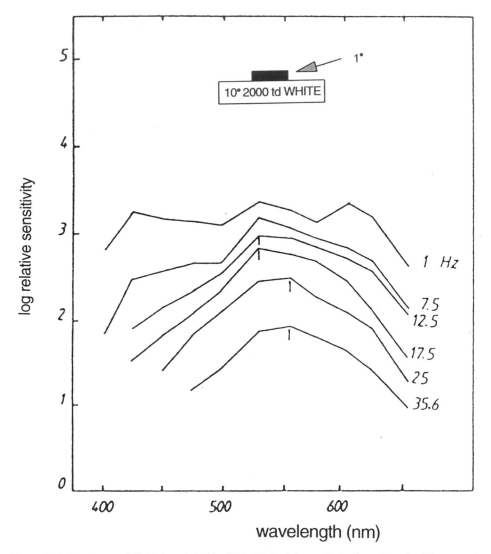

Figure 3.3.2. Spectral (1 Hz) and flicker (7.5–35.6 Hz) sensitivity functions for 1° test spots presented on large 10° 2000 td white backgrounds. The subject is AN (author).

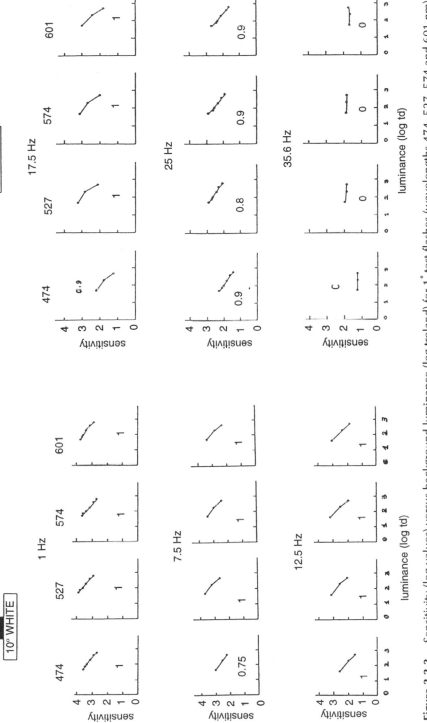

Figure 3.3.3. Sensitivity (log values) versus background luminance (log troland) for 1° test flashes (wavelengths 474, 527, 574 and 601 nm). Flicker rates are the same as in Figure 3.3.2. The numbers in each plot are calculations of the Weber fraction. The subject is AN.

This finding is often interpreted as evidence for slowness of blue cones, but it is more plausible that the blue cones contribute predominantly (if not exclusively) to colour opponency, so that the blue mechanism can practically be studied only via this channel. In any case, the idea that blue cones are particularly slow is disproved by direct recordings from blue cones (which are not much slower than the others, see Baylor *et al.*, 1987). The alternative interpretation must be substantiated with more rigorous elimination of the possible role of other mechanisms. In fact the presence of some achromatic intrusion can be detected when the temporal-frequency characteristics are band-pass with peaks around 10 Hz, and such components are indeed evident when measuring characteristics for blue and yellow spots on large white backgrounds (Figures 3.3.4c and 3.3.4d). Without the pedestal, achromatic intrusion is clearly evident. In Figure 3.3.4c there is an obvious break in the curve at around 8 Hz. The lower temporal frequencies are detected by the chromatic mechanism with the same characteristics as Figures 3.3.4a and b. Above 8 Hz the activity

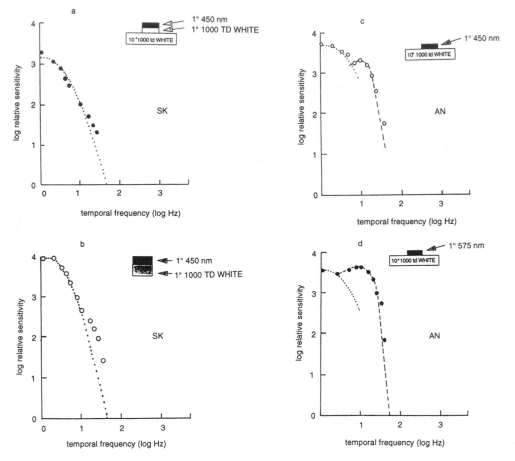

Figure 3.3.4. Flicker sensitivity plotted as a function of temporal frequency for four different test and background conditions. The dotted lines drawn through the data are fitted by eye. The subjects AN and SK are author and co-author. a: The blue test flashes (450 nm) are presented centrally on a combination of pedestal (spatially coincident with the test spot) and a large background. Both the pedestal and the background are white. b: Blue test (450 nm) on a yellow pedestal. c: Blue test (450 nm) at the centre of a large white background. d: Yellow test (575 nm) at the centre of a large white background.

of the achromatic mechanism is evident. This faster mechanism has a peak at around 10 Hz and compares favourably with achromatic mechanisms described by other authors (e.g. Burr and Ross, 1982; Kulikowski and Tolhurst, 1973). The yellow spot (575 nm) is detected by chromatic mechanisms only at very low temporal frequencies. Hence, in Figure 3.3.4d the break point between chromatic and achromatic activity occurs at a lower temporal frequency than in Figure 3.3.4c.

3.3.4.4 Can the chromatic-opponent system detect 25 Hz flicker?

At the other extreme, the fast (25 Hz) flicker is considered as activating a pure luminance mechanism. However, we find this holds true only for flicker above 33 Hz when flicker threshold solely depends on luminance change irrespective of background luminance. In some pathological cases, in which a selective loss of magnocellular function is suspected, there may be a total absence of flicker detection above 30 Hz. However, 25 Hz flicker may be detected and flicker-based spectral sensitivity then exhibits a characteristic peak around 450 nm, evidently due to some contribution of blue-cone inputs. These cases are analogous to blue cone monochromats; their flicker resolution is about 30 Hz at 1000 td as shown by Hess et al., (1989), the spectral sensitivity for flicker is reduced by about 1.5 log units, and there is a peak around 450 nm as shown in the case of multiple sclerosis illustrated in Figure 3.3.5.

Thus, the 25 Hz stimulus, although commonly used as a test of luminosity function, must be treated with caution because it may reveal residual responses of the chromatic system when the magno-system is severely damaged.

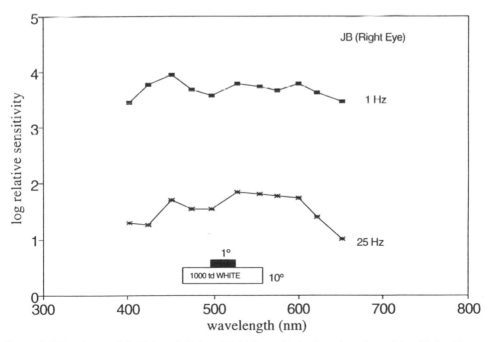

Figure 3.3.5. Spectral (1 Hz) and flicker (25 Hz) sensitivity functions for subject JB for 1° test flashes on large 10° white background. Notice the severe reduction in the 25 Hz function compared to the 1 Hz curve, which is normal. Adapted from Russell et al. (1991).

3.3.5 DISCUSSION

When a range of temporal frequencies is investigated three mechanisms are revealed in spectral sensitivity functions. The chromatic mechanism is apparent at 1 Hz, the achromatic mechanism at > 20 Hz and pure flicker at 33 Hz and above. The transition from chromatic to achromatic mechanisms is illustrated in Figure 3.3.2, and the transition from achromatic to pure flicker detection is seen in Figure 3.3.3 as a change of the slope of the threshold versus intensity (tvi) functions from −1 to 0 between 17.5 Hz and 35 Hz.

This interpretation is confirmed when stimulus conditions are manipulated to favour the operation of either chromatic or achromatic mechanisms. We can isolate the colour-opponent contribution by superimposing the stimulus on a coincident field, either with or without an extended background. In both cases, the temporal frequency characteristics are practically the same. There is a resolution limit of about 35 Hz revealing the operation of only the achromatic mechanism. It will be seen that these two curves are over 1 log unit below the spectral sensitivity at 25 Hz on a white background with no masking (when no pedestal is used to mask the test spot edges).

Without masking, two mechanisms are shown to operate (see Figures 3.3.4c and d). As might be expected, the chromatic mechanism has poorer temporal characteristics than the achromatic. The 450 nm curve is very similar to the 575 nm curve at high temporal frequencies (this wavelength is known to be detected by the achromatic mechanism). Thus normal subjects exhibit achromatic V_λ detection at 25 Hz over the range of 400–650 nm.

3.3.6 CONCLUSION

We confirm that $1°$ spectral spots on white background (1000 td) are detected by the chromatic-opponent mechanism at 1 Hz and by the achromatic non-opponent mechanism at and above 25 Hz. It is shown that 25 Hz flicker, though convenient, is not necessarily an unequivocal index of the integrity of the achromatic luminance system (identified with the V_λ function). Only above 35Hz is such selectivity attained.

3.3.7 REFERENCES

BAYLOR, D.A., NUNN, B.J. & SCHNAPF, J.L. (1987) Spectral sensitivity of cones of the monkey macaca fascicularis, *Journal of Physiology*, **390**, 145–160.

BURR, D.C. & ROSS J. (1982) Contrast sensitivity at high velocities, *Vision Research*, **23**, 3567–3569.

CIE (1978) *Light as True Visual Quantity: Principles of Measurements*, Publication CIE No 41 (TC-1.4), Paris: Bureau Central de la CIE.

FOSTER, D.H. & SNELGAR, R.S. (1983) Test and field spectral sensitivity of colour mechanisms obtained on small white backgrounds: action of unitary opponent-colour processes? *Vision Research*, **23**, 787–797.

HESS, R.F., MULLEN, K.T. & ZRENNER, E. (1989) Human photopic vision with only short wavelength cones: post-receptoral properties, *Journal of Physiology*, **417**, 151–172.

KING-SMITH, P.E. (1975) Visual detection analysed in terms of luminance and chromatic signals, *Nature*, **255**, 69–70.

KING-SMITH, P.E. & CARDEN, D. (1976) Luminance and opponent-color contributions to visual detection and adaptation and to temporal and spatial integration, *Journal of the Optical Society of America*, **66**, 709–717.

KING-SMITH, P.E. & KULIKOWSKI, J.J. (1975) Pattern and flicker detection analysis by sub-threshold summation, *Journal of Physiology*, **249**, 519–548.

KULIKOWSKI, J.J. & TOLHURST, D.J. (1973) Psychophysical evidence for sustained and transient neurones in the human visual system, *Journal of Physiology*, **232**, 149–162.

MARRÉ, M. (1973) The investigation of acquired colour vision deficiencies. In: *Colour 73*, London: Adam Hilger, pp. 99–135.

RUSSELL, M.H.A. (1991) VEP and psychophysical investigation of chromatic and achromatic visual function in humans; applications in the investigation of multiple sclerosis and optic neuritis, PhD thesis, University of Manchester.

RUSSELL, M.H.A., MURRAY, I.J., METCALFE, R. & KULIKOWSKI, J.J. (1991) Visual evoked potentials and psychophysical investigation of chromatic and achromatic visual function in humans; applications in the investigation of multiple sclerosis and optic neuritis, *Brain*, **114**, 2419–2435.

SHAPLEY, R. & ENROTH-CUGELL, C. (1984) Visual adaptation and retinal gain controls. In: N. Osborne & G. Chader (Eds) *Progress in Retinal Research (Vol. 3)*, Oxford: Pergamon Press.

SPERLING, H.G. & HARWERTH, R.S. (1971) Red-green cone interactions in the increment threshold spectral sensitivity of primates, *Science*, **172**, 180–184.

STILES, W.S. (1939) The directional sensitivity of the retina and the spectral sensitivities of the rods and cones, *Proceedings of the Royal Society, London*, **127B**, 64–105.

WESTHEIMER, G. (1966) The Maxwellian view, *Vision Research*, **6**, 669–682.

Spectral Sensitivity in Glaucoma and Ocular Hypertension

Sharanjeet-Kaur, E. O'Donoghue, I.J. Murray
and J.J. Kulikowski

3.4.1 INTRODUCTION

Patients with glaucoma are invariably asymptomatic. This means that detection of the disease relies on patient screening and at present the strategies adopted for this are remarkably inefficient. There is now strong evidence from population and epidemiological studies (Klein *et al.*, 1992; Teilsch *et al.*, 1991) that, at any one time, only about half the total number of individuals with glaucoma are actually detected. One of the main reasons for this is that the neuropathology of the disease is poorly understood.

3.4.1.1 Raised intra-ocular pressure (IOP)

The detection of glaucoma is complicated by the distribution in the normal population of IOP. Traditionally, high IOP was regarded as being inextricably linked with, if not the direct cause of, glaucoma. The advent of large-scale assessment of IOP has revealed the fallacy of this. A recent epidemiological study (Teilsch *et al.*, 1991) investigated the accuracy of IOP and ophthalmoscopy findings in the diagnosis of glaucoma. When based on IOP of greater than 21 mm Hg, only 47 per cent of cases were detected. Furthermore, only 5–10 per cent of those with IOP outside the upper range of so-called normal developed glaucoma (according to conventional criteria) after 10 years. Evidently, measuring IOP is not an efficient means of detecting glaucoma. The large numbers of patients with increased IOP, but with apparently normal visual fields, so-called ocular hypertension (OHT), has created a diagnostic smoke screen in the detection of glaucoma.

3.4.1.2 Parvo and magno-cellular pathways

In man and higher primates there exist two morphologically distinct pathways between the retina and the primary visual cortex. Briefly, these are termed parvo- and magno-cellular after the layers of the lateral geniculate nucleus to and from which they project, in the retino-geniculo-striate pathway. Parvo-cellular neurons constitute around 80 per cent of the total output of the retina. They are smaller than their magnocellular counterparts in terms of axonal diameter, soma size and receptive field size. In general, they are more sluggish in operation and have much poorer contrast sensitivity. Magno-cellular neurons seem designed to detect fast flicker; they have a faster response time course, large receptive fields and very high contrast sensitivity. It is now accepted that, although some magno cells respond to coloured targets, true chromatic vision is exclusively subserved by parvo cells. At the opposite extreme, magno cells are selectively responsive to fast flicker and Crook *et al.*, (1987) have shown convincingly that they account for the luminosity function or V-lambda curve.

3.4.1.3 Link between histology and sensitivity loss

Animal models of glaucoma in primates conducted by raising intra ocular pressure (IOP) in monkeys, suggest that large fibres are more susceptible than smaller fibres to high IOP (Quigley *et al.*, 1987; Quigley *et al.*, 1988). This is supported by psychophysical measurements on patients with glaucomatous eyes who have impaired flicker sensitivity (Tyler, 1981) and motion detection thresholds (Fitzke *et al.*, 1988). Further evidence for the idea has emerged from the use of blue targets on a yellow background to isolate blue cone pathways. Here the argument is that as there are fewer yellow-blue than red-green retinal ganglion cells then blue-on-yellow visual field defects will appear sooner than white-on white-defects. This is reinforced by the fact that ganglion cells coded for yellow-blue are larger than those coded for red-green. There is substantial experimental support for this approach. Heron *et al.* (1988) showed evidence of abnormalities in the detection of blue-on-yellow at different points across the visual field in both ocular hypertension (OHT) and in confirmed glaucoma patients.

Interpretational difficulties remain however. Although the blue-on-yellow visual field test seems more sensitive than conventional visual fields, in many cases there are those who develop white-on-white defects without any impairment of blue-on-yellow. Furthermore, blue/yellow ganglion cells constitute only a small proportion of the parvo-cellular pathway. It may be that numerical superiority rather than greater resistance to high IOP based on their size, accounts for the apparent survival of red/green ganglion cells. There are many reports of substantial fibre loss post mortem in patients who had no discernible reduction in visual function. This inherent robustness in the visual pathway creates problems for the interpretation of the histological findings in glaucoma.

3.4.1.4 Chromatic and achromatic channels

Since the pioneering work of Sperling and Harwerth (1971) and King-Smith and Carden (1976) it has been accepted that chromatic and achromatic processing in humans can be tested separately with a 1 degree spectral spot superimposed on a photopic white background. When the target is presented at 1 Hz and increment detection thresholds are measured, then the target is assumed to monitor the activity of colour opponent channels. A three-peaked function is obtained with the peaks (at 410 nm, 535 nm and 615 nm) corresponding to colour opponent mechanisms. If the target is presented at 25 Hz and flicker detection thresholds are measured, the obtained function is similar to the V-lambda curve and is a measure of the sensitivity of a luminance channel. Broadly speaking, the technique allows the selective stimulation of parvo (1 Hz stimulation) and magno (25 Hz stimulation) pathways.

In the present study we have used spectral sensitivity to compare two groups of patients; one with confirmed glaucoma and the other with OHT. This is a preliminary investigation and the numbers in each group are small. Nevertheless, the findings are compelling. In common with other studies of this type (Alvarez and Mills, 1985; Heron *et al.*, 1988) we find that some OHT patients do have reduced visual sensitivity in the fovea. Furthermore, patients with confirmed glaucoma are abnormal in that fast flicker detection is often severely impaired and chromatic processing shows reduced sensitivity.

3.4.2 METHODS

3.4.2.1 Spectral sensitivity

The spectral sensitivity apparatus used in these experments has been described in detail elsewhere (Alvarez and Mills, 1985). Briefly, the set-up comprises a two-channel optical system. One channel produces the 1 degree spectral spot via narrow band filters. The spot is seen in Maxwellian view and superimposed on a white background derived from the other channel. The same light source supplies the input to both channels. The spectral spot is obtained by passing the light beam through Balzers B40 interference filters with bandwidths of 10 nm and peak transmissions of 401, 425, 450, 474, 497, 527, 554, 574, 601, 622, and 652 nm. The brightness of the background is adjusted by neutral density filters. Increment detection thresholds (at 1 Hz) and flicker detection thresholds (at 25 Hz) are set by the method of adjustment. Observers vary the brightness of the target by adjusting the setting of an annular neutral density wedge (calibrated for non-linearity and spectral sensitivity) until they found the appropriate criterion. All observations were repeated twice.

3.4.2.2 Patients and subjects

Twenty-five patients (44 eyes) were tested. Their mean age was 60.9 years. Two patients were aged between 30 and 40 and the others were aged between 50 and 70 years. The patients had no other ocular or systemic disease, they were not taking any drugs that might induce changes in colour perception and all were colour normal. We tested patients with confirmed primary open angle glaucoma (POAG) and ocular hypertension (OHT). Ten patients had POAG in both eyes and two patients had POAG in one eye only. Seven patients had OHT in both eyes and six patients had OHT in one eye and POAG in the fellow eye. In four of these, only one eye was tested.

All eyes tested had visual acuity of 6/9 or better and none had media opacities. Visual fields were examined on all patients using an Octopus 500 E and intra-ocular pressures were measured by Goldman tonometry. All patients were diagnosed by a senior registrar at Manchester Royal Eye Hospital. Our stimulus area did not fall within a known visual field defect in the POAG patients.

A group of 10 age-matched normal observers took part in the study. The mean age was of 62.4 years. None of these individuals had any systemic or ocular pathology and all were colour normal. Their visual acuities were 6/6 or better.

3.4.3　RESULTS

3.4.3.1 OHT patients

Spectral sensitivity data are divided into four groups according to the following criteria:
Group 1. Normal 1 Hz and 25 Hz sensitivity
Group 2. Reduced 25 Hz normal 1 Hz sensitivity
Group 3. Reduced 1 Hz normal 25 Hz
Group 4. Reduced 1 Hz and 25 Hz sensitivity

3.4.3.3 POAG patients

Spectral sensitivity data are divided into the following groups:
Group 1. Normal 1 Hz and 25 Hz sensitivity
Group 2. Reduced 1 Hz sensitivity in the blue region only, normal 25 Hz.
Group 3. Reduced 1 Hz and reduced 25 Hz sensitivity.
Group 4. Reduced 1 Hz and absent 25 Hz.
Sensitivity plots were classified as abnormal if any data point was outside ± 1 SD for the age matched normal data.

3.4.3.3 Normal spectral sensitivity

The data for OHT group 1 and POAG group 1 are illustrated in Figure 3.4.1. In each case the upper curve is the 1 Hz increment threshold data and the lower curve is the 25 Hz flicker threshold data. The left-hand graph is the OHT patients' data and the right-hand graph is the POAG patients' data. Solid lines depict the mean of 10 age-matched normals and the dashed lines indicate ± 1SD.

The data show that all eyes are within normal limits.

3.4.3.4 Patients with ocular hypertension (OHT)

In Figures 3.4.2a,b and c the OHT data are illustrated. In Figure 3.4.2a there is a marked abnormality in flicker sensitivity across all wavelengths while there appears to be no abnormality in the 1 Hz data.

Figures 3.4.2b and c illustrate the data for OHT groups 3 and 4. Some patients have normal 25 Hz functions and reduced sensitivity across all wavelengths (Figure 3.4.2b). Note that the notch around 580 nm is maintained suggesting that colour opponency is not entirely abolished in these patients. Figure 3.4.2c shows the data for those OHT patients in whom there is reduction in both 1 Hz and 25 Hz sensitivity (OHT group 4). Again the notch at 580 nm is well defined.

3.4.3.5 Patients with primary open angle glaucoma (POAG)

Figure 3.4.3a shows the cases we have called POAG group 2 in which 1 Hz spectral sensitivity is reduced in the blue region and 25 Hz flicker sensitivity is normal. Figure 3.4.3b illustrates those cases in which both 1 Hz and 25 Hz sensitivities are severely

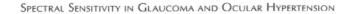

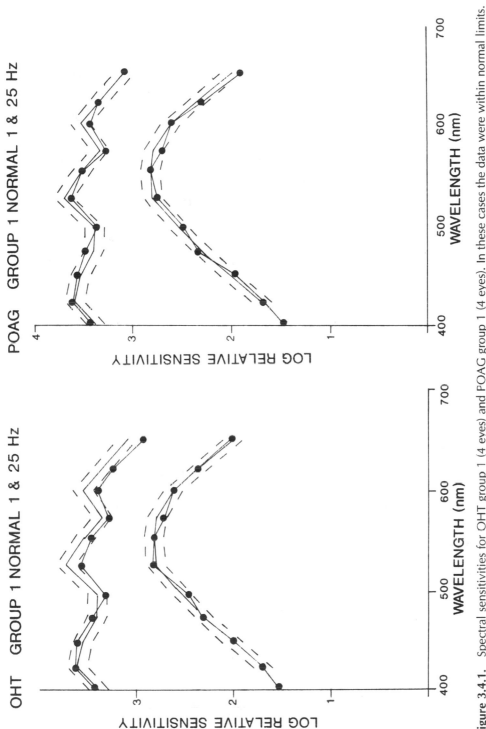

Figure 3.4.1. Spectral sensitivities for OHT group 1 (4 eyes) and POAG group 1 (4 eyes). In these cases the data were within normal limits.

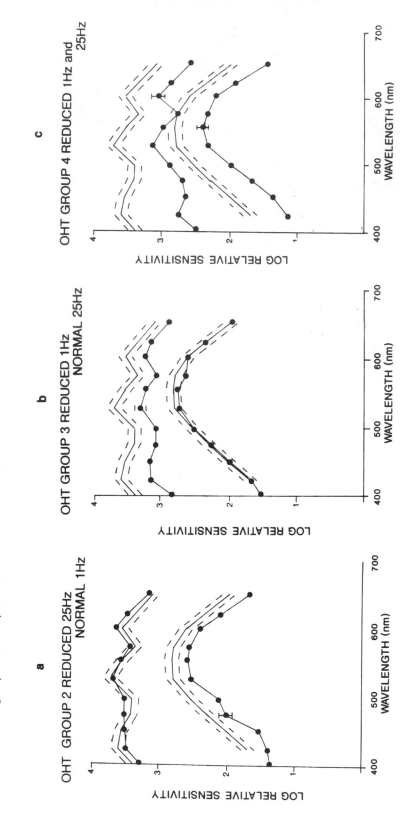

Figure 3.4.2(a) Spectral sensitivity for OHT group 2 (four eyes), 1 Hz normal, reduced 25 Hz. (b) OHT group 3 (four eyes), 1 Hz normal, reduced 25 Hz. (c) OHT group 4 (seven eyes), reduced 1 Hz and 25Hz.

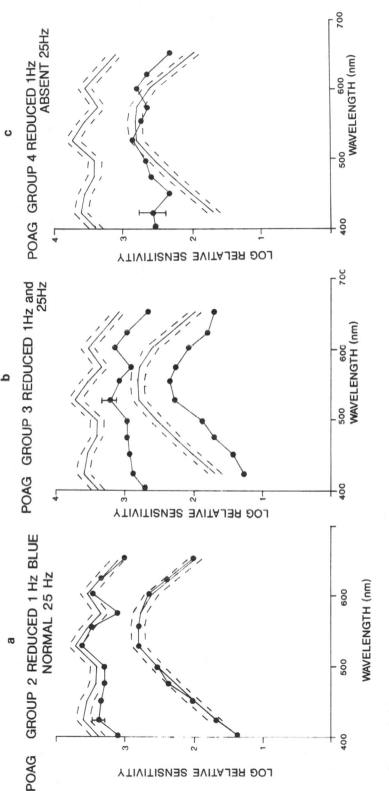

Figure 3.4.3(a) Spectral sensitivity for POAG group 2 (three eyes), reduced 1 Hz mainly blue. (b) POAG group 3 (13 eyes), both 1 Hz and 25 Hz reduced. (c) POAG group 4 (four eyes), reduced 1 Hz and absent 25 Hz.

reduced (POAG group 3). Again despite the averaging procedures that are inclined to mask such effects, the 580 nm notch in the 1 Hz data is clearly evident. Figure 3.4.4c illustrates the data in our POAG group 4; here there is a dramatic reduction in 1 Hz sensitivity and a total loss of the ability to detect flicker at 25 Hz. Where there is substantial spread in the data as in the 1 Hz patient data in group 3 and the 1 Hz patient data in group 4, error bars are indicated.

3.4.4   DISCUSSION

The above observations provide evidence that the nerve fibre damage in glaucoma is not only peripheral, but that there may be an overall loss of sensitivity that includes the fovea. This type of generalised sensitivity loss has been reported previously (e.g. Anctil and Anderson, 1984; Alvarez and Mills, 1985) and there is neurophysiological support for the idea. Glovinsky *et al.*, (1993) studied the pattern of foveal ganglion cell loss in experimental glaucoma. They showed a selective loss of larger ganglion cells in the foveal plateau and that the degree of foveal ganglion cell loss was significantly correlated to the degree of nerve fibre bundle loss in the temporal optic nerve of the same eye. The successful use of foveal fixation (with our stimulus within the central 1 degree of the visual field) implies that peripheral and foveal losses may progress in tandem and that previous studies aimed at establishing which comes first have not been sufficiently sensitive. This is not surprising; given the general levels of redundancy in the primary visual pathway it is feasible that many macular fibres could be lost before any reduction in visual acuity or sensitivity occurs. Foveal testing has many obvious advantages compared with peripheral testing and if there is a possibility of developing appropriate procedures for identifying early glaucoma sufferers without testing large areas of visual field, this deserves investigating.

3.4.4.1 Importance of testing blue-yellow and flicker mechanisms

The present investigation enabled us to examine the functions of two different non-overlapping mechanisms, namely, chromatic opponency and fast flicker detection by testing spectral sensitivity at 1 and 25 Hz respectively (Kaplan *et al.*, 1989). The 25 Hz curve represents the activity of a unitary achromatic mechanism subserved by the magno-system, whereas the 1 Hz function represents two opponent mechanisms: blue-yellow and red-green.

The data reveal that both magno- and parvo-fibres can be lost in glaucoma. It is not possible to deduce which of the two types of deficit occurs first. It is tempting to speculate that the group 4 glaucoma patients were in the most advanced stages of the disease. In this group, all patients were unable to detect the flicker of the target even at maximum intensity and therefore had severe loss of magno-fibres. How the clinical status of the patients corresponds to the spectral sensitivity changes is an issue being addressed by the next stage of the study. Suffice to say that there were only four eyes in this group whereas there were 13 in group 3 who exhibited approximately equal losses in magno- and parvo-cellular fibres. Notice that when 1 Hz sensitivity was reduced there was a greater loss in the blue region than in the red-green. This applies particularly to glaucoma group 3, but is also evident in glaucoma group 2. Hence, some patients show preferential reduction for the blue, others do not, but on average blue testing is more informative.

As far as the OHT data are concerned the findings appear, as in previous reports (Alvarez and Mills, 1985) to be similar to those in glaucoma but less extreme in magnitude. This implies that the majority of OHT patients are pre-glaucomatous with only a small number developing the visual field loss that enables them to be diagnosed as having glaucoma. As with glaucoma it is possible to have mild loss of either 1 Hz or 25 Hz sensitivity or substantial loss of both, although, in general, extreme loss of 25 Hz sensitivity is accompanied by some loss of 1 Hz sensitivity. The only feature that discriminates the two groups is that some glaucoma patients have a complete absence of 25 Hz flicker.

The OHT and POAG patients were grouped according to the severity of spectral sensitivity reduction. In this early stage of the study we have not looked at the correlation between our psychophysical findings and the clinical status of each patient. Though we have no reason to believe that our patients are not a representative sample, we are unable to generalise our observations because of the small numbers of patients included in the study.

3.4.4.2 Selectivity limits of glaucoma damage

The present demonstration of complete inability to detect 25 Hz flicker by some glaucoma patients is consistent with the studies on induced glaucoma in macaques (e.g. Glovinsky *et al.*, 1993) in which preferential damage to large ganglion cells in the monkey fovea is demonstrated. However, the presence of some sensitivity reduction for colour opponent function (1 Hz presentation) is also consistent with the observation (Zamber *et al.*, 1988) that the damage is not restricted to large ganglion cells (i.e. the magno-stream). Hence, though there is some evidence of bias towards larger ganglion cell loss in glaucoma the condition cannot be regarded as causing selective damage to a particular pathway as in the case of DIDMOAD (diabetes insipidus diabetes mellitus optic atrophy and deafness) and HOA (hereditary optic atrophies) (Alvarez & Kulikowski, 1989; King-Smith *et al.*, 1980). In both of these conditions, damage was found to be confined to thin optic nerve fibres. Glaucoma may be regarded as more selective than multiple sclerosis in which all nerve fibres appear to be affected randomly (Russell *et al.*, 1991).

3.4.5   ACKNOWLEDGEMENTS

The authors would like to pay tribute to the patients who cheerfully gave their time in the collection of the data in this project. We are also grateful to the consultants at Manchester Royal Eye Hospital who allowed us to test their patients.

3.4.6   REFERENCES

ALVAREZ, S.L. & KULIKOWSKI, J.J. (1989) Spatial resolution limits for pattern and movement detection in patients with familial optic nerve atrophies. In: Kulikowski, J.J., Dickinson, C.M. & Murray, I.J. (Eds) (1989). *Seeing Contour and Colour*, Pergamon Press: Oxford, pp. 403–408.

ALVAREZ, S.L. & MILLS K.B. (1985) Spectral and flicker sensitivity in ocular hypertension and glaucoma, *Research and Clinical Forums*, **7**, 83.

ANCTIL, J.L. & ANDERSON, D.R. (1984) Early foveal involvement and generalized depression of the visual field in glaucoma, *Archives of Ophthalmology*, **102**, 363.

CROOK, J.M., LEE. B.B. TIGWELL, D.A. & VALBERG, A. (1987) Thresholds of chromatic spots of cells in the macaque lateral geniculate nucleus as compared to detection sensitivity in man, *Journal of Physiology*, **392**, 193–211.

FITZKE, F.W., POINOOSAWMY, D., NAGASUBRAMANIAN, S. & HITCHINGS, R.A. (1988) Peripheral displacement threshold in glaucoma and ocular hypertension. In: Kriegelstein, G.K. (Ed.) *Perimetry Update*, Amsterdam: Kugler.

GLOVINSKY, Y., QUIGLEY, H.A. & PEASE, M.E. (1993) Foveal ganglion cell loss is size dependent in experimental glaucoma, *Investigative Ophthalmology & Visual Science*, **34**, 395–400.

HERON, G., ADAMS, A. & HUSTED, R. (1988) Central visual fields for short wavelength sensitive pathways in glaucoma and ocular hypertension, *Investigative Ophthalmology & Visual Science*, **29**, 64–72.

KAPLAN, E., LEE, B.B. & KULIKOWSKI, J.J. (1989) The role of P and M systems. In: Kulikowski, J.J., Dickinson, C.M. & Murray, I.J. (Eds), *Seeing Contour and Colour*, Oxford: Pergamon Press, pp. 224–237.

KING-SMITH, P.E. & CARDEN, D. (1976) Luminance and opponent colour contributions to visual detection and adaptation and to temporal and spatial integration, *Journal of the Optical Society of America*, **66**, 709–717.

KING-SMITH, P.E., ROSTEN, J.G., ALVAREZ, S.L. & BHARGAVA, S.K. (1980) Human vision without tonic ganglion cells? In: Verriest, G. (Ed.) *Colour Vision Deficiencies V*, Bristol: Adam Hilger, pp. 99–105.

KLEIN, B.E.K., KLEIN, R. AND SPONSEL, W.E. (1992) Prevalence of glaucoma; the Beaver Dam eye study, *Ophthalmology*, **99**, 1499–1504.

QUIGLEY, H.A., SANCHEZ, R.M., DUNKELBERGER, G.R., L'HERNAULT, N.L. & BAGINSKI, T.A. (1987) Chronic glaucoma selectively damages large optic nerve fibres, *Investigative Opthalmology & Visual Science*, **28**, 913–920.

QUIGLEY, H.A., DUNKELBERGER, G.R. & GREEN, W.R. (1988) Chronic human glaucoma causing selectively greater loss of large optic nerve fibres, *Opthalmology*, **95**, 357–363.

RUSSELL, M.H.A., MURRAY, I.J., METCALFE, R. & KULIKOWSKI, J.J. (1991) Visual evoked potentials and psychophysical investigation of chromatic and achromatic visual function in humans; application to the investigation of multiple sclerosis and optic neuritis, *Brain*, **114**, 2419–2435.

SPERLING, H.G. & HARWERTH, R.S. (1971) Red-green cone interactions in the increment threshold sensitivity of primates, *Science*, **172**, 180–184.

TEILSCH, J.M., KATZ, J. & SINGH, K. (1991) A population based evaluation of glaucoma screening; the Baltimore eye survey, *American Journal of Epidemiology*, **134**, 1102–1110.

TYLER, C.W. (1981) Specific deficits of flicker sensitivity in glaucoma and ocular hypertension, *Investigative Ophthalmology & Visual Science*, **20**, 204–212.

ZAMBER, R.W., MILLS, R.P., KOONTZ, M.A., PHILLIPS, J.O. & HENDRICKSON, A.E. (1988) Ganglion cell loss in laser induced primate glaucoma, *Investigative Ophthalmology and Visual Science*, **29** (suppl), 421.

Human Colour Imaging Evoked Potentials in the Inferior Parietal Lobule (IPL) and Colour Sensitive Cells in Area 7 of the Monkey Implicating the IPL System in Higher Order Colour Processing

Baruch Blum

3.5.1 INTRODUCTION

This chapter brings together evidence from human inferior parietal lobule visual evoked potentials VEP responses and microelectrode recordings in area 7 of the rhesus monkey on colour functioning in the IPL system with the assumption of homology of these. The combining of these two sources was prompted by the belief that they converge on the crucial question about posterior parietal cortex participation in higher level colour processing.

Experiments were designed to allow possible elucidation of IPL's specific involvement in processing of colour information. A special thrust was made to clarify a question that seemed of utmost importance: the possibility hinted by data that this is a high order involvement. This has been apparent from clinical sources documenting a left hemispheric IPL connection to colour anomia and colour naming/pointing (Davidoff and Ostergaard, 1984; Geschwind and Fusillo, 1966; Meadows, 1974), as well as data reported on unilateral changes in colour functioning in posterior parietal lesioned patients (Driver *et al.*, 1992).

Zeki (1980) reports that V4 cells are selectively responsive to narrow-bands of the visual spectrum so that a population of such cells taken together may cover almost the entire visual spectrum. In the present work a model is proposed that envisages that the continuation of the colour pathway from V4, at least for some aspects of colour vision e.g. the more global ones, could be the pathways to the posterior parietal cortex (Baizer *et al.*, 1991; Cavada *et al.*, 1989).

Comprehensive research undertaken on area 7 of the monkey in many laboratories, including the author's (Blum, 1991), provided evidence that the system has much to do with the integration of sensory information into behaviour. The lack of data on colour in that model had been a strong indication for the present work (see also Blum, 1995).

3.5.2   METHODS

3.5.2.1 The study in monkeys

Three adult, about 4 kg, male Macaca monkeys were prepared for study under monitored pentobarbital surgical anaesthesia. Restraint gear, silver-silver chloride pellet EOG electrodes and skull cylinder were installed for chronic microelectrode recording in the awake, attentive, fixating monkey (Blum, 1985). Single cell responses of area 7 were studied by means of platinum iridium microelectrodes, in two monkeys from the left, and in one from the right hemisphere.

The monkeys were trained on a 'fixation' paradigm (Blum, 1985) to 75 per cent correct performance. While in a primate chair, in a dimly lit room and quiet conditions a light spot appeared in the middle of a white screen, 0.57 m away from the monkey's eyes. At a prescribed time this spot started to dim, as a signal to the monkey to lift a lever. For successful trials the monkey was rewarded with a drop of water. Immobilization of the head and fixation of the eyes ensured constancy and repeated delivery of the stimulus to the same part of the retina. Maintenance of fixation by the animal was monitored by the EOG recording.

Stimuli were projector-generated rectangles (5 minutes of arc at 0.57 m distance) of white or coloured light (red, green or blue-violet), shaped by a four leaf diaphragm. The specific colour was obtained by intercepting the white light beam with Kodak gelatin colour filters: Wratten #26 for red, #98 for blue and #61 for green. Light intensities of about 1–1.5 log units above background illumination of 1 cdm^{-2} were used, the luminance adjusted by means of Wratten neutral density filters and matched to the white light stimulus by brightness judgement. Stimuli were displayed to the monkey on a screen in a dimly lit room by a PDP 11–34 computer for 16 trials each time for a period of 800 ms and the interstimulus interval randomly varied between 1 and 1.5 s. Cells were tested, first, for sensitivity to coloured light, then for colour responsiveness. The smallest area giving optimal response was defined as the cell's receptive field (RF) for the tested stimulus. Neuronal activity was recorded after amplification by a Bak unity gain amplifier, with use of a window discriminator. Post-stimulus rasters and histograms were constructed. Locations of microelectrode penetrations and of derivation of data were estimated and charted. Response or failure of response was verified statistically. Post stimulus dot displays, each composed of 16 trials, were submitted to a Wilcoxon non-parametric ('signed rank') test for matched pairs. The number of spikes in 60 ms bins for each of the 16 trial display for 600 ms period prior to stimulus presentation was calculated and compared to similar period after stimulus presentation. A 'null hypothesis' test was carried out for the occurrence at a significantly greater rate than chance in each case. A probability $p < 0.0168$ was set as the significance level for red and green light stimuli. For blue light with a weak response, $p < 0.03$ was set as the level of significance. This was based on experience with analysis of white 'no response'.

3.5.2.2 Human studies

VEPs were evoked by square-wave pattern reversal stimulation with green-red (G/R) and white-black (W/B) checkerboards delivered by a two-beam Maxwellian view stimulator. The checks (0.16 c deg^{-1} in spatial frequency (measured diagonally)) filled a circular field subtending 45° of arc and were reversed by a pivoting mirror at a rate of 2 Hz. The W/B

checkerboard was generated by superimposing a homogenous white field (tungsten filament 362 td maximum) on white (tungsten filament, 2192 td maximum) and black checks.
Maximal retinal luminance was 4.07 logphot td. The contrast of the W/B checkerboard was
90 per cent. The G/R checkerboards were produced by optically superimposing a homogenous monochromatic red field (625 nm, 106 td maximum) onto a green and black
checkerboard (500 or 510 nm, 1645 td maximum). We used 0.6 neutral density (nd) filters
to attenuate luminance from maximum. The relative output of the monochromator was
determined at each wavelength with a calibrated photodiode. The G/R checks were
adjusted by neutral density filters to be close to equiluminance as established by heterochromatic brightness matching. Consistency of the optical stimulation was achieved by
instructing subjects to fixate the centre of the checkerboard. Successful fixation could be
detected by comparing average responses elicited by left and right pattern alternations.

VEPs were recorded from skull locations estimated to overlie the left and right
supramarginal (conventional P3 and P4) respectively, and 2–2.5 cm caudal in the direction
of the occiput presumably overlying the angular gyrus. For comparison, occipital (V1)
recordings were taken from loci 1–3 cru above the inion presumably the striate cortex. Two
scalp locations were recorded from at one time. Monopolar and Laplacian methods were
used employing silver-silver chloride disc electrodes (about 10 kΩ in impedance), that
were attached to the scalp by a highly conductive electrolytic paste. In monopolar
derivations, the ear-lobe contralateral to the stimulated eye was used as reference electrode
and the ipsilateral as ground. In the Laplacian recordings, an 'active' central electrode was
surrounded by three electrodes placed in triangulation of 120°, each 2.5 cm from the central
electrode. The three surrounding electrodes were fed into a resistive network and the
average of their voltages was used to obtain a differential recording against the central
electrode. Response potentials were fed through isolation amplifiers to Princeton model
113 pre-amplifiers (10 k gain, 0.3–100 Hz bandwidth) and averaged (n = 100) by a
laboratory computer. Responses to each of the two halves of an alternation were obtained
separately and also summed together, with 500 ms duration for each half allowing the
unfolding also of late VEP waves.

A Fourier analysis program was used offline to filter from the averaged records' noise
and sporadic artefacts, the latter presumably of muscular origin. The averaged response
waveform was decomposed into a series of harmonic sine and cosine components. The first
12 harmonics, starting from the second harmonic of the stimulus temporal frequency, and
the next 11 even harmonics were then added together in proper phase relations to
reconstruct the waveform. A 'cleaner' average response waveform was thus obtained with
preservation of the correct phase relations between the several harmonic components.
Thus, latencies of response components were obtainable with fidelity.

In an experiment, first the optical stimulus, Co (the reversing checkerboards, either G/R
or W/B), was used alone as a control. It was then paired with mental imaging task, the G or
the G + C task, respectively. The imaging task used, referred to as the 'G' task, involved
imaging of colour pictures successively and mentally identifying each. The other task,
referred to as 'G + C', was the same except that it also required retrieving a colour from the
picture. In the control B/W series retrieving was of a salient feature from the picture. During
the runs, subjects were instructed to successively image a series of about 30 memorised
pictures, one in each run, and to attempt to synchronise their imaging with the checkerboard
alternation. This synchronisation was possible presumably on the basis of anticipatory
processes (Kowler, 1989). In one experiment, the pictures were colour and in another
experiment they were black and white; the experiments ran on different days. Independent
measurements of the time taken for the G task was 700 ± 125 ms and for the G + C it was

500 ± 80 ms. Recordings were made primarily from two subjects, while confirmatory records were obtained from two additional subjects. In experiments involving imaging, extensive data (86 recording runs of which 27 were complete with imaging) were obtained from one subject, a 60-year-old female painter. Eight of these experiments were of black and white imaging without colour. Thirteen experiments were black and white without imaging and with imaging in black and white carried out on a different day from the colour imaging to avoid possible interference. The rest of the experiments were divided equally for control recordings from occipital and angular. Confirmatory observations were made as follows: runs inclusive of imaging were made on another subject, 50-year-old female painter (three recordings), and 15 recordings without imaging were obtained from two male subjects.

3.5.3   RESULTS

3.5.3.1 Monkey

In extensive research on area 7a of the monkey many cells were encountered with no response to white light stimulation. Many of these cells remain still unknown, although a 'visual strip' was defined in that region 20 years ago on the basis of white light sensitivity (Hyvarinen and Poranen, 1974; Mountcastle et al., 1975).

Cells that fail to respond to white and respond to colour were found within the 'visual strip' sharing with the white sensitive cells the same PG region of area 7 (Blum, 1995). In Figures 3.5.1 and 2 a cell entity of area 7a is presented that is white light insensitive (Figure 3.5.1); the same cell (Figure 3.5.2(I)) shows incremented firing responses to green and to red, respectively, the receptive field co-extensive for the different colours and in the contralateral hemifield. Figure 3.5.2(II) illustrates another cell's failure of response to white and decremented firing responses to red, incremented followed by decremented firing responses to green and a weak, but definite response to blue-violet. Receptive field was again co-extensive for the different colours, and it occupied an area in both hemifields. From 22 cells studied, 17 had contralateral, 3 ipsilateral and 2 bilateral receptive fields. This contrasted with area V4 mainly contralateral receptive fields (Tanaka et al., 1986) and with obviously lesser range of options. The main difference, however, was the latter's showing some white light sensitivity.

A preliminary study was made on the co-extensive receptive fields for the colours. It was possible to show for two cells, presumably bichromatic, i.e. with responses shown to green and for red, that for each colour there was quick adaptation, whereas if the colours were presented in alternation within their common receptive field at about 2–3 s interval, there was a potentiation of response, and the adaptation did not set in quickly.

3.5.3.1 Human data

Figure 3.5.3 compares VEP responses to G/R and W/B checkerboards in two subjects (S1 and S2); early negativity is shown in (A) in left supramarginal (l.Su.m.) monopolar, in Laplacian derivation (B) and also in left angular monopolar recording (l ANG) (C). In these, one could observe, in response to optical stimulation with G/R and W/B reversing checkerboards, an early wave response to G/R consisting of a negativity followed by positivity. To W/B checks there was a negative wave or a negative followed by a positive wave response. Similar waveforms were obtained from the IPL leads of the right hemisphere. On the other hand, in (C) the recordings obtained from the occipital lead shows entirely different waveforms. Moreover, it could be shown in the Oz lead that the G/R and W/B checks may evoke VEPs with waveform dissimilarities. These could be made undifferentiably similar by adjusting the luminance of the G and R of G/R checks away from equiluminance. This was unattainable with the IPL leads, which shows the independence of response to the G/R of the luminance and colour components. Furthermore, responses were obtained in the parietal leads with start latency of about 60 ± 5 ms with no significant difference between the individual leads. On the other hand, the occipital VEPs to G/R and to W/B were only slightly different in waveforms, consisting of large positive waves, the earliest appearing at wave onset latency of 70 ± 10 ms, i.e. of comparable order of magnitude to parietal latencies ($p = 0.09$ at 16 degrees of freedom).

Parietal negativity obtained with simple optical stimulation, i.e. G/R alternating checkerboards, is shown to be modifiable with pairing of this stimulus with imaging. In Figure 3.5.4, it is shown that with such paradigms differentiation within IPL is obtainable. Extensive data from one, female, painter (86 experiments) with confirmatory work from another (three experiments) done with pairing of optical stimulation and imaging paradigms have shown the following.

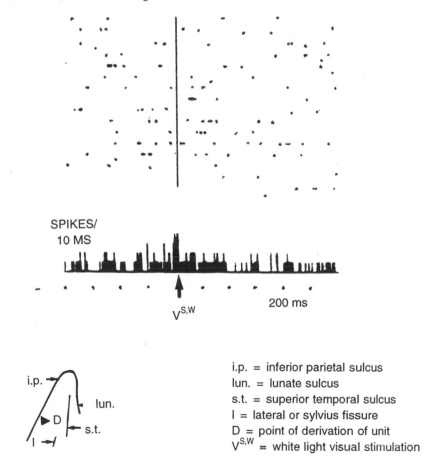

SPIKES/
10 MS

$V^{S,W}$

200 ms

i.p. = inferior parietal sulcus
lun. = lunate sulcus
s.t. = superior temporal sulcus
l = lateral or sylvius fissure
D = point of derivation of unit
$V^{S,W}$ = white light visual stimulation

Figure 3.5.1 Monkey area 7 cell, no response to white light stimulation.

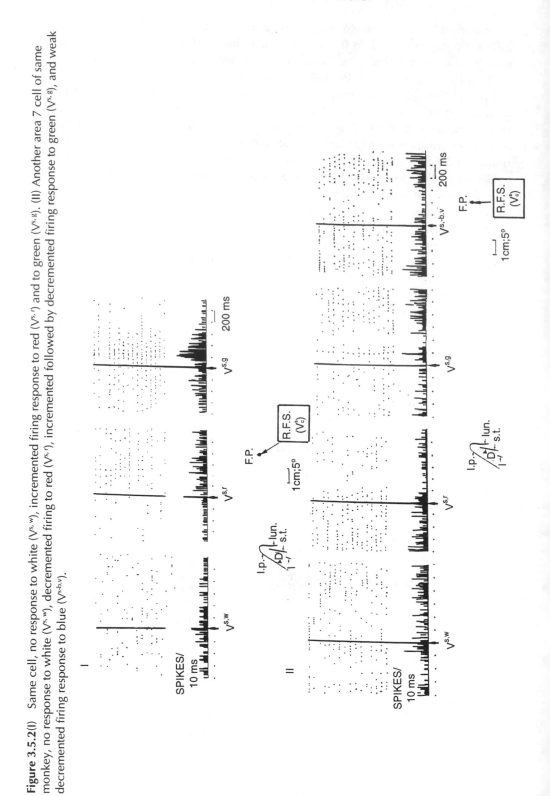

Figure 3.5.2(I) Same cell, no response to white ($V^{s,w}$), incremented firing response to red ($V^{s,r}$) and to green ($V^{s,g}$). (II) Another area 7 cell of same monkey, no response to white ($V^{s,w}$), decremented firing to red ($V^{s,r}$), incremented followed by decremented firing response to green ($V^{s,g}$), and weak decremented firing response to blue ($V^{s,b,v}$).

In the G + C imaging task there was observed, in more than 80 per cent of trials, a modification in the VEPs recorded from the left Su.m., i.e. there was annulling of the early negativity, a positive wave component appearing at a longer latency (Figure 3.5.4; $p = 0.00007$). These waveform changes were shown in the left Su.m. in relation to the pairing of the imaging tasks; they were not shown in the right Su.m. and also not in the ANG of either hemisphere (Figure 3.5.4(A)) that showed only amplitude changes. As illustrated in Figure 3.5.4, the G imaging task as well modified the VEPs of the left Su.m., annulling the second positive component wave, whereas the latency changed only slightly and insignificantly. The G imaging, like the G + C task, did not cause an obviously significant effect in the other leads. In Figure 3.5.4(B) mean values are illustrated for the G + C task from eight

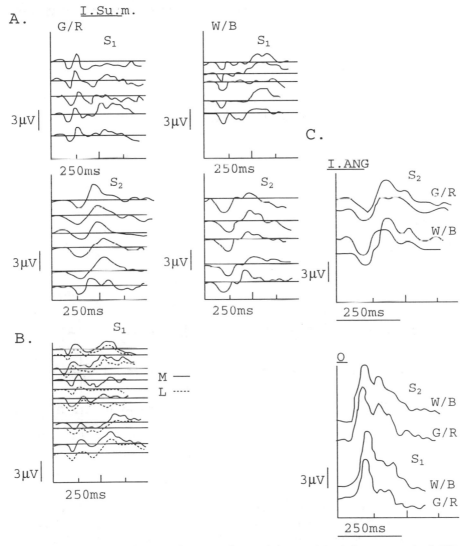

Figure 3.5.3 VEPs recorded from human subjects. (A) S1 and S2, left supramarginal G/R and W/B; (B) R/G responses, comparing six records monopolar versus Laplacian paired derivations. In (C), left angular of S2 is compared with S2 supramarginal, both G/R and W/B and also occipital records of S1 and S2 W/B and G/R.

experiments showing again in left supramarginal the changes described earlier, in comparison to left angular and right supramarginal that show only amplitude changes and no waveform changes.

Similar tests to the G and G + C carried out in W/B showed no similar changes to those described above; the Laplacian derivations also failed to show such changes with imaging. No changes were observed in the occipital lead with the mental tasks.

3.5.4   DISCUSSION

A model is proposed on the basis of the data that postulates a linkage between colour and spatial vision; it assumes a high order early vision orientational response towards an object

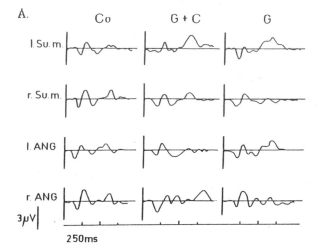

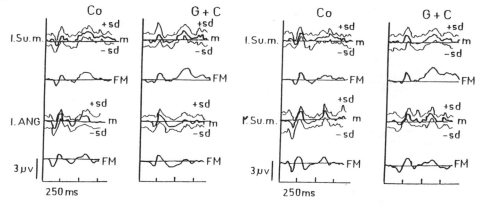

Figure 3.5.4(A)   The pairing of a simple optical stimulus (Co = R/G checkerboard reversal) with cognitive-spatial tasking, i.e. imaging of pre-learnt colour pictures (G) and with a task inclusive of the same protocol as the G task with addition of retrieval of colour from the picture (G + C) is illustrated. Left and right supramarginal and left and right angular leads are compared. (B) Mean and standard deviations (FM = fourier mean), derived from eight experiments over half a year for the G + C task; the illustration compares left supramarginal and left angular leads.

that appears in the visual scene, and that part of this initial response is a generalised colour attribute response (Damasio, 1990). The IPL, which is widely believed to play central roles in spatial processing (Andersen, 1987), is assumed to involve in the colour aspect one of its specialised networks.

This hypothesis also claims that this system plays a central role in enabling the use of integrated sensory inputs in behaviour. In an attempt to account for the characteristics observed in the colour responses of the presumably homologous area 7a of the monkey and in the human IPL VEPs to colour imaging, examination was made whether and how these can subserve in the above-mentioned functioning.

The colour cells found in monkey area 7a show trichromacy, and bichromacy, both with co-extensive receptive fields, i.e. with a propensity for a multi-duty mode of operation. As the IPL system responsiveness is known to be modulated by a variety of inputs (Blum, 1991), it may be conjectured that with the manifested characteristics these colour responses may subserve in generalised colour response at one time, and, conversely, under other conditions with the individuality of the colour response preserved.

Adaptation can occur in a channel at any of its 'levels'. Thus, the finding of a cell entity in area 7 that responds to red and also to green, respectively, but rapidly adapting unless the colours are presented alternately when response potentiation occurs instead of adaptation, satisfies a primary requirement for the hypothesised network, i.e. of a conditional probability mode of operation.

The receptive field characteristics of area 7 colour cells, including bilaterality of some, are shared with the white sensitive cells (Blum, 1985). This is compatible with a model that is conducive to the functioning of the two sub-modalities cooperatively in orientation reaction.

The observation in the human left supramarginal, not in the other leads, of color imaging relatable VEP changes, detectable by monopolar but not by Laplacian derivation hints that these may result from interactions in the depth of this massive gyrus, presumably a high level spatial processing linking colour picture imaging with simple optical stimulus (green/red checks alternation). It is significant that the interaction occurs in the early wave in a way reminiscent of the 'enhancement' phenomenon in the monkey (Blum, 1985; Robinson et al., 1978). This actually ties the observations in the monkey and in the human in such a way that the homology hypothesis is substantially bolstered.

The human observations have important clinical implications. Anatomically (Kappers et al., 1967), a deep cortical region of occipito-temporo-parietal confluence may be defined. It is evolutionarily high in development in the primates and is suggested to have spatial vision function. It includes parts of peristriatum, of the occipito-temporal convolution and parieto-occipital transitional convolutions, gyrus angularis, part of the gyri fusiformis and lingualis, possibly also deep portion of supramarginalis that extends in this direction. Of some interest in this connection is the report of Wright et al. (this volume) showing linkage between spatial and colour processing dysfunction in patients with fusiform and lingual gyri lesions. Our data agrees by showing VEP changes relatable to these anatomical structures and also combining colour and spatially linked responses.

These data, from man and monkey are counter-current to the Ungerleider-Mishkin hypothesis which regards the posterior parietal to be achromatic (see the critical paper of Goodale and Milner, 1992). These concepts must be adapted to conform with the phenomena observed.

3.5.5   SUMMARY

The trichromaticity and dichromaticity of the cells defined in area 7a of the monkey and also the VEP records from the human showing interaction between simple optical colour stimulus (G/R checks) with colour picture imaging are consistent with human clinical data on the relationship of the posterior parietal cortex to colour vision. The observations in the human IPL of interaction of imaging colour pictures with simple optical colour stimuli, which has similarity to the enhancement phenomenon observed in monkey area 7, supports the contention of homology of these brain regions. Most of the responses to colour that were obtained in monkey area 7a were of decremented firing, but some showed incremented or biphasic firing, i.e. increment followed by decrement firing. It was also observed that the changes in these responses, i.e. their modulations, were similar, and therefore may be assumed equivalent in signal value. Supportive of this is the observation that alternation of two colours, red and green, enhanced the responses. Furthermore, responses to colour have shown similarities to previously described responses to white light sensitive cells. The special properties revealed for these colour cells suggest, first, separate channels for white and for colour in area 7 and, second, that these may be relevant when chromaticity is of generalised import, e.g. in an animal's orienting response.

3.5.6   ACKNOWLEDGEMENTS

The part of this work dealing with human VEPs was derived from joint work carried out with Dr Marcus Bearse Jr at the Department of Psychology, Northeastern University, Boston, MA, USA. It benefited greatly from sagacious advice of Professors John Armington and Adam Reeves. The monkey study was done in part when the author held a senior research fellowship of the USA National Research Council at AFFRI, Bethesda, MD, USA, and in part at Tel Aviv University Sackler School of Medicine with the aid of The Schouder Fund for Medical Research and The Charles Smith Family Israel National Institute for Psychobiology.

3.5.6   REFERENCES

ANDERSEN, R.A. (1987) Inferior parietal lobule function in spatial perceptions and micromotor integration. In: *Handbook of Physiology. The Nervous system. Higher functions of the Brain*, Bethesda, MD: American Physiology Society, pp 83–518.

BAIZER, J.S., UNGERLEIDER, L.G. & DESIMONE, R. (1991) Organization of visual inputs to the inferior temporal and posterior parietal cortex in macaques, *Journal of Neuroscience*, **11**, 168–190.

BLUM, B. (1985) Enhancement of visual responses of area 7 neurones by electrical pre-conditioning stimulation of LP-Pulvinar nuclei of the monkey, *Experimental Brain Research*. **59**, 434–440.

BLUM, B. (1991) An experimentally-supported model for inferior parietal lobule high order visual function. In: Blum, B. (Ed.) *Channels in the Visual Nervous System. Neurophysiology, Psychophysics and Models*, London and Tel Aviv: Freund.

BLUM, B. (1995) Responses to colour of neurones in area 7a of the inferior parietal lobule of the rhesus monkey, *Ophthalmic and Physiological Optics*, **15**, 145–151.

CAVADA, C. & GOLDMAN-RAKIC, P. (1989) Posterior parietal cortex in rhesus monkey. I. Parcellation of areas based on distinctive limbic and sensory corticortical connections, *Journal of Comparative Neurology*, **287**, 393–421.

DAMASIO, A.R. (1990) Category-related recognition defects as a clue to the neural substrates of knowledge, *Trends in Neuroscience*, **13**, 95–98.

DAVIDOFF, J.B. & OSTERGAARD, A.L. (1984) Colour anomia resulting from weakened short-term colour memory. A case study, *Brain*, **107**, 415–431.

DRIVER, J., BAYLIS, G.C. & RAFAL, R.D. (1992) Preserved figure-ground segregation and symmetry perception in visual neglect, *Nature*, **360**, 73–75.

GESCHWIND, N. & FUSILLO, M. (1966) Colour-naming defects in association with alexia, *Archives of Neurology*, **15**, 137-146.

GOODALE, M.A. & MILNER, D.A. (1992) Separate visual pathways for perception and action, *Trends in Neuroscience*, **15**, 20–25.

HYVARINEN, J. & PORANEN, A. (1974) Function of the parietal associative area 7 of the monkey, *Brain*, **97**, 673– 692.

KAPPERS, C.U.A., HUBER, G.C. & CROSBY, E.C. (1967) *The Comparative Anatomy of the Nervous System of Vertebrates including Man*, New York: Huner, p. 1654.

KOWLER, E. (1989) Cognitive expectations, not habits, control anticipatory smooth oculomotor pursuit, *Vision Research*, **29**, 1049–1057.

MEADOWS, J.C. (1974) Disturbed perception of colours associated with localized cerebral lesions, *Brain*, **97**, 615–632.

MICHAEL, C.J. (1978) Colour-sensitive complex cells in monkey striate cortex, *Journal of Neurophysiology*, **41**, 1250–1266.

MOUNTCASTLE, V.B., LYNCH, J.C., GEORGOPOULOS, A.P., SAKATA, H. & ACUNA, C. (1975) Posterior parietal association cortex of the monkey: command functions for the operations within the extrapersonal space, *Journal of Neurophysiology*, **38**, 871-908.

ROBINSON, D.L., GOLDBERG, M.E. & STANTON, G.B. (1978) Parietal association cortex in the primate: sensory mechanisms and behavioural modulations, *Journal of Neurophysiology*, **41**, 910–932.

TANAKA, M., WEBER, H. & CREUTZFELDT, O.D. (1986) Visual properties and spatial distribution of neurones in the visual association area on the prelunate gyrus of the awake monkey, *Experimental Brain Research*, **65**, 11–37.

ZEKI, S.M. (1980) The representation of colours in the cerebral cortex, *Nature*, **284**, 412–418.

Chromatic Visual Evoked Potentials: Special Requirements for Blue

A.G. Robson, D.J. McKeefry and J.J. Kulikowski

3.6.1 INTRODUCTION

Low spatial frequency achromatic gratings elicit positive VEPs that are similar for stimulus onset, offset and reversal; that is, they depend solely on a transient change in contrast (Kulikowski, 1974; 1977; 1991). Such transient response characteristics are consistent with the involvement of the magnocellular system. Conversely, the onset of low contrast, low spatial frequency isoluminant chromatic gratings elicits a response that is different from the reversal response (predominantly negative) and consistent with a sustained contribution from the parvocellular system (Berninger and Arden, 1991; Carden et al., 1985; Kulikowski et al., 1989; Murray et al., 1987). Such a dichotomy of VEPs is consistent with the deoxyglucose labelling of the corresponding magno- and parvo-pathways (Tootell et al., 1988) and is, therefore, likely to prove useful in the monitoring of pathological conditions, which selectively affect specific achromatic or chromatic pathways.

Most studies have utilised gratings modulated along the red-green axis to generate chromatic-specific responses. Responses generated using stimuli modulated along the blue-yellow axis have received less attention for at least three reasons:

1. The blue-yellow system relies on blue cones that are less numerous than the other long- and medium-wavelength sensitive cones and are particularly rare in the foveola (Marc and Sperling, 1977; Williams et al., 1981), which therefore requires a minimum area of stimulation.
2. There are less blue-yellow than red-green units in the primary visual cortex V1 (Livingstone and Hubel, 1984; Ts'o and Gilbert, 1988), hence smaller potentials are expected.
3. Chromatic aberration is greater for blue-yellow than for red-green pairs of hues (Bedford and Wyszecki, 1957).

In this study, blue-yellow VEPs were first generated using a system that eliminated chromatic aberration by focusing different wavelengths (tritanopic pairs of hues) on the same plane (Mullen, 1985). The VEPs generated by this stimulus provide a reference for the second study, which uses a flat screen and stimulation along a non-tritanopic, maximum blue-yellow axis. In the clinical setting this axis would allow the greatest latitude in detecting abnormalities in the retino-cortical pathway (Grigsby *et al.*, 1991). The limitations of flat screen stimulation (gratings generated on a TV monitor) were examined by eliciting VEPs using simple blue-yellow square wave gratings of different sizes.

Two measures of specificity of chromatic stimulation were used:

1. Chromatic VEPs generated by a blue-yellow grating onset should be substantially different from that of the offset or reversal reflecting a sustained (tonic) response component (Kulikowski, 1977; 1978; 1991). This difference should be maximal at isoluminance (minimal for luminance-contrast coarse gratings).
2. VEPs generated by the phase reversal of a blue-yellow grating at a frequency of 12.5 Hz should drop to a minimum at isoluminance (Kulikowski *et al.*, 1991).

3.6.2   METHOD

3.6.2.1 Aberration-free apparatus

Sinusoidal gratings generated on two Joyce DM2 displays were placed at right angles to each other, their chromatic images (hues: tritanopic or red/green) were superimposed and viewed monocularly at different distances. The contrast of the chromatic gratings was defined as being equivalent to the Michelson contrast of the constituent monochromatic gratings namely:

$$C = (Lmax-Lmin)/(Lmax + Lmin)$$

For details see McKeefry and Kulikowski, this volume (pp. 163–172).

3.6.2.2 Flat screen stimulation

Isoluminant blue-yellow square wave gratings were generated on a Grundig TV monitor using a BBC microcomputer and purpose built interface. The blue and yellow elements were non-tritanopic and chosen according to a recommendation by Grigsby *et al.*, (1991) in which the axis coincided with the blue phosphor and yellow resulting from a red/green mixture. These blue and yellow components were linked reciprocally, so that their relative intensities (luminance) could be adjusted without varying mean luminance. The system was calibrated with a Photo Research PR1500 photometer. Binocular viewing was used.

3.6.2.3 Stimulus presentation

Isoluminance of the blue-yellow pattern was determined using heterochromatic flicker photometry with adjacent stripes alternating at 12.5 Hz. Stimulus presentation was either on-off or reversal. In on-off mode the pattern was replaced by a uniform field with no accompanying change in mean hue and luminance. When contrast reversal was used, contrast was reduced by a factor of 0.5 to produce the same contrast change as in on-off presentation.

3.6.2.4 Recording technique and electrode montage

VEPs were recorded using a Medelec 'Sensor' system and stored on an Apple 11e microcomputer. Filter bandwidth was 0.3–30 Hz for slow (2 Hz) presentations and 10–60

Hz for fast (12.5 Hz) presentations. Silver/silver chloride electrodes were placed on Oz and referred to either linked ears or a mid-frontal (Fz) electrode (International 10/20 system, Jasper, 1958). Each part of the experiment was repeated on at least one other subject.

3.6.3   RESULTS AND COMMENTS

3.6.3.1 Low-rate on-off presentations

Aberration-free apparatus

At the lowest contrasts (0.05 and 0.1) both the blue-yellow (tritan) and red-green chromatic VEPs have similar waveforms and both are substantially different from the corresponding (much larger) achromatic VEPs (Figure 3.6.1). Note that both chromatic onset VEPs are dominated by strong negative waves peaking at about 300 ms, whereas the chromatic reversal presentations (of the same change in contrast) elicit only residual responses. This is consistent with the sustained nature of chromatic responses in which standing (onset) contrast determines the response. Conversely, the corresponding achromatic VEPs are characterised by shorter latency positive waves, which are similar when evoked by either onset, offset or reversal presentations. Thus, a transient change in contrast (either from 0 to C, from C to 0 or from –C/2 to + C/2) elicits responses consistent with the 'purely transient' nature of achromatic VEPs at low spatial frequencies.

At a higher contrast of 0.2, new components appear in the red-green VEP, mainly the earlier negative wave (time to peak of about 130 ms) as reported previously (see Murray *et al.*, 1987 and the Discussion below). The blue-yellow onset VEP maintains its shape and this was found to hold for other spatial frequencies and stimulus sizes (McKeefry, 1992). Thus, the blue-yellow VEP waveform illustrated in Figure 3.6.1 can be regarded as a standard, reflecting specific stimulation of the blue-yellow pathway.

Television monitor

Gratings generated on a flat screen (sine- or square-wave) are subject to chromatic aberration, which turns them into partly achromatic patterns (Charman, 1991). In agreement with this expectation, only gratings containing few spatial cycles generate VEPs resembling the standard despite some inter-subject variations.

Figure 3.6.2 shows the VEPs elicited by gratings of 1 c/deg, at which maximal amplitude was obtained for subject JS. The onset of a 3-cycle blue-yellow grating elicits a simple negative waveform (latency to peak about 200 ms) that is substantially different from the equivalent reversal response. In spite of the use of crude square wave gratings this negative wave is qualitatively similar to that seen following aberration-free stimulation and can therefore be considered a chromatic VEP. Onset of larger gratings (e.g. 6 or 10 cycles) generate more complex waveforms in which chromatic components (negative waves peaking at about 130 and 250 ms) are swamped by positive waves (latency to peak approximately 120 ms), which are very similar to those generated by chromatic offset and reversal stimulation; this similarity is a hallmark of transient responses, characteristic of achromatic intrusions. At 15 cycles, almost identical VEPs are elicited by on-off and reversal stimulation, thereby showing no discernible chromatic components.

For subject FE the greatest differences between chromatic onset and reversal responses (i.e. sustained components) were seen when gratings containing three or six spatial cycles were used at a spatial frequency of 2 c deg^{-1} (Figure 3.6.3). Grating onset resulted in predominantly negative potentials peaking between 130 and 210 ms. Increasing field size

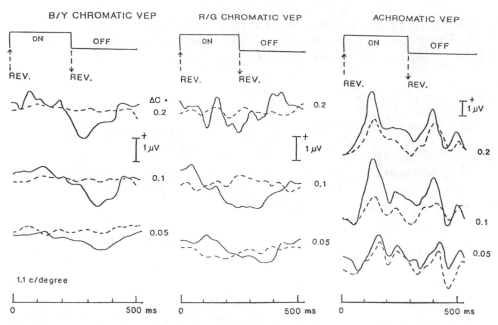

Figure 3.6.1. VEPs elicited by the onset (solid lines) and phase reversal (broken lines) of aberration-free blue-yellow, red-green and achromatic gratings at different levels of contrast change (ΔC). Mean luminance was kept constant (25 cd m⁻²), screen subtended 4.5° (5 spatial cycles), subject DM (normal vision, corrected myope).

further resulted in the introduction of positive waves resembling the offset and reversal responses (indicating achromatic intrusions).

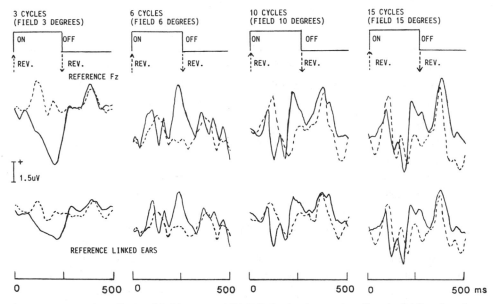

Figure 3.6.2. The effects of field size on VEPs elicited using onset-offset (solid lines) and reversal (broken lines) presentations of blue-yellow square wave gratings on a TV monitor. Stimulus repetition rate: 2 Hz, spatial frequency: 1 c deg⁻¹, Lo = 30 cd m⁻², ΔC = 0.3, subject JS (normal vision, corrected myope).

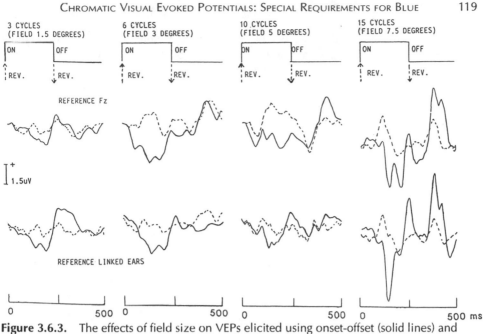

Figure 3.6.3. The effects of field size on VEPs elicited using onset-offset (solid lines) and reversal (broken lines) presentations of blue-yellow square wave gratings on a TV monitor. Stimulus repetition rate: 2 Hz, spatial frequency: 2 c deg^{-1}, Lo = 30 cd m^{-2}, ΔC = 0.3, subject FE (normal vision, corrected myope).

3.6.3.2 Fast contrast reversal at 12.5 Hz

Figure 3.6.4 illustrates the effects of stimulus size over a range of blue-yellow ratios. The maximum relative attenuation of the VEP occurred around isoluminance when large gratings (30 or 15 spatial cycles) were used as these contained achromatic components which generate the largest VEPs. For moderate fields (six spatial cycles), the VEP

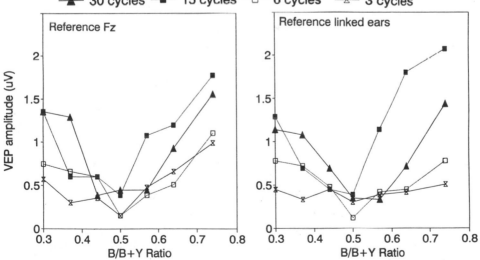

Figure 3.6.4. The effects of field size and recording montage on VEPs elicited by the phase reversal of blue-yellow square wave gratings at a repetition rate of 12.5 Hz. Spatial frequency: 2 c deg^{-1}, Lo = 30 cd m^{-2}, ΔC = 0.3, subject FE.

amplitude was significantly reduced, but only at the isoluminant point. For gratings containing three cycles, the change was too small to indicate isoluminance electro-physiologically.

3.6.4   DISCUSSION

3.6.4.1 Low-rate presentations

Aberration-free apparatus

Low contrast, aberration-free, red-green and blue-yellow gratings produce VEPs with dominant negative waves suggesting a chromatic-specific source (Figure 3.6.1). Note that contrary to expectations, both aberration-free chromatic VEPs have similar shapes and sizes, as though the most sensitive (R-G and B-Y) units were matched in properties and numbers. Differences between R-G and B-Y VEPs occur at contrasts above 0.1, partly because the magnocellular system responds to isoluminant red-green borders in a non-linear, on-off manner (Lee *et al.*, 1988). There is at least one distinct positive component superimposed upon the negative wave, which resembles reversal and offset components, thereby being 'achromatic-like' in spite of purely chromatic stimulation. Conversely, the magno-responses to blue-yellow patterns are either much smaller or non-existent at low contrasts.

Television monitor

Bearing in mind the selectivity limitations outlined above it is rather surprising that flat screen blue-yellow gratings (containing few cycles) can generate VEPs that resemble the selective chromatic VEPs obtained under aberration-free conditions. These non-transient responses reflect the sustained characteristics of visual cortical cells involved in processing colour information (Kulikowski and Walsh, 1993) whose retinal origins are tonic ganglion cells. Chromatic selectivity is lost when gratings containing large numbers of spatial cycles are used. This has unfortunate consequences in that the signal-to-noise ratio of such selective stimuli is low.

Some inter-subject differences, revealed by recording with different reference electro-des, suggest that optimisation of VEP recordings requires a flexible approach. For subject JS stimuli containing six cycles abolished the clear onset negativity and generated positive waves. As the number of spatial cycles was increased these luminance (transient) compo-nents predominated. For subject FE selective stimulation was lost when stimuli contained 10 or more cycles.

Offset always elicited a response similar to that of the chromatic reversal VEP suggest-ing that these responses contain substantial achromatic elements.

Therefore, in spite of precautions, some achromatic contamination must nearly always be present following low-rate stimulation. In the case of aberration-free gratings, intrusion is indirect, due to a magno-cellular response to isoluminance (especially in red-green chromatic onset VEPs), whereas flat stimuli are prone to chromatic aberration (see below). These achromatic intrusions are easily recognised by being transient and of a non-linear, on-off type (the same for onset, offset and reversal). In either case achromatic contamination is readily revealed by comparing the VEPs to onset versus offset/reversal.

3.6.4.2 Fast reversal presentations

The temporal frequency characteristics of achromatic and chromatic responses reflect the manner in which the respective parvo- and magno-systems operate. Chromatic reversal VEPs decrease with temporal frequency and at a repetition rate of 12.5 Hz should be a minimum (low pass characteristic with a cut-off at 3–5 Hz reflecting the sustained nature of the chromatic response). Conversely achromatic VEPs to coarse gratings peak around 5 Hz (band-pass response dominated by transient components) and the drop at 12.5 Hz is smaller (Kulikowski, 1991; Regan, 1989). Thus, isoluminance may be objectively determined at a luminance ratio of two chromatic components at which minimum 12.5 Hz reversal VEP is obtained, assuming that the residual responses to isoluminant patterns are small (as they should be for blue-yellow patterns).

The results show that gratings containing three spatial cycles are not large enough to generate reversal VEPs of sufficient magnitude to specify isoluminance (Figure 3.6.4). VEPs elicited by large and moderate sized blue-yellow gratings can indicate isoluminance, thereby forming the electrophysiological basis of heterochromatic flicker photometry. However, the largest gratings (15 or 30 spatial cycles) generate residual VEPs which, although substantially reduced, are greater at isoluminance than those generated by small gratings (evidence of achromatic intrusion). This resembles the VEPs elicited by red-green stimuli (Kulikowski et al., 1991), which also have elevated residual levels at isoluminance. As mentioned earlier, red-green patterns elicit additional responses of the magno-system around isoluminance that produce 'false nulling' of VEPs at red-green ratios either side of isoluminance. The blue-yellow patterns minimally activate the magno-system, hence only residual achromatic responses are left at the isoluminant point.

3.6.4.3 The sources and effectiveness of achromatic contamination

Thus the above-mentioned factors that contribute to achromatic intrusion have different effects on red-green and blue-yellow VEPs elicited by slow onset and fast reversal presentations.

Onset blue-yellow VEPs are particularly sensitive to achromatic contamination. The most likely explanation is that longitudinal chromatic aberration (different focus for different colours) and particularly transverse chromatic aberration (different magnification of different parts of the spectrum) result in the introduction of significant achromatic elements from blue-yellow gratings. It has been estimated that a five per cent departure of a blue-yellow grating from isoluminance results in the development of characteristic positive components (Berninger et al., 1989; Carden et al., 1985). Consequently the principle of using only three spatial cycles seems a useful guide to future applications of VEPs in clinical testing.

However, in spite of greater chromatic aberration for blue and yellow stripes, the non-selective responses to fast reversal of large red-green gratings are more conspicuous (Kulikowski et al., 1991) than evaluated for blue-yellow at present. This suggests that the fast reversal VEP, elicited by large gratings, contains components of different temporal phases than the blue-yellow VEP, evidently due to additional response components, e.g.

those of chromatic-texture (see Kulikowski, this volume, pp. 133–146) and/or due to greater variations of isoluminance with eccentricity (Zrenner, 1983).

3.6.4.4 Non-tritan stimuli and the blue-yellow system

Simple blue-yellow VEPs to square wave gratings generated on the flat screen closely resemble the selective chromatic VEPs generated by tritan-pairs in an aberration-free system. Computations of the S-cone contrast (McKeefry, 1992) indicate that little reduction of contrast occurs with this seemingly non-optimal stimulus. The main disadvantage of this arrangement is that the contributions from long-wavelength and medium-wavelength cones are not eliminated. However, this disadvantage may be offset if blue-yellow stimuli prove more informative than tritan stimuli in revealing central deficiencies. The present data justify the use of simple flat TV monitors for collection of clinical data. Moreover, it is convenient to use the blue-phosphor to the full and employ the stimulation suggested by Grigsby et al., (1991). In any case, our preliminary experiments suggest that stimulation using tritan pairs of hues on a flat TV produces similar results.

3.6.5   CONCLUSION

Generation of VEPs specific to blue-yellow stimulation requires careful monitoring of artefacts caused by chromatic aberration. Simple TV monitors can be used in clinical testing as chromatic stimulators generating blue-yellow gratings provided that chromatic aberration is adequately controlled by restricting the number of spatial cycles contained within a grating.

3.6.7   ACKNOWLEDGEMENTS

We thank Dr N.R.A. Parry and John Simpson for their help.

3.6.8   REFERENCES

BEDFORD, R.E. & WYSZECKI, G. (1957) Axial chromatic aberration of the human eye, *Journal of the Optical Society of America*, **47**, 564–565.

BERNINGER, T.A. & ARDEN, G.B. (1991) Visual evoked cortical potential with chromatic stimuli. In: Heckenlively, J.R. & Arden G.B. (Eds) *Principles and Practice of Clinical Electrophysiology of Vision*, pp. 147–150, St Louis: Mosby Year Book.

BERNINGER, T.A., ARDEN, G.B., HOGG, C. & FRUMKES, E. (1989) Colour vision defect diagnosed by evoked potentials, *Investigative Ophthalmology and Visual Science*, **30**, 299.

CARDEN, D., KULIKOWSKI, J.J., MURRAY, I.J. & PARRY, N.R.P. (1985) Human occipital potentials evoked by the onset of equiluminant chromatic gratings, *Journal of Physiology*, **369**, 44P.

CHARMAN, W.N. (1991) Limits on visual performance set by the eye's optics and the retinal cone mosaic. In: Kulikowski, J.J., Walsh, V. & Murray, I.J. (Eds) *Vision and Visual Dysfunction, Vol 5, Limits of Vision*, London: Macmillan.

GRIGSBY, S.S., VINGRYS, A.J., BENES, S.C. & KING-SMITH, P.E. (1991) Correlation of chromatic, spatial, and temporal sensitivity in optic nerve disease, *Investigative Ophthalmology and Visual Science*, **32**, 3252–3262.

JASPER, H.H. (1958) Report to the committee on methods of clinical examination in electro-encephalography, *Electroencephalography and Clinical Neurophysiology*, **10**, 370–375.

KULIKOWSKI, J.J. (1974) Human averaged occipital potentials evoked by pattern and movement, *Journal of Physiology*, **242**, 70–71P.

KULIKOWSKI, J.J. (1977) Separation of occipital potentials related to the detection of pattern and movement. In: Desmedt, J.E. (Ed.), *Visual Evoked Potentials in Man: New Developments*, pp. 184–196, Oxford: Clarendon Press.

KULIKOWSKI, J.J. (1978) Pattern and movement detection in man and rabbit: separation and comparison of occipital potentials, *Vision Research*, **18**, 183–189.

KULIKOWSKI, J.J. (1991) On the nature of evoked potentials, unit responses and psychophysics. In: Valberg, A. & Lee, B.B. (Eds) *From Pigments to Perception*, pp. 197–209, New York: Plenum Press.

KULIKOWSKI, J.J. & WALSH, V. (1993) Colour vision: Isolating mechanisms in overlapping streams. In: Hicks, T.P., Molotchnikoff, S. & Ono, T. (Eds.), *Progress in Brain Research*, New York: Elsevier.

KULIKOWSKI, J.J., MURRAY, I.J. & PARRY, N.R.A. (1989) Electrophysiological correlates of chromatic opponent and acromatic stimulation in man. In: Drum, B. & Verriest, G. (Eds), *Colour Vision Deficiencies IX*, pp. 145–153, Dordrecht: Kluwer.

KULIKOWSKI, J.J, MURRAY, I.J. & RUSSELL, M.H.A. (1991) Effect of stimulus size on chromatic and achromatic VEPs. In: Drum, B., Moreland, J.D. & Serra, A. (Eds) *Colour Vision Deficiencies X*, pp. 51–56, Dordrecht: Kluwer.

LEE, B.B., MARTIN, P.R. & VALBERG, A. (1988) The physiological basis of heterochromatic flicker photometry demonstrated in the ganglion cells of the macaque retina, *Journal of Physiology*, **414**, 223–243.

LIVINGSTONE, M.S. & HUBEL, D.H. (1984) Anatomy and physiology of a colour system in the primate visual cortex, *Journal of Neuroscience*, **4**, 309–356.

MARC, R.E. & SPERLING, H.G. (1977) Chromatic organisation of primate cones, *Science*, **196**, 454–456.

McKEEFRY, D.J. (1992) A psychophysical and electrophysiological study of the spatio-temporal characteristics of the blue/yellow and red/green colour opponent systems. PhD thesis, UMIST, Manchester.

MULLEN, K.T. (1985) The contrast sensitivity of human colour vision to red-green and blue-yellow chromatic gratings, *Journal of Physiology*, **359**, 381–400.

MURRAY, I.J., PARRY, N.R.A., CARDEN, D. & KULIKOWSKI, J.J. (1987) Human visual evoked potentials to chromatic and achromatic gratings, *Clinical Vision Science*, **1**(3), 231–244.

REGAN, D. (1989) *Human Brain Electrophysiology: Evoked Potentials and Evoked Magnetic Fields in Science and Medicine*, New York: Elsevier.

TOOTELL, R.B.H., HAMILTON, S.L. & SWITKES, E. (1988) Functional anatomy of Macaque striate cortex. IV. Contrast and magno-parvo streams, *Journal of Neuroscience*, **8**, 1594–1609.

TS'O, D.Y. & GILBERT, C.D. (1988) The organisation of chromatic and spatial interactions in the primate striate cortex, *Journal of Neuroscience*, **8**, 1712–1727

WILLIAMS, D.R., MACLEOD, D.I.A. & HAYHOE, M.M. (1981) Punctate sensitivity of the blue cone mechanism, *Vision Research*, **21**, 1357–1375.

ZRENNER, E. (1983) *Neurophysiological Aspects of Colour Vision in Primates*, Berlin: Springer-Verlag.

Latency of Transient Chromatic Response Revealed with Temporal Isoluminant Double-pulse Method

Tatsuya Yoshizawa and Keiji Uchikawa

3.7.1 INTRODUCTION

In previous studies concerning the temporal characteristics of chromatic channels (Brindley *et al.*, 1966; Green, 1969; Breton, 1977; Bowen, 1981; Uchikawa and Yoshizawa, 1993), it has been debated whether these are different between the different chromatic channels. Brindley *et al.* (1966) and Green (1969) reported that the CFF of the blue mechanism was different from that of the red and green mechanisms. Bowen (1981) found that the onset latency of chromatic response depended on wavelength of stimuli. Uchikawa and Yoshizawa (1993) also reported the temporal integration property of the r-g opponent channel to be similar to that of y-b opponent channel.

In this study, as an approach to clarify this problem we measured temporal characteristics, especially latency, of transient chromatic response by isoluminant double-pulse method and compared these between chromatic channels. This method is an excellent technique that is able to extract the responses of chromatic channels to chromatic stimuli without activating an achromatic channel. Chromatic pulses were presented successively with a stimulus onset asynchrony (SOA) and were alternated with an equal-luminance reference white stimulus. The luminance of the chromatic pulses was equal to that of the references. The color of the chromatic pulse changed by varying the ratio of the primaries so that there was a luminance difference of the primary in the chromatic pulse compared to the white. This stimulus makes a chromatic channel active and makes an achromatic channel silent because this stimulus had a chromatic change, but not luminance change. By the above method which measures temporal integration of the response to chromatic pulses, we compared latency of response between chromatic channels. If response to one chromatic pulse A and that to another B have a latency L^1 and L^2, respectively, and then pulse A presents after pulse B, temporal integration of responses to their pulses as a function of SOA will differ from that of responses to pulses whose presented order is inverted, that is, pulse B presents after pulse A. Thus, we could infer a difference of latency between responses to the pulses by comparing temporal integration functions obtained with the two opposite pulses' orders.

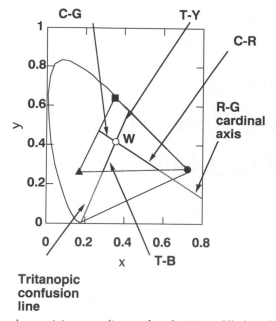

Figure 3.7.1. A xy chromaticity co-ordinate of each LED. A filled circle, a filled square, a filled triangle and an open circle represent co-ordinates of red, green, blue LED and the white, respectively. Our apparatus can present stimuli within the dashed triangle.

3.7.2 METHOD

3.7.2.1 Apparatus

We used a six channel Maxwellian-view optical system (Yoshizawa *et al.*, 1993) using red, green and blue high-luminant LEDs as light sources. As shown in Figure 3.7.1, the coordinates of red, green and blue LED were (0.723, 0.276), (0.363, 0.632) and (0.156, 0.231), respectively. Luminance of each LED was controlled by changing duty ratio of 10

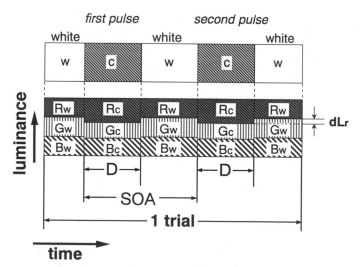

Figure 3.7.2. Time course of luminances of three LEDs in presenting isoluminant double pulses.

kHz flicker light, to avoid the varying chromaticity of LEDs due to changing spectral distribution at different current levels (Watanabe *et al.*, 1992).

3.7.2.2 Stimulus

T-B and T-Y stimuli changed from the reference white (0.355, 0.416) along the tritanopic confusion line (Smith and Pokorny, 1975) on xy chromaticity diagram and C-R and C-G stimuli changed from the white along the R/G cardinal axis (Krauskopf *et al.*, 1982), as shown in Figure 3.7.1. We chose two of these stimuli and presented the pair as first and second pulses: T-B and C-R, C-R and C-G, and T-B and T-Y were presented as three pairs in this or reversed order. These conditions are abbreviated to T-B/C-R (or C-R/T-B), C-R/ C-G (or C-G/C-R) and T-B/T-Y (or T-Y/T-B), respectively. Each chromatic pulse and white were made by mixture of three LEDs primaries and were changed by varying the mixture ratio. The luminance of these stimuli was set by flicker photometry so that they were equivalent to that of the white for each observer. The retinal illuminance was 100 td. The stimulus was a 1.5 degree diameter without surround. Duration of chromatic pulses was 10 ms and SOAs were up to 2000 ms.

3.7.2.3 Procedure

Observers responded when a change in stimulus was detected during the trial in which the starting and the ending beep sound from a computer in multi staircase method. The heads of the three observers, TY(27), TS(24), and YN(30), were fixed by a dental bite board.

3.7.3 RESULTS

We determined dL_e and dL_s of 50 per cent of psychometric probability function as the threshold value of each SOA and that of single pulse, respectively, for each stimulus condition. The dL was defined as a luminance difference between the chromatic pulse and the white as shown in Figure 3.7.2. These functions were obtained by Probit analysis (Finney, 1971). We expressed the degree of temporal integration of responses to two different pulses as the summation index described the equation (1).

$$\text{summation index} = -\text{Log}\{(dL_{e1}/dL_{s1} + dL_{e2}/dL_{s2}/2\} \tag{1}$$

where dL_{e1} and dL_{e2} are threshold values of first and second pulses, respectively, for each SOA, and dL_{s1} and dL_{s2} are those of presenting only first pulse and only second pulse, respectively. The dL was obtained for each luminance of three LEDs. The summation index was calculated using one of three dLs is the same as others.

Figures 3.7.3, 3.7.4 and 3.7.5 show the respective summation index functions of subject TY obtained in C-R and T-B, C-R and C-G, and T-B and T-Y conditions. In Figure 3.7.3, both summation index functions are about 0.3 at SOA of shorter than 30 ms; the functions decrease as SOA increases up to 150 ms and then they increase up to 300 ms again. As SOA increases more, the functions decrease, and then they are constant at longer than 600 ms. Other observers' functions had the same trend. In Figure 3.7.4, the summation index functions increase as SOA increases up to 200 ms. The negative values at SOA of shorter than 100 ms indicate that responses to C-R and C-G cancel each other. The functions decrease as SOA increases up to 600 ms and they reach an asymptote at SOA of longer than

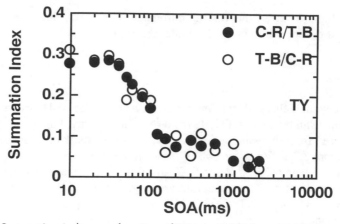

Figure 3.7.3. Summation index as a function of SOA in C-R/T-B and T-B/C-R conditions, for subject TY.

600 ms. The results of other observers indicate that the function in C-R/C-G is similar to that in C-G/C-R. In Figure 3.7.5, when SOA is shorter than 200 ms, the summation index

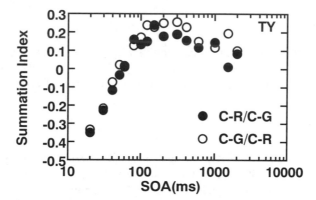

Figure 3.7.4. Summation index as a function of SOA in C-R/C-G and C-G/C-R conditions, for subject TY.

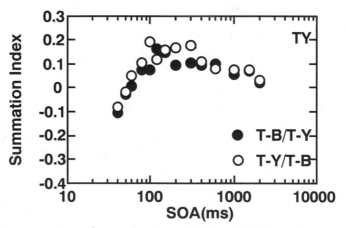

Figure 3.7.5. Summation index as a function of SOA in T-B/T-Y and T-Y/T-B conditions for subject TY.

functions decrease. The negative values in this range of SOA indicate that the response to T-B pulse cancels that to T-Y pulse. As SOA increases, the functions decrease and reach an asymptote by 600 ms. The summation index function of T-B/T-Y condition corresponds with that of T-Y/T-B condition.

In all figures, the two functions that were obtained in the two conditions by exchanging the order of chromatic pulses have the same trend. This indicates that latencies of responses to these pulses are not different.

3.7.4   DISCUSSION

We have shown that latencies of response to the chromatic pulse that stimulate a chromatic channel alternatively were not different among chromatic channels in our experimental conditions. However, previous studies concerning the latency of chromatic systems (Cushman and Levinson, 1983; Mollon and Krauskopf, 1973; Swanson *et al.*, 1987, 1988) reported that reaction times or latencies were affected by the wavelength of the stimulus. We think that this difference can be attributed to the difference of stimulus condition.

3.7.4.1 Color vision model

We derived a colour vision model from our data. We assumed that the chromatic response was produced through the colour vision system as shown in Figure 3.7.6. This model consists of three processing levels; the first and the second levels are cone and opponent mechanisms, respectively; and the third level is higher order mechanism. In this figure, each solid line between levels represents the excitatory connection and dashed lines for inhibitory inputs from cones to opponent systems. The connection (Boynton, 1979; Ingling,

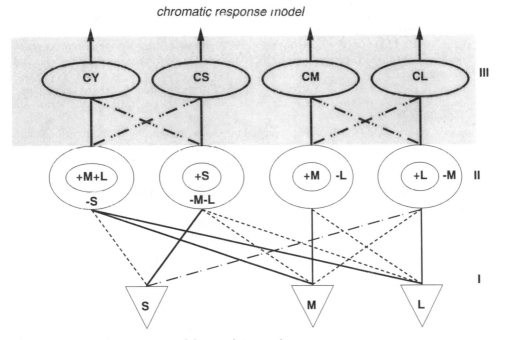

chromatic response model

Figure 3.7.6.   Colour vision model to explain our data.

1977) from S to L-M is represented by single dotted line. Double dotted lines represent that the output from level II transmits to level III with its absolute amplitude and a time delay of its output relative to the output of the excitatory connection. Our model is the same as Boynton's model (1979) from first to second level. All summation index functions have the bump that reaches the peak at SOA of 300 ms. This cannot be explained by Boynton's model. We therefore suggested this colour vision model as one of the models that can explain our data.

3.7.5   REFERENCES

BOWEN, R.W. (1981) Latencies for chromatic and achromatic visual mechanisms, *Vision Research*, **21**, 1457–1466.

BOYNTON, R.M. (1979) *Human Color Vision*, New York: Holt-Rinehart-Winston.

BRETON, M.E. (1977) Hue substitution: Wavelength latency effects, *Vision Research*, **17**, 435–443.

BRINDLEY, G, DU CROZ, J.J. & RUSHTON, W.A.H. (1966) The flicker fusion frequency of the blue-sensitive mechanism of colour vision, *Journal of Physiology*, **183**, 497–500.

CUSHMAN, W.B. & LEVINSON, J.Z. (1983) Phase shift in red and green counterphase flicker at high frequencies, *Journal of the Optical Society of America*, **73**, 1557–1561.

FINNEY, D.J. (1971) *Probit Analysis*, Cambridge: Cambridge University Press.

GREEN, D.G. (1969) Sinusoidal flicker characteristics of the color-sensitive mechanisms of the eye, *Vision Research*, **9**, 591–601.

INGLING, C.R (1977) The spectral sensitivity of the opponent-color channels, *Vision Research*, **17**, 1083–1089.

KRAUSKOPF, J., WILLIAMS, D.R. & HEELEY, D.W. (1982) Cardinal directions of color space, *Vision Research*, **22**, 1123–1131.

MOLLON, J.D. & KRAUSKOPF, J. (1973) Reaction time as a measure of the temporal response properties of individual colour mechanisms, *Vision Research*, **13**, 27–40.

SMITH, V.C. & POKORNY, J. (1975) Spectral sensitivity of the foveal cone photopigments between 400 and 500 mm, *Vision Research*, **15**, 161–171.

SWANSON, W.H., POKORNY, J. & SMITH, V.C. (1987) Effects of temporal frequency on phase-dependent sensitivity to heterochromatic flicker, *Journal of the Optical Society of America*, A **4**, 2266–2273.

SWANSON, W.H., POKORNY, J. & SMITH, V.C. (1988) Effects of chromatic adaptation on phase-dependent sensitivity to heterochromatic flicker, *Journal of the Optical Society of America*, A **5**, 1976–1982.

UCHIKAWA, K & YOSHIZAWA, T. (1993) Temporal responses of chromatic and achromatic changes inferred from temporal double-pulse integration, *Journal of the Optical Society of America*, A **10**, 1697–1705.

WATANABE, T., MORI, N. & NAKAMURA, F. (1992) A new superbright LED stimulator: photodiode-feedback design for linearing and stabilizing emitted light, *Vision Research*, **32**, 953–961.

YOSHIZAWA, T., NAKANO, Y. & UCHIKAWA, K. (1993) Rapid visual stimulator using color mixture of red, green and blue LEDs, *Japanese Journal of Optics*, **22**, 630–634.

Section 4 – Spatial and Temporal Aspects of Colour Vision

Spatial and Temporal Properties of Chromatic Processing: Separation of Colour from Chromatic Pattern Mechanisms

J.J. Kulikowski

4.1.1 INTRODUCTION

The pathway processing colour information in vision is seemingly easy to trace as it begins with three cone types, whose signals are sent to a distinct parvo-pathway with cone-opponent cells, reaching ultimately the visual cortex and the colour constancy centre, V4 (Wild *et al.*, 1985; Zeki, 1980). Long- and medium-wavelength cones are used in both chromatic and achromatic processing pathways. The two pathways have different spatio-temporal properties and both have lower spatio-temporal resolution than the cone mosaic (Schnapf *et al.*, 1990). The early post-receptoral stages also have higher spatial and temporal resolution limits than revealed psychophysically (Crook *et al.*, 1987; 1988; Lee *et al.*, 1989). In fact, the only spatio-temporal correlates of human colour psychophysics can be found among the cells with clear opponency in the primary (striate) cortex (V1) of macaques (Dow and Vautin, 1987; Kulikowski, 1991a; Kulikowski and Walsh, 1993; Kulikowski *et al.*, 1989; Ts'o and Gilbert, 1988; Vautin and Dow, 1985).

Considerable controversy exists as to the number of chromatic mechanisms (Krauskopf, this volume, pp. 431–440; Krauskopf *et al.*, 1982; Webster and Mollon, 1991) and their spatio-temporal properties. This chapter deals only with the principal red-green (R/G) and blue-yellow (B/Y) mechanisms because they provide the basis for discrimination of hues in four spectral ranges at detection threshold (Jordan and Kulikowski, this volume, pp. 421–430; Mullen and Kulikowski, 1990).

The aim of this study is twofold. First, to re-examine spatial and temporal properties of chromatic mechanisms, mainly red-green and blue-yellow. Second, to develop a range of selective chromatic stimuli, capable of isolating colour-related responses from the others, which may partly involve achromatic mechanisms and which will be tentatively labelled 'chromatic-pattern', or chromatic-texture mechanisms. Chromatic opponency was tested using two psychophysical methods. The psychophysical data is then compared with electrophysiological recordings from macaque V1.

It is observed that a colour-labelled system, properly isolated at the detection thresholds, is blind to pattern, motion and stereopsis. However, these sub-modalities are well served by another mechanism that is almost as sensitive as the colour mechanism to contour-rich isoluminant red-green stimuli.

4.1.2 METHODS

4.1.2.1 Maxwellian view

A spectral spot (diameter 1°) was presented on a white background (1000 Td, colour temperature 2700 K); the experimental paradigm is basically the same as described by King-Smith and Carden (1976; see also Nacer *et al.*, this volume, pp. 83–91), except that the spot can be blurred (with approximately Gaussian profile in Figure 4.1.1(B)). Presentation in time was either sinusoidal or flashed in a square-wave manner and the subjects task was to detect step increments, or sinusoidal modulation, expressed in radiometric units by the method of adjustment.

4.1.2.2 Aberration-free system

Two gratings of a sinusoidal luminance profile and of different spectral contents can be added in spatial anti-phase, thereby forming a chromatic grating. Both the spectral components, blue-yellow (B/Y) or red-green (R/G) of a grating were generated on separate screens positioned at different distances (Regan, 1973) to minimise chromatic aberration, viewed monocularly and with head immobilised. Gratings were made isoluminant when both components were balanced using the minimum flicker (12.5 or 25 Hz) method. Mean hues were kept constant in all presentations (see McKeefry and Kulikowski, this volume, pp. 163–172). The data were collected for mean luminance kept constant (60 td) and with narrow-band filters – hue pairs: R/G: 600/540 nm and B/Y: 439/568 nm. B/Y gratings were close to the tritanopic confusion line for the subjects, as indicated by the minimum border effect. The small departure from the theoretical tritan line (which originates at $x = 0.169$; $y = 0$, instead of about $x = 0.165$; $y = 0.1$ for 439 nm) had a negligible effect compared with experimental errors and inter-subject variations (Fry, 1989).

The minimum stimulation area (diameters of 1° or 2°) was chosen in order to stimulate both B/Y and R/G patterns (as S-cones are missing in the very central foveola – Williams *et al.*, 1981); otherwise gratings consisted of only three spatial cycles (which additionally minimises chromatic aberration).

Chromatic contrast was defined according to physical parameters when both component gratings are of the same luminance profile:

$$C = (L_{max} - L_{min})/(L_{max} + L_{min})$$

where L_{max}, L_{min} are respectively luminance of light and dark stripes. Alternatively, cone contrast can be computed using Smith and Pokorny (1975) fundamentals (see Mullen, 1990).

Temporal presentations used here were square-wave, either in the on-off or contrast reversal modes; if the waveforms are similar for both modes this suggests detection of sustained contrast, whereas a twofold increase in sensitivity shows that transient changes in contrast are detected (Kulikowski and Tolhurst, 1973). The experimental subject was J.K., a normally sighted presbyope aged 56 years.

4.1.3   RESULTS AND COMMENTS

4.1.3.1 Spectral sensitivity and temporal responses

Figure 4.1.1(A) shows the standard spectral sensitivity curve (Sperling and Harwerth, 1971; King-Smith and Carden, 1976) for the detection of 1° spectral spot flashed on a white background at a frequency of 1 Hz. The curve has three peaks, characteristic of contribution from colour opponent mechanisms, in spite of luminance increments. Kranda and King-Smith (1979) fitted to these data a model based on difference of weighted cone-opponent inputs. The blue-yellow and red-green components are clearly discernible, although the envelope of these discrete mechanisms is a nearly flat curve, covering all the spectrum.

For backgrounds of a relatively low colour temperature (2700 K) the yellow branch of the blue-yellow opponency has about 0.25 log unit lower sensitivity than the luminosity mechanism (LUM). Consequently, the detection of yellow is carried out by the achromatic mechanism, which may also contribute to the detection of green. Blue and red show best separation from the luminosity mechanism, but testing with blue-yellow and red-green stimuli may involve achromatic intrusions, due to the poor separation of yellow and green.

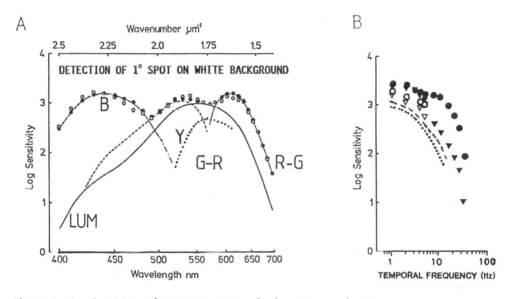

Figure 4.1.1.   Sensitivity of cone-opponent and achromatic mechanisms.
(A) Spectral sensitivity for the detection of a 1° spectral spot on a white (about 2700 K) background (1000 td). Data points are shown by open circles, filled circles and lines are the prediction of the model (after Kranda and King-Smith, 1979 and Crook et al., 1987). G-R and R-G represent weighted differences of cone-opponent inputs. Y is a yellow branch of the blue-yellow (+ B-G-R) opponency; its peak sensitivity is about 0.25 log unit below the achromatic (LUM = luminosity) curve for 500 ms on-off presentations.
(B) Temporal sensitivity for spectral spots 450 nm (triangle) and 622 nm (circles) that are modulated either sinusoidally (open symbols) or in a square-wave mode (filled symbols). Note that the curve for 622 nm diverges at high frequencies. The temporal sensitivity data for 0.85 c deg^{-1} aberration-free gratings blue-yellow (dots) and red/green (dashes) are given for comparison (log sensitivity is arbitrary).

Figure 4.1.1(B) shows temporal characteristics of the chromatic components best separated from the achromatic mechanism: blue (450 nm) and red (622 nm), both for sinusoidal and square-wave presentations. In spite of using luminance increments (which might favour achromatic detection) detection sensitivity of the defocused 1° spot is constant at low frequencies for both sine and square-wave modulation (the latter shifted up by about 0.1 log unit or 4/pi, as originally observed by de Lange). This low-pass detection (no attenuation at low temporal frequencies) is characteristic of chromatic-opponent mechanisms.

Achromatic contributions become conspicuous at high frequencies, especially in the 'red' sensitivity characteristic. Not only is 'red' temporal resolution greater (than for blue), but a separate 'branch' is noticeable. This branch with a local sensitivity peak at about 8 Hz is a hallmark of achromatic contributions at high temporal frequencies (see Swanson et al., 1987); more intrusions of this kind were observed for green and yellow whose detection thresholds were less separated from achromatic thresholds (see also Nacer et al., this volume, pp. 83–91).

For comparison, the temporal sensitivity characteristic of a 0.85 c deg^{-1} isoluminant grating is sketched in Figure 4.1.1(B), showing that blue-yellow, (B/Y) and red-green, (R/G), grating detection is basically similar to blue (but not red) spot detection. Both the B/Y and R/G curves are 'low-pass' and differ from each other only marginally at high frequencies. However, both are different from the 'red' curve with its 'branch' at high frequencies, which, not surprisingly, suggests greater selectivity of isoluminant gratings as compared with flashed spots at high frequencies.

4.1.3.2 Spatial contrast sensitivity for colour detection

Chromatic isoluminant gratings can be used to evaluate both spatial and temporal characteristics of colour vision. However, certain precautions are necessary, because such gratings do not always selectively stimulate colour-related cells, for the following reasons:

1. Chromatic gratings cannot be strictly isoluminant over their whole area mainly due to chromatic aberration.
2. Even perfectly isoluminant, aberration-free, R/G gratings stimulate magno-cells (Lee et al., 1989).
3. Long stripes (more than spots) can readily stimulate simple or complex cells in V1, due to both residual chromatic aberration and sensitivity of input magno-cells to red-green isoluminant stimuli.
4. The experiment illustrated in Figure 4.1.2(B) demonstrates an additional factor augmenting achromatic-like intrusions, namely the number of spatial cycles in a grating.

Hence chromatic gratings should consist of pairs of opponent components which are known to optimally stimulate colour vision. Red-green and blue-yellow gratings with chromatic components close to peaks of spectral sensitivity (Figure 4.1.1(A)) are an obvious choice; these spectral components are preferred to the non-spectral cardinal axis (red-green, or pink-cyan of Krauskopf et al., 1982) because chromatic aberration can readily be minimised. In addition, the use of square-wave presentations makes it possible to test whether or not the detection process is 'sustained' (i.e. 'low-pass'),, or 'transient' (i.e. 'band-pass').

Figure 4.1.2(A) shows chromatic contrast sensitivity for aberration-free gratings. Two features are apparent:

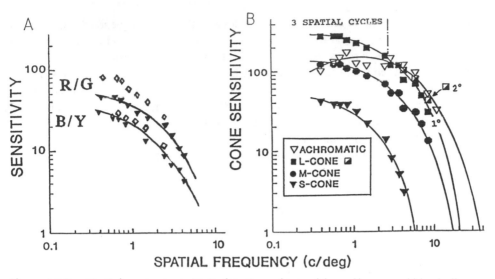

Figure 4.1.2. Spatial contrast sensitivity functions obtained for red/green and blue/yellow gratings (R/G, B/Y). Subjects DMcK (A) and JJK (B).
(A) On/off (filled triangles) and reversal (open diamonds) are illustrated. Mean retinal illuminance = 60 photopic trolands, temporal presentation rate = 1 Hz.
(B) Cone contrast sensitivity for S-cone (blue-yellow detection, triangles), M- and L-cones (red-green detection, circles and squares). Note the highest sensitivity of the L-cone. Coarse gratings consist of only three cycles. However, grating finer than 3 c deg^{-1} have a fixed area of usually 1°; half-filled squares show the data for 2°.

1. *Similarities*: sensitivities to B/Y and R/G stimuli, presented on-off, do not differ much; both curves are 'low-pass' against spatial frequency. This confirms Mullen's (1985) data for similar conditions, but, not surprisingly, is different from the data collected in presence of chromatic aberration (van der Horst and Bouman, 1969).
2. *Differences*: Sensitivity to B/Y gratings is virtually the same for on-off and reversal presentations, demonstrating that the contrast-detecting, sustained systems cannot take advantage of a transient change that is twice as large at reversal than at on-off. Conversely, sensitivity for a contrast-reversing R/G grating is higher than for on-off presentations, but less than twice. This suggests that the detection mechanism for on-off presentation of a grating is sustained, but there must be another mechanism just below threshold, which contributes to the detection when doubled contrast increments are introduced by the reversal mode.

4.1.3.3 Cone contrast sensitivity

Physical chromatic contrast does not reveal how cones are stimulated. Hence, another measure of sensitivity is cone contrast sensitivity. This correction for cone-contrast affects only L- and M-cones, for which effective contrast is reduced due to a large overlap in their spectral characteristics (Mullen, 1990).

Figure 4.1.2(B) shows that L-cone chromatic contrast sensitivity is highest over the range of low spatial frequencies; the M-cone sensitivity is obviously the same curve (shifted down) as both are derived from one experiment. Note that the achromatic contrast sensitivity (for luminance modulation) dominates at high spatial frequencies, but characteristically drops at low spatial frequencies. For a screen of 1° the L and achromatic curves clearly intersect which means that they represent different mechanisms.

Conversely, when the 2° screen is used, both the curves almost merge, as though the L-cones determined the sensitivity envelope of both chromatic opponent and achromatic channels (consistent with the data of Mullen, 1990, for similar conditions). An alternative explanation, based on the present experiments, is that the high spatial frequency branch belongs to another mechanism: larger numbers of spatial cycles in a chromatic grating may stimulate residually the achromatic system, or another partly-chromatic process (as the gratings still appear chromatic).

4.1.3.4 Perceptual observations

Granger and Heurtley (1973) were first to report differences between the threshold detection and hue discrimination of gratings; the resolution of colour gratings exceeds the resolution for identification of component colours; the latter corresponds to the resolution of aberration-free stripes (Figure 4.1.2). However, if the resolution enhancement was entirely due to residual stimulation of achromatic channels, fine chromatic gratings should be seen as achromatic, not partly-chromatic. On the other hand, the temporal characteristics indicate clear achromatic-like intrusion with its approximately 8 Hz peak, which leaves open the possibility of some chromatic-achromatic interactions.

4.1.4   DISCUSSION

4.1.4.1 Matched chromatic contrast sensitivities of B/Y and R/G mechanisms

The main finding of this study is that the B/Y and R/G opponent mechanisms are basically matched in both spatial and temporal sensitivity when viewing conditions minimise achromatic intrusions due to chromatic aberration and residual magno-stimulation. In the spatial domain, Mullen (1985) was first to demonstrate such matching, although her B/Y gratings contained hues closer to maximum blue-yellow categories than to tritanopic pairs of hues. The 'sensitivity matching' is not self-explanatory for the underlying morphology of retinal ganglion cells has been reported as different: B/Y retinal ganglion cells are 'bistratified', whereas R/G are midgets (Dacey and Lee, 1994). Hitherto there is no evidence for the previous model of separate colour channels based solely on bistratified cells (Rodieck, 1991).

One of the explanations of this, rather mysterious, matching of two dissimilar systems is that they have evolved as an attempt of the colour-labelled visual system to analyse veridically physical hues. It is tempting to postulate that a substantial overlap in spectral sensitivity of long- and medium- wavelength cones forces the cone opponent R/G system to make use of over-sampling of L-/M-cones (that is present due to the demand on achromatic acuity) in order to maintain similar physical chromatic contrast sensitivity. In other words, the R/G opponent system must be more sensitive than B/Y in order to detect similar chromatic contrasts (Figure 4.1.2).

4.1.4.2 Dual use of L and M cones in chromatic processing

The L/M cones are used in achromatic processing, which requires high acuity and, therefore, similar spectral properties. The L/M spectral overlap requires obviously high sensitivity of R/G opponent mechanisms (possibly achieved by the over-sampling of R/G opponent cells) in order to balance the B/Y and R/G systems and analyse hues veridically. The mechanism that carries out veridical colour analysis is probably based on a distinct system (see Neural correlates, below). This distinctness is supported by the finding that colour identification thresholds are not affected by chromatic aberration, which otherwise affects grating detection thresholds (see McKeefry and Kulikowski, this volume, pp. 163–172). What happens when the achromatic intrusion prevails? Under such conditions colours of stripes are not perceived veridically, but they are not colourless either (various phenomena of distorted colour perception have been reported).

Colour analysis is only one aspect of vision. Probably most vital for survival is detection of shapes, which may be camouflaged. In such cases the detection of outlines, or borders, i.e. seeing the difference between two adjacent surfaces, is more immediately important than proper identification of their colours, which can be done at leisure. Fast shape detection may take priority over colour fidelity. It is tempting to speculate that chromatic aberration is not a detriment to vision, but facilitates detection of isoluminant (camouflaged) shapes by making them luminance-modulated. It is strongest for B/Y and smaller for R/G patterns. The R/G patterns, however, can stimulate residually the achromatic (magno) system. As a result, some involvement of the achromatic system exists in all but very specific conditions and this involvement increases the sensitivity of pattern detection. This still fails to explain why such patterns, detected due to achromatic intrusions, are not colourless, and that spurious colours are seen. The proposed explanation is in terms of involvement of another chromatic mechanism, tentatively called the chromatic-pattern, or chromatic-texture system.

4.1.4.3 Chromatic stimuli for the chromatic pattern/texture system

The main feature of this postulated system is strong sensitivity imbalance in favour of R/G compared with Y/B opponency, owing to input from many R/G opponent units (utilising numerically superior L/M cones). Another feature is that its response depends on contour-rich stimuli. In fact the first observations, leading to the formulation of this hypothesis, were made with chromatic texture patterns which produce stereoscopic effects when rich in contours (Kulikowski, 1992; Kulikowski and Walsh, 1995).

An elegant example of using texture to detect forms is provided by McIlhagga and Mullen, this volume, pp. 187–196; it is significant that the reported phenomena are much stronger for R/G than B/Y contours.

The existence of such chromatic-texture analysis can explain several other effects, including seeing illusory colours. A Benham wheel provides such an example, because fast moving achromatic contours differently activate R/G and B/Y peripheral units. Such illusions may be a penalty for over-utilising the peripheral opponent system for the benefit of sensitive detection.

It may be assumed as a rule of thumb that, whenever any chromatic effect shows significant asymmetry with respect to R/G versus B/Y patterns, a chromatic texture system is involved (because the veridical colour opponent system is balanced).

4.1.4.4 Colour and spatio-temporal channels: perception and physiology

Colour analysis is both slow and best implemented under static presentations. This feature is the basis of heterochromatic flicker photometry. It is now established that three temporal filters can be identified for threshold stimuli (King-Smith and Kulikowski, 1975; Kulikowski and Tolhurst, 1973; Mandler and Makous, 1984): sustained (low-pass), and two transient (band-pass) filters. Many phenomena, and the present data, suggest that isolated colour analysers have only access to one (low-pass or sustained) temporal filter (e.g. Livingstone and Hubel, 1987; Mullen and Boulton, 1992; Ramachandran and Gregory, 1978). Isolation of colour is obviously artificial (chromatic aberration is normally insepar-able), but it demonstrates that colour analysis relies on a distinct mechanism. Hence, less selective methods of stimulation bring about more contributions from other temporal filters. In particular, the secondary peaks in temporal sensitivity (Figure 4.1.1(B)) have been reported since de Lange and correctly associated with residual contribution of the 'luminance-like' mechanisms (Swanson et al., 1987). In the temporal domain, the 'tran-sient' contribution is shown by shorter integration times (e.g. Eskew et al., 1994). Figure 4.1.2(A) demonstrates that for on-off presentations R/G gratings are detected by the sustained (low-pass) mechanism, but that the transient (low-pass) detection is only slightly less sensitive. For reversal presentations, transient detection takes over (sensitivity is almost, but not quite, doubled). Information about motion can be signalled when two temporal filters are activated, but still chromatic gratings activate transient filters less than their achromatic equivalents, hence they are not perceived as mobile. Note that a similar situation occurs for fine achromatic gratings which poorly, or fail to, activate the transient filter, hence their mobility is low (see stopped motion, Kulikowski, 1991b). It is proposed that the mechanisms associated with transient filters belong to another processing system (see Figure 4.1.3). In this figure, three main classes of retinal ganglion cells are described: bistratified (cone inputs + S–L–M), midget (cone inputs + L–M and + M–L) and parasol (cone inputs + L + M). Bistratified and midget cells with chromatic opponency project to parvo-LGN layers and are used in two systems. Parasol cells project to the magno-LGN layers to form the basis of the achromatic luminosity system; these cells are also stimulated by chromatic red/green isoluminant contours in a non-linear manner and can signal the presence of a red/green border, or residual isoluminant flicker, but not the description of the constituent colours (Lee et al., 1989). The primary visual cortex, V1, is the site of basic reorganisation of parvo/magno inputs, where some of them mix (Lund et al., 1994). However, both the colour mechanism and the achromatic luminosity mechanism respon-sive to fast flicker remain segregated in terms of parvo and magno inputs.

The colour mechanism integrates signals using filters that are low-pass in both spatial and temporal frequency domains (the latter due to eye movements?). Owing to spatial summation of signals from the LGN cells, the V1 blue/yellow and red/green receptive fields are large, show clear double opponency in the centre and relatively weak opponency in the surround (not shown); their temporal response properties are slower than in LGN. The colour mechanism responds best to isoluminant stimuli; blue/yellow and red/green opponency are balanced, and of comparable chromatic contrast sensitivity.

The chromatic pattern mechanism, based on joint magno/parvo projections, is organised in channels that are specific to orientation, spatial frequency and binocular disparity. The red/green projection from the LGN cells is both dominant and its spatio-temporal resolution higher than that of weak inputs from blue/yellow LGN cells. Consequently, trichromacy is not balanced and colour is not signalled reliably (e.g. temporal modulation may signal false colours). This mechanism can also signal brightness of objects by integrating signals of the parvo-division with luminance signals of the magno-division. Isoluminant patterns are not optimal, but are often sufficient to elicit responses.

The model postulates an inhibitory interaction between the colour mechanism and the chromatic-pattern sub-division (inferred from 'chromatic-rivalry' experiments, Kulikowski and Walsh, 1995).

The 'luminosity' system (exclusively magno) can signal luminance of fast flicker only,

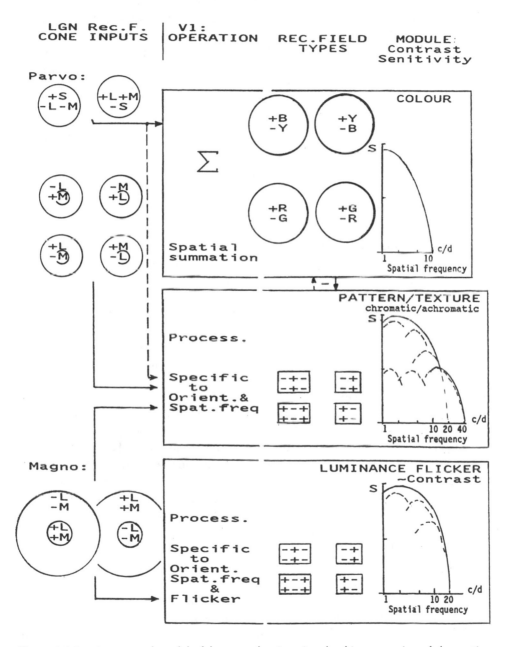

Figure 4.1.3. A proposed model of three mechanisms involved in processing of chromatic stimuli.

for slow temporal modulation of suprathreshold patterns favours brightness signals (of the pattern/texture system).

The same arguments apply to the spatial channels, although spatial filters are more numerous and more difficult to separate. Critical re-examination of interactions between chromatic and achromatic mechanisms (Switkes *et al.*, 1988) revealed that they are largely independent at threshold (Mullen and Losada, 1994). But, somewhat surprisingly, spatial channels revealed by masking are virtually identical for chromatic and achromatic channels (Losada and Mullen, 1994). However, masking is shown (Kulikowski, 1991b) to reveal characteristics of interactions between channels (not of channels themselves) and by its very nature, masking is a supra-threshold process. Humanski and Wilson, 1992, showed that there are only two very broad-band spatial frequency channels in the B/Y mechanism; the B/Y and R/G asymmetry is inconsistent with colour analysis data, but consistent with chromatic-texture analysis (Eskew *et al.*, 1994).

The presence of a separate system analysing chromatic texture is also consistent with the demonstrations of stereopsis of contour-rich patterns (Kulikowski, 1992; Kulikowski and Walsh, 1995; Simmons and Kingdom, 1994).

4.1.4.5 Neuronal correlates

The early discoveries of cone opponent cells in various vertebrates were interpreted as evidence for Hering's colour opponency (for review, see De Valois and De Valois, 1988). Later, it has become clear that the properties of pre-cortical cells do not account quantitatively for properties of colour vision (e.g. Derrington *et al.*, 1984; Lee *et al.*, 1989); these cells respond to sub-threshold stimuli. Worse still, single-unit properties in the monkey striate cortex show considerable variations (e.g. Lennie *et al.*, 1990) from chromatic double-opponent cells (practically not responding to achromatic contrast, e.g. Kulikowski and Vidyasagar, 1984) to partly chromatic cells (for discussion, see Valberg and Lee, 1991). Most recent studies (Gegenfurtner *et al.*, 1994) challenged the orderly model of the cortical (V2) chromatic pathway.

However, global recordings using multi-unit or visual evoked responses and near-threshold stimuli, showed that psychophysical thresholds and VEPs are related quantitatively (Kulikowski, 1991a,b). Combined with the finding that the cells in V1 with double opponency (within one region of the concentric receptive field, e.g. +r/–g) are monocularly driven and have properties similar to the psychophysical (low-pass in terms of spatial and temporal frequencies, Kulikowski and Walsh, 1993), this suggests that only the most sensitive units can signal colour veridically near threshold. Potentials evoked by near threshold stimuli are similar for aberration-free B/Y and R/G gratings (Robson *et al.*, this volume, pp. 115–123), and, thus, consistent with the psychophysics.

Varieties of partly chromatic cells, many of them oriented, simple-like with clear spatial frequency tuning, can be recorded in V1 (Kulikowski and Vidyasagar, 1986). It is proposed that they belong to another system (Figure 4.1.3), processing chromatic patterns or textures. Further, it is tempting to associate this system with the inter-blob to thin-stripe projection from V1 to V2 (Livingstone and Hubel, 1987, 1988), which is parvo-dominated, but the contribution of the magno-inputs cannot be ruled out (note that many cells in laminae 4C have mixed parvo/magno inputs; Lund *et al.*, 1994).

Thus, data on the organisation of colour processing should be collected afresh, paying particular attention to quantitatively evaluated chromatic contrast sensitivity; the previously observed order of connections (e.g. Hubel and Livingstone, 1990; Livingstone and Hubel, 1988) may then be restored.

4.1.4.6 Do selective stimuli exist and are they helpful?

A sceptical reader who follows the methods of isolating distinct mechanisms outlined above may conclude that these attempts are almost in vain. However, we have to understand the difficulties of isolating mechanisms against the rule of nature: the visual system has not evolved to have clearly separated modules, especially in its peripheral parts (which must transmit signals through a bottleneck of the optic nerve). Hence, peripheral components must be shared by several sub-systems and the segregation of signals is carried out in the visual cortex. It also seems probable that this selection is not only due to an overall averaging of the strongest signals, but is most likely 'sharpened' by selective attention, which allows the selection of responses from particular groups of cells and treats others as noise. Many experiments, including those reported by McKeefry and Kulikowski (this volume, 163–172), show that the visual system can extract veridical information about colour in the presence of confusing signals, e.g. due to chromatic aberration. Whatever the precise mechanisms of tuning of higher-order perceptual stages, the experiments on both normal and deficient brains indicate selectivity of percepts, or perceptual deficiencies (see Zeki et al., 1991), and this makes the attempts to find selective stimuli worthwhile. In particular, selective stimuli make it possible to demonstrate properties of fundamental mechanisms, such as the matched, low-pass characteristics of colour vision described here.

4.1.4.7 Applications

Colour vision is a sub-modality served by a relatively isolated pathway of the visual system, which in its initial stages relies on thin (parvo-) nerve fibres. It consists of two distinct opponent mechanisms whose responses can be isolated near threshold, namely red-green and blue-yellow. As each of them has a different neuroanatomical basis, they show different vulnerability in acquired colour deficiencies.

Of particular clinical interest is the blue-yellow mechanism because S-cones are easily damaged by over-exposure to light. Furthermore this mechanism has a unique neuroanatomical substrate being subserved only by bistratified retinal ganglion cells. In a sense the blue-yellow mechanism operates as a canary in a coal-mine showing early susceptibility to many forms of ocular pathology. Thus S-cone specific (tritan) responses, when properly isolated, are of great diagnostic and probably prognostic importance. However, proper isolation very often does not depend on adherence to the tritanopic confusion line: as shown in Figure 4.1.1, S-cone stimulation can be achieved over a range of wavelengths up to 470 nm for large spots, particularly if mean adaptation backgrounds are of low colour temperatures. For space-periodic patterns, some departures from the tritanopic confusion line (e.g. Mullen, 1985) have negligible effects, as compared with substantial achromatic intrusions caused by chromatic aberration. In this respect polychromatic displays with continuously adjustable pairs of isoluminant hues to coincide with the tritan line (Krauskopf et al., 1982) do not guarantee exclusive S-cone stimulation for achromatic intrusions are substantial in a grating with several spatial cycles. Such a possibility of artefactual stimulation has recently been shown in a study by Rabin *et al.*, (1994) in which S-cone VEPs with band pass properties are misleadingly reported. Identification of limits of selective stimulation forestalls such misconceptions (see Robson *et al.*, this volume, pp. 115–123).

4.1.5   CONCLUSIONS

Various experiments suggest that threshold detection of isolated colour patches is sub-served by red-green and blue-yellow colour-opponent mechanisms matched in their sensitivity and low-pass spatio-temporal resolution. These colour mechanisms are blind to form, motion or depth. However, vision of patterns, motion and depth can also be served by chromatic texture mechanisms that utilise chromatic aberration and residual sensitivity of the magno-system to isoluminant patterns, especially red-green. Many perceptual phenomena can be explained by involvement of other chromatic mechanisms or chromatic-achromatic interactions, these are tentatively named chromatic, texture channels.

4.1.6   REFERENCES

Crook, J.M., Lee, B.B, Tigwell, D.A. & Valberg, A. (1987) Thresholds to chromatic spots of cells in the macaque geniculate nucleus as compared to detection sensitivity in man, *Journal of Physiology*, **392**, 193–211.

Dacey, D.M & Lee, B.B. (1994) The blue-on opponent pathway in primate retina originates from a distinct bistratified ganglion cell type, *Nature*, **367**, 731–735.

Derrington, A.M., Krauskopf, J. & Lennie, P. (1984), Chromatic mechanisms in the Lateral Geniculate Nucleus of the macaque, *Journal of Physiology*, **357**, 241–265.

De Valois, R.L. & De Valois, K.K. (1988) *Spatial Vision*, New York: Oxford University Press.

Eskew, R.T., Stromeyer, C.F. & Kronauer, R.E. (1994) Temporal properties of the red-green chromatic mechanisms, *Vision Research*, **34**, 3127–3138.

Fry, G.A. (1989) Koenig models of colour vision. In: Drum, B. & Verriest, G. (Eds) *Colour Vision Deficiencies IX*, Dordrecht: Kluwer Academic Publishers, pp. 117–24.

Gegenfurtner, K.R., Kiper, D.C. & Fenstemaker, S.B. (1994) Processing of colour information in area V2 of macaque, *Perception*, **23**, S30–31.

Granger, E.M. & Heurtley, J.C. (1973) Visual chromaticity-modulation transfer function, *Journal of the Optical Society of America*, **63**, 1173–1174.

Hubel, D.H. & Livingstone, M.S. (1990) Colour and contrast sensitivity in the lateral geniculate body and the primary visual cortex of the macaque monkey, *Journal of Neuroscience*, **10**, 2223–2237.

Humanski, R.A. & Wilson, H.R. (1992) Spatial frequency mechanisms with short wavelength sensitive cone inputs, *Vision Research*, **32**, 549–560.

King-Smith, P.E. & Kulikowski, J.J. (1975) Pattern and flicker detection analyzed by subthreshold summation, *Journal of Physiology*, **249**, 519–548

King-Smith, P.E. & Carden, D. (1976) Luminance and opponent colour contributions to visual detection and adaptation and to temporal and spatial integration, *Journal of the Optical Society of America*, **66**, 709–717.

Kranda, K. & King-Smith, P.E. (1979) Detection of coloured stimuli by independent linear systems, *Vision Research*, **19**, 733–745.

Krauskopf, J., Williams D.R. & Heeley D.M. (1982) The cardinal directions of colour space, *Vision Research*, **22**, 1123–1131.

Kulikowski, J.J. (1991a) On the nature of visual evoked potentials, unit responses and psychophysics. In: Valberg, A. & Lee, B.B. (Eds), *From Pigment to Perception*, New York: Plenum Press, pp. 197–209.

KULIKOWSKI, J.J. (1991b) What really limits vision. In: Kulikowski, J.J., Walsh, V. & Murray, I.J. (Eds), *Limits of Vision*, London: Macmillan Press, pp. 286–329.

KULIKOWSKI, J.J. (1992) Binocular chromatic rivalry and single vision, *Ophthalmic and Physiological Optics*, **12**, 168–170.

KULIKOWSKI, J.J. & TOLHURST, D.J. (1973) Psychophysical evidence for sustained and transient detectors in human vision, *Journal of Physiology*, **232**, 149–162.

KULIKOWSKI, J.J. & VIDYASAGAR, T.R. (1984) Macaque striate cortex: pattern movement and colour processing, *Ophthalmic amd Physiological Optics*, **4**, 77–81.

KULIKOWSKI, J.J. & VIDYASAGAR, T.R. (1986) Space and spatial frequency: Analysis and representation in the macaque striate cortex, *Experimental Brain Research*, **64**, 5–18.

KULIKOWSKI, J.J. & WALSH, V. (1993) Colour vision: isolating mechanisms in overlapping streams, *Progress in Brain Research*, **95**, 417–426.

KULIKOWSKI, J.J., DICKINSON, C.M. & MURRAY, I.J. (Eds) (1989) *Seeing Contour and Colour*, Oxford: Pergamon Press.

LEE, B.B., MARTIN, P.R. & VALBERG, A. (1989) Sensitivity of macaque retinal ganglion cells to chromatic and luminance flicker, *Journal of Physiology*, **414**, 223–244.

LENNIE, P., KRAUSKOPF, J. & SCLAR, G. (1990) Chromatic mechanisms in the striate cortex of the macaque, *Journal of Neuroscience*, **10**, 649–669.

LIVINGSTONE, M.S. & HUBEL, D.H. (1987) Psychophysical evidence for separate channels for the perception of form, colour, movement and depth, *Journal of Neuroscience*, 7, 3416–3468.

LIVINGSTONE, M.S. & HUBEL, D.H. (1988) Segregation of form, colour, movement and depth: anatomy, physiology and perception, *Science*, **240**, 740–750.

LOSADA, M.A & MULLEN, K.T. (1994) The spatial tuning of chromatic mechanisms identified by simultaneous masking, *Vision Research*, **34**, 331–341.

LUND, J.S., YOSHIOKA, T. & LEVITT, J.B. (1994) Substrates for interlaminar connections in area V1 of macaque monkey cerebral cortex. In: Peters, A. & Rockland, K.S. (Eds) *Cerebral Cortex*, Vol.10, New York: Plenum Press, pp. 37–60.

MANDLER, M.B. & MAKOUS, W. (1984) A three channel model of temporal frequency perception, *Vision Research*, **24**, 1881–1887.

MULLEN, K.T. (1985) The contrast sensitivity of human colour vision to red/green and blue/yellow gratings, *Journal of Physiology*, **395**, 381–400.

MULLEN, K.T. (1990) The chromatic coding of space. In: Blakemore, C. (Ed.), *Vision: Coding and Efficiency*, Cambridge: Cambridge University Press, pp. 150–158.

MULLEN, K.T. & KULIKOWSKI, J.J. (1990) Wavelength discrimination at detection threshold, *Journal of Optical Society of America*, A **7**, 733–742.

MULLEN, K.T. & BOLTON, J.C. (1992) Absence of smooth motion perception in colour vision, *Vision Research*, **32**, 483–488.

MULLEN, K.T. & LOSADA, M. (1994) Evidence for separate pathways for colour and luminance detection, *Journal of Optical Society of America*, A **11**, 3136–3151.

RABIN, J., SWITKES, E., CROGNALE, M., SCHNECK, E. & ADAMS, A.J. (1994) Visual evoked potentials in three dimensional colour space: correlates of spatio-chromatic processing, *Vision Research*, **34**, 2657–2671.

RAMACHANDRAN, V.S. & GREGORY, R.L. (1978) Does colour provide an input to human motion perception?, *Nature*, **275**, 55–57.

REGAN, D. (1973) Evoked potentials specific to spatial patterns of luminance and colour, *Vision Research*, **13**, 2381–2402.

RODIECK, R.W. (1991) Which cells code for colour? In: Valberg, A. & Lee, B.B. (Eds) *From Pigment to Perception*, New York: Plenum Press, pp. 83–93.

SCHNAPF, J.L., NUNN, B.J., MEISTER, M. & BAYLOR D.A. (1990) Visual transduction in cones of the monkey, *Journal of Physiology*, **427**, 681–713.

SIMMONS, D.R & KINGDOM, F.A.A. (1994) Contrast thresholds for stereoscopic depth identification with isoluminant stimuli, *Vision Research*, **34**, 2971–2983.

Smith, V.C. & Pokorny, J. (1975) Spectral sensitivity of the foveal cone pigments between 400 and 500 nm, *Vision Research*, **15**, 161–171.

Sperling, H.G. & Harwerth, R.S. (1971) Red-green interactions in the increment threshold spectral sensitivity of primates, *Science*, **172**, 180–184.

Swanson, W.H., Uueno, T., Smith, V.C. & Pokorny, J. (1987) Temporal modulation sensitivity and pulse-detection thresholds for chromatic and luminance perturbations, *Journal of Optical Society of America*, **A 4**, 1992–2005.

Switkes, E., Bradley, A. & De Valois, K.K. (1988) Contrast dependence and mechanisms of masking interactions among chromatic and luminance mechanisms, *Journal of Optical Society of America*, **A 5**, 1149–62.

Ts'o, D.Y. & Gilbert, C.D. (1988) The organisation of chromatic and spatial interactions in the primate striate cortex., *Journal of Neuroscience*, **8**, 1712–1728.

Valberg, A. & Lee, B.B. (Eds) *From Pigment to Perception*, New York: Plenum Press.

van der Horst, G.J.C. & Boumnan, M.A. (1969) Spatio-temporal chromaticity discrimination, *Journal of Optical Society of America*, **59**, 1482–1488.

Vautin, R.G. & Dow, B.M. (1985) Color cell groups in foveal striate cortex of the behaving macaque, *Journal of Neurophysiology*, **54**, 273–292.

Webster, M.A. & Mollon, J.D. (1991) Changes in colour appearance following post-receptoral adaptation, *Nature*, **349**, 235–238.

Wild, H.M., Butler, S.R., Carden, D. & Kulikowski, J.J. (1985) Primate cortical area V4 important for colour constancy, but not wavelength discrimination, *Nature*, **313**, 133–35.

Williams, D.R., MacLeod, D.I.A. & Hayhoe, M.M. (1981) Foveal tritanopia, *Vision Research*, **21**, 1341–1356.

Zeki, S. (1980) The representation of colours in the visual cortex of rhesus monkey, *Nature*, **284**, 412–418.

Zeki, S.M., Watson, J.D.G., Lueck, C.J., Friston, K.J., Kennard, C. & Frackowiak, R.S.J. (1991) A direct demonstration of functional specialisation in human visual cortex, *Journal of Neuroscience*, **11**, 641–649.

Spatial and Temporal Contrast Sensitivity During Saccades: Evidence for Suppression of the Magnocellular Visual Pathway

David C. Burr, M. Concetta Morrone and John Ross

4.2.1 INTRODUCTION

A long standing puzzle to visual scientists is why the world appears to remain stable during *saccades*, the ballistic eye-movements that cause continual sporadic displacements of the retinal image. Saccadic velocities are fast (around 300 deg s^{-1}), but not beyond the resolution limit of human vision. Image motion (at least up to 10,000 deg s^{-1}) does not reduce sensitivity, but merely shifts the range of spatial frequencies to which we are most sensitive (Burr and Ross, 1982). As the Fourier power spectrum of natural visual scenes varies inversely with spatial frequency (Field, 1987), there will generally be considerable energy of low spatial frequency moving across the retina during a saccade, that should elicit a powerful sense of motion.

An early idea was that vision is actively interrupted during saccades by a 'central anaesthesia', thereby eliminating the sense of motion (Dodge, 1900). Efforts to measure the magnitude of this anaesthesia (now referred to as 'saccadic suppression') have produced variable results (e.g. Krauskopf *et al.*, 1966; Latour, 1962; Riggs *et al.*, 1974), leading to the conclusion by Matin (1974) and others that any central suppression must be negligible compared with masking suppression. However, strong saccadic suppression (of an order of magnitude) has been reported, but only for patterns of low spatial frequency (Burr *et al.*, 1982). This result led to the suggestion that motion sensitivity is selectively damped during saccades, thereby eliminating the otherwise disconcerting sense of image motion (reinforced by more recent studies of Shiori and Cavanagh, 1989; and Ilg and Hoffmann, 1993). Here we extend the previous study by investigating colour sensitivity during saccades. The results suggest that the magno visual pathway is selectively blocked during saccades, probably at the level of the lateral geniculate nucleus, while the parvo pathway continues to function normally. A brief report of some of these findings has been published (Burr *et al.*, 1994).

4.2.2   METHODS

Contrast sensitivity for detection of briefly presented horizontal gratings was measured for normal vision and during large horizontal saccades. As the saccades ran parallel to the gratings, there was no effective image motion of the gratings. Stimuli were generated by framestore and displayed on the face of a Mitsubishi colour monitor at 120 Hz, 600 lines/frame at a mean luminance of 10 cd m^{-2}. The 40 × 30 cm display subtended 67° by 53° at a 30 cm viewing distance, and was surrounded by white card floodlit by two lateral projectors. The gratings were modulated either in chromaticity (equiluminant red-green by standard flicker-photometry criteria) or in luminance (yellow-black of the same average chromaticity as the equiluminant gratings). The equiluminant point did not change during saccades.

Voluntary saccadic eye-movements were recorded with electrodes positioned near the outer canthus of each eye (earth on forehead), connected to the computer A/D after suitable amplification and filtering. On reaching a voltage threshold, the computer initiated presentation at the beginning of the next frame. The contrast of each presentation was near the estimated threshold (as determined by the Bayesian QUEST procedure of Watson and Pelli, 1983), and final thresholds calculated by fitting cumulative Gaussian curves to the probability of seeing data. For the data of Figure 4.2.1, observers indicated whether they saw the grating or not (yes-no procedure), while for that of Figure 4.2.2 they were required to discriminate the position of a briefly presented (8 ms) horizontally oriented grating patch centred 6.6° above or below the centre of the screen. This experiment employed a test and mask pattern. The test was a grating of 0.075 c deg^{-1} vignetted within a Gaussian patch with horizontal space constant of 16.7° and vertical space constant 13.2°. The mask was a sinusoidal grating of the same spatial frequency and phase as the test, displayed for one frame (8 ms).

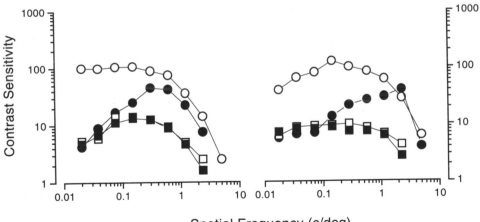

Figure 4.2.1.   Contrast sensitivity (inverse of contrast at threshold) for detecting briefly presented (17 ms) horizontal gratings of variable spatial frequency, modulated either in luminance (circles) or colour (squares). Measurements were made both in free viewing conditions (open symbols) and during large (40°) horizontal saccades (filled symbols). Standard errors, calculated by repeated estimates with partial data, were on average 0.05 log-units (less than symbol size).

4.2.3   CONTRAST SENSITIVITY TO LUMINANCE AND CHROMATIC CONTRAST DURING SACCADES

Figure 4.2.1 shows contrast sensitivity for luminance and chromatic patterns, briefly presented during normal viewing (open symbols) and during saccades (closed symbols). For luminance contrast (circles), there was strong reduction in sensitivity during saccades at low spatial frequencies, while sensitivity at high spatial frequencies was virtually unchanged (confirming Burr et al., 1982). However, for equiluminant stimuli, sensitivity during saccades was at least as high at all spatial frequencies as that in free viewing, and in some cases even higher. It should also be pointed out that at threshold, both during saccades and in free viewing, the colour of the chromatic gratings was resolvable, suggesting that the gratings were detected by chromatically sensitive mechanisms.

As it is generally agreed that the magno-system conveys no useful information about colour (see Merigan, 1991; Merigan et al., 1991), these results suggest that the magnocellular, but not the parvocellular pathway is suppressed during saccades. The reduced sensitivity for low spatial frequencies is consistent with suppression of the magno pathway that spans a lower range of low spatial frequencies than the parvo pathway.

4.2.4   SITE OF SACCADIC SUPPRESSION

We next sought to identify the level of visual analysis at which the suppression of low-frequency luminance stimuli occurs, using a *contrast masking* paradigm. Either the test or the mask (or both) were presented during saccades (see illustrations in Figure 4.2.2). Here observers were required to discriminate in a two-alternative forced choice paradigm the position of a briefly displayed (8 ms) horizontally oriented low-frequency grating vignetted by a Gaussian patch centred above or below the centre of the screen. A *mask* grating (also displayed briefly) followed the test after 90 ms (backward masking), or preceded it by 90 ms (forward masking), or followed immediately after it ('simultaneous' masking).

With normal viewing (open symbols of Figure 4.2.2) masks reduced sensitivity in all three masking conditions as has been previously documented in many laboratories. Saccadic viewing (filled symbols) changed the results in a quantitatively consistent way. With the backward masking condition, saccades reduced sensitivity at all contrasts by a factor of three (half a log-unit), suggesting that the test was suppressed before the site of contrast masking: suppression after masking would act on the 'masked' test, and hence would depend on mask contrast. With the forward masking paradigm, the saccade-triggered sensitivities were systematically higher than those in free viewing, and well fit by displacing the normal threshold curve by half a log-unit *horizontally* along the mask contrast axis. This also implies that saccadic suppression precedes contrast masking, as later suppression could not influence the masking process. The simultaneous masking results were also consistent with early suppression, as sensitivities during saccades were well predicted by displacing the normal results both vertically and horizontally by half a log unit, modelling the early attenuation of both test and mask.

These results suggest that saccadic suppression occurs early in visual processing, before the site of contrast masking. As much evidence suggests that contrast masking occurs mainly in primary visual cortex (Bonds, 1992; Ohzawa et al., 1982; Schlar et al., 1990), saccadic suppression that precedes masking must occur at a very early visual site, making the lateral geniculate nucleus (LGN) a likely candidate.

4.2.5   TEMPORAL IMPULSE RESPONSE DURING SACCADES

To occur within the duration of a saccade, stimuli must be brief, giving them a broad temporal spectrum, unsuitable to measure temporal frequency selectivity directly. However, it is possible to obtain an estimate of the impulse response function by a two-pulse summation technique (e.g. Burr and Morrone, 1993; Roufs, 1972; Uchikawa and Ikeda, 1986; Watson and Nachmias, 1977). As before, the stimuli were 8 ms horizontal gratings, but this time displayed twice, with variable stimulus-onset-asynchrony, either with the same or opposite contrast. Using the technique detailed in Burr and Morrone (1993), impulse responses were derived from these data and shown in Figures 4.2.3(a) and 4.2.3(c). As reported in the earlier paper, the impulse response during normal viewing is di-phasic for luminance contrast and mono-phasic for chromatic contrast. During saccades, the impulse response for luminance vision remains di-phasic, but becomes accelerated, with a time-to-peak of 12 ms compared with 20 ms in normal viewing. The impulse response for chromatic contrast remains mono-phasic during saccades, and quite similar to that of normal viewing, except for a slight increase in sensitivity and time-to-peak for subject MCM.

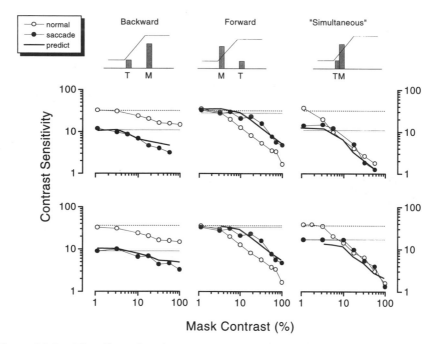

Figure 4.2.2.   The effect of masking on contrast sensitivity during saccadic and normal viewing conditions for two observers, DCB (upper curves) and MCM (lower curves). The open symbols represent measurements in free viewing, and the closed symbols measurements when the sequence was triggered by a 20° saccade. The dashed lines show un-masked thresholds in normal viewing, and the dotted lines during saccades. The thick lines show the predicted result if saccades attenuated contrast-gain before the site of masking: the normal-viewing curves are displaced vertically by half a log-unit (attenuating test contrast) for backward masking, horizontally by the same amount (attenuating mask contrast) for forward masking and in both directions (attenuating both contrasts) for simultaneous masking.

The temporal frequency tuning curves, derived by Fourier transform of the impulse response functions, are reported in Figures 4.2.3(c) and 4.2.3(d). For both normal and saccadic viewing the tuning curves for colour are low-pass, while those for luminance are band-pass. For the luminance condition, the gain is reduced by more than a factor-of-three for low temporal frequencies, but less at higher temporal frequencies, causing the peak to occur at higher temporal frequencies in the saccadic condition. At the very highest temporal frequencies, the curves are virtually coincident.

At first glance this result certainly seems to be at odds both with the suggestion that motion is suppressed during saccades and that the suppression is selective for the magno pathway, which has a higher temporal response to gratings (e.g. Derrington and Lennie, 1984). However, closer consideration reveals that the result is not completely unexpected. Detectors of the human visual system vary in spatial frequency selectivity over a very wide range, down to at least 0.003 c deg^{-1} (Anderson et al., 1991), with receptive field size varying inversely with preferred spatial frequency (Anderson and Burr, 1987). Our results show that the mechanisms selective to low-spatial-frequency luminance-contrast are suppressed during saccades, leaving only those of higher spatial frequency tuning, above 0.3 c deg^{-1} (Figure 4.2.1). Thus the low frequency gratings (0.07 c deg^{-1}) used for the two-pulse summation may have been of optimal spatial frequency for the best responding unit of normal vision, but about four times lower than the preferred spatial frequency of the best responding unit during saccades, and therefore stimulate both the centre and surround of the detector together. As there exists a difference in response latency of the centre and surround

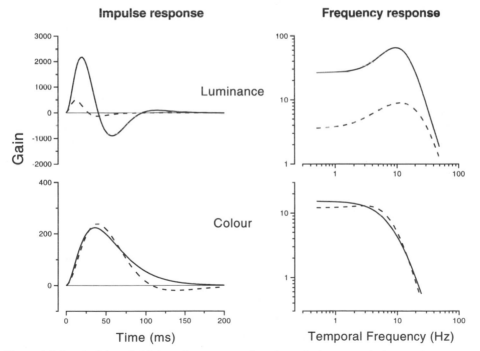

Figure 4.2.3. *Left-hand side* Impulse response functions during normal viewing (continuous curves) and saccades (dashed curves), derived from the two-pulse summation data (not shown), using the technique described in Burr and Morrone (1993); *Right-hand side*: temporal tuning functions during normal viewing (continuous curves) and saccades (dashed curves), obtained by Fourier transform of the impulse response functions.

of retinal and geniculate cells (Zrenner, 1983), simultaneous stimulation will cause a faster impulse response.

It should also be pointed out that while the temporal resolution of retinal and geniculate P-cells (or 'tonic' cells) is certainly low for chromatic modulation, it is much higher for luminance modulation (Lee *et al.*, 1989, 1990). In response to large field flicker, the temporal frequency tuning curves of P-cells (to luminance modulation) have a very similar form to those of M-cells after scaling for absolute sensitivity (Lee *et al.*, 1990, Figure 3). Furthermore, if the argument of the previous paragraph is accepted, then the impulse response during normal vision should be determined by an M-cell in response to a stimulus of preferred spatial frequency (consistent with the fact that M-cells prefer lower spatial frequencies than P-cells), while that during saccades by the response of a P-cell to stimulus of spatial frequency much lower than preferred, hence stimulating both centre and surround together. Unfortunately, this comparison is not available in the literature, but theoretical considerations would suggest that the P-cell response should be further accelerated.

4.2.6   CONCLUDING REMARKS

The results of this study support earlier suggestions (Burr *et al.*, 1982; Ilg and Hoffmann, 1993; Shiori and Cavanagh, 1989) that motion mechanisms are selectively suppressed during saccades. The suppression should attenuate the potentially disturbing sense of motion of low spatial frequency components that otherwise would be highly visible at saccadic speeds (Burr and Ross, 1982). In natural viewing conditions, this suppression could be supplemented by separate visually-driven mechanisms (Mackay, 1970; Matin, 1974) to attenuate further any residual visual signals generated by the saccade. Interestingly, effects of this type also seem to be confined to low-frequency patterns modulated in luminance (Derrington, 1984).

It is now clear that visual information is processed through the functionally separate M- and P-pathways. The division is established in the retina, well-preserved at the LGN, and continues (with some crosstalk) through to associative cortex (e.g. DeYoe and Van Essen, 1988; Merigan and Maunsell, 1993). Our results strongly suggest that saccades suppress selectively the M-pathway, probably at the level of the LGN, while sparing or even enhancing the P-pathway. This suggestion is also supported by recent measurements of increment thresholds for large monochromatic patches against a white background (Uchikawa and Sato, 1995). For brief presentations, thresholds follow the V_λ sensitivity curve, determined primarily by the M-pathway (Lee *et al.*, 1988; Zrenner, 1983). During saccades, however, the curves become double-peaked, indicating chromatical opponency, similar to the response of P-cells (Zrenner, 1983). There is also evidence that displacement thresholds for equiluminant stimuli are unaffected during saccades, while those for luminance defined stimuli increase by 50 per cent (Macknick *et al.*, 1991).

As the M-pathway provides the major input to the putative motion centres (Maunsell *et al.*, 1990), suppression of this pathway would explain why motion perception is dampened during saccades. The M-pathway also provides the predominant input to the associative areas of the parietal visual cortex (Ungerleider and Desimone, 1986) thought to be highly implicated in visual attention (see, for example, Grüsser and Landis, 1991). Suppression of this input may account for the fact that large-field motion during saccades does not command *attention* as it does in normal vision (Burr *et al.*, 1982), and that observers are unaware of changing letter case during saccades (McConkie and Zola, 1979). The unimpaired or even enhanced function of the parvo pathway during saccades may in some way help to preserve the continuity of vision during saccades.

4.2.7   ACKNOWLEDGEMENTS

This work was supported by the Australian Research Council and the Italian *Consiglio Nazionale delle Ricerche*, targetted grant PF Robotica 93.00926.PF67.

4.2.8   REFERENCES

ANDERSON, S.J. & BURR, D.C. (1987) Receptive field sizes of human motion detectors, *Vision Research*, **27**, 621–635.

ANDERSON, S.J., BURR, D.C. & M.C. MORRONE (1991) The two-dimensional spatial and spatial frequency properties of motion sensitive mechanisms in human vision, *Journal of the Optical Society of America*, A **8**, 1340–1351.

BONDS, A.B. (1992) Spatial and temporal nonlinearities in receptive fields of the cat striate cortex. In: Pinter, R.B. & Nabet, B. (Eds) *Nonlinear Vision: Determination of Neural Receptive Fields, Functions and Networks*, CRC Press, pp. 329–352.

BURR, D.C. & MORRONE, M.C. (1993) Impulse response functions for chromatic and achromatic stimuli, *Journal of the Optical Society of America*, A **10**, 1706–1713.

BURR, D.C. & ROSS, J. (1982) Contrast sensitivity at high velocities, *Vision Research*, **22** 479–484.

BURR, D.C., HOLT, J., JOHNSTONE, J.R. & ROSS, J. (1982) Selective depression of motion sensitivity during saccades, *Journal of Physiology*, **333**, 1–15.

BURR, D.C., MORRONE, M.C. & ROSS, J. (1994) Selective suppression of the magnocellular visual pathway during saccadic eye movements, *Nature*, **371**, 511–513.

DEYOE, E.A. & VAN ESSEN, D.C. (1988) Concurrent processing streams in the visual cortex, *TINS*, **11**, 219–226.

DERRINGTON, A.M. (1984) Spatial frequency selectivity of remote pattern masking, *Vision Research*, **24**, 1965–1968.

DERRINGTON, A.M. & LENNIE, P. (1984) Spatial and temporal contrast sensitivities of neurones in lateral geniculate nucleus of macaque, *Journal of Physiology*, **357**, 219–240.

DODGE, R. (1900) Visual perception during eye movements, *Psychological Review*, 7, 454–465.

FIELD, D.J. (1987) Relations between the statistics of natural images and the response properties of cortical cells, *Journal of the Optical Society of America*, A **4**, 2379–2394.

GRÜSSER, O-J. & LANDIS, T. (1991) In: Cronly-Dillon, J.R. (Ed.) *Vision and Visual Dysfunction: Visual Agnosias and Other Disturbances of Visual Perception and Cognition*, London: MacMillan.

ILG, U.J. & HOFFMANN, K-P (1993) Motion perception during saccades, *Vision Research*, **33**, 211–220.

KRAUSKOPF, J., GRAF, V. & GAARDNER, K. (1966) Lack of inhibition during involuntary saccades, *American Journal of Psychology*, **79**, 73–81.

LATOUR, P.L. (1962) Visual threshold during eye movements, *Vision Research*, **2**, 261–262.

LEE, B.B., MARTIN, P.R. & VALBERG, A. (1988) The physiological basis of heterochromatic flicker photometry demonstrated in the ganglion cells of the macaque retina, *Journal of Physiology*, **404**, 223–243.

LEE, B.B., MARTIN, P.R. & VALBERG, A. (1989) Amplitude and phase of responses of macaque retinal ganglion cells to flickering stimuli, *Journal of Physiology*, **414**, 245–263.

LEE, B.B., POKORNY, J., SMITH, V., MARTIN, P.R. & VALBERG, A. (1990) Luminance and chromatic modulation sensitivity of macaque ganglion cells and human observers, *Journal of the Optical Society of America*, A **7**, 2223–2236.

MACKAY, D.M. (1970) Elevation of visual threshold by displacement of visual images, *Nature*, **225**, 90–92.

MACKNIK, S.L., BRIDGEMAN, B. & SWITKES, E. (1991) Saccadic suppression of displacement at isoluminance, *Investigative Ophthalmology and Visual Science*, **32** (Suppl.), 899.

MATIN, E. (1974) Saccadic suppression: a review and an analysis, *Psychological Bulletin*, **81**, 899–917.

MAUNSELL, J.H.R., NEARLY, T.A. & DePRIEST, D.D. (1990) Magnocellular and parvocellular contributions in the middle temporal visual area (MT) of the macaque monkey, *Journal of Neuroscience*, **10**, 3323–3334.

McCONKIE, G.W. & ZOLA, D. (1979) Is visual information integrated across successive fixations in reading? *Perception and Psychophysics*, **25**, 221–224.

MERIGAN, W.H. (1991) P and M pathway specialization in the macaque. In: Valberg, A. & Lee, B.B. (Eds) *From Pigments to Perception*, New York: Plenum Press, pp 117–126.

MERIGAN, W.H. & MAUNSELL, J.H.R. (1993) How parallel are the primate visual pathways? *Annual Review Neuroscience*, **16**, 369–402.

MERIGAN, W.H., KATZ, L.M. & MAUNSELL, J.H.R. (1991) The effects of parvocellular lateral geniculate lesions on acuity and contrast sensitivity of macaque monkeys, *Journal of Neuroscience*, **11**, 994–1001.

OHZAWA, I., SCHLAR, G. & FREEMAN, R.D. (1982) Contrast gain control in the cat's visual cortex, *Nature*, **298**, 5871–5873.

RIGGS, L.A., MERTON, P.A. & MORTON, H.B. (1974) Suppression of visual phosphenes during saccadic eye movements, *Vision Research*, **14**, 997–1011.

ROUFS, J.A.J. (1972) Dynamic properties of vision-II. Theoretical relationships between flicker and flash thresholds, *Vision Research*, **12**, 279–292.

SCHLAR, G., MAUNSELL, J.H.R. & LENNIE, P. (1990) Coding of image contrast in central visual pathways of the macaque monkey, *Vision Research*, **30**, 1–10.

SHIORI, S. & CAVANAGH, P. (1989) Saccadic suppression of low-level motion, *Vision Research*, **29**, 915–928.

UCHIKAWA, K & IKEDA, I. (1986) Temporal integration of chromatic double pulses for detection of equal-luminance wavelength changes, *Journal of the Optical Society of America*, **A 3**, 2109–2115.

UCHIKAWA, K. & SATO, M. (1995) Saccadic suppression of achromatic and chromatic responses measured by increment-threshold spectral sensitivity, *Journal of the Optical Society of America*, **A 12**, 661–666.

UNGERLEIDER, L.G. & DESIMONE, R. (1986) Cortical projections of visual area MT in the macaque, *Journal of Comparative Neurology*, **248**, 147–163.

WATSON, A.B. & NACHMIAS, J. (1977) Patterns of temporal interaction in the detection of gratings, *Vision Research*, **17**, 893–902.

WATSON, A.B. & PELLI, D.G. (1983) QUEST: A Bayesian adaptive psychometric method, *Perceptive Psychophysics*, **33**, 113–120.

ZRENNER, E. (1983) Neurophysiological aspects of colour vision mechanisms in the primate retina. In: Mollon, J.D. & Sharpe, L.T. (Eds) *Colour Vision: Physiology and Psychophysics*, London: Academic Press, pp. 195-210.

Effects of Colour Difference on Perceptual Fading

Hiroyasu Ujike, K. Yokoi and Keiji Uchikawa

4.3.1 INTRODUCTION

When a small low contrast stimulus is seen peripherally with strict fixation, it tends to fade within several seconds and the region of the stimulus is filled in by the surround. Recently, this fading was shown to be facilitated by dynamic noise backgrounds (Ramachandran *et al.*, 1993; Spillmann and Kurtenbach, 1992). Ramachandran *et al.* (1993) suggested that the fading occurred by the selective fatigue of neural detectors for edges and neural representation of the surround in the stimulus region.

The importance of the edge information has been discussed for filling-in of colour and brightness information to a region defined by edge information (Grossberg and Mingolla, 1985; Paradiso and Nakayama, 1991). Yokoi *et al.* (1994) found that when the luminance difference between a target and the surround became larger, the time for a target to disappear got longer. This may be explained by the selective fatigue of edge detectors taking longer for a higher luminance edge.

The edge information can be provided not only by luminance but also by texture, motion and colour. Although the border defined only by colour (equiluminant with surround) is often said to be weak, the target does not disappear instantaneously. Tansley *et al.* (1983) argued that the border defined only by colour is elicited by the difference of responses of L cone and M cone.

Our concern in this study was to investigate what determines the time for fading of a target defined only by colour, and if dynamic noise backgrounds defined by luminance difference or colour difference facilitate the fading.

4.3.2 EXPERIMENT 1

4.3.2.1 Method

Figure 4.3.1(a) shows the stimulus configuration. The stimuli were generated by a Macintosh IIci computer and presented on an Apple Color 13-inch High Resolution Monitor with eight bit luminance levels for each of the red, green and blue phosphors. The stimulus was viewed binocularly at a distance of 60 cm. The size of the stimulus was 23.6

(a)   **(b)**

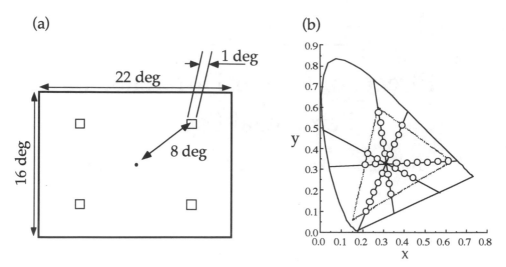

Figure 4.3.1. (a) Stimulus configuration and (b) the chromaticity co-ordinates of the target colours.

× 17.0 cm or 22.2 × 16.1 deg. A small target (1.0 × 1.0 deg) was presented at one of four possible positions, shown in the figure, at 7.9 deg eccentricity from a black fixation point (20 arc min in diameter). The surround of the target was white with a luminance of 16.0 cdm^{-2}. The chromaticity coordinates of the white background were $x = 0.31$ and $y = 0.33$.

Thirty different colours of the target were used; the chromaticities of those colours are shown as small open circles in Figure 4.3.1(b). In this figure a region surrounded by dotted lines indicates the chromaticities of colours that the monitor could generate. The luminance of each colour target was determined by flicker-photometry for each observer so that the target and the surround had the same luminance. In flicker photometry, the stimulus configuration was the same as in Figure 4.3.1(a).

The observers' task was to respond immediately when the target faded and was filled in by the surround. After adapting to a white uniform field for three minutes, the first trial started. Between every trial, the white adapting field was again presented for 15 seconds to reduce the effect of adapting to the target. In each trial, the observer indicated readiness for the trial, and then a target stimulus was presented. The observer fixated on the central black dot and responded using a keyboard when the target disappeared and was filled in by the background. Observers were instructed to reduce eye blinks. Each observer redid the trial if he thought necessary because of his eye movements or eye blinks.

In this experiment each target colour was presented twice for each stimulus position for each observer. Thus, the total of the trials from an observer was 240, which was done in four sessions. The order of the stimuli was randomised.

4.3.2.2 Results

Figure 4.3.2 shows examples of results of fading time as a function of distance from the surround white on the chromaticity diagram. The left-hand plot was obtained from targets of which colours were yellowish green on a tritanopic confusion line, and the right-hand plot from targets of which colours were orange on the line between white and chromaticity coordinates of R phosphor of the monitor. The solid line in each graph is a best fit to the results. From this graph we can see that the fading time increases as the distance from white increases; however, the inclination of the line is steeper in the right-hand than in the left hand plot. In order to see the difference of the inclination between the dominant wavelengths, in the chromaticity diagram of Figure 4.3.3 we plotted the point for fading times of 5, 10, 15 second and so on, which were determined by the fitted line in Figure 4.3.2. Solid ellipses, which are contours of equal fading time, in the graph were fitted by eye for each fading time. From this graph we can confirm the above finding of an increase of fading time with the increase of distance from the surrounding white.

To make clear what determines the fading time, the data shown in Figure 4.3.3 are

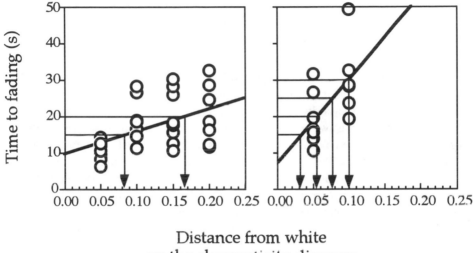

Distance from white
on the chromaticity diagram

Figure 4.3.2. Example results of fading time as a function of distance from white.

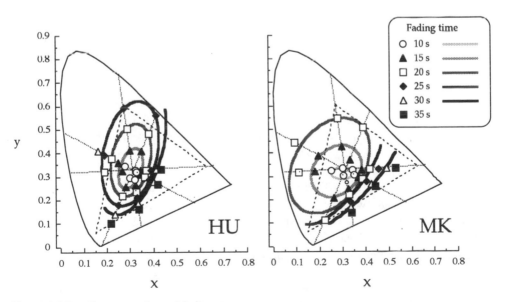

Figure 4.3.3. Contours of equal fading time.

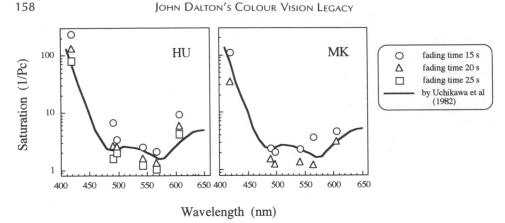

Figure 4.3.4.   Saturation corresponding to fading time.

transformed to the scale of purity, and plotted in Figure 4.3.4. The abscissa represents the dominant wavelength, and the ordinate represents the saturation, which is just the reciprocal value of colorimetric purity. We compared these plotted values with the saturation function derived by Uchikawa *et al.* (1982). The saturation function is shown as solid line. This function was derived by equating the various dominant wavelengths for saturation in a suprathreshold method. The data we got is well fit to that saturation function. Although the well-known saturation discrimination function of Priest and Brickwedde (1938) is not shown here, it seems a poorer fit to our data than that of Uchikawa *et al.* The feature of Uchikawa's saturation function that is different from Priest's is that the saturation values between 480 and 590 nm are almost the same, even though the value of 570 nm is the smallest. This might come from using a suprathreshold method rather than a discrimination method. As all the target colours in our experiment are discriminable from white, it is reasonable that our data corresponds to Uchikawa's saturation function.

4.3.3   EXPERIMENT 2

4.3.3.1 Method

The apparatus and the stimulus configuration, except the dynamic random noise (DRN) surrounds, used in this experiment were the same as Experiment 1. There are three different kinds of surrounds: (a) DRN that consisted of small squares defined by two different luminance (dark and light), (b) DRN that consisted of small squares defined by two different opponent colours (red and green), and (c) uniform white field of the chromaticity co-ordinates $(x, y) = (0.32, 0.33)$ with the luminance of 16.0 cdm^{-2}. The random noises of (a) or (b) were squares with the size of 20×20 min arc, and were randomly distributed on the surround field with 50 per cent dark (or red) and 50 per cent light (or green). The luminance or colour of each square in the dynamic random noise backgrounds was randomly changed: the temporal frequency will be described below.

The luminances of dots in surround (a) were 9.6 and 22.4 cdm^{-2}; thus, the mean luminance was 16.0 cdm^{-2}, and the contrast 40 per cent. The two colours in surround (b) were chosen in the following way. One colour, green, was chosen as the chromaticity co-ordinates $(x, y) = (0.22, 0.38)$. And then the other colour, red, was determined so that the spatially additive mixture colour of the two became nearly the same as the white of surround (c). In this procedure, the luminances of all the colour stimuli were equated by flicker photometry with the white.

This experiment consisted of two parts. In part 1, nine different colours of the target were used; all the colours were on the tritanopic confusion line through white, and were used also in Experiment 1. The surrounds were three kinds mentioned above, and the frequency of the dynamic noise backgrounds was 10 Hz. In part 2, three different colours (greenish yellow, purple and orange) of the target were used; the chromaticity co-ordinates of those were $(x, y) = (0.37, 0.47), (0.27, 0.24)$ and $(0.46, 0.34)$. The first two colours were included in the target colours in part 1. Only the DRN of luminance and colour were used, and the frequencies of those were varied in seven steps between 1 and 30 Hz.

The procedure in this experiment is the same as that of Experiment 1. In part 1, all the stimulus conditions (the combinations of nine target colours, three different backgrounds and four target positions) were randomised and divided into two sessions. This was done twice; thus, a total of 216 trials were performed.

In part 2, all the stimulus conditions (the combinations of three target colours, seven different frequencies of the backgrounds and four target positions) were randomised and divided into two sessions. This was done twice; thus, the total of 168 trials were performed for observer HU. For observer MK, only two stimulus positions were performed twice; thus, the total of 126 trials were done.

4.3.3.2 Results

Figure 4.3.5 shows the results of part 1. The abscissa represents the distance from the white on the chromaticity diagram; positive values mean the colour of yellowish green side, and negative values mean the colour of purple side. The ordinate represents the time for the target to disappear. The symbols show the background conditions: open circle means the white surround, filled triangle the DRN of luminance, and open square the DRN of colour.

The graph shows that the fading time increases with the absolute value of the distance, as shown in Experiment 1. Moreover, the fading time with the white surround was largest, while the fading time of luminance DRN was slightly larger than that of colour DRN. This result indicates that the dynamic random noise backgrounds of luminance difference and colour difference facilitate the perceptual fading of equiluminance colour target.

Figure 4.3.6 shows the results of part 2. The abscissa represents the frequency of dynamic noise backgrounds. The ordinate represents, again, the time for the target to disappear. The symbols show the target colour conditions: open circle means the greenish yellow, the open triangle the purple, and the open square the orange.

We can see in this graph that the fading time decreases as the frequency increases with the luminance DRN surround while the fading time was almost constant with colour DRN surround. Moreover, the fading times for the three different targets were different with the luminance DRN surround while the fading time did not depend on the target colours with the colour DRN surround. These results indicate that the dynamic random noise surrounds of luminance difference and colour difference have different effect on the perceptual fading of equiluminance colour target.

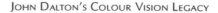

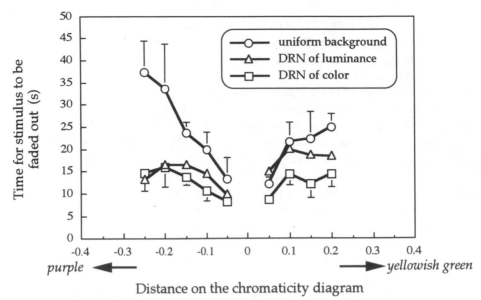

Figure 4.3.5.   Fading time with three different surrounds as a function of distance from white.

4.3.4   DISCUSSION

The detecting boundary in visual field is the basis of our visual perception, and might be related to perceptual fading. The boundary is usually determined by discontinuities of the amount of light, especially by luminance difference. The boundary determined by colour has also been investigated by several authors (e.g. Kaiser *et al.*, 1971; Tansley and Valberg, 1979). Kaiser *et al.* suggested that the distinctness of chromatic borders is related to the saturation difference, while Tansley and Valberg argue that only L and M cones contributed to the chromatic border perception. The difference of their arguments is in the contribution

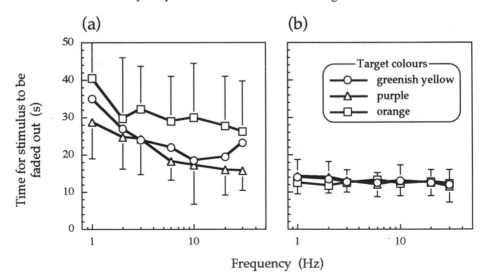

Figure 4.3.6.   Fading time as a function of the frequencies of dynamic random noise of luminance (a) and colour (b).

of S cone. Kaiser and Boynton (1985) reported that a small contribution of S cone for chromatic border can be seen by changing the observer's criteria. Moreover, Kimura (1991) showed that the contribution of S cone to the saturation discrimination function changes with luminance level. Thus, the perception of chromatic borders may be derived by saturation differences.

As for the perceptual fading, our results suggested that the fading time of equiluminance colour target surrounded by white field is determined by the saturation of the target. Considering Ramachandran's idea that the fading occurred by the selective fatigue of edge detectors, the results are consistent with the above discussion of the chromatic border perception. The increase in saturation difference makes the chromatic border clearer, and therefore the fatigue of the edge detectors may be harder to occur.

The saturation function, well fit to our data, derived by Uchikawa *et al.* (1982) is somehow different from the well-known saturation discrimination function in light of the fact that Uchikawa's function has a larger dip near 500nm. This difference is similar to that of the saturation discrimination functions under higher and lower luminance conditions reported by Kimura (1991); thus, there may be the contribution of S cone in our results. However, we do not know if that contribution in our study is derived because the saturation difference is suprathreshold, or because the target was observed peripherally.

The results in Experiment 2 showed: (a) the fading times of different equiluminant colour targets were almost the same with colour DRN, (b) while those depended on the target colours with luminance DRN, and (c) the fading time was almost constant across the frequencies of colour DRN, while that was smaller with the higher frequencies of luminance DRN. The above two seem to reveal the different mechanisms: chromatic and achromatic channels. However, the (a) may depend on target colours, because Figure 4.3.5 shows that under colour DRN condition, there is a small increase of fading time as the distance from white on the chromaticity diagram increases.

Although the results in Experiment 2 are far from conclusions, we speculate that the (a) may be due to the two colours of the colour DRN: red and green on the deuteranopic confusion line. The reason is that saturation is determined by the opponent system of L and M cone with small contribution of S cone. We also speculate that the (b) may be due to the different saturations between the colour targets. Frome *et al.* (1981) reported that perception of borders is derived by luminance and colour difference independently. Thus, the saturation effect on fading time may not be reduced by the luminance DRN.

4.3.5 REFERENCES

FROME, F. S., BUCK, S. L. & BOYNTON, R. M. (1981) Visibility of borders: separate and combined effects of color differences, luminance contrast, and luminance level, *Journal of the Optical Society of America*, **71**, 145–150.

GROSSBERG, S. & MINGOLLA, E. (1985) Neural dynamics of perceptual grouping: Textures, boundaries, and emergent segmentations, *Perception and Psychophysics*, **38**, 141–171.

KAISER, P. K. & BOYNTON, R. M. (1985) Role of the blue mechanism in wavelength discrimination, *Vision Research*, **25**, 523–529.

KAISER, P. K., HERZBERG, P. A. & BOYNTON, R. M. (1971) Chromatic border distinctness and its relation to saturation, *Vision Research*, **11**, 953–968.

KIMURA, E. (1991) Effects of luminance level on the saturation function: Sensitivities based on saturation discrimination, *Color Research and Application*, **16**, 289–296.

PARADISO, M. A. & NAKAYAMA, K. (1991) Brightness perception and filling-in, *Vision Research*, **31**, 1221–1236.

PRIEST, I. G. & BRICKWEDDE, F. G. (1938) The minimum perceptible colorimetric purity as a function of dominant wave-length, *Journal of the Optical Society of America*, **28**, 133–139.

RAMACHANDRAN, V. S., GREGORY, R. L. & AIKEN, W. (1993) Perceptual fading of visual texture borders, *Vision Research*, **33**, 717–721.

SPILLMANN, L. & KURTENBACH, A. (1992) Dynamic noise backgrounds facilitate target fading, *Vision Research*, **32**, 1941–1946.

TANSLEY, B. W. & VALBERG, A. (1979) Chromatic border distinctness: Not an index of hue or saturation differences, *Journal of the Optical Society of America*, **69**, 113–118.

TANSLEY, B. W., ROBERTSON, A. W. & MAUGHAN, K. E. (1983) Chromatic and achromatic border perception: A two-cone model accounts for suprathreshold border distinctness judgments and cortical pattern-evoked response amplitudes to the same stimuli. In: Mollon, J. D. & Sharpe, L. T. (Eds) *Colour Vision*, London: Academic Press, pp. 445–453.

UCHIKAWA, K., UCHIKAWA, H. & KAISER, P. K. (1982) Equating colors for saturation and brightness: the relationship to luminance, *Journal of the Optical Society of America*, **72**, 1219–1224.

YOKOI, K., UCHIKAWA, K., UJIKE, H. & NAKANO, Y. (1994) 'Effects of dynamic noise on filling-in', presentation at The 41st Spring Meeting of The Japan Society of Applied Physics and Related Societies, Kanagawa, March.

Spatial and Temporal Sensitivities of Colour Discrimination Mechanisms

D.J. McKeefry and J.J. Kulikowski

4.4.1 INTRODUCTION

Functional segregation is a strategy employed by the visual system whereby the parallel and simultaneous analysis of various attributes of a visual scene such as colour, form and movement, can take place (Livingstone and Hubel, 1988). In the case of colour vision it is the parvocellular (P) system, the constituent neurones of which possess tonic or sustained response properties, which forms the conduit of information from the retina to parvo-recipient layers of the striate cortex (Merigan, 1989; Schiller *et al.*, 1990). Within the striate cortex the cytochrome oxidase blobs appear to be a major locus for colour processing (Livingstone and Hubel, 1984) and these areas project to the thin stripes of area V2, which in turn project to the extra-striate area, V4 (Shipp and Zeki, 1985).

Colour vision in the primate visual system is ultimately based upon the responses of three cone types; the long, medium and short wavelength sensitive cones (L, M and S cones). The S cones have a much sparser population than either the L or M cones, comprising only 3–10 per cent of the total cone population in macaques and humans (Ahnelt *et al.*, 1987; Curcio *et al.*, 1991).

Each of the cone types have different but largely overlapping spectral sensitivities and, therefore, chromatic contrast detection is enhanced by the opponent interaction of the cone outputs at some post-receptoral stage. As predicted by Hering (1878) a red-green colour opponent channel is formed by the opponent interaction of L and M cones (L/M) and a blue-yellow channel by the opponent interaction of S cones and an additive L and M cone output (S/(L + M).

The paucity of S cones is reflected in the ganglion cell layer of the primate retina where the numbers of colour opponent ganglion cells receiving S cone input are reduced in comparison to those receiving L and M cone inputs (Creutzfeldt *et al.*, 1979; DeMonasterio and Gouras, 1975; Malpeli and Schiller, 1978; Valberg *et al.*, 1986; Zrenner and Gouras, 1981). This domination of input to chromatically sensitive neurones by the red-green (L/M) system over the blue-yellow (S/L + M) system continues at the level of the striate cortex. Livingstone and Hubel (1984) report that a majority of chromatic neurones in the blobs in the upper layers of V1 receive L/M inputs. In addition Ts'o and Gilbert (1988) found that they could characterise blobs upon the basis of whether they were involved in red-green or blue-yellow analysis, the former outnumbering the latter by a ratio of 3:1.

In view of the fact that a larger proportion of the neurones in the colour processing stream appear to be devoted to the red-green colour opponent system, it was perhaps not surprising that results from psychophysical studies tended to promote the system receiving input from the S cones as a system of low sensitivity and low resolution (Brindley *et al.*, 1966; Green, 1969; Van der Horst and Bouman, 1969). However, contradicting this view is evidence to suggest that the spatio-temporal properties of the L/M and S/(L + M) colour mechanisms are more closely matched than at first realised (Mullen, 1985; Smith *et al.*, 1984).

This study aims to examine the spatio-temporal properties of the blue-yellow colour opponent system compared to those of the red-green system. Employing selective stimulation of the two opponent systems, we propose to examine the nature of chromatic contrast detection and determine whether the red-green and blue-yellow systems are fundamentally different in terms of their psychophysical properties. The selective stimulation of the colour opponent pathways is achieved by the use of isoluminant, chromatic stimuli that modulate along the cardinal colour axes of Krauskopf *et al.* (1982) and are free from the confounding effects of chromatic aberrations. The use of the blue-yellow cardinal axis provides an additional benefit in the search for increased selectivity as it constitutes stimulation of the S-cone recipient system along a tritanopic confusion line. This precludes any involvement from the L and M cones in the detection of such stimuli.

4.4.2   METHODS

Sinusoidal, isoluminant bichromatic gratings were produced by the optical combination, in anti-phase, of two monochromatic gratings produced on separate Joyce cathode ray tube displays. In addition, achromatic or luminance gratings could be generated simply by the combination of the two gratings in-phase.

One of the two displays could be placed at varying distances from the observer's eye, thus allowing for the correction of longitudinal chromatic aberration between specific colour combinations. Transverse chromatic aberration, which introduces spatial frequency differences between two colours, was eliminated by the adjustment of the time base and raster size of one of the displays.

The colours of the two constituent monochromatic gratings were produced by the introduction of broadband filters into the paths of the two displays. In order to produce appropriate hues for stimulation along the cardinal axes of Krauskopf *et al.* (1982) in CIE colour space, it was often necessary to use combinations of Lee broadband filters; for blue (165 + 180), yellow (104 + 121), red (148) and green (165 + 174 + 122). Isoluminance of the chromatic stimuli was checked by empirical equalisation of the luminances of the constituent coloured gratings, employing a Photo Research PR1500 photometer. Further verification of isoluminance was achieved by the subjective technique of heterochromatic flicker photometry.

The subjects, both colour normals, DMcK a 26-year-old myope and JJK a 58-year-old presbyope (both with 6/5 corrected acuity), viewed the stimulus monocularly through a 5 mm artificial pupil. Pupil dilatation was achieved by the instillation of 1% Tropicamide. Steady fixation of the stimulus was facilitated by the presence of central fixation spots placed in the centre of each Joyce display screen. The strict maintenance of the alignment of these two spots throughout the experiment was further aided by means of a dental bite-bar, which minimised head movements.

Detection thresholds were set by method of adjustment for chromatic and achromatic gratings presented in pattern onset/offset and pattern reversal modes. Contrast was expressed in terms of the Michelson contrast ($L_{max} - L_{min}/L_{max} + L_{min}$) of the constituent monochromatic gratings.

The stimuli viewed consisted of a minimum of three cycles with a mean luminance of either 60, 480 or 600 photopic trolands. However, for the spatial contrast sensitivity assessments, as the spatial frequency of the grating increased, the visual angle subtended by the stimulus was never less than one degree. This was so as not to encroach upon the region of foveal tritanopia (Williams *et al.*, 1981), a region from which the S cones are absent. For the temporal modulation sensitivity experiments, the spatial frequency of the stimulus was a constant 0.85 cycles per degree producing a field size of 4.3 degrees.

4.4.3   RESULTS

Figures 4.4.1 and 4.4.2 illustrate spatial and temporal contrast sensitivity functions, obtained for blue-yellow and red-green stimulation for subjects DMcK and JJK. The utilisation of isoluminant, chromatic aberration-free gratings enables the observers to set colour detection thresholds, where the component colours of the red-green and blue-yellow gratings are identifiable close to threshold.

Examination of the on/off presentation sensitivity (filled triangles) reveals a close degree of similarity between the L/M and S/(L + M) systems in both the spatial and temporal domains. When linear regression lines are fitted to the data points and extrapolated to 100 per cent modulation on semi-logarithmic co-ordinates, an estimate of resolution is possible. Employing this technique, both spatial and temporal resolutions were also found to be comparable for the two opponent systems. In the case of subject DMcK, the value of spatial resolution obtained for the L/M system is approximately 11 cdeg^{-1} compared to 10 cdeg^{-1} for the S/(L + M) system; the values of temporal resolution are 25 Hz and 20 Hz for the L/M and S/(L + M) systems, respectively. Thus, there appears to be a close match between the spatio-temporal properties of the L/M and S/(L + M) colour opponent systems in terms of their sensitivity and resolution limits.

The comparison of on/off and reversal sensitivity allows the assessment of the contribution of transient and sustained mechanisms to the detection of grating stimuli (Kulikowski and Tolhurst, 1973). For tritanopic blue-yellow stimuli, onset and reversal sensitivity are equal, indicating that sustained mechanisms, dependent upon standing levels of contrast, subserve detection. For red-green stimuli reversal sensitivity is observed to be greater than that for onset presentations. An increase of a factor of two is indicative of transient mechanisms, dependent upon contrast change, subserving detection (Kulikowski and Tolhurst, 1973). However, for red-green reversal presentation the increase in sensitivity is less than a factor of two times greater than onset sensitivity. This implies that the detection of red-green isoluminant gratings is largely of a sustained nature for on/off presentations, but that the threshold of some transient mechanism is very close, hence its contribution to reversal detection is noticeable.

Figures 4.4.3 and 4.4.4 illustrate what happens to the spatial and temporal chromatic contrast sensitivity functions when chromatic aberration is not corrected. As may be observed from Figure 4.4.3, on/off sensitivity for spatial frequencies less than 3 cdeg^{-1} is comparable to the sensitivity obtained for aberration-free gratings (Figure 4.4.3b). Reversal sensitivity, however, is increased, indicating a greater contribution from transient mechanisms to the detection of such stimuli. At higher spatial frequencies, the introduction of chromatic aberration appears to increase the sensitivity and the resolution of the visual system above that attainable by the colour opponent system. It was observed that within this region of higher sensitivity, induced via the introduction of chromatic aberrations, the

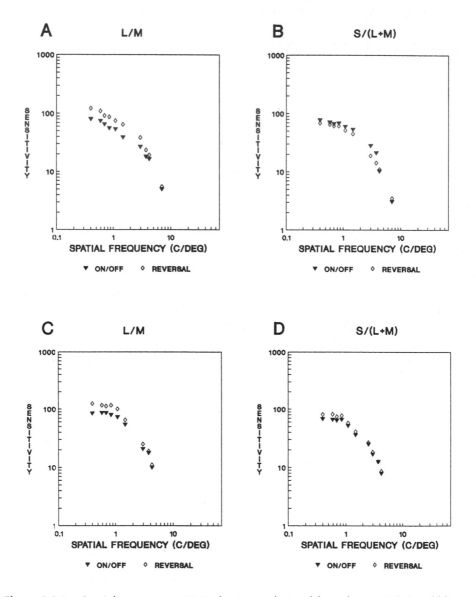

Figure 4.4.1. Spatial contrast sensitivity functions obtained for red-green (L/M) and blue-yellow (S/(L + M)) gratings for subjects DMcK (A and B) and JJK (C and D). On/off (filled triangles) and reversal (open diamonds) are illustrated. Mean retinal illuminance = 600 photopic trolands, temporal presentation rate = 1 Hz.

constituent colours of gratings were not identifiable close to threshold (as in the case of the detection thresholds set for aberration-free chromatic stimuli). Instead, the gratings appeared 'pseudochromatic', i.e. there did appear to be a coloured pattern present but the component colours of the stimulus could not be correctly identified.

Figure 4.4.4 illustrates a similar phenomenon in the temporal domain. Sensitivity (in this case for reversal presentations) is observed to be markedly increased at temporal fre-

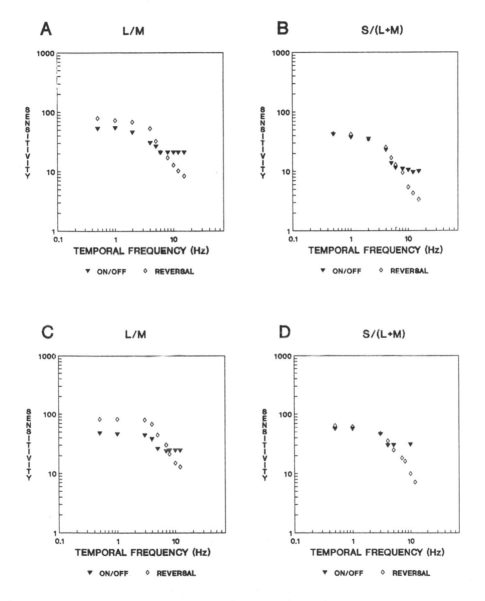

Figure 4.4.2. Temporal contrast sensitivity functions obtained for red-green (L/M) and blue-yellow (S/(L + M)) gratings for subjects DMcK (A and B) and JJK (C and D). On/off (filled triangles) and reversal (open diamonds) are illustrated. Mean retinal illuminance = 480 photopic trolands, spatial frequency = 0.85 cdeg^{-1}.

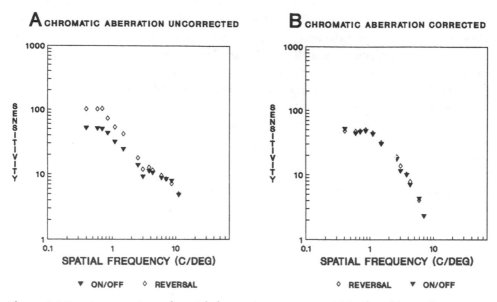

Figure 4.4.3. A comparison of spatial chromatic contrast sensitivity for a blue-yellow grating under conditions when chromatic aberrations are uncorrected (A) and when the stimulus is chromatic aberration-free (B). Mean retinal illuminance = 60 photopic trolands, temporal presentation rate = 1 Hz. Subject JJK.

quencies greater than 4 Hz when chromatic aberration is not corrected. Between 5 Hz and 8 Hz the pseudochromatic function exhibits a localised maxima, similar to that which is

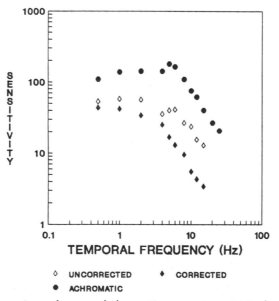

Figure 4.4.4. A comparison of temporal chromatic contrast sensitivity for a blue-yellow grating under chromatic aberration-free (filled diamonds) conditions and when chromatic aberration is uncorrected (open diamonds). Only reversal sensitivities are illustrated in addition to the achromatic temporal function (filled circles). Mean retinal illuminance = 480 photopic trolands, spatial frequency = 0.85 cdeg^{-1}. Subject DMcK.

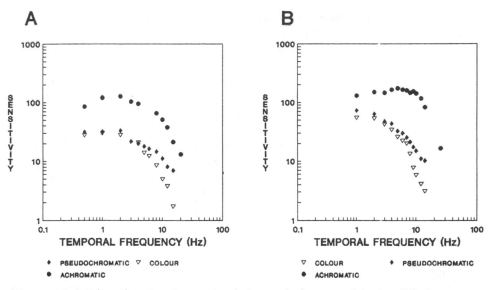

Figure 4.4.5. Colour detection (open triangles), pseudochromatic detection (filled diamonds) and achromatic detection (filled circles) thresholds for a 0.85 cdeg⁻¹ blue-yellow grating. (A) Subject DMcK, 60 photopic trolands. (B) Subject JJK, 480 photopic trolands.

exhibited by the achromatic function also illustrated. Colour detection thresholds, on the other hand, exhibit no such peak.

Following these experiments we re-examined the detection of aberration-free stimuli and found that separable colour detection and pseudochromatic thresholds could also be set for these stimuli. Figure 4.4.5 illustrates the results of such an experiment performed with a temporally modulated stimulus. At low temporal frequencies the sensitivity of the colour and pseudochromatic functions appear to be similar. It is again at higher frequencies (> 4 Hz) where the two functions appear to diverge, the pseudochromatic function possessing a greater sensitivity and resolution limit than the colour opponent function. The colour detection function remains low-pass in nature and has a steeper fall-off at high temporal frequencies.

In marked difference to the pseudochromatic function obtained in the presence of chromatic aberrations, the function obtained under these conditions exhibits no localised maxima between 5 Hz and 8 Hz.

4.4.4 DISCUSSION AND CONCLUSIONS

The detection, at threshold, of chromatic aberration-free isoluminant gratings is subserved by mechanisms which allow the identification of veridical colours. Presumably it is the colour opponent channels that subserve this detection. When such chromatic aberration-free, isoluminant stimuli modulate the colour opponent systems along the cardinal red-green and blue-yellow axes, systems with closely matching spatio-temporal properties are revealed.

This matching of sensitivity and resolution between the L/M and S/(L + M) colour opponent systems occurs in spite of the disadvantages imposed upon the S cone system right from the level of the retina (e.g. Ahnelt *et al.*, 1987) to the striate cortex (e.g. Ts'o and Gilbert, 1988). The similarity between the spatio-temporal properties of these two colour opponent systems runs counter to the idea of the S cone recipient system as a system of low resolution and low sensitivity (Brindley, 1954; Brindley *et al.*, 1966; Kelly, 1974).

However, matched properties of the opponent systems are in keeping with the work of Schnapf *et al.* (1990) who have found that the temporal responses of the L, M and S cones, which form the inputs to the colour opponent mechanisms, are similar. Moreover, a study by Lennie *et al.* (1990) of the chromatic properties of neurones receiving L/M and S/ (L + M) inputs, in contrast to neurones in the striate cortex failed to reveal a simple bimodal distribution of neurones in the lateral geniculate nucleus (Derrington *et al.*, 1984). Instead, cells appeared to be tuned to a variety of different colour axes other than the L/M and S/ (L + M) cardinal axes. Such a finding may represent a reorganisation of colour analysis in the striate cortex away from the traditional opponent model, a suggestion to which psychophysical studies have also alluded (Krauskopf *et al.*, 1986; Webster and Mollon, 1991). The equality between the red-green and blue-yellow systems, therefore, may also be a reflection of such a neural re-organisation. The surplus of neurones receiving L and M cone inputs may be used to generate a number of mechanisms along differently orientated colour axes, each with similar spatio-temporal properties. However, this is as yet highly speculative and merits further psychophysical investigation.

In addition to the veridical colour detection threshold a separable pseudochromatic detection threshold may also be set for chromatic stimuli. At such a threshold coloured patterns can be observed but the component colours of the grating cannot be identified. The functions that describe pseudochromatic sensitivity appear to be similar to the colour opponent functions at low spatial and temporal frequencies. At higher frequencies, however, pseudochromatic detection possesses a greater sensitivity and has a higher limit of spatial and temporal resolution. Figure 4.4.6 represents a schematic representation of the interaction between the colour opponent systems and the pseudochromatic system in the spatial and temporal domains.

The presence of a pseudochromatic function with a higher spatio-temporal resolution than the colour opponent mechanism, implies that it may constitute another separate chromatic channel other than that which is responsible for the detection of veridical colours. The suggestion that this pseudochromatic system is due simply to luminance intrusion, is refuted by the fact that the chromatic aberration-free temporal function (Figure

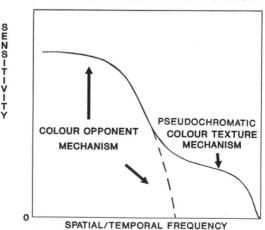

Figure 4.4.6.   A schematic representation of the spatio-temporal properties of the proposed pseudochromatic channel and its interaction with the colour opponent system.

4.4.5) exhibits no localised maxima between 5 Hz and 8 Hz. Such a maxima is indicative of luminance system involvement in detection and is evident in the achromatic functions and in the pseudochromatic functions obtained when chromatic aberrations are present (Figure 4.4.4).

The identity of this additional putative chromatic channel is uncertain. One may speculate that it constitutes a parallel pathway involved in the analysis of colour additional to the colour opponent pathways that subserve veridical colour detection. In such a case the anatomical pathway subserving this channel may differ from the parvo–blob–V2 thin stripe–V4 pathway associated with such traditional colour processing. Certainly it possesses properties very different from the colour opponent pathways. It would seem a likely candidate for the mechanism that facilitates the fusion and stereopsis of high frequency chromatic stimuli (Kulikowski, 1991) and may represent a separable processing stream involved in the processing of colour-plus-luminance or chromatic texture information.

4.4.5   SUMMARY

1. The spatial and temporal properties of the blue-yellow and red-green colour opponent systems appear to be closely matched in terms of their sensitivity and resolution limits.
2. Separable chromatic and pseudochromatic thresholds can be set for isoluminant chromatic gratings.
3. The pseudochromatic function possesses spatio-temporal properties different from the colour opponent system, and as such, it may constitute an additional chromatic channel.
4. The increased sensitivity and resolution of this putative pseudochromatic channel suggests that it could subserve the fusion and stereopsis of high spatial frequency chromatic stimuli, thus facilitating the analysis of chromatic texture.

4.4.6   REFERENCES

AHNELT, P.K., KOLB, H. & PFLUG, R. (1987) Identification of a sub-type of photoreceptor, likely to be blue sensitive, in the human retina, *Journal of Comparative Neurology*, **255**, 18–34.

BRINDLEY, G.S. (1954). The summation areas of the human colour receptive mechanisms at increment threshold, *Journal of Physiology*, **124**, 400–408.

BRINDLEY, G.S., DuCROZ, J.J. & RUSHTON, W.A.H. (1966) The flicker fusion frequency of the blue sensitive mechanism of colour vision, *Journal of Physiology*, **183**, 497–500.

CREUTZFELDT, O.D., LEE, B.B. & ELEPFANDT, A. (1979) A quantitative study of chromatic organisation and receptive fields of cells in the lateral geniculate body of the rhesus monkey, *Experimental Brain Research*, **35**, 527–545.

CURCIO, C.A., ALLEN, K.A., SLOAN, K.R., LEREA, C.L., HURLEY, J.E., KLOCK, I.B. & MILAM, A.H. (1991) Distribution and morphology of the human photoreceptors stained with anti-blue opsin, *Journal of Comparative Neurology*, **312**, 610–624.

DeMONASTERIO, F.M. & GOURAS , P. (1975) Functional properties of ganglion cells of the rhesus monkey retina, *Journal of Physiology*, **251**, 167–195.

DERRINGTON, A.M., KRAUSKOPF, J. & LENNIE, P. (1984) Chromatic mechanisms in the Lateral Geniculate Nucleus of the macaque, *Journal of Physiology*, **357**, 241–265.

GREEN, D.G. (1969) Sinusoidal flicker characteristics of the colour sensitive mechanisms of the eye, *Vision Research*, **9**, 591–601.

KELLY, D.H. (1974) Spatio-temporal frequency characteristics of colour vision mechanisms, *Journal of the Optical Society of America*, **64**, 983–990.

KRAUSKOPF, J., WILLIAMS D.R. & HEELY, D.M. (1982) The cardinal directions of colour space, *Vision Research*, **22**, 1123–1131.

KRAUSKOPF, J., WILLIAMS, D.R., MANDLER, M.B. & BROWN, A.M. (1986) Higher order colour mechanisms, *Vision Research*, **26**, 23–32.

KULIKOWSKI, J.J. (1991). Binocular chromatic rivalry and single vision, *Ophthalmic and Physiological Optics*, **12**, 168–170.

KULIKOWSKI, J.J. & TOLHURST, D.J. (1973) Psychophysical evidence for sustained and transient detectors in human vision, *Journal of Physiology*, **232**, 149–162.

LENNIE, P., KRAUSKOPF, J. & SCLAR, G. (1990) Chromatic mechanisms in the striate cortex of the macaque, *Journal of Neuroscience*, **10**, 649–669.

LIVINGSTONE, M.S. & HUBEL, D.H. (1984) Anatomy and physiology of a colour system in the primate visual cortex, *Journal of Neuroscience*, **4**, 309–356.

LIVINGSTONE, M.S. & HUBEL, D.H. (1988) Segregation of form, colour, movement and depth: anatomy, physiology and perception, *Science*, **240**, 740–750.

MALPELI, J.G. & SCHILLER, P. (1978) Lack of blue off-centre cells in the visual system of the monkey, *Brain Research*, **141**, 385–389.

MERIGAN, W.H. (1989) P and M pathway specialisation in the macaque. In: Valberg, A. & Lee, B.B. (Eds) *From Pigments to Perception: Advances in Understanding Visual Processes*, New York: Plenum Press, pp. 117–126.

MULLEN, K.T. (1985) The contrast sensitivity of human colour vision to red-green and blue-yellow gratings, *Journal of Physiology*, **395**, 381–400.

SCHILLER, P.H., LOGOTHETIS, N.K. & CHARLES, E.R. (1990) Functions of the colour opponent and broad-band channels of the visual system, *Nature*, **343**, 68–70.

SCHNAPF, J.L., NUNN, B.J., MEISTER, M. & BAYLOR, D.A. (1990) Visual transduction in cones of the monkey, *Journal of Physiology*, **427**, 681–713.

SHIPP, S.D. & ZEKI, S.M. (1985) Segregation of pathways leading from V2 to areas V4 and V5 of the macaque visual cortex, *Nature*, **315**, 322–325.

SMITH, V.C., BOWEN, R.C. & POKORNY, J. (1984) Threshold temporal integration of chromatic stimuli, *Vision Research*, **24**, 653–660.

TS'O, D.Y. & GILBERT, C.D. (1988) The organisation of chromatic and spatial interactions in the primate striate cortex, *Journal of Neuroscience*, **8**, 1712–1728.

VALBERG, A., LEE, B.B. & TRYTI, J. (1986) Neurones with strong inhibitory S-cone inputs in the macaque lateral geniculate nucleus, *Vision Research*, **26**, 1061–1064.

VAN DER HORST, G.J.C. & BOUMAN, M.A. (1969) Spatio-temporal chromaticity discrimination, *Journal of the Optical Society of America*, **59**, 1482–1488.

WEBSTER, M.A. & MOLLON, J.D. (1991) Changes in colour appearance following post-receptoral adaptation, *Nature*, **349**, 235–238.

WILLIAMS, D.R., MacLEOD, D.I.A. & HAYHOE, M.M. (1981) Foveal Tritanopia, *Vision Research*, **21**, 1341.

ZRENNER, E. & GOURAS, P. (1981) Characteristics of the blue sensitive cone mechanism in the primate retinal ganglion cells, *Vision Research*, **21**, 1605–1609.

Temporal Characteristics of Colour Discrimination

Hirohisa Yaguchi, Yasuaki Mohri, Masaki Ishiwata and Satoshi Shioiri

4.5.1 INTRODUCTION

There are a number of studies (e.g. King-Smith and Carden, 1976; Thornton and Pugh, 1983; Sperling and Harwerth, 1971) showing that the mechanism of visual detection may be described in terms of parallel luminance and opponent-colour channels. Recently, Cole *et al.* (1993) obtained detection thresholds for a 2° Gaussian-blurred spot flash of 200 ms on a white adapting field, and found that the threshold detection data were well described by the probability summation of three sets of mechanisms: L + M, L − M, and S − (L + M), each having linear cone contrast inputs. Chaparro *et al.* (1994) measured detection thresholds for foveal small flashes of 200 ms duration on a bright yellow field. They found that the most sensitive mechanism was not a luminance mechanism, but rather a red-green mechanism that responds to the linear difference of equally weighted L and M cone contrasts. Metha *et al.* (1994) measured the detection and direction discrimination thresholds using moving stimuli, and found that the luminance mechanism is directionally sensitive at detection threshold. On the other hand, there are also many studies (e.g. Kelly, 1974; Kelly and van Norren, 1977; Noorlander and Koenderink, 1983) showing that the temporal contrast sensitivity function for chromatic modulation differs from that for luminance modulation in showing no low temporal frequency attenuation and in having a lower high temporal frequency cut. These findings suggest that the colour-discrimination thresholds vary with the temporal configurations of stimulus presentation. There are, however, few studies concerned with the temporal character-istics of colour discrimination.

In the present study, we have measured colour-discrimination thresholds for various temporal conditions. The discrimination threshold data are represented in a red-, green-, and blue-primary luminance contrast space, an L-, M-, and S-cone contrast space, and the CIE 1976 $L^*a^*b^*$ (CIELAB) space.

4.5.2 METHOD

The experiments were done using a computer-controlled colour monitor. The colour of pattern components was controlled by a colour map that has 12 bits of resolution of each primary, that is, there are 4096 discrete colours between the minimum and the maximum output of each primary colour. Determination of the discrimination threshold employed here was originally developed by Cowan *et al.* (1984). In the experiment, the observer saw a brief flash of the test stimulus with a colour slightly different from a steady background colour. The background field was a square of $6° \times 6°$. The test stimulus and the background were separated with a black gap of 6 min arc width. The idea behind employing this gap is that the observer cannot use a criterion of detecting edges between the test colour and the background colour as a cue of colour discrimination. The test stimulus was presented in any one of four panes, each of them $1° \times 1°$, aligned as a 2×2 matrix with a fixation point in its centre. The observer's task was to report which of the four panes contained the test stimulus. The test patterns were presented in four different temporal conditions: a 50 ms rectangular pulse, a 200 ms rectangular pulse, a Gaussian profile with 200 ms in half width, and a 200 ms rectangular pulse preceded and succeeded by 200 ms dark rectangular blanks that we call temporal gaps. Among these temporal conditions, a 50 ms condition consists of a high temporal frequency component, a 200 ms Gaussian condition has a relatively low temporal frequency component, and a 200 ms condition is an intermediate condition. In the temporal gap condition, the observer cannot see any transient change of the background colour to the test colour.

We employed five background colours: white, red, green, yellow and blue, which the CIE has recommended for the colour difference evaluation. The CIE 1931 (x, y) chromaticity co-ordinates and the luminance of background colours are shown in Table 4.5.1.

Test stimuli are expressed in terms of the luminance contrast, that is, the increment or decrement luminance of the primary-component of test stimulus $(\Delta R, \Delta G, \Delta B)$ is divided by the luminance of the primary-component of background colour (R, G, B). Thresholds for the test stimuli along 26 different directions away from each background colour were determined. When measuring the threshold for a given direction in a colour space, the red/green/blue ratio of the test stimulus was kept constant. Thresholds were determined by the interleaved staircase method, in which the test stimuli along four different directions were presented in a random order in a single session.

4.5.3   RESULTS AND DISCUSSIONS

We plotted the discrimination threshold data in the luminance contrast space. Figure 4.5.1. shows discrimination thresholds plotted on a $\Delta R/R–\Delta G/G$ plane (upper graphs) and a $\Delta R/R–\Delta B/B$ plane (lower graphs) in the luminance contrast space. Graphs from left to right indicate the results obtained by the observer YM for five background colours, white, red, green, yellow and blue, respectively. The origin of each graph corresponds to each background colour. The straight line shows the isoluminance line for each background

Table 4.5.1. The CIE 1931 (x, y) chromaticity co-ordinates and luminance of the background colour.

Background colour	x	y	L (cd m^{-2})
white	0.314	0.331	30.0
red	0.484	0.342	14.1
green	0.248	0.362	24.0
yellow	0.388	0.428	30.0
blue	0.219	0.216	8.8

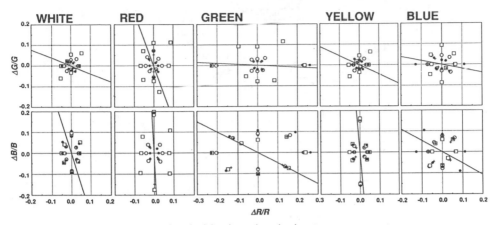

Figure 4.5.1. Discrimination thresholds plotted in the luminance-contrast space.

condition. Different symbols indicate different temporal conditions of the stimulus presentation. The experimental results show that the discrimination thresholds for a Gaussian condition (open circles) and those for a temporal gap condition (open squares) increased toward the direction of change of luminance. On the other hand, a 50 ms pulse condition (dots) shows the threshold elevation along the isoluminance plane where only colour changes. Crosses indicate the 200 ms pulse condition.

We also analysed the obtained data in the cone-contrast space ($\Delta L/L$, $\Delta M/M$, $\Delta S/S$), where ΔL, ΔM and ΔS, are the change in cone excitation in the L-, M- and S-cones due to the increment or decrement of test stimulus, and L, M and S are the cone excitation due to the background colour. The excitations of L-, M-, and S-cone for each test stimulus are calculated by the following equations,

$$L = \int E(\lambda)l(\lambda)d\lambda \tag{1}$$
$$M = \int E(\lambda)m(\lambda)d\lambda \tag{2}$$
$$S = \int E(\lambda)s(\lambda)d\lambda \tag{3}$$

where $E(\lambda)$ is the spectral radiance of the stimulus, and $l(\lambda)$, $m(\lambda)$, and $s(\lambda)$ are the spectral sensitivity functions for L-, M-, and S-cone, respectively, derived by Smith and Pokorny (1975). Figure 4.5.2 shows discrimination thresholds projected on the $\Delta L/L$–$\Delta M/M$ plane (upper graphs) and on the $\Delta L/L$–$\Delta S/S$ plane (lower graphs) for a 50 ms rectangular (left), a 200 ms Gaussian (centre) and a temporal gap condition (right). Thresholds for all background colours are plotted altogether. Different symbols indicate the different background colour; white (open circles), red (closed circles), green (open squares), yellow (crosses), and blue (open triangles). The discrimination threshold contours in the cone-excitation contrast space, particularly on the $\Delta L/L$–$\Delta M/M$ plane, vary little with the background colour but much with the temporal profile of test stimulus presentation. Discrimination thresholds for a temporal gap condition elongate toward a slope of 45°, which corresponds to pure luminance change without colour change. It is clearly shown that the discriminability along the direction of the excitation of S-cone is poorer than those of M- and L-cone.

Finally, we plotted the discrimination threshold data obtained here in the CIELAB space. Upper graphs of Figure 4.5.3. show the discrimination thresholds for a 50 ms condition (open circles) and those for a temporal gap condition (dots) projected on the Δa^*-Δb^* plane for five background colours, and lower graphs are the projections on the Δa^*-ΔL^* plane.

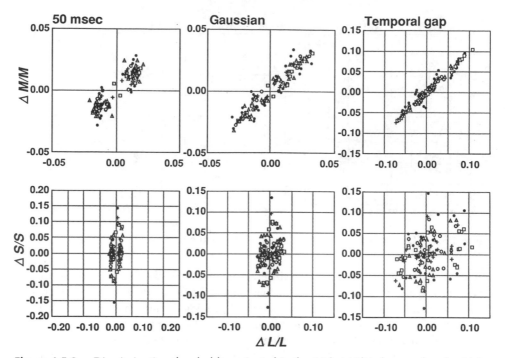

Figure 4.5.2. Discrimination thresholds projected to the ΔL/L-ΔM/M plane and to the ΔL/L-ΔS/S plane in the cone-contrast space.

These figures clearly show that the CIELAB space is not uniform in terms of colour discrimination. The differences of L^* between test stimuli and a background colour at discrimination thresholds are less than those of a^*, which means that the value of L^* is underestimated for colour discriminations. Among 26 directions of the test stimulus in the luminance contrast space, we chose three directions that are the closest to the L^*-, a^*- and b^*- axes in order to obtain the cross sections of the discrimination threshold contour and each axis of the CIELAB. Figure 4.5.4 shows ΔL^*, Δa^* and Δb^* at discrimination threshold

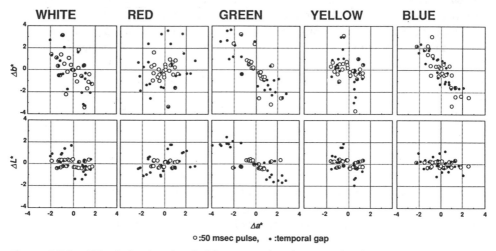

○ :50 msec pulse,   • :temporal gap

Figure 4.5.3. Discrimination thresholds projected to the Δa*-Δb* plane and to the Δa*-ΔL* plane in the CIELAB space.

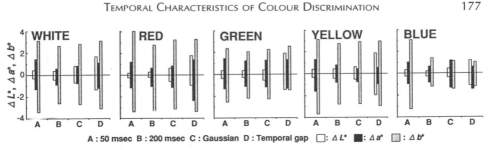

Figure 4.5.4. Differences of *L**, *a** and *b** *between* the test and the background colour at discrimination threshold near *L**-, *a**- and *b**-axis in the CIELAB space, respectively.

near *L**-, *a**- and *b**-axis, respectively. If we compare ΔL^* for different temporal conditions, discrimination thresholds for the test stimuli consisting of a low temporal frequency component such as a temporal gap condition and a Gaussian condition increase toward the *L** direction. On the other hand, discrimination thresholds along the *a**- or *b**-axis were not much affected by changing temporal profile of the test stimulus except for the blue background. Discrimination thresholds for a 50 ms condition with the blue background show an extremely large Δb^* compared with the other conditions. As the deviation of *b** roughly corresponds to changing colour between yellow and blue, the elevation of threshold for a short duration condition seems to reveal the phenomenon of transient tritanopia.

The present study will give a great role in establishing a new formula for evaluation of small colour differences.

4.5.4 REFERENCES

CHAPARRO, A., STROMEYER III, C.F., KRONAUER, R.E. & ESKEW JR, R.T. (1994) Separable red-green and luminance detectors for small flashes, *Vision Research*, **34**, 751–762.

COLE, G.R., HINE, T. & MCILHAGGA, W. (1993) Detection mechanisms in L-, M-, and S-cone contrast space, *Journal of the Optical Society of America*, A **10**, 38–51.

COWAN, W.B, WYSZECKI, G. & YAGUCHI, H. (1984) Probability summation among color channels, *Journal of the Optical Society of America*, A **1**, 1307.

KELLY, D.H. (1974) Spatio-temporal frequency characteristics of color-vision mechanisms, *Journal of the Optical Society of America*, **64**, 983–990.

KELLY, D.H. & VAN NORREN, D. (1977) Two-band model of heterochromatic flicker, *Journal of the Optical Society of America*, **67**, 1081–1091.

KING-SMITH, P.E. & CARDEN, D. (1976) Luminance and opponent-color contributions to visual detection and adaptation and to temporal and spatial integration, *Journal of the Optical Society of America*, **66**, 709–717.

METHA, A.B., VINGRYS, A.J. & BADCOCK, D.R. (1994) Detection and discrimination of moving stimuli: the effects of color, luminance, and eccentricity, *Journal of the Optical Society of America*, A **11**, 1697–1709.

NOORLANDER, C. & KOENDERINK, J.J. (1983) Spatial and temporal discrimination ellipsoids in color space, *Journal of the Optical Society of America*, **83**, 1533–1543.

SMITH, V.C. & POKORNY, J. (1975) Spectral sensitivity of the foveal cone photopigments between 400 and 500 nm, *Vision Research*, **15**, 161–171.

SPERLING, H.G. & HARWERTH, P.S. (1971) Red-green cone interactions in the increment-threshold spectral sensitivity of primates, *Science*, **172**, 180–184.

THORNTON, J.E. & PUGH JR, E.N. (1983) Red/green color opponency at detection threshold, *Science*, **219**, 191–193.

Opponent Mechanisms Revealed by Chromatic Modulation Threshold

Yasuhisa Nakano, Mitsuo Ikeda and Keiji Uchikawa

4.6.1 INTRODUCTION

Chromatically opponent mechanisms play an important role in human colour vision. Much psychophysical data, such as increment threshold (Cole *et al.*, 1993; Kalloniatis and Harwerth, 1990, 1991; Kranda and King-Smith, 1979; Sperling and Harwerth, 1971), heterochromatic brightness matching (Guth and Lodge, 1973; Ikeda and Nakano, 1986; Nakano *et al.*, 1988; Yaguchi and Ikeda, 1983; Yaguchi *et al.*, 1993), and colour discrimination (Boynton and Kambe, 1980; Romero *et al.*, 1993) show significant contributions from the opponent mechanisms. Physiological opponent mechanisms frequently found in monkey retina and LGN (Lateral Geniculate Nucleus) are chromatically-opponent ganglion and LGN cells of L-M (L-cone on-centre M-cone off-surround) and M-L (M-cone on-centre L-cone off-surround) types (Valberg *et al.*, 1987; Zrenner, 1983). The mechanisms assumed in psychophysical models of the increment threshold (Cole *et al.*, 1993; Kranda and King-Smith, 1979; Sperling and Harwerth, 1971) and the heterochromatic brightness matching (Nakano *et al.*, 1988; Tamura *et al.*, 1988) seem to correlate to such physiological mechanisms fairly well. Although the colour discrimination models (Boynton and Kambe, 1980; Guth, 1991; Knoblauch, 1993; Romero *et al.*, 1993) also assume opponent mechanisms, correlations to physiology seem weaker than former examples.

It is interesting if all these data can be explained with mechanisms based on physiology, although these might not necessarily be explained at the level of ganglion or LGN cells. The purpose of this study is to collect psychophysical colour discrimination data that evidently show contributions from opponent mechanisms and to analyse the data using a model closely related to physiological mechanisms.

4.6.2 METHODS

4.6.2.1 Chromatic Modulation Threshold (CMT)

We used the Chromatic Modulation Threshold (CMT) as a task of colour discrimination. The CMT is a detection threshold of spatial inhomogeneity in chromaticity. Figure 4.6.1 schematically illustrates an idea of the CMT. Two sinusoidally modulated colours were superposed with phase shift of 180°. Their average retinal illuminances were equal so that the stimulus became spatially equiluminant. When modulation equalled zero, two colours were mixed in the same ratio over the whole stimulus (Figure 4.6.1(a) top), and the stimulus appeared homogeneous (Figure 4.6.1(a) bottom). As the modulation increased, the mixture ratio changed from place to place (Figure 4.6.1(b) top, and the stimulus began to appear inhomogeneous (Figure 4.6.1(b) bottom). The CMT is the modulation when the inhomogeneity is just noticeable. The modulation in this case is:

$$\text{modulation} = \frac{I_{\lambda,\,max} - I_{\lambda,\,min}}{I_{\lambda,\,max} + I_{\lambda,\,min}} \tag{1}$$

where $I_{\lambda,\,max}$ is a maximum intensity of monochromatic light at a position labelled + in Figure 4.6.1(b) and $I_{\lambda min}$ is a minimum intensity at a position labelled − in the same figure.

4.6.2.2 Stimulus

In the actual stimulus, the two colours were modulated along a perimeter of a circle to form an annular shaped stimulus which extended about 2° of arc. Spatial frequency of the stimulus was two cycles per round. Inner and outer edges of the annulus were blurred by Gaussian function to prevent high spatial frequency components. One of the colours was fixed as white having xy-chromaticity co-ordinates of (0.43, 0.45). The other colour was monochromatic light produced by an interference filter. We used 25 interference filters with peak wavelength ranging from 437 to 679 nm. Average retinal illuminances of the white and the monochromatic light were set to 50 td for both resulted in a 100 td equiluminant stimulus.

4.6.2.3 Procedure

The CMT was measured as a function of wavelength using 25 monochromatic lights. After five minutes of dark adaptation, one of the 25 stimuli was presented in random order. Stimulus duration was one second and it was repeatedly presented with one second intervals. A subject started to adjust the chromatic modulation of the stimulus from homogeneous position and adjusted until the stimulus appeared just inhomogeneous using a method of adjustment. The adjustment was repeated four times for each monochromatic light in succession. In a session, this process was repeated until all 25 monochromatic lights were tested. Eight sessions were repeated for each subject. Three colour normal subjects participated in the experiment.

4.6.3   RESULTS

Figure 4.6.2 shows the results of the experiment. Logarithm of the modulation at just noticeable inhomogeneity for each monochromatic light was plotted as a function of wavelength. The results for subjects YN (top), JI (middle) and HU (bottom) are shown with standard deviations. Each graph was vertically shifted 0.6 log unit but correct scales appear on the axes indicated by arrows.

The CMT is highest at 584 nm for all subjects. The CMT decreases as wavelength becomes either longer or shorter than 584 nm. These features clearly correlate with saturation of the monochromatic lights. That is, the CMT function is inversely related to the saturation function. This explanation is not quantitative but qualitative. Quantitative analysis of the data using physiologically significant model will be discussed in the next section.

4.6.4   DISCUSSION

Our hypothesis is that some kinds of opponent mechanisms determine CMT. We assume that the response of the opponent mechanisms is calculated as follows:

$$R = \alpha \log L + \beta \log(k_M M) + \gamma \log(k_S S), \tag{2}$$

where L, M and S are the cone tristimulus values for L-, M- and S-cones based on Smith and Pokorny cone fundamentals (Smith and Pokorny, 1975). In the Smith and Pokorny system, peak sensitivity of S-cone is not defined. One of the Vos-Judd modified colour matching functions (Vos, 1978) $\bar{z}'(\lambda)$ was used as an S-cone sensitivity conventionally, and peak sensitivities of M- and S-cone are adjusted so as to fit the data. Constants k_M and k_S adjust peak sensitivities of M- and S-cone relative to the L-cone. Coefficients α, β and γ determine positive or negative amounts of contributions from three kinds of cones to the opponent mechanism. Logarithmic non-linearity was assumed here to represent response non-

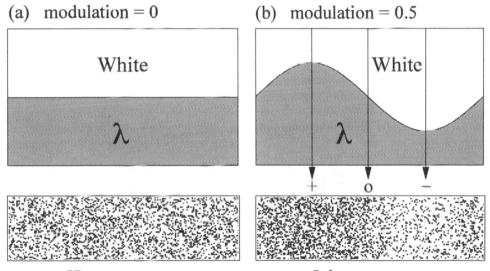

Figure 4.6.1.   Schematic illustration of Chromatic Modulation Threshold (CMT). (a) When two colours, white and monochromatic light λ in this case, are superposed without spatial modulation, the stimulus appears homogeneous. (b) When the two colours are sinusoidally modulated with phase shift of 180° while keeping their average retinal illuminances equal, the stimulus begins to appear inhomogeneous beyond certain point of the modulation. The CMT is the modulation when the inhomogeneity is just noticeable. Responses of opponent mechanisms at positions labelled +, o and − are calculated using equation (2) to analyse the CMT data. See text for details.

linearity of the cones. The non-linearity plays an important role in the following analysis of the data. We tried a linear version of equation (2) but no good result was obtained.

At the first stage, we tested the simplest opponent mechanism, that is,

$$R = \log L - \log M \tag{3}$$

To analyse the data using this mechanism, we calculated the following quantities. Response to spatial mean of the stimulus R_0 and a difference of responses at two most distinct positions of the stimulus $\Delta R = R_+ - R_-$ where R_+ is the response at a position where the monochromatic component is maximum and R_- is that at a position where the monochromatic component is minimum (see positions labelled + and − in Figure 4.6.1(b)). If this mechanism determines the CMT, it is expected that ΔR will be a monotonous function of R_0. If $\Delta R/R_0$ = constant, for example, this means Weber's law and replotted data on R_0 - ΔR diagram will be a linear function. Figure 4.6.3(a) shows the results of the calculation using the data for subject YN. Data points were plotted in different symbols in different wavelength regions to explain segmentation of the graph. Labelled points correspond to those wavelengths. A solid line was drawn by eye to fit the data points. As this graph shows, the function is far from monotonous. There exist a scatter of the data points at short wavelength region and a sudden jump at around 570 nm. The scatter is supposed to happen because of S-cone intrusion. The jump is supposed to happen because the mechanism that

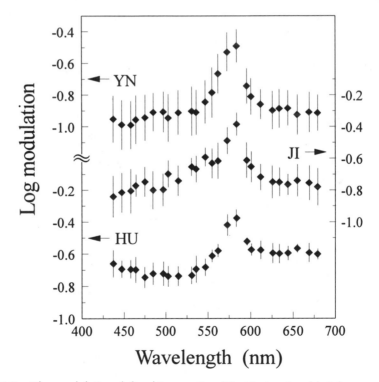

Figure 4.6.2. The modulation defined in equation (1) at just noticeable inhomogeneity was plotted in logarithmic scale as a function of wavelength. The results (diamonds) for subjects YN (top), JI (middle) and HU (bottom) are shown with standard deviations (bars). Each graph was vertically shifted 0.6 log unit for clarity, but correct scales appear on the axes indicated by arrows. All subjects show highest threshold at 584 nm and the threshold decreases as wavelength becomes either longer or shorter than 584 nm.

determines CMT changes from M-L type opponent to L-M type opponent at around 570 nm. It is, therefore, necessary to divide the data into several segments and to fit individual mechanism for each segment.

We divided the data into three segments, that is, 437–485 nm (filled circles), 497–562 nm (open squares), and 584–679 nm (open circles), and applied individual opponent mechanism for each segment. The criterion to choose an opponent mechanism for each segment was to fit all the data points into single monotonous function when plotting the data on R_o $-\Delta R$ diagram using individual mechanism for each segment. The following mechanisms were obtained as a result.

$$R = -2\log L + 3.2\log(2M) - 0.2\log(0.6S) \qquad \text{for 437–485 nm} \quad (4)$$
$$R = -3\log L + 4\log(2M) \qquad \text{for 497–562 nm} \quad (5)$$
$$R = 2.3\log L - 1.3\log(2M) \qquad \text{for 584–679 nm} \quad (6)$$

Figure 4.6.3 (right-hand plot) shows the results of the recalculation using an individual mechanism for each segment. Symbols are the same as in Figure 4.6.3 (left-hand plot). As shown in this graph, all the data points locate along a single monotonous function. An exponential function was used to approximate the function shown as a solid line.

Finally, we predicted the CMT curve using three opponent mechanisms and an approximated exponential function. Figure 4.6.4 shows the results. The data points were replotted from Figure 4.6.2 and solid curves represent the theoretical curves. L-M-S, L-M and M-L types of opponent mechanisms determine the CMT at short, middle and long wavelength regions, respectively, and the theoretical curves fit to the data points fairly well.

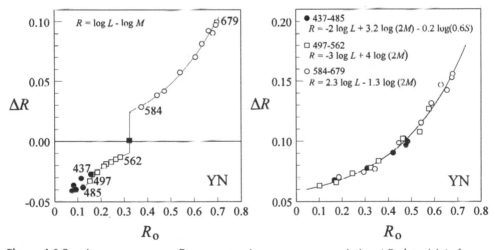

Figure 4.6.3. Average response R_o versus maximum response variation ΔR plots. (a) *Left-hand plot* Response of each opponent mechanism was calculated using equation (3). Maximum response variation $\Delta R = R_+ - R_-$, where R_+ and R_- are the responses at positions labelled + and − respectively, was plotted against average response R_o that is the response at a position labelled o in Figure 4.6.1(b). Data for subject YN in Figure 4.6.2 were used. This graph does not appear monotonous but seems to be separated into three segments. Different symbols represent different segments, 437–485 nm (filled circles), 497–562 nm (open squares) and 584–679 nm (open circles), respectively. A solid line was drawn by eye to fit the data. (b) *Right-hand plot* The same plot but an individual opponent mechanism, equation (4), (5) or (6), was applied to each segment. All points lie on exponential function (solid line) fairly well.

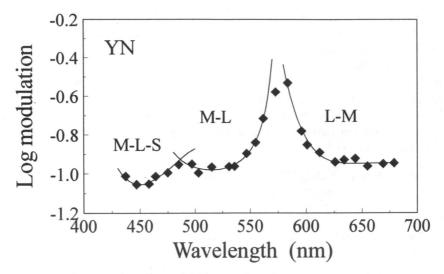

Figure 4.6.4. Theoretical prediction of the CMT for subject YN. Equations (4), (5) and (6) were applied to respective wavelength regions. At each wavelength, R_o was calculated using Equation (4), (5) or (6) at first, and then ΔR was obtained using the exponential function in Figure 4.6.3(b). Then a modulation to produce this ΔR was calculated using Equation (4), (5) or (6) again. The theoretical curves (solid lines) fit to the data fairly well. Three types of opponent mechanisms, M-L-S, M-L and L-M, operating in short, middle and long wavelength regions, respectively, were revealed by this analysis.

4.6.5   CONCLUSIONS

We obtained colour discrimination data that show clear evidence of contributions from opponent mechanisms, and proposed a way to analyse the data using specific opponent mechanisms. We found at least three opponent mechanisms contribute to colour discrimination, that is, L-M-S, L-M and M-L type opponent mechanisms. These mechanisms can be related to physiological evidence easily.

4.6.6   REFERENCES

BOYNTON, R. M. & KAMBE, N. (1980) Chromatic difference steps of moderate size measured along theoretically critical axes, *Color Research and Application*, **5**, 13–23.

COLE, G. R., HINE, T. & MCILHAGGA, W. (1993) Detection mechanisms in L-, M-, and S-cone contrast space, *Journal of the Optical Society of America*, **A10**, 38–51.

GUTH, S. L. (1991) Model for color vision and light adaptation, *Journal of the Optical Society of America*, **A8**, 976–993.

GUTH, S. L. & LODGE, H.R. (1973) Heterochromatic additivity, foveal spectral sensitivity, and a new color model, *Journal of the Optical Society of America*, **63**, 450–462.

IKEDA, M. & NAKANO, N. (1986) The Stiles summation index applied to heterochromatic brightness matching, *Perception*, **15**, 765–776.

KALLONIATIS, M. & HARWERTH, R. S. (1990) Spectral sensitivity and adaptation characteristics of cone mechanisms under white-light adaptation, *Journal of the Optical Society of America*, **A7**, 1912–1928.

KALLONIATIS, M. & HARWERTH, R. S. (1991) Effects of chromatic adaptation on opponent interactions in monkey increment-threshold spectral-sensitivity functions, *Journal of the Optical Society of America*, **A8**, 1818–1831.

Knoblauch, K. (1993) Theory of wavelength discrimination in tritanopia, *Journal of the Optical Society of America*, **A10**, 378–381.

Kranda, K. & King-Smith, P. E. (1979) Detection of coloured stimuli by independent linear systems, *Vision Research*, **19**, 733–745.

Nakano, Y., Ikeda, M. & Kaiser, P. K. (1988) Contributions of the opponent mechanisms to brightness and nonlinear models, *Vision Research*, **28**, 799–810.

Romero, J. R., García, J. A., del Barco, L. J. & Hita, E. (1993) Evaluation of color-discrimination ellipsoids in two-color spaces, *Journal of the Optical Society of America*, **A10**, 827–837.

Smith, V. C. & Pokorny, J. (1975) Spectral sensitivity of the foveal cone photopigments between 400 and 500 nm, *Vision Research*, **15**, 161–171.

Sperling, H. G. & Harwerth, R. S. (1971) Red-green cone interactions in the increment-threshold spectral sensitivity of primates, *Science*, **172**, 180–184.

Tamura, T., Ikeda, M. & Uchikawa, K. (1988) The effect of stimulus duration on the luminous efficiency functions for brightness, *Color Research and Application*, **13**, 363–368.

Valberg, A., Lee, B. B. & Tryti, J. (1987) Simulation of responses of spectrally-opponent neurones in the macaque lateral geniculate nucleus to chromatic and achromatic light stimuli, *Vision Research*, **27**, 867–882.

Vos, J. J. (1978) Colorimetric and photometric properties of a 2° fundamental observer, *Color Research and Application*, **3**, 125–128.

Yaguchi, H. & Ikeda, M. (1983) Subadditivity and superadditivity in heterochromatic brightness matching, *Vision Research*, **23**, 1711–1718.

Yaguchi, H., Kawada, A., Shioiri, S. & Miyake, Y. (1993) Individual differences of the contribution of chromatic channels to brightness, *Journal of the Optical Society of America*, **A10**, 1373–1379.

Zrenner, E. (1983) *Neurophysiological Aspects of Color Vision in Primates*, Berlin: Springer-Verlag.

The Contribution of Colour to Contour Detection

W. McIlhagga and K.T. Mullen

4.7.1 INTRODUCTION: THE USES OF COLOUR

It is obvious, if one looks at a black and white photograph, that colour is not needed to perceive objects. But when colour is added, those same objects become more distinct, and instead of seeming to be formed from the same greyness, take on the aspects of grass, skin, and sky. Colour adds much to our perception of the world, but what exactly is added is a subject of some speculation. Two ideas are commonly advanced. The first is that colour 'promotes the perception of contrast and hence, visibility' (Walls, quoted in Jacobs, 1981). The second idea suggests that, by encoding the spectral reflectance of surfaces, colour provides information about the material of objects (e.g. Rubin and Richards, 1982, 1988).

Consider the first idea, which can be stated formally as follows. The light incident at two points x and y on the retina has power distributions $i_x(\lambda)$ and $i_y(\lambda)$. The total difference in intensity is $\int (i_x(\lambda) - i_y(\lambda))^2 d\lambda$. If this light is absorbed by a univariant mechanism with sensitivity $s(\lambda)$, for example the luminance channel, the quantal catches are $q_x = \int s(\lambda)i_x(\lambda)d\lambda$ and $q_y = \int s(\lambda)i_y(\lambda)d\lambda$. The intensity difference measured by this mechanism is $(q_x - q_y)^2$, which is less than the total difference between i_x and i_y. A second mechanism with a different spectral sensitivity will recover more of the total difference, and it will be useful for contrast detection if a significant amount of the total difference cannot be detected by the first mechanism. If one considers the Munsell spectra (Parkkinen et al., 1989) a luminance channel, however defined, accounts for 98 per cent of the variation in L, M and S cone catches (Figure 4.7.1). A colour channel based on L, M and S cone catches, therefore, will increase the recovered contrast between Munsell patches by only about two per cent on average. (This is true whether the colour channel is a simple difference of cone responses, or whether it is some more complicated function, for example a chromaticity measure). Given that natural scenes (Burton and Moorhead, 1986) are more restricted in colour than the Munsell chips, it is unlikely that such a small effect can be useful for promoting the perception of contrast in everyday vision. We must postulate a subsequent amplification of the colour signal to account for the extreme sensitivity of the colour channel (Chaparro et al., 1993). As an equal amplification of the luminance system would improve contrast detection far more, the amplification of the colour signal must serve a purpose other than that of merely detecting contrast.

According to the second theory, colour is a source of information about the material of objects, because different materials reflect light differently. The light i_x reaching point x on the retina is a product of surface reflectance and illuminant light, so changes in i_x could be due to a change in either of these. A measure of reflectance must therefore be invariant to changes in the illuminant. The chromaticity c_x at point x on the retina is the ratio of quantal catches (or of power) measured by two mechanisms with sensitivities $s_1(\lambda)$ and $s_2(\lambda)$:

$$c_x = \frac{\int s_1(\lambda) i_x(\lambda) d\lambda}{\int s_2(\lambda) i_x(\lambda) d\lambda}$$

If the illuminant intensity changes, this will merely scale i_x by a factor that appears in both the numerator and denominator of this equation. This cancels, leaving the chromaticity

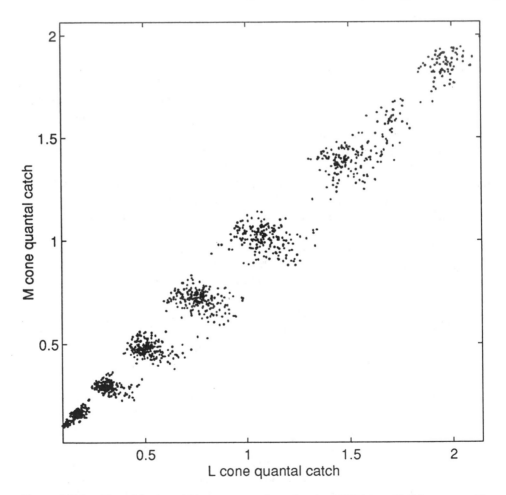

Figure 4.7.1.   Plot of the L and M cone quantal catches for 1250 Munsell chip spectra. The cone fundamentals are those of Vos *et al.* (1990). Note the high correlation between the L and M cone catches. This means that the intensity differences between different Munsell chips are best captured by a luminance (L + M) channel.

unchanged. Hence the chromaticity can yield some information about the surface reflectance. If the chromaticities c_x and c_y at two points x and y are equal, both the illuminant spectrum and the reflectance are likely to be the same at these points. Conversely, if the chromaticities are different, then either the reflectance or the illuminant spectrum has changed. Provided that the illuminant tends to change more slowly than the reflectance across an image, sudden changes in chromaticity – in effect, colour contrast – are a strong cue to reflectance changes, and if objects tend to have similar reflectance across their surface, different chromaticities c_x and c_y imply that retinal points x and y are projections of different objects. Reality is more complicated, because interreflections from near objects and light from the sky will mean that the effective illuminant will often change its spectral power as well as intensity, but it is nevertheless clear that colour contrast can be a powerful cue for image segmentation. Furthermore, the importance of this cue is not very dependent on the magnitude of colour contrast. By allowing the visual system to distinguish shadows and shading from changes in surface reflectance, colour vision aids the interpretation of image boundaries and contours.

4.7.2 COLOUR IN IMAGE SEGMENTATION

We can suggest two simple models of how colour could be involved in image segmentation. One model, which we will call the 'colouring-book' model, is similar to that proposed by Livingstone and Hubel (1987), and gives colour a subordinate role in object perception. In this model, illustrated in Figure 4.7.2a, all luminance edges are extracted and they are used to divide the image into a number of non-overlapping areas. Each object in the image is composed of one or more of these areas. The colour of each of these luminance-defined areas is then extracted, and describes the reflectance within that area. Finally, regions with a similar colour are linked to form objects. This model implies that the colour system should have two properties. First, the colour detectors should have localised, low-pass receptive fields. Second, as the colour system is subordinate to the luminance system, it should be incapable of seeing form by itself.

The other model will be called 'intrinsic images' after Barrow and Tennenbaum (1978) who described a computer vision system that computes a series of 2D overlaid maps, or 'intrinsic images', each of which plots a parameter intrinsic to the three-dimensional scene (e.g. texture or depth). Our version of intrinsic images is illustrated in Figure 4.7.2b. In this, the luminance system extracts edges from the image and uses them to divide the image into non-overlapping areas. In this model, the colour system also extracts edges. These chromatic edges, which localise a sudden change in colour, also divide the image into non-overlapping areas. Thus, both the luminance and colour systems perform the same computation, but on different data. The colour edges are then matched to luminance edges, and mark these luminance edges as being due to object boundaries. Any unmatched luminance edges are due to changes in the intensity of the illuminant. This model implies two properties of the colour system. First, the colour detectors should be band-pass to detect edges. Although these detectors need not be oriented, it would be useful. Second, as the colour system independently finds object boundaries, it should be able to support form perception without the luminance system.

Neither model is expected to be perfect, but we can see how the evidence stacks up in their favour. The spatial low pass characteristics of the colour system (Mullen, 1985) favour the colouring-book model. However, evidence suggests that the low pass chromatic contrast sensitivity function is probably an envelope of a number of band-pass colour channels (Losada and Mullen, 1994, 1995; Switkes *et al.*, 1988), which supports the idea of intrinsic images. Our ability to group by colour, in say the Ishihara tests or as illustrated by Morgan *et al.* (1992), is a component of the colouring book model, and so tends to favour this idea.

There is mounting evidence that the colour system can detect all the characteristics of edges that are encoded by the luminance system, such as orientation (Webster *et al.*, 1983) and disparity (Scharff and Geisler, 1992; Simmons and Kingdom, 1994). This supports the intrinsic images model for the colour system which must match its boundaries to those of the luminance image, and any shared characteristic of edges is helpful in this regard. Border capture (Gregory and Heard, 1989) supports both models.

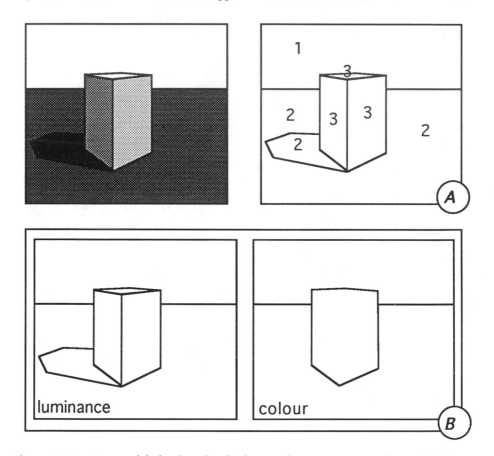

Figure 4.7.2. Two models for the role of colour in object segregation. The top left diagram shows a line drawing of a cylinder of one colour on a ground of another. The top right diagram (A) shows the segmentation performed by the colouring-book model. Edges are delineated by the luminance system. Each region is marked as a particular colour by the colour system (the numbers 1,2,3 indicate different colours), and objects are segregated by combining regions with the same colour. The lower two diagrams (B) depict the intrinsic images model. Here, both colour and luminance systems detect edges, and the edges form the perimeters of non-overlapping regions. A comparison of the luminance and colour edge maps indicates which luminance edges are due to shading (these have no corresponding colour edge).

Form perception is sometimes said to be lost at isoluminance. For example, if a black and white shaded picture is converted into a red/green isoluminant image so that all the luminance borders become isoluminant colour borders, the forms it contains become difficult to see (Gregory and Heard, 1989; Livingstone and Hubel, 1987). However, this effect is not contrary to the intrinsic images model. All that has happened in these demonstrations is that the set of edges appropriate to the luminance system has been sent instead to the colour system. It should be no surprise (indeed, something of a relief) that the colour system interprets the edges in an entirely different way from the luminance system. Thus, this effect simply demonstrates that shape-from-shading computations are impossible in a system that does not know what shading is. The form perception that persists at isoluminance (Gregory and Heard, 1989) favours an intrinsic images model.

The evidence presented favours the intrinsic images model, although not to the exclusion of the colouring-book model. The intrinsic image model raises a number of interesting questions:

1. How do the colour and luminance border-detecting systems work and how do they compare in performance?
2. How are colour and luminance borders integrated?
3. Are colour borders really intensity independent?

4.7.3   COLOUR AND LUMINANCE BORDERS

A crucial component of the intrinsic image model is the extraction of colour and luminance borders. Previously, this process has largely been studied in terms of the detection and discrimination of sinusoidal variations in colour and/or luminance contrast. In this chapter, we discuss a different experimental approach to this issue. The visual system at the early cortical level encodes the local orientation in an image. A percept of a continuous border, by contrast, requires the integration, or grouping, of the outputs of many of these local detectors. The Gestalt psychologists have described many figural grouping processes. However, when the task is to group oriented features into continuous boundaries there are relatively few relevant parameters. These include the proximity of the features, the relative orientations of the features, their spatial scale, and their colour and luminance contrast. We have been looking at the importance of these factors in the detection of colour and luminance contours.

Continuous contours are by themselves so easy to see that we need to make the task harder in order to study it. We have used an experimental stimulus introduced by Field et al. (1992), illustrated in Figure 4.7.3 (see also McIlhagga and Mullen, 1995). A 2-alternative forced choice paradigm was used. One stimulus, called the contour stimulus, consisted of ten oriented gabor elements aligned along a winding contour or path, surrounded by 186 randomly scattered gabor elements, as in Figure 4.7.3. The difference in orientation of adjacent contour elements determined the contour's straightness (see Figure 4.7.3, inset). A difference of zero generated a perfectly straight contour, whereas the largest difference used (45 degrees) generated a very winding contour. The other stimulus contained no contour and consisted only of 196 oriented gabor elements randomly scattered in a 14 x 14 degree square. We used gabor elements with a relatively low spatial frequency (1.5 cycles per degree) in order to match the receptive fields of single cells, and to reduce chromatic aberration. The task was to decide whether a contour was present or absent in the stimulus. Note that the only cue for detecting the contour was the common alignment of those elements comprising it. Thus, if the orientation of elements in the contour was randomised, the contour could not be detected, even with extended viewing. The gabor elements of the contour are separated by a distance equal to the inter-element spacing of the random elements, so providing no additional cues to the presence of a contour. Only the red and green guns of the monitor were used with the blue gun intensity at zero. Each stimulus is displayed for one second.

We have investigated the effects of the contrast magnitude and type of element contrast on contour detection. The probability of correct responses as a function of the orientation difference between adjacent elements of the contour was measured and the results for a luminance stimulus are shown in Figure 4.7.4 (left panel). Results are for a range of element contrasts. As found previously (Field *et al.*, 1993), performance deteriorates with increasing contour angle. The contrast of the elements, however, has little effect until it falls below 12 per cent, when performance deteriorates. We repeated the experiment using isoluminant red/green gabor elements. Contour detection performances for the isoluminant stimuli are shown in Figure 4.7.4 (right panel). At 50 per cent colour contrast, the observer's performance is identical to their best performance with the luminance stimulus. Thus, given

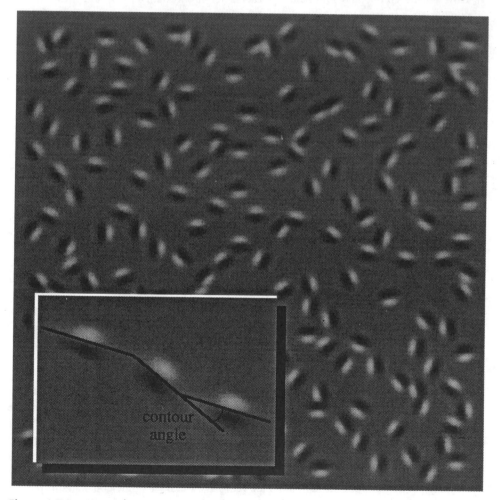

Figure 4.7.3.　Monochrome image of a typical contour stimulus. The contour runs horizontally above the inset. There are 10 elements in the contour. The inset shows how the contour angle is defined.

a high enough contrast, the colour and luminance systems are capable of integrating contours equally well.

The similar performance found for contour integration by the colour and luminance systems may arise through a number of different mechanisms. On the one hand, the visual system may ignore the type of contrast, luminance or colour, when the contour is detected. This hypothesis includes the possibility that only the luminance system can extract contours, but that it has a partial sensitivity to 'isoluminant' stimuli. On the other hand, the colour and luminance systems may be wholly separate, with each performing similarly for contour integration. We tested these two hypotheses using a mixed colour and luminance stimulus. Consider the luminance stimulus shown in Figure 4.7.3, and imagine making every second element in the contour an isoluminant gabor, for example by replacing the light area with isoluminant red and the dark area with isoluminant green. Half the background elements are replaced in the same way. If the first hypothesis is correct, changing the type of contrast will not affect contour detection, for the contour detection process is insensitive to contrast type. If the second hypothesis is correct, however, both colour and luminance systems will attempt to detect a contour in a stimulus that, to each, appears to have half the density of elements. Thus the detection probability will be the probability summation of detection in the colour and luminance systems. When we measure detection with this kind of mixed colour/luminance stimulus, we find that performance is never as good as detection of a pure colour or pure luminance stimulus. Thus the first hypothesis is ruled out. However, detection is rather better than the probability summation prediction. (We found that erasing all elements of one type of contrast, colour or luminance, reduced detection to near-chance levels.) Thus, the second hypothesis is also ruled out. Apparently, the contour extraction mechanism prefers contours to have the same colour along their length, but will, albeit more reluctantly, also find

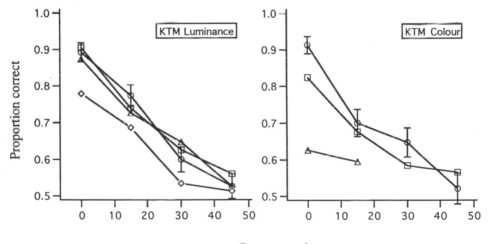

Figure 4.7.4. Contour detection results for one observer. The *x* axis gives the contour angle; the *y* axis gives the proportion of correct responses. Each curve shows results for a different element contrast (contrast is defined as the Michelson contrast of the gabor carrier): circles, 50 per cent contrast; squares, 25 per cent; triangles, 12 per cent; diamonds, 6 per cent. The left graph gives results with luminance stimuli. The right graph shows results for red-green isoluminant stimuli. Isoluminance for the gabor carrier was determined by a motion-nulling technique (Anstis and Cavanagh, 1983), and the colour contrast is taken to be the Michelson contrast of the red gun image.

contours where the contrast type varies. This would be useful in realistic situations where we cannot guarantee that the colour of an object is uniform. It does, however, argue for more interaction between the colour and luminance systems than the intrinsic images model permits.

Earlier, we noted that colour is relatively invariant to changes in illuminant intensity. We might expect, therefore, that detection of a colour-defined contour should be unaffected by changes in the luminance contrast of the elements. Certainly, this appears to be the case for small random variations in luminance, such as in the Ishihara plates. We assessed the effect of variations in contrast luminance on the detection of a colour path, using elements in which the luminance contrast reversed between successive elements. In Figure 4.7.5, probability correct for this stimulus is plotted against the probability correct for an isoluminant stimulus of the same colour contrast and contour angle, over a range of combined colour and luminance contrasts and contour angles. If detection of the colour contour is invariant to luminance contrast, we would expect this plot to be a straight line. For two subjects, however, (including WHM) adding variable luminance contrast to a colour path caused a reduction in performance. For a third subject (KTM), there was no consistent effect. In all cases the results do not support the hypothesis that luminance variations have no effect on the detection of a colour path.

4.7.4   DISCUSSION

It is clear that colour perception plays a role in object perception, but how it is involved remains an open question. Our experiments have shown that the colour system is as capable as the luminance system at extracting and integrating contours, at least with our stimuli. These results provide added support for a model of object segregation, which we have called 'intrinsic images', in which the colour and luminance systems make a similar

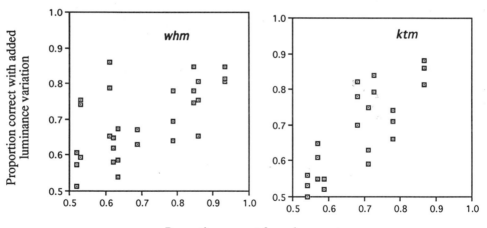

Figure 4.7.5. Comparison of contour detection of a purely colour contour, and a colour contour with added variations in luminance contrast. The *x* axis gives the probability correct for an isoluminant contour at a particular setting of contrast and contour angle. The *y* axis gives the probability correct of a colour contour with the same colour contrast and angle, but with added luminance contrast variations (see text for details). For observer WHM, the added luminance variations generally reduce detection of the contour; for KTM, they have no consistent effect.

contribution to the identification of object boundaries. Support for the intrinsic images model, however, does not invalidate the 'colouring-book' model. Although they differ with regard to colour's role, they are not logical complements, and both may be true.

We expected, on the basis of the definition of chromaticity, that any colour-based contour would be equally visible regardless of luminance variation. The result of the final set of experiments was therefore surprising. We found that adding varying luminance contrast to a colour contour did affect the contour visibility. However, we did not consider the role that the luminance system must play in identifying the albedo of surfaces. Changes in the surface albedo are also changes in surface reflectance, and provide another cue for object segregation. Surface albedo is signalled, albeit ambiguously, by the luminance system, so if the observers interpreted luminance variations as variations in albedo, then these would be as disruptive of contour perception as changes in element colour.

4.7.5   REFERENCES

ANSTIS, S. & CAVANAGH, P. (1983) A minimum motion technique for judging equiluminance. In: Mollon, J. D., & Sharpe, L. T. (Eds) *Color Vision: Physiology and Psychophysics*, London: Academic Press.

BARROW, H. G. & TENNENBAUM, J. M. (1978) Recovering intrinsic scene characteristics from images. In: Hanson, A. & Riseman, E. (Eds) *Computer Vision Systems*, New York: Academic Press.

BURTON, G. J. & MOORHEAD, I. R. (1986) Color and spatial structure in natural scenes, *Applied Optics*, **26**, 157–169.

CHAPARRO, A., STROMEYER, C. F., HUANG, E. P., KRONAUER, R. E. & ESKEW R. T. (1993) Colour is what the eye sees best, *Nature*, **361**, 348-350.

FIELD, D., HAYES, A., & HESS, R. (1993) Contour integration by the human visual system: Evidence for a local 'Association field', *Vision Research*, **33**, 173–193.

GREGORY, R. L. & HEARD, P. F. (1989) Some phenomena and implications of isoluminance. In: Kulikowski, J. J., Dickinson, C. M. & Murray, I. J. (Eds) *Seeing Contour and Colour*, Oxford: Pergamon Press.

JACOBS, G. H. (1981) *Comparative Color Vision*, New York: Academic Press.

LIVINGSTONE, M. S. & HUBEL, D. H. (1987) Psychophysical evidence for the perception of form, color, movement, and depth, *Journal of Neuroscience*, **7**, 3416–3468.

LOSADA, M. A. & MULLEN, K. T. (1994) The spatial tuning of chromatic mechanisms identified by simultaneous masking, *Vision Research*, **34**, 331–341.

LOSADA, M. A. & MULLEN, K. T. (1995) Colour and luminance spatial tuning estimated by noise masking in the absence of off-frequency looking, *Journal of the Optical Society of America*, **A12**, 250–260.

MCILHAGGA, W.H. & MULLEN, K.T. (1995) The detection of colour and luminance contours, *Vision Research*, (in revision).

MORGAN, M. J., ADAM, A., & MOLLON, J. D. (1992) Dichromats detect colour-camouflaged objects that are not detected by trichromats, *Proceedings of the Royal Society of London*, **B 248**, 291–295.

MULLEN, K. T. (1985) The contrast sensitivity of human color vision to red-green and blue-yellow chromatic gratings, *Journal of Physiology*, **359**, 381–409.

PARKKINEN, J. P. S., HALLIKAINEN, J. & JAASKELAINEN, T. (1989) Characteristic spectra of Munsell colors, *Journal of the Optical Society of America*, **A 6**, 318–322.

RUBIN, J. M. & RICHARDS, W. A. (1982) Color vision and image intensities: when are changes material?, *Biological Cybernetics*, **45**, 215–226.

RUBIN, J. M. & RICHARDS, W. A. (1988) Color vision: material categories. In: Richards, W. A. (Ed.) *Natural Computation*, Cambridge: MIT Press, pp. 194–213.

SCHARFF, L. V. & GEISLER, W. S. (1992) Stereopsis at isoluminance in the absence of chromatic aberrations, *Journal of the Optical Society of America*, **A** 9, 868–876.

SIMMONS, D. R. & KINGDOM, F. A. A. (1994) Contrast thresholds for stereoscopic depth identification with isoluminant and isochromatic stimuli, *Vision Research*, **34**, 2971– 2982.

SWITKES, E., BRADLEY, A. & DEVALOIS K. K. (1988) Contrast dependency and mechanisms of masking interactions among chromatic and luminance mechanisms, *Journal of the Optical Society of America*, **A** 5, 1149–1162.

VOS, J. J., ESTEVEZ, O., & WALRAVEN, P. L. (1990) Improved color fundamentals offer a new view on photometric additivity, *Vision Research*, **30**, 937–944.

WEBSTER, M. A., DEVALOIS, K. K. & SWITKES, E. (1983) Orientation and spatial frequency discrimination for luminance and chromatic gratings, *Journal of the Optical Society of America*, **A** 7, 1034–1049.

Chromatic Contribution to Shape Perception is Revealed in a Non-temporal Detection Task Using Distance

Thomy Nilsson and Kevin Connolly

4.8.1 INTRODUCTION

What colours should be used to make symbols visually effective? Other than artistic considerations and recommended standards, there is surprisingly little empirical data from which to answer this question. At high ambient luminance Boff and Lincoln (1988) find some evidence that red symbols produce faster response times than greens and yellows. Perhaps colour effects are primarily cognitive, and this precludes any general guidelines on what colours to use for symbols. For more data on general effects of colour, we had to look at the effects of colour on legibility.

Recent research by Knoblauch *et al.* (1991), Legge and Rubin (1986) and Pastoor (1990) leaves little doubt that it is the luminance contrast of letter colour with respect to the background that determines legibility. Yet the recent research used stimuli produced on colour video monitors. A comparative study of reading video and printed text reveals there are some systematic differences in these tasks (Jorna and Snyder, 1991). For research using coloured text printed on coloured paper, we had to go back to Tinker and Patterson (1931). They found black/white to be most legible, closely followed by green/white, blue/white, black/yellow, and red/yellow. Red/green and black/purple were the least legible. All these results seem consistent with research on the effects of colour on the detection of edges and gratings (DeValois and DeValois, 1988). It appears that legibility is determined only by luminance contrast, and colour doesn't matter.

However, all these studies on legibility have something in common. They all defined legibility in terms of reading speed. Recognition speed is not the only criterion for the visual effectiveness of words or symbols in many applications. Evidence of different time constants of different colour mechanisms (Courtney and Buchsbaum, 1991) and of changes in colour as a function of viewing time (Nilsson, 1972) leave room for doubt as to whether the final decision on these matters should be based on recognition speed.

Pastoor (1990) also had subjects rate the different colour combinations for legibility. This produced statistically significant preferences: White/dark-blue was best; followed by light-blue/dark-blue, light-blue/black, red/black, and then black/white. Though Pastoor used either light letters on dark backgrounds or dark letters on light backgrounds, there was evidence here of preferences that were not wholly determined by luminance contrast. For legibility data not involving reading speed with printed materials, there was a study by Preston et al. (1932). They measured the maximum distance at which various coloured text printed on various coloured papers could be read. Using the same materials as Tinker and Patterson (1931), they found three colour combinations: blue/white, black/yellow, and green/white that were more legible than black/white.

We had also used words printed in colour backed by coloured paper to measure the distance at which various colour combinations could be read (Nilsson and Connolly, 1993). Green/white, black/yellow, and green/yellow were significantly more legible than black/white. Colour photometry of the letters and backgrounds revealed that chroma also contributed to legibility distance. Inability to exactly match the colours of the LetraSet letters to the Pantone backgrounds prevented more precise determination of the effects of colour contrast. In the present study, a colour printer permitted an exact match between symbol and background colour.

4.8.2   METHOD

Five hired subjects plus the second author made the observations. They were between 20 and 26 years old with normal or corrected acuity and normal colour vision as determined by the Dvorine Test. All had participated in a previous study of the legibility of coloured words and were familiar with the apparatus and procedure.

From a reference book on standard symbols (Dreyfuss, 1972), 10 symbols were selected on the basis of approximately equal complexity, colour neutrality, and some unfamiliarity to minimise colour expectancy. They included symbols for a picnic table, children running, a row boat, a rock slide. The symbols were scanned, coloured, scaled and printed using a Canon CJ10 colour copier interfaced to a computer running a Postscript interpreter and Adobe Illustrator. The exact shade of the six primary colours tested was obtained by visual match to the red, yellow, green, blue, black and white of LetraSet letters. The CIE $L^*u^*v^*$ colour characteristics of the printed inks are provided in Table 4.8.1. The final stimuli were 2.5×2 cm prints mounted on a 12.5×17.5 cm flat-black backing.

The stimuli were mounted in a viewing box lined with black velvet to minimize stray light. They were illuminated from 45° by 100 watt General Electric 'Soft White Delux' bulbs at a distance of 60 cm on each side. These two lamps produced a luminance of 110 cdm^{-2} with a colour temperature of 2700K on a calcium carbonate test plate at the stimulus

Table 4.8.1. Colour specifications of the printed inks used to produce the symbols and background

Colour		L*	u*	v*
Black	(K)	0	0	0
White	(W)	99	−7	7
Red	(R)	52.4	98	−1.2
Yellow	(Y)	92	37	32
Green	(G)	50	−52	11
Blue	(B)	38	−23	−29

position. Lamp housings and lensless, baffled projection tubes produced a light beam whose residual struck the back wall of the viewing box outside the subject's field of view. Viewed in a black, light-proof room, the visual effect was that of a bright symbol floating in empty space.

The viewing box was mounted on a 7 metre track (Figure 4.8.1). A 15 N-m stepping motor moved the box via chain drive at an acceleration of 19 cms^{-2} to and from a maintained velocity of 19 cms^{-1}. Preliminary testing found that this moderate walking speed was optimal for producing consistent results without rushing or boring the subjects. Box position was measured independently of the drive using an optical encoder driven by a miniature toothed belt. A computer conducted the measurement procedure by telling the experimenter which stimulus to test, controlling the motor, obeying the subject's commands, monitoring box position, and recording data. The subject was seated at one end of the track and used a chin rest to maintain eye position. Independent safety switches operating an electric clutch and brake system protected the subject and apparatus from overrunning.

The method of limits was used to measure recognition distance with the subjects instructed to judge when they could just recognise or no longer recognise the symbol. Each symbol was first presented close to the subject. Fixed plus random increments in position were made after each response. For each stimulus, 10 measurements were made, but the highest and lowest were not used. The stimuli were tested in sequences that changed the

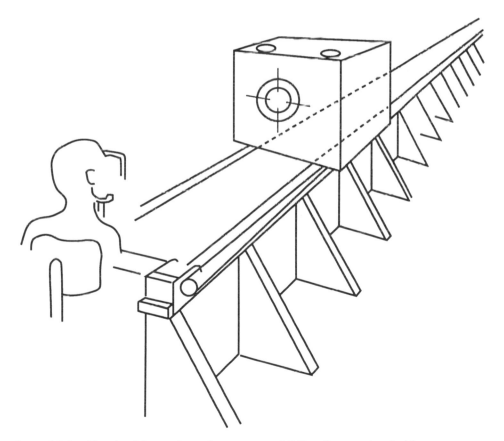

Figure 4.8.1. Sketch of the track used to measure visibility distance thresholds.

symbol and colours on each trial. The sequences were counterbalanced across subjects. The 300 combinations of symbol, symbol colour and background colour were tested in 15 one-hour sessions of 20 symbols with each subject.

4.8.3 RESULTS

The data were analysed from the running averages of each subject's back and forth responses. The mean standard deviation of the subjects' running averages per stimulus was 11 cm. Mean recognition distance varied from 224 to 442 cm depending on symbols and colour combination. Averaged across symbols and subjects, black/red and black/yellow were recognised furthest away; white on yellow had to be brought closest. The mean results are shown in Table 4.8.2.

Table 4.8.2. Relative mean threshold distance (cm), standard deviation, Duncan's ranges, and relative visibility of coloured symbols printed with coloured backgrounds – averaged across symbols and subjects

Symbol	Background	Threshold Distance	SD	Significantly different ranges					Relative visibility
Black	Yellow	442	11	1					100
Black	Red	442	12	1					100
White	Blue	433	11	1	2				96
Black	White	427	11		2	3			93
Blue	Yellow	423	13		2	3	4		92
Red	Black	423	11		2	3	4	5	91
Green	Yellow	422	11			3	4	5	91
Yellow	Green	421	12			3	4	5	91
Black	Green	418	10	6		3	4	5	89
Blue	White	418	11	6		3	4	5	89
Red	Yellow	415	12	6	7		4	5	88
White	Red	414	11	6	7		4	5	88
White	Green	414	12	6	7		4	5	88
Green	White	413	12	6	7	8	4	5	87
Yellow	Red	411	11	6	7	8		5	86
Yellow	Blue	408	11	6	7	8			85
Green	Black	407	10	6	7	8			85
Yellow	Black	407	9	6	7	8			85
White	Black	403	10		7	8	9		83
Red	White	402	11			8	9		83
Blue	Red	401	12			8	9		82
Red	Blue	394	11				9	10	79
Black	Blue	389	11					10	77
Blue	Black	376	11		11				72
Blue	Green	375	13		11				72
Green	Red	369	10		11				70
Green	Blue	357	10			12			65
Red	Green	354	10			12			64
Yellow	White	235	9				13		28
White	Yellow	224	9					14	26

Duncan's test indicates 18 significantly different ranges of recognition distance. Not only are two combinations (black/red and black/yellow) significantly better than black/white, but seven combinations (white/blue, blue/yellow, red/black, green/yellow, yellow/green, black/green, blue/white) did not differ significantly from black/white. Though a precise equating of lightness contrast was not possible with printed colours, it appears that recognition distance was not determined solely by lightness contrast.

4.8.4   DISCUSSION

To relate threshold distance to the effort required for recognition, one should take into account that retinal area decreases with the square of the distance. Assuming a parallel processing of visual information, the retinal area needed to recognise a symbol mirrors the amount of processing or 'effort' required for recognition to occur. 'Relative visibility' in Table 4.8.2 inversely scales recognition distances in terms of retinal area relative to the retinal area subtended by the most distantly recognised stimulus. It is simply a ratio of a symbol's threshold distance squared to the threshold distance squared of the symbol that could be recognised furthest away.

Figure 4.8.2 shows the average relative visibility of the symbols as a function of symbol/background colour together with the lightness contrast as a function of those colours. For some colour combinations visibility and lightness contrast were closely related, but for others that clearly was not the case. The correlation between visibility distance and lightness contrast is + 0.64. This compares with a correlation of + 0.15 for chroma contrast, −0.19 for hue contrast and + 0.34 for colour contrast. It was difficult to discern any pattern

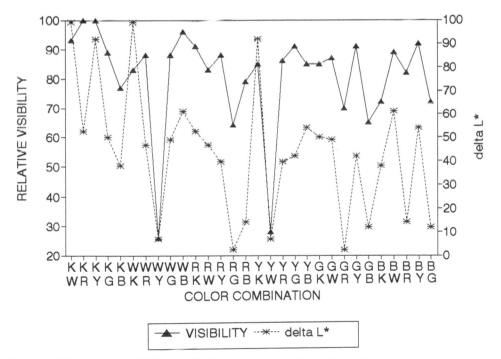

Figure 4.8.2.   Relative visibility and lightness contrast (delta L*) as a function of symbol/background colours.

in these data until they were rearranged in order of increasing difference between relative visibility and lightness contrast as shown in Figure 4.8.3.

Figure 4.8.3 shows a prevalence of combinations that include black, and white and yellow colours towards the left side where relative visibility and lightness contrast were closely related. Towards the right where visibility was higher than contrast, the colours red, green, and blue were prevalent. Combinations with higher chroma were less closely related to visibility than combinations with lower chroma. Adding to the lightness contrast a factor that represented the total amount of chroma in symbol and background, the root-mean-square of the symbol and background chroma, improved the correlation with visibility to +0.78. Evidently, chroma contributes substantially to how far a symbol can be seen.

The data were rearranged in terms of increasing difference between the visibility and colour functions as shown in Figure 4.8.4. This revealed a lot of blue in the combinations that were more visible than was predicted by the lightness-contrast-plus-rms-chromaticity factor. For a characteristic that would increase the predicted contribution of blue in particular, v* in Table 4.8.1 had a salient though negative value for blue. Subtracting its mean value for symbol and background increased the correlation further. Giving this average v* factor a weight of –0.7 maximised the correlation between relative visibility and colour at +0.85. Evidently, the presence of blue improved visibility by more than was predicted by its lightness contrast and chromaticity.

Again the data were rearranged in terms of difference between visibility and the new colour function. This revealed that when both symbol and background colours were red, green and blue, the colour function tended to exceed the visibility function. Subtracting a small amount of chroma contrast, –0.3 delta C*, maximised the correlation at +0.88. Evidently strong chromatic contrast somewhat hampered symbol recognition.

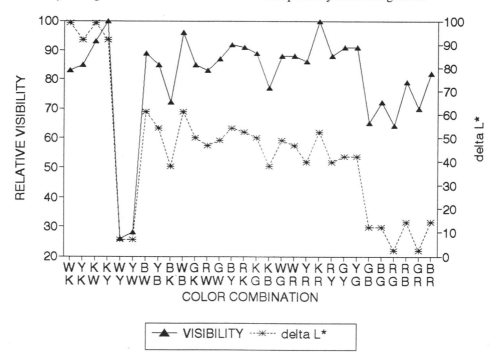

Figure 4.8.3.   The data in Figure 4.8.2 rearranged in terms of increasing difference between the visibility and contrast functions.

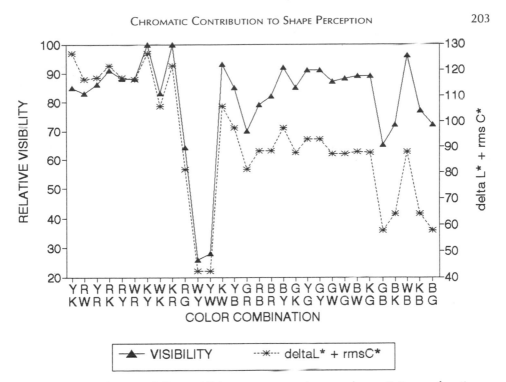

Figure 4.8.4. Relative visibility and lightness-contrast-plus-rms-chromaticity as a function of symbol/background colours.

Could the correlation between visibility and colour characteristics be still further improved by another colour factor? Replotting in terms of increasing difference showed that the visibility of colour combinations that included green tended to be underestimated. As the u* characteristic of our green ink had a salient negative value, its average value was subtracted from the other factors. The weight of the v* factor then had to be reduced because u* also had a substantial negative value for the blue ink. The following weights produced a maximum correlation with visibility of +0.95:

$$0.8 \text{ dL*} + \text{rmsC*} - 0.4 \text{ avg u*} - 0.4 \text{ avg v*} - 0.05 \text{ dC*}$$

Figure 4.8.5 shows the values of the above formula as a function of colour combination together with relative visibility.

Figure 4.8.5 and Table 4.8.2 show some colour combinations that changed markedly in visibility when symbol and background colours were inverted. Most prominent are black/yellow, black/white, and blue/yellow with relative visibilities of 100, 93 and 92. Inversely, yellow/black, white/black, and yellow/blue had significantly lower visibilities at 85, 83 and 85 respectively. The more visible versions tended to be darker symbols on lighter backgrounds. Similarly, dark letters on light background are slightly more legible than light letters on dark background (Sanders and McCormick, 1991). The visibility equation was slightly improved by adding a 'lightness of background' factor. Its weight was only +0.02, and it improved the correlation by only one per cent. Furthermore, other differences in the visibility of opposite colour combinations were not attributable to a lighter background. Perhaps the colour pathways for processing foreground information are proportioned slightly differently from those for background. Attempts to develop a visibility function using initially separate symbol and background characteristics were not as successful. That

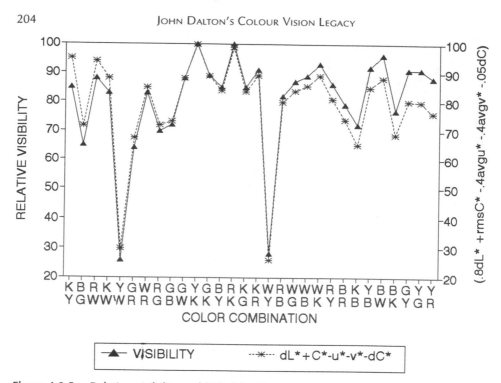

Figure 4.8.5.   Relative visibility and (0.8 delta L* + rms C* – 0.4 u* – 0.4 v* – 0.05 delta C*) as a function of symbol/background colour.

might be due to lack of patience in working with twice as many factors, and the issue remains open.

4.8.5   CONCLUSION

When the visibility of coloured stimuli on coloured backgrounds was measured in terms of distance, chroma characteristics contributed substantially to visibility. This contradicts what is generally believed and the findings of most previous studies. Our results differed because our measure of visibility was not time dependent. The visual pathways mediating colour information are slower than those mediating lightness contrast (DeValois and DeValois, 1988). Therefore, time-dependent measures of visibility do not reveal what the chromatic pathways contribute when more time is allowed for perception.

Overall chroma of our stimuli was measured as the root mean square (rms) of the chroma C* of symbol and background. Based on an equation that predicted the relative visibility of our stimuli with a correlation of +0.95, chroma was the largest determining factor with a weight of 1.0. Lightness contrast, delta L* was the second largest factor with a weight of 0.8. The delta L* factor was equalled by the combined influence of two factors derived from the average u* and v* characteristics of the stimuli. That the best weights of the u* and v* factors were equal and negative suggests that blue contributes to shape perception as much as other colours in the final analysis. As this contradicts previous research, which clearly shows a predominance of red-green pathways in early visual processing for edges (DeValois and DeValois, 1988), the 'final analysis' must incorporate some magnification factor that equalises colour information. Other evidence of equal contributions by long-, medium- and short-wavelength pathways has been reported by Webster *et al.* (1990) in the perception of gratings and their orientation.

Though we averaged our results across symbols, we do not doubt that shape and cognitive factors affected visibility. What we sought was evidence of general colour characteristics that affected visibility. These clearly were found to exist. Therefore, it is possible to have general guidelines for colour combinations to improve the visibility of symbols. These guidelines can now be based on more than just lightness contrast, delta L*, and should also include the chromatic properties, u* and v*.

4.8.6   ACKNOWLEDGEMENTS

This research was supported by a cooperative development contract 9F006 from the Canadian Space Agency and the Province of Prince Edward Island to Triad Design. The test facility was developed under Health and Welfare contract H4078 to T. Nilsson. Glenda Clements-Smith of Triad Design prepared the stimuli.

4.8.7   REFERENCES

BOFF, K.R. & LINCOLN, J.E. (1988) *Engineering Data Compendium: Human Perception and Performance*, Wright-Patterson AFB.

COURTNEY, S.M. & BUCHSBAUM, G. (1991) Temporal differences between colour pathways within the retina as a possible origin of subjective colours, *Vision Research*, **31**, 1541–1548.

DEVALOIS, R.L. & DEVALOIS, K.K. (1988) *Spatial Vision*, New York: Oxford University Press.

DREYFUSS, H. (1972) *Symbol Sourcebook*, New York: McGraw-Hill.

JORNA, G.C. & SNYDER, H.L. (1991) Image quality determines differences in reading performance and perceived image quality with CRT and hard copy images, *Human Factors*, **33**, 456–69.

KNOBLAUCH, K., ARDITI, A. & SZLYK, J. (1991) Effects of chromatic and luminance contrast on reading, *Journal of the Optical Society of America*, A **8**, 428–39.

LEGGE, G.E. & RUBIN, G.S. (1986) Psychophysics of reading IV. Wavelength effects in normal and low vision, *Journal of the Optical Society of America*, A **3**, 40–51.

NILSSON, T.H. (1972) The effects of pulse rate and pulse duration on hue of monochromatic stimuli, *Vision Research*, **12**, 1907–21.

NILSSON, T.H. & CONNOLLY, G.K. (1993) 'Colour (not just contrast) affects legibility distance of printed words', presentation at the 37th Annual Meeting of the Human Factors and Ergonomics Society, Seattle, October.

PASTOOR, S. (1990) Legibility and subjective preference for colour combinations in text, *Human Factors*, **32**, 157–71.

PRESTON, K., SCHWANKL, H.P. & TINKER, M.A. (1932) The effect of variations in colour of print and background on legibility, *Journal of General Psychology*, **6**, 459–61.

SANDERS, M.S. & MCCORMICK, E.J. (1993) *Human Factors in Engineering and Design*, New York: McGraw-Hill.

TINKER, M.A. & PATTERSON, D.G. (1931) Studies of typographical factors influencing speed of reading, *Journal of Applied Psychology*, **45**, 471–79.

WEBSTER, M.A., DEVALOIS, K.K., & SWITKES, E. (1990) Orientation and spatial-frequency discrimination for luminance and chromatic gratings, *Journal of the Optical Society of America*, A **7**, 1034–1049.

Reading Performance of Low Vision Observers for Equal Luminance Coloured Text

Kelley L. Jacobs, Susan J. Leat and Jeffery K. Hovis

4.9.1 INTRODUCTION

The study of acquired colour vision defects occurring in different disease processes has been extensively studied by many researchers. It is well known that individuals suffering from conditions such as optic atrophy, diabetic retinopathy and age-related macular degeneration (ARM) can develop acquired colour discrimination losses. Blue-yellow defects are common in early stages of ARM with red-green defects occurring as visual acuity worsens (Campbell and Rittler, 1972; Cox, 1961; Verriest, 1964). Cox (1961) found that both blue-yellow and red-green colour vision defects occur in optic atrophy. In diabetic retinopathy, both blue-yellow and red-green colour vision defects occur with blue-yellow being the most common (Lakowski et al., 1973; Trick et al., 1988).

Along with colour discrimination losses there may also be selective losses in spectral sensitivity. In ARM, a severe loss of blue sensitivity occurs along with a loss in the longer wavelengths (Alvarez et al., 1983a; Cox, 1961). Alvarez et al. (1983b) concluded that both short- and long-wavelength sensitivity losses occur in optic atrophy. Cox (1961) found a loss of short wavelength sensitivity in patients with diabetic retinopathy. With the increasing use of video display terminals (VDTs) as low vision aids, these spectral sensitivity losses may be important in selecting the appropriate VDT colour.

Determining the spectral sensitivity of low vision patients and relating it to reading performance has not been widely researched. Legge and Rubin (1986) studied the effects of wavelength on reading performance in normal and low vision subjects and concluded that, for normal subjects under photopic levels, the wavelength does not affect reading performance when the text is luminance matched. Results from the low vision subjects were mixed. While 75 per cent of the subjects did not show a significant wavelength effect 25 per cent did. For these six subjects, who had degenerative photoreceptor disorders, reading performance was better for green and grey text and worst for red when the text was luminance matched using the normal observer spectral sensitivity function. Jacobs (1990) concluded that the reading performance using a VDT for low vision individuals was not affected by the screen colour.

The purpose of this study was to measure the contrast sensitivity of patients with diabetic retinopathy, optic atrophy and disciform ARM and to relate it to reading performance of

207

coloured text to determine if there is an optimum colour that should be used for VDT and closed circuit television (CCTV) low vision aids. These diseases represent the three most common conditions in the Centre for Sight Enhancement (CSE), University of Waterloo, Canada, which require a CCTV or VDT for reading. In the present chapter, we present reading performance data for green, yellow and red texts.

4.9.2   METHODS

4.9.2.1 Subjects

There were 24 low-vision subjects recruited from the patient files at the CSE, University of Waterloo. Nine had diabetic retinopathy, eight had various types of optic atrophy, and seven had disciform ARM. The age of the subjects ranged from 14 to 89 years. Table 4.9.1 shows the mean ages and visual acuities along with the standard deviations for each group of subjects. Visual acuity was measured with a Bailey-Lovie logMAR chart through the optimal refractive correction determined prior to the trials. This spectacle correction was used during all testing procedures. An additional lens was used for presbyopic subjects to correct for the viewing distance.

4.9.2.2 Procedure

Contrast sensitivity for a one c deg^{-1} sinusoidal grating was measured using a two alternative forced choice parameter estimation sequencing technique (PEST). The gratings were generated using the Cambridge Research Systems VSG stimulus generator (Kent, England) and displayed on a Hitachi 19-inch colour monitor. The gratings were oriented horizontally and displayed on either the left or the right side of the screen. The vertical drift frequency of the grating was 0.5 Hz. The targets subtended a circular area of four degrees at a one metre viewing distance. The luminance of the background and average luminance of the gratings for each colour were set to 18 cdm^{-2} using a Minolta CS-100 luminance meter. The colours were white, red, green and yellow. A response box with buttons corresponding to the left and right side of the screen was used by the subjects to indicate their choice of where the grating was presented. Each trial consisted of 40 presentations beginning with a suprathreshold grating. The threshold value in per cent contrast for each subject was determined from the last contrast presented. The following PEST parameters were used: initial step size equalled five per cent, maximum step size equalled ten per cent, minimum step size equalled 0.01, Wald limit equalled 1, Findlay constant equalled 1, response probability equalled 0.5.

Reading rates were measured for stationary and rapid serial visual presentation (RSVP) modes using the four different colours presented on the Hitachi monitor screen. The

Table 4.9.1.   Mean ages and visual acuities of subjects with the various conditions.

	Diabetic retinopathy	Optic atrophy	ARM
Mean age	59	42	81
(SD)	(15.2)	(20.1)	(4.3)
Mean visual acuity: logMAR	0.72	0.80	1.07
(SD)	(0.37)	(0.50)	(0.20)

character size was six degrees. This size was selected because it provides optimum reading rates for most low vision subjects (Legge and Rubin, 1985). The green, yellow, red, and white texts were luminance matched to 18 cdm^{-2} by placing the appropriate neutral density filter over the subject's eye. The text was presented as coloured letters on a dark background. Subjects read aloud for both presentation modes.

The reading rate for the stationary mode was determined by presenting a sentence consisting of four lines (average 3 words per line) on the monitor. The sentences were taken from the Minnesota Low-Vision Reading Test (Legge and Rubin, 1989) and were balanced with words of equal frequency in the English language. For the RSVP mode, a paragraph of text was presented to the subject one word at a time in the centre of the screen. The paragraphs were selected from grade four reading texts and were previously checked for equal difficulty by measuring the reading rates of normal subjects. Reading rates were calculated in correct words per minute for each colour in both the stationary and RSVP mode. In using this method, the text presentation rate had to be fast enough so that errors were made. This rate was determined for each colour by initially presenting the text at a rate well within most subject's ability and gradually increasing the speed until the subject made at least one error. This rate of presentation was then used for the trials.

Testing for all conditions was done with either the subject's preferred eye or the eye with the better visual acuity. The colour of the text or grating was chosen in random order. The stationary reading test was performed first, followed by the RSVP and contrast sensitivity tests. Two trials were done for each testing procedure.

4.9.3   RESULTS

The results of the different tests were all normalised to the white condition so that any differences between the relative spectral sensitivity of the low vision observer and the standard observer function used in the luminance meter would be reflected as values equal to, greater than, or less than one. Figure 4.9.1 shows the relative correct words per minute plotted against the colour of the text displayed on the monitor for the stationary reading mode. For the subjects as a whole, reading performance was best for the yellow text (30 per cent better than red or white) followed by green (12 per cent faster than red or white). Red text resulted in the minimal reading speed. These differences were significant at the $p \leq 0.05$ level. The better reading performance using the yellow text was mainly due to the ARM subjects whose reading speed showed an appreciable increase when yellow was used. The trend for the RSVP mode was similar to the stationary in that reading rates were slightly better for the yellow and green text; however, these results were not significant (rejection level $p \leq 0.05$).

Reading rate versus visual acuity for the different colours of the stationary and RSVP modes were also analysed. The general trend between normalised reading performance and visual acuity was that, as visual acuity decreased, relative performance using the red text decreased. These results were significant for only the RSVP mode. Because the ARM subjects had fairly similar visual acuities, the relatively poorer reading performance as a function of acuity for the red text is mainly due to subjects with optic atrophy and diabetic retinopathy.

Figures 4.9.2 and 4.9.3 show reading rate versus visual acuity using RSVP mode for the diabetic retinopathy and optic atrophy patients respectively. The correlation coefficients were significantly different from zero ($p \leq 0.05$).

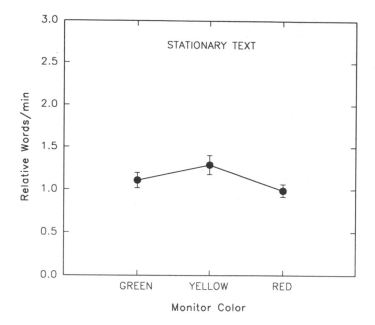

Figure 4.9.1. Relative reading rate in correct words per minute as a function of monitor colour using stationary mode. Reading rates have been normalised to the rate for white.

No association was found between the normalised contrast sensitivity values for the different colours and reading performance.

4.9.4 DISCUSSION

The general results of our study, though not dramatic, are consistent with those of Legge and Rubin (1986) who found that some low vision subjects performed poorest with red text. Our results may not be as obvious as theirs because we used broader band spectral stimuli and different subject groups. In our sample of subjects with advanced diseases, spectral sensitivity is probably reduced in both the short and long wavelengths, although ARM and diabetic subjects may have a greater loss in the shorter wavelengths (Alvarez *et al.*, 1983a, b; Cox, 1961). To estimate the impact of these losses on reading performance with our broad band colours, we determined the relative effective luminance to white for the green, yellow, and red text using spectral sensitivity functions with just a short wavelength sensitivity loss, just a long wavelength sensitivity loss, equal losses in sensitivity at short and long wavelength spectral regions, and losses in the short and long wavelengths but with a greater loss in the short. The magnitude of these losses was based on the long wavelength losses seen in protanopes (Pitt, 1935). The emission spectrum of the four monitor colours was measured with a Li-1800 spectroradiometer (Li-Cor, Lincoln, NE) in 5 nm intervals.

Our calculations showed that a combined loss of both short and long wavelength sensitivity results in the effective luminance of red being approximately half that of white, whereas the effective luminance of green is approximately 10 per cent greater than white, and yellow is approximately equal to white. This trend is present whether the short wavelength loss is equal to the sensitivity loss at the longer wavelengths or the short wavelength sensitivity loss is greater. Whether the yellow is effectively dimmer or brighter than white is dependent on the luminance ratio of the red and green phosphors. That is, reddish yellows will be dimmer whereas greenish yellows will be brighter. If the spectral sensitivity loss is just at the shorter wavelengths, then the effective luminance of the green is equal to white, while the red and yellow are about 10 per cent brighter. Except for the red colour, when losses occur just at long wavelengths the changes relative to white are small and would probably have negligible effects on reading speed.

Although we are uncertain as to whether subjects in our sample have spectral sensitivity functions identical to the ones used in our calculations, our estimations illustrate that selective losses in spectral sensitivity will have marginal effects on the relative luminances of broad band white, green and yellow stimuli. These marginal effects probably would not influence reading speed with text luminance greater than 10 cdm^{-2} (Legge and Rubin, 1986). These two factors partially explain why Jacobs (1990) did not find any significant effect on reading speed with screen colours of white, green and amber when using a luminance level of 100 cdm^{-2}.

The predicted marginal changes in the green and yellow relative to white also partially explain the lack of significant results found for contrast sensitivity. Although there may be

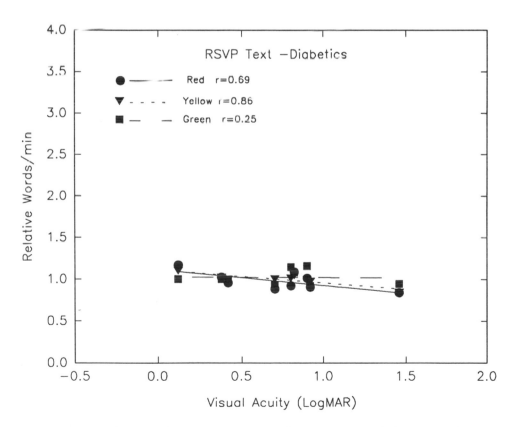

Figure 4.9.2. Relative reading rate in correct words per minute, for diabetic retinopathy subjects, as a function of visual acuity using RSVP mode. Reading rates have been normalised to the rate for white.

a loss in effective luminance of the red, this decrease in luminance is not enough to affect contrast sensitivity for a one c deg^{-1} target. Even if there is a drop in effective luminance of 50 per cent, the dimmer luminance is still in the range where Weber's Law holds and as a result contrast sensitivity would not be affected (Van Nes and Bouman, 1967).

The practical implications of this study are, given that the luminance range of the colours of the display are equal, the monitor colour for low vision patients with ARM, optic atrophy or diabetic retinopathy should not be red. A text of yellow or green should be tried first, especially for ARM patients. However, selective losses at a particular spectral region can be compensated for by increasing the luminance of that colour. For a red or white display our results suggest that the upper limit of this luminance range should be at least 30 per cent greater than the yellow or green display in order to compensate for spectral sensitivity losses we have reported. In practice this compensation is possible with white text, but not red because the dynamic range of the red phosphors is small. However, at luminance levels typically used by low vision patients, a 30 per cent increase in luminance may not make a dramatic change in reading performance, so other factors such as magnification, maximum luminance and maximum contrast of a monitor are probably more important.

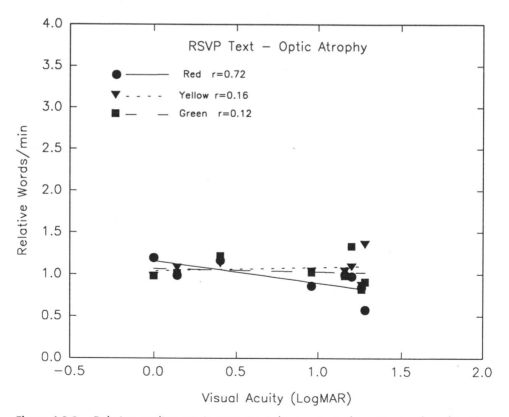

Figure 4.9.3.   Relative reading rate in correct words per minute for optic atrophy subjects, as a function of visual acuity using RSVP text. Reading rates have been normalised to the rate for white.

4.9.5 ACKNOWLEDGEMENTS

We thank Bob Mansfield of Optilec US Inc. for providing the text presentation software. This project was partially funded by the National Science and Engineering Research Council of Canada.

4.9.6 REFERENCES

ALVAREZ, S.L., KING-SMITH, P.E. & BHARGAVA, S.K. (1983a) Spectral thresholds in macular degeneration, *British Journal of Ophthalmology*, **67**, 504–507.

ALVAREZ, S.L., KING-SMITH, P.E. & BHARGAVA, S.K. (1983b) Spectral threshold measurement and clinical applications, *British Journal of Ophthalmology*, **67**, 508–511.

CAMPBELL, C.J. & RITTLER, M.C. (1972) Colour vision in retinal pathology, *Modern Problems in Ophthalmology*, **11**, 98–105.

COX, J. (1961) Colour vision defects acquired in diseases of the eye, *British Journal of Physiological Optics*, **18**, 3–32, 67–89.

JACOBS, R.J. (1990) Screen colour and reading performance on closed circuit television, *Journal of Visual Impairment and Blindness*, **84**, 569–572.

LAKOWSKI, R., ASPINALL, P.A. & KINNEAR, P.R. (1973) Association between colour vision losses and diabetes mellitus, *Ophthalmological Research*, **4**, 145–159.

LEGGE, G.E., PARISH, D.H., LUEBKER, A. & WURM, L.H. (1990) Psychophysics of reading IX. Comparing colour contrast and luminance contrast, *Journal of the Optical Society of America*, **A7**, 2002–2010.

LEGGE, G.E., & RUBIN G.S. (1986) Psychophysics of reading. IV. Wavelength effects in normal and low vision, *Journal of Optical Society of America*, **A 3**, 40–51.

LEGGE, G.E., RUBIN, G.S., PELLI, D.G. & SCHLESKE, M.M. (1985) Psychophysics of reading II. Low vision, *Vision Research*, **25**, 253–266.

PITT, F.H.G. (1935), *Characteristics of Dichromatic Vision*, Medical Research Council, Report of Committee on Physiology of Vision, No. XIV, London: HMSO.

TRICK, G.L., BURKE, R.M., GORDON, M.O., SANTIAGO, J.V. & KILO, C. (1988) The relationship between hue discrimination contrast sensitivity deficits in patients with diabetes mellitus, *Ophthalmology*, **95**, 693–698.

VAN NES, F.L. & BOUMAN, M.A. (1967) Spatial modulation transfer function in the human, *Journal of the Optical Society of America*, **57**, 401–406.

VERRIEST, G. (1964) Les deficiences acquises de la discrimination chromatique, *Mem. Acad. R. Med.*, Belgium **II/IV**, 5.

Section 5 – Development and Colour Vision Defects

The Development of Colour Vision in Infants

Davida Y. Teller

5.1.1. INTRODUCTION

Colour vision is relatively well-understood in adults. There is consensus that there are four photoreceptor types (L-cones, M-cones, S-cones, and rods) with sensitivity maxima in differing locations across the visible spectrum. There is also consensus that, early in visual processing, signals from the three cone types are combined additively to form a luminance channel, and subtractively to form two chromatic channels. Modellers of this early opponent stage commonly posit a red/green channel formed from a subtractive interaction of L- and M-cone-initiated signals, and a tritan channel formed from a subtractive interaction of S- versus L- and M-cone-initiated signals (e.g. Boynton, 1979; Krauskopf *et al.*, 1982). The need for a later opponent stage, making explicit the red-green and blue-yellow channels suggested by classical opponent process theory (Jameson and Hurvich, 1955) is also broadly acknowledged. Moreover, the partially separate processing of colour and motion signals is well accepted, although there is currently debate on the degree to which the chromatic channels eventually contribute to motion processing (e.g. Cavanagh and Anstis, 1991; Dobkins and Albright, 1994, 1995).

Given the advanced status of our understanding of adult colour vision, study of the development of colour vision is an attractive option. We say this because in the literature certain spectral signatures are taken as evidence of the presence of particular well-defined physiological or theoretical entities. For example, a spectral sensitivity curve with a λ_{max} near 440 nm is an unmistakable signature for the presence of S cones. A Sloan notch indicates both the presence of L and M cones and their opponent interaction: a luminous efficiency curve corresponding to V_λ signals the presence of a classical luminance mechanism. Data from human infants rarely allow this level of certainty of interpretation.

Moreover, evidence from other paradigms is at least provisionally accepted as providing signs for the presence of other specific mechanisms. For example, the capacity to make chromatic discriminations is usually taken to signal the presence of chromatic channels. The cardinality or independence of particular pairs of chromatic axes (Krauskopf *et al.*, 1982) is taken to signal the form of the chromatic code at a particular stage of processing, and the capacity to code the direction of motion for isoluminant stimuli is taken as a sign of the contribution of chromatic channels to motion processing (e.g. Cavanagh and Anstis, 1991; but see Dobkins and Albright, 1994, 1995).

A promising approach to the study of infant colour vision, therefore, is to look for these particular signs and signatures in infant colour vision, and use them as evidence that particular mechanisms are present and functional. In principle, one should be able to use these signs and signatures to establish the presence, or absence, of each receptor type and each post-receptoral channel, the cardinality of particular chromatic axes, and the contribution of colour to motion, over the course of early postnatal life.

5.1.1.1 Interesting versus uninteresting outcomes

Of course, the answers found by a programme of research can turn out to be relatively more or less interesting. It might be that all aspects of colour vision are adult-like in young infants, or that all of the mechanisms of colour vision simply increase in absolute sensitivity in step with each other. Such an outcome, while worth knowing, might be considered to be relatively uninteresting and have little theoretical impact. Alternatively, some aspects of colour vision might be adult-like in early infancy, while others might be absent or differentially immature. If so, the development of colour vision might provide the fodder for new theorising about the mechanisms of visual development, and possibly even about colour vision in general.

We provide a very brief review of the current state of knowledge about infant colour vision. More extensive reviews and theoretical treatments may be found in Teller and Bornstein (1987), Brown (1990) and Teller and Lindsey (1993). The present discussion is organised around the question of which of the signs and signatures of particular adult colour vision mechanisms have been sought, and either found or not found, in infants of various ages. We believe that potentially interesting immaturities have been found; these are emphasised under each section.

5.1.2   PHOTORECEPTORS

The foveae of infants are very immature at birth (Yuodelis and Hendrickson, 1986). The packing density of the cone outer segments is less than that of adults, the rod-free area is larger, and the outer segments of infant foveal cones are extremely short. These immaturities limit the quantum-catching ability of infant foveal cones, and may have other consequences for infant colour vision.

Nonetheless, by two to three months postnatal, if not before, infants are known to have functional photoreceptors of all four types. The presence of functional rods is shown conclusively by the presence of a spectral luminous efficiency curve that conforms to V'_λ in infants as young as one month of age (Powers et al., 1981; Werner, 1982). The presence of functional S cones is suggested by the fact that infants can make tritan discriminations (Clavadetscher et al., 1988; Varner et al., 1985; but see Brown, 1990), and conclusively established by the existence of a peak in sensitivity at about 440 nm under yellow-adapted conditions (Volbrecht and Werner, 1987).

Early suggestive evidence for functional L and M cones came from demonstrations that photopic spectral sensitivity varied with adaptation and test conditions, but was broader than could be accounted for by a single cone mechanism. Moreover, photopic spectral sensitivity was shown to be similar in infants and adults when both were tested under the same conditions (e.g. Dobson, 1976; Peeples and Teller, 1978). The next line of evidence

was provided by demonstrations that two-month-old infants can make Rayleigh discriminations (Hamer *et al.*, 1982; Packer *et al.*, 1984). More recent evidence comes from the
demonstration of a Sloan notch in three-month-olds (Brown and Teller, 1989), and of a high
degree of similarity between infant and adult flicker-based photopic luminous efficiency
curves in two and four-month-olds (Bieber *et al.*, in press). And finally, Knoblauch *et al.*
(1995) have used null plane analysis to show conclusively the contribution of isolated L and
M cones to visual evoked potentials.

5.1.2.1 Interesting immaturities

Two interesting questions arise from our current understanding of photoreceptor
development.

Foveal immaturities and metameric matches

Given the very short outer segments of infant foveal cones (Yuodelis and Hendrickson,
1986), one would expect that the effective optical density of the infant's photoreceptor
would be substantially reduced (Banks and Bennett, 1988; Brown, 1990). In consequence,
one might expect to see changes in the metameric matches of infants. To our knowledge
this question has never been studied, probably in part because infants' chromatic discrimination is so poor (see below) that metameric match ranges might be too broad to allow
a clear test of the predicted match points.

Immaturity of processing of S cone signals

Functional S cones are unquestionably present in infancy (Volbrecht and Werner, 1987).
However, the S-cone signature has failed to reveal itself in two-month-old infants in at least
one behavioural chromatic adaptation study (Pulos *et al.*, 1980). This result provides an
early hint (there are more to come) of a possible differential loss of absolute sensitivity of
S cones, or of S-cone-initiated signals, at some later post-receptoral stage.

5.1.3 PHOTOPIC LUMINOUS EFFICIENCY

As noted above, early investigations showed variations of infant photopic spectral sensitivity across studies, but strong similarities between infants and adults tested under similar
conditions (e.g. Dobson, 1976; Peeples and Teller, 1978). More recently, techniques more
like those classically used to define photopic luminous efficiency have been developed and
used with infants. Analogs to both motion photometry (Maurer *et al.*, 1989; Teller and
Lindsey, 1989) and flicker photometry (Bieber *et al.*, in press) have been used. After
appropriate corrections for lens and macular pigment density, these studies all reveal close
similarity of the infant data to adult data and to standard adult photopic luminous efficiency
curves. Thus, there can be little doubt that infants have an adult-like photopic luminance
mechanism at an early age.

5.1.3.1 A possibly interesting immaturity: rod intrusion at mesopic levels?

Infants clearly have both scotopic and photopic mechanisms. However, there are at least
two reasons to suspect that infants' mesopic vision might be more rod dominated than that

of adults. The first is the immaturity of the infant's fovea (Yuodelis and Hendrickson, 1986), which could lead to a possibly increased reliance on extra-foveal retinal regions in which rods are more prevalent. The second comes from a chromatic discrimination study carried out at low photopic levels (Clavadetscher *et al.*, 1988). In that study, infants' discrimination failures and performance minima unexpectedly followed V'$_\lambda$ rather than a photopic curve over the short to middle wavelength range.

Of course, the finding of rod dominance at mesopic levels might be ultimately uninteresting. That is, it might stem simply from relatively equal elevations of absolute thresholds for both rod and cone mechanisms, with rods left to dominate at mesopic levels. On the other hand, this finding could be an indicator of some more interesting developmental change in visual processing. Studies of the transition from rod to cone vision are needed to sort out this question.

5.1.4   CHROMATIC DISCRIMINATIONS

Most studies of chromatic discrimination to date have been done on a pass-fail basis, using the largest available chromatic differences. Tested behaviourally, most one-month-olds have so far failed to make chromatic discriminations (with the partial exception of discriminating long-wavelength lights from lights of other spectral compositions). Two-month-olds can unquestionably make at least some chromatic discriminations when chromatic differences are large; but they also fail in some cases, particularly in the discrimination of yellows, yellow-greens and mid-purples from white (Allen *et al.*, 1988; Clavadetscher *et al.*, 1988; Hamer *et al.*, 1982; Peeples and Teller, 1975; Teller *et al.*, 1978; Varner *et al.*, 1985). Larger field sizes enhance infants' chromatic discrimination capabilities (Packer *et al.*, 1984).

Recent visual-evoked potential (VEP) studies from two different laboratories provide contradictory evidence for the onset times of VEP responses to red/green chromatic modulation. One recent report (Allen *et al.*, 1993) suggests that chromatic stimuli generate measurable VEP responses as early as five weeks, while another (Morrone *et al.*, 1993) suggests that chromatic signals are rare before about two months. The basis of these differences remains to be sorted out.

5.1.4.1. Interesting immaturities

The chromatic discrimination data raise interesting questions concerning the presence and maturation of chromatic channels.

Chromatic channels or luminance-channel 'artefacts'?

One would like to conclude that infants make chromatic discriminations via functional post-receptoral chromatic channels. However, to prove this conclusively, one would need to show that infants are not using 'artefactual' signals in a luminance channel. The potential sources of such 'artefactual' signals include chromatic aberration, variation in isoluminance points across the population of cells that constitutes the luminance channel, and possible transient signals generated by eye-movements (for discussion, see Cavanagh and Anstis, 1991; Dobkins and Albright, 1994, 1995).

What chromatic channels?

Moreover, even if chromatic channels mediate infants' chromatic discriminations, infants' chromatic channels might differ from those of adults. The channels that mediate infants' chromatic discriminations might be more rod-dominated, or even have different cone input weights. In addition, there are no data to address the question of whether infants show the signs of independent cardinal directions in colour space; or if so, whether their cardinal directions coincide with the red-green and tritan axes identified by Krauskopf and colleagues in adults (e.g. Krauskopf *et al.*, 1982). Although the possible existence of juvenile chromatic channels that differ from those of adults seems remote, there is little evidence to rule out these options.

Uniform versus differential loss

As indicated above, chromatic discrimination is poor in early infancy; but so is luminance discrimination (reviewed in Brown, 1990). It has not been clear, therefore, whether infants should be said to show a (relatively uninteresting) uniform loss of sensitivity to both chromatic and luminance differences, or a (much more interesting) differential loss of sensitivity to chromatic with respect to luminance differences, or of one chromatic channel with respect to another (Banks and Bennett, 1988; Brown, 1990; Teller and Lindsey, 1993).

In an extensive, ideal-observer-based analysis of behavioural data from our laboratory, Banks and his colleagues (Banks and Bennett, 1988; Banks and Shannon, 1993) have concluded that infants show a uniform loss of sensitivity for red-green versus luminance differences, but a differential loss of sensitivity for tritan differences. The conclusion of a differential tritan loss is consistent with the earlier hints of a differential loss of S-cone absolute sensitivity (see above).

Recent VEP studies have raised controversy concerning losses of sensitivity to red/green differences. Data from Allen *et al.* (1993) support the uniform loss model, while those from Morrone *et al.* (1993) support the differential loss model. Tritan losses have not been extensively studied with VEP techniques.

Better discrimination at higher luminance levels?

Finally, as stated above, the foveal cones of infants are very immature (Yuodelis and Hendrickson, 1986), and their outer segments are poorly designed to catch quanta (Banks and Bennett, 1988; Brown, 1990). It is possible that some of the difficulty one-month-olds have with chromatic discrimination could stem from this factor alone. New studies of chromatic contrast thresholds at higher light levels are needed to address this issue.

5.1.5 COLOUR AND MOTION

Our laboratory has recently undertaken studies of the question of whether or not infants code the direction of motion for moving isoluminant chromatic stimuli. The infant's opto-kinetic-nystagmus-like, or directionally-appropriate eye movements (DEMs) are used as the response measure. Under the conditions tested to date, two-month-olds (but not one-month-olds) make DEMs to moving red-green stimuli (Teller and Lindsey, 1993). Motion nulling experiments between red-green and luminance-modulated stimuli (Teller and Lindsey, 1993; Teller and Palmer, 1996) reveal a relatively constant equivalent luminance contrast between infants and adults, and are thus consistent with the uniform loss hypothesis for moving red-green versus luminance stimuli. In contrast, neither two-month-olds nor four-month-olds make DEMs to moving tritan stimuli (Teller *et al.*, 1994).

We (Dobkins *et al.*, 1995) have also undertaken studies of infants' motion/detection (M/D) ratios for red-green and luminance-modulated stimuli. In classical psychophysical theory (Graham, 1989), M/D ratios near 1 provide evidence that detection mechanisms are coded for the direction of motion, while M/D ratios greater then 1 provide evidence that they are not. In adults, M/D ratios are approximately 1 for luminance-modulated stimuli (Graham, 1989) but larger than 1 for chromatic stimuli (e.g. Cavanagh and Anstis, 1991; Lindsey and Teller, 1990). In infants, our preliminary and unexpected result is that M/D ratios are near 1 for both kinds of stimuli.

5.1.5.1 Interesting immaturities of chromatic motion processing

These new experiments on chromatic motion processing suggest two potentially interesting immaturities.

M/D ratios near 1 for chromatic stimuli

The preliminary finding of M/D ratios near 1 for chromatic stimuli in infants suggests that, surprisingly, infants' chromatic detection mechanisms may be coded for the direction of motion. Whereas adults detect red-green stimuli with one set of detectors and code their direction of motion with another, it is as though infants use the same detectors for both tasks. If these data and theoretical notions are correct, then either the infant's chromatic detectors for red-green stimuli are differentially delayed, or the infant's chromatic motion analysers for red-green stimuli are differentially precocious.

No DEMs to tritan stimuli

The finding that infants do not make directionally-appropriate eye movements in response to moving tritan-modulated stimuli (Teller *et al.*, 1994) provides yet another hint of a differential loss of sensitivity to tritan stimuli. Whether there is one loss for static tritan stimuli, and an additional loss for tritan motion processing, or just one loss that applies equally to both, remains to be sorted out.

5.1.6   SUMMARY

In summary, much has been learned about infant colour vision over the past 20 years. But many old questions remain, and new ones have been raised. Infants show the spectral signatures of functional photoreceptors of all four types. They also have a photopic spectral luminous efficiency function that conforms well to standard adult photopic spectral luminous efficiency; that is, they show the signature of an adult-like luminance channel.

Infants also make chromatic discriminations, and therefore could be said to show clear signs of chromatic channels. It seems likely, a priori, that these discriminations are made with an immature but otherwise standard version of adult chromatic channels. However, to date, the ruling out of other options has not been vigorously pursued. Moreover, there are as yet no direct studies demonstrating the cardinality of red-green and tritan chromatic axes in infants. Finally, studies of chromatic motion processing reveal interesting possible differences between infants and adults.

Can the study of infant colour vision tell us anything interesting about colour vision in general? Maybe: it is interesting to entertain the argument that the differential loss of a mechanism in development is itself evidence for the existence and independence or separability of that element in the adult visual system. Arguments of exactly this kind led historically to the use of the confusion lines of colour deficient observers as a basis for estimating the action spectra of the cone fundamentals. On this argument, differential losses of sensitivity to tritan stimuli during development would provide further evidence of the cardinality of the tritan versus red-green channels in the adult colour vision system. If sensitivity to tritan stimuli can be truly differentially lost, the tritan channel must be an independent entity, somehow susceptible to independent maturational manipulation. If this argument is accepted, then studies of infant colour vision, as they progress, may well contribute to advances in our understanding of colour vision in general.

5.1.7   REFERENCES

ALLEN, D., BANKS, M.S. & SCHEFRIN, B. (1988) Chromatic discrimination in human infants, a re-examination, *Investigative Ophthalmology and Visual Science*, **29** (Suppl.), 25.

ALLEN, D., BANKS, M.S. & NORCIA, A.M. (1993) Does chromatic sensitivity develop more slowly than luminance sensitivity? *Vision Research*, **33**, 2553–2562.

BANKS, M.S. & BENNETT, P.J. (1988) Optical and photoreceptor immaturities limit the spatial and chromatic vision of human neonates, *Journal of the Optical Society of America*, A **5**, 2059–2079.

BANKS, M.S. & SHANNON, E. (1993) Spatial and chromatic visual efficiency in human neonates. In: Granrud, C. (Ed.), *Visual Perception and Cognition in Infancy*, pp. 1–46, Hillsdale, NJ: Lawrence Erlbaum.

BIEBER, M., VOLBRECHT, V. & WERNER, J. HFP spectral efficiency is similar for 2-and 4-month old human infants and adults, *Vision Research*, in press.

BOYNTON, R. (1979) *Human Color Vision*, New York: Holt, Rinehart and Winston.

BROWN, A.M. (1990) Development of visual sensitivity to light and color vision in human infants: A critical review, *Vision Research*, **30**, 1159–1188.

BROWN, A. & TELLER, D.Y. (1989) Chromatic opponency in 3-month-old human infants, *Vision Research*, **29**, 37–46.

CAVANAGH, P. & ANSTIS, S. (1991) The contribution of color to motion in normal and colour-deficient observers, *Vision Research*, **31**, 2109–2148.

CLAVADETSCHER, J.E., BROWN, A.M., ANKRUM, C. & TELLER, D.Y. (1988) Spectral sensitivity and chromatic discriminations in 3-and 7-week-old human infants, *Journal of the Optical Society of America*, A **5**, 2093–2105.

DOBKINS, K.R. & ALBRIGHT, T.D. (1994) What happens if it changes color when it moves?: The nature of chromatic input to macaque visual area MT, *Journal of Neuroscience*, **14**, 4854–4870.

DOBKINS, K.R. & ALBRIGHT, T.D. (1995) Behavioral and neural effects of chromatic isoluminance in the primate visual motion system, *Visual Neuroscience*, **12**, 321–332.

DOBKINS, K.R. LIA, B, & TELLER, D.Y. (1995) Infant motion:detection (M:D) ratios for color-defined and luminance-defined moving gratings, *Investigative Ophthalmology and Visual Science*, **36**, 5443.

DOBSON, V. (1976) Spectral sensitivity of the 2-month infant as measured by the visually evoked cortical potential, *Vision Research*, **16**, 367–374.

GRAHAM, N. (1989) *Visual Pattern Analyzers*, New York: Oxford University Press.

HAMER, R.D., ALEXANDER, K.R. & TELLER, D.Y. (1982) Rayleigh discriminations in young human infants, *Vision Research*, **22**, 575–587.

JAMESON, D. & HURVICH, L.M. (1955) Some quantitative aspects of an opponent-colors theory: 1. Chromatic responses and spectral saturation, *Journal of the Optical Society of America*, **45**, 546–552.

KNOBLAUCH, K., BIEBER, M. & WERNER, J.S. (1995) Assessing dimensionality in infant color vision. In: Vital-Durand, F., Atkinson, J. and Braddick, O. (Eds), *Infant Vision*, Oxford: Oxford University Press.

KRAUSKOPF, J., WILLIAMS, D.R. & HEELEY, D.W. (1982) Cardinal directions in color space, *Vision Research*, **22**, 1123–1131.

LINDSEY, D.T. & TELLER, D.Y. (1990) Motion at isoluminance: Discrimination/detection ratios for moving isoluminant gratings, *Vision Research*, **30**, 1751–1761.

MAURER, D., LEWIS, T., CAVANAGH, P. & ANSTIS, S. (1989) A new test of luminous efficiency for babies, *Investigative Ophthalmology and Visual Science*, **30**, 297–303.

MORRONE, M.C., BURR, D.C. & FIORENTINI, A. (1993) Development of infant contrast sensitivity to chromatic stimuli, *Vision Research*, **33**, 2535–2552.

PACKER, O., HARTMANN, E.E. & TELLER, D.Y. (1984) Infant color vision: The effect of test field size on Rayleigh discriminations, *Vision Research*, **24**, 1247–1260.

PEEPLES, D.R. & TELLER, D.Y. (1975) Color vision and brightness discrimination in two-month-old human infants, *Science*, **189**, 1102–1103.

PEEPLES, D.R. & TELLER, D.Y. (1978) White-adapted photopic spectral sensitivity in human infants, *Vision Research*, **18**, 49–53.

POWERS, M.K. SCHNECK, M & TELLER, D.Y. (1981) Spectral sensitivity of human infants at absolute visual threshold, *Vision Research*, **21**, 1005–1016.

PULOS, E., TELLER, D. & BUCK, S. (1980) Infant color vision: a search for short-wavelength-sensitive mechanisms by means of chromatic adaption, *Vision Research*, **20**, 485–493.

TELLER, D.Y. & BORNSTEIN, M. (1987) Infant color vision and color perception. In Salapatek, P. & Cohen, L. (Eds), *Handbook of Infant Perception, I: From Sensation to Perception*, New York: Academic Press.

TELLER, D.Y. & LINDSEY, D.T. (1989) Motion nulls for white versus isochromatic gratings in infants and adults, *Journal of the Optical Society of America*, **A 6**, 1945–1954.

TELLER, D.Y. & LINDSEY, D.T. (1993) Infant color vision: OKN techniques and null plane analysis. In: Simons, K. (Ed.), *Infant Vision: Basic and Clinical Research*, New York: Oxford University Press, pp. 143–162.

TELLER, D.Y. & PALMER, J. (1996) Infant color vision: Motion nulls for red/green- vs. luminance-modulated stimuli in infants and adults, *Vision Research*, **36**, 955–974.

TELLER, D.Y., PEEPLES, D.R. & SEKEL, M. (1978) Discrimination of chromatic from white light by two-month-old human infants, *Vision Research*, **18**, 41–48.

TELLER, D.Y., BROOKS, T.W. & SIMS, J.D. (1994) Moving tritan stimuli do not drive directional eye movements in infants, *Investigative Ophthalmology & Visual Science*, **35**, 1643.

VARNER, D., COOK, J.E., SCHNECK, M.E., McDONALD, M. & TELLER, D.Y. (1985) Tritan discriminations by 1- and 2-month-old human infants, *Vision Research*, **25**, 821–831.

VOLBRECHT, V.J. & WERNER, J.S. (1987) Isolation of short-wavelength-sensitive cone photoreceptors in 4–6-week-old human infants, *Vision Research*, **27**, 469–478.

WERNER, J.S. (1982) Development of scotopic sensitivity and the absorption spectrum of the human ocular media, *Journal of the Optical Society of America*, **72**, 247–258.

YUODELIS, C. & HENDRICKSON, A. (1986) A qualitative and quantitative analysis of the human fovea during development, *Vision Research*, **26**, 847–855.

Do Congenital Colour Vision Defects Represent a Selective Advantage?

Pia Grassivaro Gallo, Luigi Romana, Franco Viviani and
Andrea Camperio Ciani

5.2.1 INTRODUCTION

The lack of a general map of the incidence of congenital colour vision defects in Italy
(which exists for other European countries (such as England and France; see Kherumian
and Pickford, 1959) has stimulated the present work, which started in 1987.

5.2.2 METHOD

A thorough investigation of colour blindness in subjects attending compulsory junior and
high schools was carried out in the following Italian regions: Veneto (1367 students from
the Venetian lagoon and 834 from Padua); Emilia-Romagna (841 students); Liguria (1645
subjects from the coastal region and 1479 inland); in Apulia (907 subjects), and in Sicily
(968 students from the Eastern coastal regions and 1977 from the central-Western inland
regions). In total, 11,642 subjects from coastal regions, and 7398 subjects from inland areas
were examined. The survey was carried out by means of the Ishihara (1973) and Farnsworth
D15 (1957) tests.

Information furnished by other authors, who have worked in Italy using the same
methodology and who have checked no less than 500 individuals, has been added to these
data. These additional data concern Lazio (3285 subjects), Calabria (2207 subjects from
coastal and 1360 subjects from inland regions), and Sardinia (1990 subjects from the
coastal area of the island).

5.2.3 RESULTS

We are now able to present the complete classification of colour vision defects in Italy
(Table 5.2.1). In classifying data, Farnsworth's suggestions were followed (1957). In
particular, in some of the samples, the number of subjects classified as being doubtful cases

Table 5.2.1. Classification of the specific categories of colour vision defect in Italy.

Region	Total subject	Doubtful cases	Protans Anopes	Protans Anomals	Deutans Anopes	Deutans Anomals	Tritans Anopes	Tritans Anomals	Total dyschromates	σ	Total Protans Deutans Tritans	%
Veneto-Inland (Pallaro & Grassivaro Gallo, 1987)	834	6	10	8	13	4			41	0.69	35	4.20
%		14.63	24.39	19.51	31.70	9.76						
Veneto-Lagoon (Grassivaro Gallo & Malfitano, 1994)	1367	3	12	10	16	40			81	0.62	78	5.70
%		3.7	14.46	12.05	19.28	48.19						
Emilia Romagna (Grassivaro Gallo, & Posceddu, 1991)	841	13	7	8	6	14			48	0.68	35	4.16
%		27.1	14.6	16.7	12.5	29.2						
Liguria-Coast (Grassivaro Gallo & Panza, 1994)	1645	14	21	6	21	36			98	0.54	84	5.10
%		14.2	21.4	6.1	21.4	36.7						
Liguria-Inland (Grassivaro Gallo & Panza, 1994)	1479	23	13	6	27	22			91	0.54	68	4.59
%		25.2	14.2	6.5	29.6	24.1						
Lazio (Malaspina et al. 1986)	3285	10							211	0.41	201	6.12
%		4.7										

Population	N								Total	σ	n	%
Puglia (Grassivaro Gallo & Folin, 1990)	907	3	7	3	22	6			41	0.66	38	4.19
Calabria-Inland (Tagarelli, personal communication)	1360	9	2	2	43	16			72	0.56	63	4.63
%		7.32	17.07	7.31	53.65	14.63						
Calabria-Coast (Tagarelli, personal communication)	2207	18	-	-	122	56			196	0.57	178	8.06
%		12.5	2.8	2.8	59.7	22.2						
Central-Western Sicily (Grassivaro Gallo & Romana, 1993)	1977	48	34	5	31	15	1	1	135	0.46	87	4.40
%		9.2			62.2	28.6						
South-East Sicily (Grassivaro Gallo & Cannizzo, 1993)	968	7	11	7	17	26	1		69	0.78	62	6.40
%		35.56	25.18	3.70	22.96	11.11	0.74					
Sardinia (Siniscalco, 1963)	1990								141	0.57	141	7.0
%		10.14	15.94	10.14	24.63	37.68	1.45					

The frequency percentage for each category refers to the total number of colour defectives in each sample. σ is calculated by means of the following formula: $\sigma = \sqrt{p*q/N}$

may seem high, but this is due to the age range (11–13 years) from which the sample was selected. Among the 11-year-olds, subjects with trichromatic vision, but making errors (because of inattention, or explicable on the basis of perceptual effects such as closeness, narrowness or similarity; see Kanizsa *et al.*, 1985), were frequently found. In the Ishihara test, for example, the number 3 was read as 8; the 6 in place of 5; the 2 instead of 7; 9 in place of 0.

The Sardinian sample (Siniscalco, 1963) was comprised of subjects living in nine municipalities: seven in the coastal (n = 1521; 8.5 per cent) and two in the inland part (n = 469; 2.1 per cent). For this reason, the latter sample cannot be considered as being representative of the inland regions, and it is shown in the map (Figure 5.2.1), but not in Table 5.2.2.

In the statistical analysis carried out (χ^2 calculations), doubtful cases were eliminated. We would like to point out that the expected frequencies have been calculated on the minimal

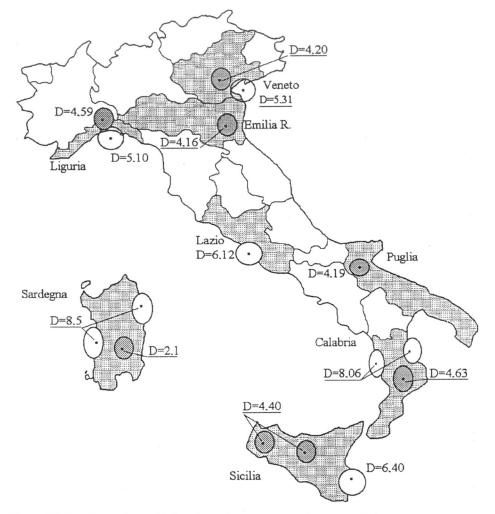

Figure 5.2.1.   The regions of Italy where the present survey was carried out.
○ Samples taken from populations living in coastal areas.
◉ Samples taken from populations living in inland areas.
D Percentage of colour vision defectives found.

Table 5.2.2. The significance of the differences in the incidence of colour vision defects among the various Italian regions

Region	χ^2	1	2	3	4	5	6	7	8	9	10	11
1 Veneto-Inland (Pallard & Grassivaro Gallo, 1987)	**0.08**											
2 Veneto-Lagoon (Grassivaro Gallo & Malfitano, 1994)	9.95	10.03										
3 Emilia Romagna (Grassivaro Gallo & Posceddu, 1991)	**0.05**	**0.13**	9.99									
4 Liguria-Coast (Grassivaro Gallo & Panza, 1994)	5.03	5.11	14.97	5.08								
5 Liguria-Inland (Grassivaro Gallo & Panza, 1994)	**1.32**	**1.40**	11.26	**1.37**	6.35							
6 Lazio (Malaspina, et al., 1986)	36.87	36.95	46.81	36.92	41.90	38.19						
7 Puglia (Grassivaro Gallo & Folin, 1990)	**0.08**	**0.16**	10.02	**0.13**	5.11	**1.40**	36.94					
8 Calabria-Inland (Tagarelli, personal communication)	**1.36**	**1.44**	11.30	**1.41**	6.39	**2.68**	38.22	**1.44**				
9 Calabria-Coast (Tagarelli, personal communication)	91.18	91.26	101.1	91.23	96.21	92.50	128.0	91.26	92.54			
10 Central-Western Sicily (Grassivaro Gallo & Romana, 1993)	**0.79**	**0.87**	10.73	**0.84**	5.82	**2.11**	37.65	**0.87**	**2.15**	91.97		
11 South-East Sicily (Grassivaro Gallo & Cannizzo, 1993)	14.00	14.08	23.94	14.05	19.03	15.32	50.86	14.08	15.36	105.1	14.79	
12 Sardinia (Sinisalco, 1963)	47.36	47.44	57.30	47.41	52.39	48.68	84.22	47.44	48.72	138.54	8.15	61.35

In the calculation of χ^2, $(f_o - f_a)^2/f_a$, the frequencies observed (f_o) do not include doubtful cases. The expected frequencies (f_a) have been calculated taking into account the lowest frequency of colour vision defects on a European level: 0.040, multiplied by the number of subjects in each sample. The first column shows the χ^2 of each sample with respect to the expected values. The following columns show the comparison of χ^2 among the samples. The figures in bold type show $\chi^2 \leq 3.84$ ($\alpha = 0.05$) and 1 df.
The samples with no significant differences are: Inland-Veneto, Emilia Romagna, Inland-Liguria, Puglia, Inland-Calabria and Central-Western Sicily.
The samples that maintain significant differences with respect to the preceding samples are: Veneto-Lagoon, Coastal-Liguria, Lazio, Coastal-Calabria, South-East Sicily and Sardinia.

frequencies of colour vision defect found at a European level: 0.040 (Kalmus, 1965). On doing this for the whole set of data available for Italy, the statistical analysis distinguishes two distinct groups:

1. data from the coastal regions, with an average of colour defective subjects of 6.39 per cent ($\sigma = 0.74$);
2. the values of the inland regions, with an average incidence of colour vision defects of 4.27 per cent ($\sigma = 0.41$).

In Table 5.2.2 the significance of the differences among the incidence of colour vision defects in the various Italian regions has been drawn up, and Figure 5.2.1 depicts the regions where the survey was carried out.

5.2.4   DISCUSSION

At first sight the authors have followed the common idea that congenital colour vision defects have a high incidence in Northern Europe (7–9 per cent) and a low one in Southern (3–5 per cent) and Mediterranean Europe (Floris et al., 1988). This idea was supported by Post's hypothesis (1982, originally published 1962) based on selection release and on the analysis of data found from 1922 and 1962, according to which it was possible to distinguish three groups of populations:

1. those who were still hunter/gatherers, with an average of 2 per cent colour vision deficiency out of 7712 subjects;
2. those who were hunter/gatherers until a short time ago: 3 per cent colour vision defects out of 9443 subjects;
3. those who were hunters a very long time ago: 5 per cent of colour defectives out of 436,943 subjects.

We share the genetics student's criticisms regarding Post since a sufficiently precise idea of the disadvantages brought about by colour blindness in a hunter/gatherer community is lacking. Selection relaxation does not completely explain the phenomenon of the origin of colour deficiency; furthermore, it has been calculated that, taking into account the mutation mechanisms, frequency levels similar to the highest ascertained until now could be reached (Curtoni et al., 1991). Cavalli-Sforza and Bodmer (1971), when commenting on Post's hypothesis, were also not convinced either by selection release, or by the above-cited mutation mechanisms. They believed that '. . . we must imagine that today colour blindness has a slight selective advantage for males and perhaps also for heterozygote females . . .' (p. 178). They thus preferred to wait for further experimental proof that would permit a more convincing hypothesis on these two X-linked polymorphisms to be formulated.

In accordance with some other authors, we deliberated on the advantages of a colour vision defect. For example, during the field administration of the Ishihara test, we were impressed by the disconcertion that orthochromates revealed when dyschromates showed a good reading ability for the camouflaged plates for orthochromates contained in the test: this represents an advantage in comparison with 'normal' subjects. Morgan et al. (1992) carried out an experimental design by using camouflaged symbols and, in effect, colour defective subjects showed a higher performance level than trichromats. Discussing their results, these authors hypothesised that ortho- and dyschromate polymorphisms are maintained in a parental-type selection within genetically kindred groups. For example, the groups who cooperate in the gathering of food could obtain advantages from the presence of members able to discover objects or camouflaged forms that are usually hidden for normals.

Recent genetic discoveries regarding colour vision defects have highlighted the positive aspects of recombination: the possibility of obtaining new genetic types and a new system of colour vision within the next thousand years (quadrichromia) (Lethuillier, 1986). The positive side-effects of recombination for a species are considered from the fitness viewpoint.

Polyak (1957) hypothesised that trichromatism developed in concomitance with the appearance of coloured fruits. This idea has recently been reconsidered in order to shed light on the types of vision of some monkeys and apes, taking into account their environment and nutrition. Frugivor monkeys have trichromatic vision, while the colour vision possessed by leaf-eating Catarrhines is not well known. The New World monkeys are dyschromates, but heterozygote females could be trichromatic: this is caused by inactivation of the X chromosome. Because of this, different pigments are expressed in the two rethinical photoreceptors. It is possible that heterozygote females lead their group when looking for ripe fruits (Mollon, 1989).

With the use of microspectrophotometry, Bowmaker et al. (1991) examined energy light photoreceptor absorption in eight different species of monkeys and apes of the Old World, from different geographical regions and ecological niches. Among the eight examined species, the λ_{max} is very similar and a fruit-based nutrition was ascertained.

In less evolved animal groups, environment-related modifications of the chromatic perception system are found. For example, fish change the proteins of photoreceptor pigments on the basis of the typology of light that effuses the environment in which they find themselves. Bridges and Delisle (1974) found that salmon change their blue-sensitive pigments into red-sensitive ones when they move from the sea to rivers (where long wavelengths predominate). The same authors examined the pigments of salmon-like fish trapped in the Quebec lakes (formed by glaciations 17 000–20 000 years ago) and compared them to salmon currently living in the Atlantic Ocean. The former possess rodopsines (which have maximal absorption at 512 ± 1nm), whereas the latter utilise porphynopsines (with a maximum absorption at 542 ± 1nm).

Birds have more photoreceptors per rethinic unit than other vertebrates, also possessing exceptionally acute vision and quick accommodation. In some falcons the photoreceptors of the foveal region are eight times longer than those found in man. Diurnal birds have excellent chromatic vision that makes use of a special structure in their photoreceptors: between the external and internal segment a coloured (red, orange, yellow) or uncoloured oil droplet exists, and its oozing or shading function favours the visual pigments (Storer et al., 1982). Bowmaker (1980) believes that, in birds, the main visual function is connected to food-gathering strategies. We would like to point out that diurnal and nocturnal vegetarian species possess about 50–80 per cent of the orange and red oil droplets. Light reflected from leaves has a peak between 540 and 570 nm, due to chlorophyll. Sea fish-eating birds, on the other hand, are divided into two distinct groups: those that feed or capture prey at or near the surface of the water (with about 50–80 per cent of red and orange oil droplets) and those that dive into deep waters, possessing only 20 per cent of red and orange oil droplets. This could be an adaptation permitting them to discover the fish through the water where sensitivity to short wavelengths could be advantageous (Bowmaker, 1980).

As far as our results are concerned, in interpreting the incidence of colour vision defects in the various Italian regions, at first we considered valid the hypothesis that on the basis of its high incidence in the coastal regions, a psycho-perceptual component would act as follows: colour defectives would tend to shift towards coastal areas because of the prevailing colours (azure/blue) found. This is because these colours would be better appreciated than those prevailing in the inland areas, i.e. generally green. This could also be experimentally verified, but it would certainly not be the only prevailing factor. Later on we added other ergonomic considerations. If we deliberate upon the occupation exclusively practised among the coastal populations (fishing), the idea spontaneously arises that a colour vision defect probably better suits fishermen, who are individuals working in a sea environment, where the prevailing light colours are blue/green. We must bear in mind that 70 per cent of defectives are deutans. Green blindness permits a reduced colour vision; thus chromatic perception has an advantage. Because of the lack of one of the primary colours, in fact, a green-blind subject can discriminate in a simplified colour system. The colour of the background of the environment can vary from blue to azure, while the colour of the object to be discriminated – the fish – is grey/black.

At this point it appears unavoidable to enquire about the length of time that man has lived near the sea and has fished? Nowadays some populations practise hand-fishing, this being presumably the original form. We state that a hand-fisherman must have sufficiently keen vision as to distinguish blue/grey colours. The situation in which he is put could represent that of experimental camouflage, where a task is performed much better by dyschromates than by orthochromates.

Some archaeological observations can be added, dating back to the Pleistocene, when the diet of human groups living close to the sea was composed of both meat and fish. In the Upper Cave Man (near Peking, China) the remnants of a human group were found, along with food remains. Among the latter, the vertebrae of a carp emerged (Anon, 1980), and radiocarbon dating dated the finds to about 18 500 years ago.

Evidence of organised fishing (that is of primary importance for feeding) is clearly documented as far back as 3000 BC in Mesopotamia and Egypt in artistic paintings and in lithographic writings. Fish-pots and nets already existed, and some other fishing devices (such as hooks, harpoons and hand-lines) were in use; the latter demonstrate that the fishermen looked attentively into the seas, rivers or marsh waters (Zaccagnini et al., 1976).

If it is possible to hypothesise that trichromacy developed thanks to a frugivor diet, it would be possible to affirm that dichromacy could probably be maintained as an advantageous specificity for fishing populations. People living in the inland areas (generally peasants or artisans) were not completely isolated from the coastal areas and marriages between the daughter of a fisherman and a peasant were certainly the main agent for the genes responsible for colour deficiency transferring towards the inland areas of a region. It appears, therefore, that a colour defective is disadvantaged as a peasant, but not as a fisherman (Grassivaro Gallo and Romana, 1993).

In conclusion, it is reasonable to believe that many populations travelled by sea along the coasts of entire continents, looking for hospitable places and seas full of fish, or along the rivers that, in the past, served as privileged communication ways. If communication between the coast and the inland area of a region occurred, the diffusion of the gene would be favoured; furthermore, in this way, the differences in gene frequency between the inland and the coastal parts would be reduced to a minimum. Other genetic mechanisms (i.e. genetic drift, which could be responsible for the high percentage of colour defectives in some isolated regions) must be added to the climatic and historical circumstances, that together with the geographical characteristics of a region, are more or less propitious for communication. Perhaps the ecological-ergonomic interpretation based on nutrition and on the prevailing lighting of an environment, as an attempt to explain the distribution of genes responsible for colour vision defects, could seem less persuasive or fanciful; nonetheless, we are convinced that the underlying data demonstrating clear geographical variations should be taken into account when considering future work on the incidence of colour vision defects.

5.2.5 REFERENCES

Anon (1980) *Atlas of Primitive Man in China*, Peking: Science Press.

Bowmaker, J.K. (1980) Color vision in birds and the role of oil droplets, *Trends in Neuroscience*, 3, 196–199.

Bowmaker, J.K., Astell, S., Hunt, D.M. & Mollon, J.D. (1991) Photosensitive and photostable pigments in the retinae of old world monkeys, *Journal of Experimental Biology*, 156, 1–19.

Bridges, C.D.B. & Delisle, C.E. (1974) Evolution of visual pigments, *Experimental Eye Research*, 18, 323–332.

Cavalli-Sforza, L.L. & Bodmer, W.F. (1971) *The Genetics of Human Populations*, San Francisco: Freeman & Co.

Curtoni, E.S., Dallapiccola, B., De Marchi, M., Mattiuz, P., Momigliano Riccardi, P. & Piazza, A. (1991) *Manuale di Genetica*, Turin: UTET.

Farnsworth, D. (1957) The Farnsworth Dichotomous test for colour blindness – panel D15, New York: The Psychological Corporation.

Floris, G., Murgia, E. & Sanciu, M.G. (1988) Further data on the frequency of color blindness in Sardinia, *International Journal of Anthropology*, 3(2), 181–183.

Grassivaro Gallo, P. & Cannizzo, M.G. (1993) *Unpublished data*.

Grassivaro Gallo, P. & Folin, M. (1990) Rilevamento delle discromatopsie nella popolazione in eta scolare del Veneto e della Puglia, *Antropologia Contemporanea*, 13(2/3), 209–214.

Grassivaro Gallo, P. & Malfitano, F. (1994) *Unpublished data*.

Grassivaro Gallo, P. & Panza, M. (1994) *Unpublished data*.

Grassivaro Gallo, P. & Pusceddu Nardella, M. (1991) Colour vision deficiencies in secondary school students in Italy. In: Drum, B., Moreland, J.D. & Serra, A. (Eds) Colour Vision Deficiences X, *Documenta Ophthalmologica Proceedings Series*, 54, 429–439, Dordrecht: Kluwer Academic.

Grassivaro Gallo, P. & Romana, L. (1993) *Unpublished data*.

Ishihara, S. (1973) *Tests for Color Blindness*, Tokyo: Kanehara Shuppan.

Kalmus, H. (1965) *Diagnosis and Genetics of Defective Color Vision*, London: Pergamon Press.

Kanizsa, G., Legrenzi, P. & Sonino, M. (1985) *Percezione, Linguaggio, Pensiero*, Bologna: Il Mulino.

Kherumian, R. & Pickford, R.W. (1959) *Heredité et Fréquence des Anomalies Congénitales du sens Chromatique (Dyschromatopsies)*, Paris: Vigot Frères.

Lethuillier, A. (1986) La découverte des genes du daltonisme, *La Recherche*, 180, 1126–1127.

Malaspina, P., Ciminelli, B.M., Pelosi, E., Santolamazza, P., Modiano, G., Santillo, C., Lofoco, G., Talone, C., Gatti, M. & Parisi, P. (1986) Colour blindness distribution in the male population of Rome, *Human Heredity*, 36, 263–265.

Mollon, J.D. (1989) 'Tho she kneel'd in that place where they grew . . .', The use and the origins of primate colour vision, *Journal of Experimental Biology*, 146, 21–38.

Morgan, M.J., Adam, A. & Mollon, J.D. (1992) Dichromats detect colour-camouflaged objects that are not detected by trichromats, *The Royal Society, Proceedings Biological Sciences*, 248, 291–295.

Pallaro, P. & Grassivaro Gallo, P. (1987) Il rilevamento del daltonismo negli adolescenti. Un contributo metodologico, *Antropologia Contemporane*, 10, 265–270.

Polyak, S.L. (1957) *The Vertebrate Visual System*, Chicago: University of Chicago Press.

Post, H.R. (1982) Population differences in red and green colour vision deficiency: A review and a query on selection relaxation, *Social Biology*, 29(3–4), 299–315.

SINISCALCO, M. (1963) Linkage data for G6PD deficiency in Sardinian villages. In: Goldsmith, E. (Ed.) *The Genetics of Migrant and Isolate Populations*, New York: Williams & Wilkins Co., pp. 106–113.

STORER, T.I., USINGER, R.L., STEBBINS, R.C. & NYBAKKEN, J.W. (1982) *Zoologia* (Italian Edition) Bologna: Zanichelli.

ZACCAGNINI, C., FALES, F.M. & LIVERANI, M. (1976) L'alba della civiltà, società economia e pensiero nel vicino oriente antico. In: Zaccagnini, C. (Ed.) *Le Techniche e le Scienze*, Turin: UTET.

Some (But Only A Few) Colour Vision Defectives Have No Difficulty With Colour

Barry L. Cole and Judy M. Steward

5.3.1 INTRODUCTION

There have been surprisingly few surveys of the difficulties with colour experienced by people with defective colour vision. We conducted one such survey several years ago (Steward and Cole, 1989) and reported on the proportion of respondents who had difficulties with a wide range of vocational and avocational tasks that involved the recognition or discrimination of colour.

The proportion reporting difficulties varied considerably depending on the task. Although three-quarters of the respondents reported difficulty with the selection of coloured goods, such as clothes, paints and cosmetics, etc., in general only one-quarter to one-third of the respondents said they had difficulty with colour in each of the 27 tasks and activities about which we asked questions.

An issue we did not consider in our original paper was whether it was the same 25–30 per cent who had difficulty with colour in each of the 27 tasks and activities, with the remainder having no difficulties; or whether across the range of tasks and activities about which we asked questions, all or most colour vision defectives had some difficulties.

This paper reports on the number of difficulties with colour reported by individuals with defective colour vision.

5.3.2 METHOD

One hundred and two subjects with defective colour vision were given a comprehensive questionnaire asking about their experiences with colour. The subjects were consecutively presenting patients to an optometric practice who had attended for a reason unrelated to their colour vision. Their defective colour vision was identified by the Ishihara test (four or more errors) and a diagnosis of the kind of defect was made using Nagel anomaloscope supplemented by other tests such as the Farnsworth D15. There were 17 protanomals, 48 deuteranomals, 19 protanopes and 18 deuteranopes in the sample.

The questionnaire was also given to 102 subjects with normal colour vision who presented in the same way. The subjects with normal colour vision reported no difficulties with colour, except two who said they had difficulty adjusting the colour of TV and two who reported confusing traffic signal lights with street lights on occasions.

The questionnaire was divided into five sections: the first section dealt with their personal awareness of their defect and when and how they first became aware of it: three sections asked questions about difficulties with colour in every day activities, at work and when driving; and the last section asked about their personal reaction to knowing they had a defect of colour vision.

The questionnaire was administered verbally so that responses could be explored in some depth. A subject was recorded as having difficulty only when there was a clear and consistent pattern of difficulty with colour for a particular task or activity.

5.3.3 RESULTS

Table 5.3.1 gives the proportion of colour vision defective subjects who reported difficulty with colour for various tasks and activities that involve colour recognition or discrimination.

As expected, the proportion experiencing difficulty depends on the type and severity of the colour vision defect. This is illustrated in Figure 5.3.1, which gives the proportions of protanomals, deuteranomals, protanopes and deuteranopes having difficulty with traffic signal lights. More detail about the occurrence of difficulties with colour for each type of colour vision defect is given in our original paper.

Table 5.3.1. Percentage of colour vision defective subjects reporting difficulty with colour[1]

Task or activity	% reporting difficulty
Every day activities	
Selecting coloured goods (clothes, paints, interior decoration items, cosmetics, etc)	74
Working at crafts or hobbies (colours of wires, threads, wools, paints, etc)	39
Identification of flowers (because of colour)	32
Judging the ripeness of fruit	28
Judging when meat is cooked	25
Watching or playing sport (difficulty because of colour)	22
Adjusting colour TV	22
Recognising skin rashes and sunburn	17
Taking wrong medicine (because of colour)	2
Driving	
Distinguishing traffic signal colours	29
Confusing street lights with traffic lights	26
Difficulty seeing brake lights	13
Difficulty reading road signs	9
Occupational	
Defective colour vision affected career choice	34
Difficulty with colour experienced at present work	25
Difficulty with colour at work in previous jobs	23

[1]Data from Steward and Cole (1989)

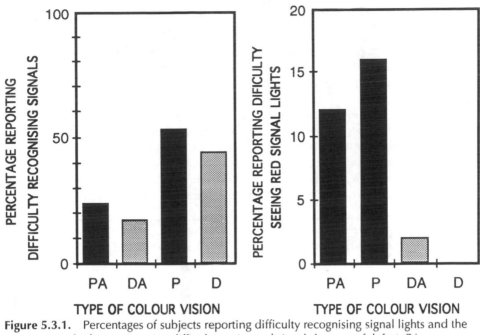

Figure 5.3.1. Percentages of subjects reporting difficulty recognising signal lights and the percentage of subjects reporting difficulty seeing red signals by type of defect. PA = protanomal, DA = deuteranomal, P = protanope and D = deuteranope.

The frequency distribution of the number of difficulties experienced by individual subjects is given in Figure 5.3.2. Figure 5.3.3 gives the frequency distributions of the number of difficulties experienced by individuals by type of colour vision defect.

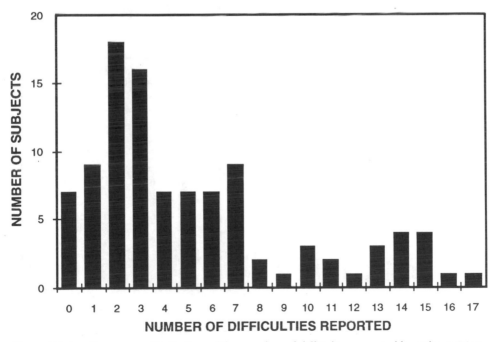

Figure 5.3.2. Frequency distribution of the number of difficulties reported by colour vision defective subjects.

5.3.4 DISCUSSION

Only seven subjects (seven per cent) reported no difficulties at all and all seven were deuteranomals. On average, deuteranomals reported three difficulties and protanomals 4.6 and, as expected, the dichromats, on average, reported a greater number of difficulties (D 7.2, P 6.5).

About 30 per cent of subjects with defective colour vision reported three or fewer difficulties, a similar proportion to the proportion who were unaware of their colour vision defect on entry into the study. Twenty-five per cent of anomalous trichromats and 5 per cent of dichromats were previously unaware that they had defective colour vision.

It is not possible with any degree of certainty to identify those who will have no or few difficulties with colour by conventional clinical assessment. There is a significant correla-

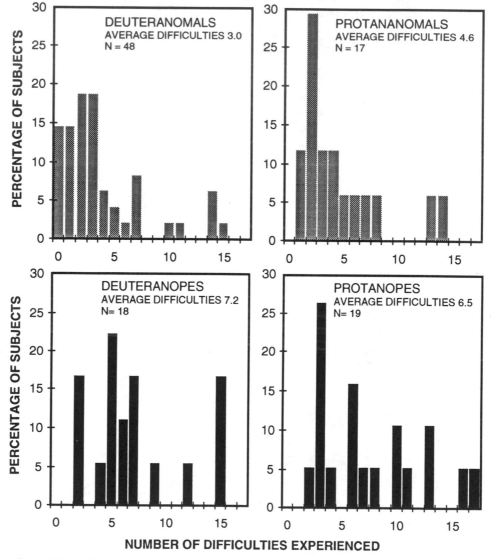

Figure 5.3.3. Frequency distributions of the number of difficulties reported by colour vision defective subjects by type of colour vision defect.

tion between the range at the Nagel anomaloscope and the likelihood of experiencing difficulty with selection of coloured goods ($r_s = 0.70$, $p < 0.01$) and the likelihood of difficulty with the colours of signal lights ($r_s = 0.80$, $p < 0.01$), but the Nagel range for the seven deuteranomals varied from 5 to 46 (average 23, median 16) and was not significantly different from that of all anomals (average 25, median 22). Likewise their anomaloquotients did not differentiate them from those anomalous trichromats who experienced difficulties.

The Farnsworth D15 test was no more certain in predicting those who had no or few difficulties. One of the seven deuteranomals with no difficulties failed the D15 (two or more diametrical crossings) and 27 of the 44 deuteranomals who had difficulties passed the D15. Of those 16 subjects who reported no or only one difficulty, five failed the D15. Nevertheless, it should be noted that most of the subjects who reported many difficulties failed the D15. Eighty-six per cent of those who reported eight or more difficulties failed the D15.

All that can be said is that a few colour vision defectives, about seven per cent, will have no difficulties with colour and these are likely to be deuteranomals. However, about one-third of colour vision defectives, including a few dichromats will have few (less than three) difficulties. This proportion will include a few dichromats.

Of course, the likelihood of difficulties will depend both on the severity of the defect and the extent to which lifestyle and occupation make demands on colour vision. It is possible that the variation in the degree of difficulty experienced among those with a defect of similar severity is due to these differences in lifestyle and occupation. On the other hand, it is possible, even probable, that there are variations in the ability to recognise and discriminate colour among persons with the same colour vision defect.

For example, there is considerable variation in the ability to recognise signal light colours among individuals with defective colour vision (Cole and Vingrys, 1983; Vingrys and Cole, 1988). Some simple deuteranomals have great difficulty with signal colours while others do not, and even some dichromats make surprisingly few errors with signal colours. It is known that some dichromats appear to have residual ability to distinguish colours along their confusion loci (Alpern et al., 1968; Scheiber and Boynton, 1968; Smith and Pokorny, 1977). We may simply need different clinical tests of colour vision to better identify those colour vision defectives who will or will not have difficulties with colour.

5.3.5 REFERENCES

ALPERN, M., MINDEL, J. & TORII, S. (1968) Are there two types of deuteranope? *Journal of Physiology*, **199**, 443–456.

COLE, B.L. & VINGRYS, A.J. (1983) Who fails lantern tests? *Documenta Ophthalmologica*, **55**, 157–173.

SCHEIBER, H.M.O. & BOYNTON, R.M. (1968) Residual red-green discrimination in dichromats, *Journal of the Optical Society of America*, **58**, 1151–1158.

SMITH, V.C. & POKORNY, J. (1977) Large-field trichromacy in protanopes and deuteranopes, *Journal of the Optical Society of America*, **67**, 213–220.

STEWARD, J.M. & COLE, B.L. (1989) What do colour vision defectives say about everyday tasks? *Optometry & Vision Science*, **66**, 288–295.

VINGRYS, A.J. & COLE, B.L., (1988) Are colour vision standards justified for the transport industry? *Ophthalmic and Physiological Optics*, **8**, 257–274.

Visualisation of Congenital Colour Vision Deficiencies with a VDU

Gunilla Derefeldt, Björn Modéer, Urban Persson and Tiina Swartling

5.4.1 INTRODUCTION

Colour video display units (VDUs) have during the last decade come into use for the testing of visual performance of colour-defective and normal trichromatic subjects (Arden *et al.*, 1988; Chioran *et al.*, 1985; Derefeldt *et al.*, 1991, 1994; Mieno *et al.*, 1986; Verriest *et al.*, 1985). The results from these studies show that VDUs might be useful devices in screening colour vision deficiencies. Although further data are needed, this notion has recently been substantiated. Reaction times of anomalous trichromats to colours presented on a VDU deviate from normals according to Cavonius *et al.* (1990). Moreover, colour defective observers may have difficulties in information acquisition from colour VDUs (Bergman and Duijnhouwer, 1980; Cole and Macdonald, 1988).

Derefeldt *et al.* (1991, 1994) have compared current methods of testing congenital colour vision deficiencies with tests designed to employ colour VDUs. Their comparisons of chromaticity coordinates of colour stimuli of colour vision tests and of a colour VDU show the potentialities of a colour VDU in studying colour vision deficiencies. Colour stimuli along chromaticity-confusion lines (Judd, 1945; Lakowski, 1966, 1969, 1971; Pitt, 1935, 1944–45) are used in testing with anomaloscopes, pseudo-isochromatic plates, and the Farnsworth 100-hue and D-15 tests. These tests are all constructed so that they present colour stimuli simultaneously from one or more closely related colour confusion lines. As shown in Figure 5.4.1, a full-colour VDU has a larger chromaticity gamut than the pseudo-isochromatic plates or the Farnsworth D-15 test. It can thus be a powerful tool for screening dichromats from normals and for illustrating the difficulties persons with colour deficiency will have in discriminating colours. VDUs may also simplify the selection and visualisation of colours that will enable a colour-deficient user to perform certain tasks efficiently.

Lakowski (1966) has shown that the chromaticity coordinates of the standard tests: the Ishihara, the Dvorine, the H-R-R, the Tokyo Medical College pseudo-isochromatic plates, the Farnsworth 100-hue and D-15 tests, all use 'the central part of the CIE space, utilizing less saturated colours than those used in tests based on the spectral principle' (Lakowski, 1969). The chromaticity coordinates of the standard tests lie within the chromaticity gamut of the colour VDU. This means that a colour VDU simulation of the pseudo-isochromatic plates could clearly be useful for revealing at least moderate-to-severe colour vision deficiencies. The red, green, and yellow colour stimuli (for deutan and protan tests) of the Nagel and Pickford-Nicolson anomaloscopes, cannot be reproduced on the VDU. Thus it is impossible to use a VDU to differentiate deuter- and protanomalous observers from deuteranopes and protanopes with the same set of chromaticity coordinates used in anomaloscopes. However, the same set of chromaticity coordinates as in anomaloscope testing might be used with a colour VDU when screening for the tritan defects, for in the Pickford-Nicolson anomaloscope the chromaticity coordinates (resulting from additive mixing) of the colour filters for tritan tests lie within the boundary of the colour VDU.

In the study by Derefeldt *et al.* (1994), 12 persons with congenital colour vision deficiencies were asked to judge and match colours presented on a full-colour VDU. Four persons with normal colour vision participated as controls. As shown in Figure 5.4.2, colour stimuli were selected from different 'chromaticity-confusion lines' within the CIE 1931 chromaticity diagram; colours were chosen from one tritan, three protan, and three deutan confusion lines.

Their results show that the ability to discriminate VDU colour stimuli is greatly impaired in protanopes and deuteranopes, compared with both normal and deuteranomalous observers. When pairs of colour stimuli lay on a protan and deutan confusion line, protanopes

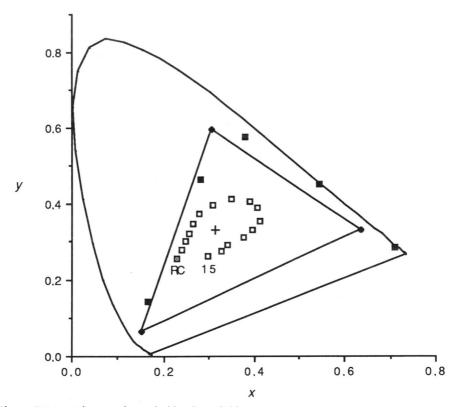

Figure 5.4.1. The area bounded by the solid line represents the gamut of chromaticities for the colour VDU on the CIE 1931 x, y chromaticity diagram. The chromaticity coordinates for the filters of the Pickford-Nicolson anomaloscope (■) and the chromaticity coordinates for the colour samples of the Farnsworth D-15 test (□) are also plotted. RC represents the Reference Cap (⊡) and the figure 15 the last sample of the Farnsworth D-15 test. The standard illuminant D white point is indicated by (+) (from Derefeldt *et al.*, 1994).

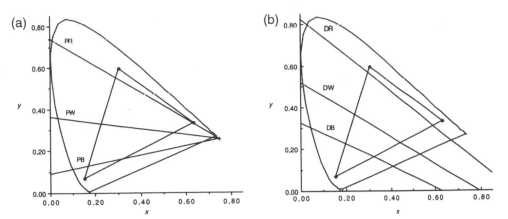

Figure 5.4.2. (a) Three protan lines plotted in the CIE 1931 x, y chromaticity diagram. The lines pass from the protanopic convergence point (x = 0.7465; y = 0.2535) through each of the three points x = 0.3101; y = 0.3162 (the standard illuminant C white point), x = 0.3200, y = 0.1600 (a point on the line representing colours from red to blue), and x = 0.3986, y = 0.5121 (a point on the line representing colours from red, yellow to green); these lines are denoted PW, PR and PB respectively. (b) Three deutan lines plotted in the CIE 1931 x, y diagram. The lines pass from the deuteranopic convergence point (x = 1.4, y = −0.40) through the same three points as given in (a); the lines are denoted DW, DR and DB respectively (from Derefeldt *et al.*, 1994).

and deuteranopes frequently accepted them as equivalent even when the stimuli were separated by large distances in the chromaticity diagram. Protanopes performed slightly better on colour stimuli from deutan lines than on those from protan lines. Similarly, deuteranopes showed better performance on protan than on deutan pairs. Deuteranomalous

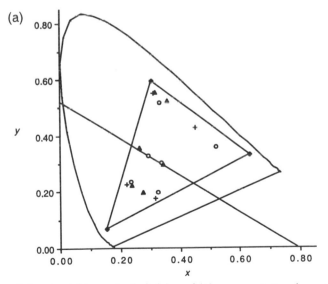

Figure 5.4.3. Colour matching pairs (+), (o), and (Δ), representative from colour matching from (a) a dichromatic, (b) a deuteranomalous, and (c) a normal observer, plotted in the CIE 1931 x, y diagram. Note: in Figure 3c, the colours within each pair lie so close that the symbols (o) representing them overlap (from Derefeldt *et al.*, 1994). (Parts (b) and (c) are overleaf.)

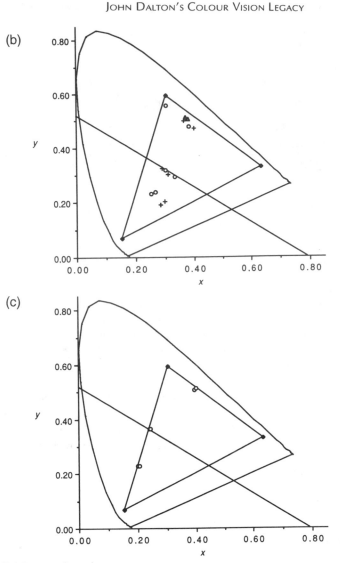

Figure 5.4.3 *continued*

observers performed better than dichromats but less well than normals. Representative data from dichromatic, deuteranomalous, and normal colour matching are illustrated in Figures 3a, 3b and 3c.

To relate their data to other data on normal colour discrimination, Derefeldt *et al.* (1994) also plotted the data for one dichromatic and one deuteranomalous subject in relation to the MacAdam discrimination ellipses (MacAdam, 1942). In the original figure presented by MacAdam (1942, Figure 48), every discrimination ellipse is drawn ten times its correct size with relation to the coordinate scale of the chromaticity diagram. The centres of the ellipses are placed at their proper locations in the chromaticity diagram. To compare their data from the deuteranomalous and the dichromatic subject with MacAdam's data, Derefeldt *et al.* (1994) plotted the lengths of the distances between two colour confusion pairs enlarged ten times actual scale on the CIE 1931 x, y-chromaticity diagram as an over-lay on MacAdam's discrimination ellipses. As shown in Figure 5.4.4, this gives very enlarged plots. For the deuteranomalous subject, the length representing the distance extends almost over the whole chromaticity diagram. For the dichromat, it extends over the whole chromaticity and even outside the diagram. The comparison illustrated in Figure 5.4.4 shows that the distances between the colour matching pairs for both the deuteranomalous and the dichromatic subject are much greater than for normal subjects as illustrated by the lengths of the axis of the discrimination ellipses. A comparison according to normal scale was also made. In Figure 5.4.5, three MacAdam ellipses are plotted in normal scale together with the data from the dichromatic subject and the deuteranomalous, also in the same scale.

Figure 5.4.5 shows that in actual scale on the CIE 1931 x, y-chromaticity diagram, the data from MacAdam are hardly discriminable because the chromaticity coordinates for each pair lie very close. Figures 5.4.3, 5.4.4 and 5.4.5 indicate that the dichromats, the deuteranomalous, and the normal subjects represent three separate groups with respect to the distances between matched colour stimuli within the CIE diagram. The poor global performance in wavelength discrimination of anomalous trichromats compared to normal observers (Birch and Wright, 1961) suggests that devices with the ability to display and vary many colour stimuli in small steps in all parts of the colour space will be of value for the screening of colour vision deficiencies. Desired colour stimuli in many parts of the colour space can be produced with a full-colour VDU (Derefeldt and Hedin, 1989; Derefeldt *et al.* 1989; Hedin and Derefeldt, 1990).

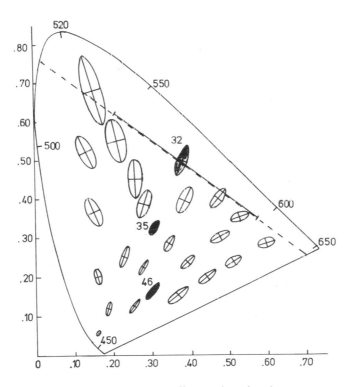

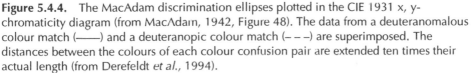

Figure 5.4.4.   The MacAdam discrimination ellipses plotted in the CIE 1931 x, y-chromaticity diagram (from MacAdam, 1942, Figure 48). The data from a deuteranomalous colour match (———) and a deuteranopic colour match (– – –) are superimposed. The distances between the colours of each colour confusion pair are extended ten times their actual length (from Derefeldt *et al.*, 1994).

5.4.2   METHOD

To illustrate the difficulties observers with congenital colour vision deficiencies have in colour discrimination for different parts of the colour space, one deuteranopic observer was extensively tested with colours chosen from 13 deutan and 10 protan chromaticity-confusion lines within the CIE 1976 u', v'-chromaticity diagram (CIE, 1986). One deuteranomalous observer was tested for four deutan and three protan lines. Figure 5.4.6 shows the lines plotted in the CIE u', v'-chromaticity diagram. The protanopic and deuteranopic convergence points used by Vos and Walraven (1970), Nimeroff (1970), and Thomson and Wright (1953) were used. For every chromaticity-confusion line, colour stimuli within the whole range of lightness (L*) possible to present on the VDU screen were tested.

5.4.2.1 Apparatus

The colour video display system which is used to display the colour stimuli is a microVAX with an image memory by Raster Technologies, Inc. Model One/80. It has also been described elsewhere (Derefeldt *et al.*, 1991, 1994). With the Raster, 256 of 16.7 million

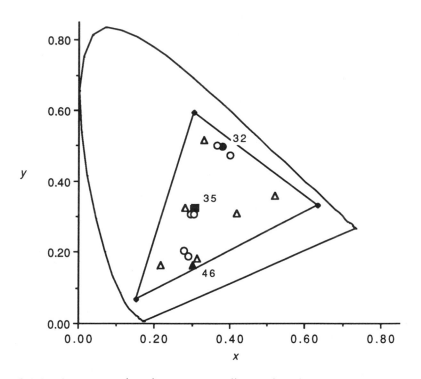

Figure 5.4.5.   Some MacAdam discrimination ellipses plotted in actual scale in the CIE 1931 x, y-chromaticity diagram together with the chromaticity coordinates of the colours from deuteranomalous and dichromatic colour matches. Note: the two symbols representing each of the three MacAdam discrimination ellipses: No. 32 (●); No. 35 (■); and No. 46(▲) overlap. Colour matching pairs for the dichromatic subjects are indicated by (Δ); and for the deuteranomalous colour by (O) (from Derefeldt *et al.*, 1994).

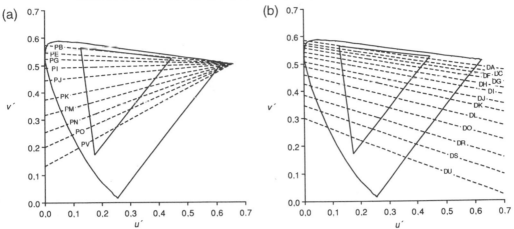

Figure 5.4.6.   (a) Ten protan lines PB, PE, PG, PI, PJ, PK, PM, PN, PO, and PV plotted in the CIE 1976 u', v'-chromaticity diagram. The lines pass from the protanopic convergence point; u' = 0.6564, v' = 0.5.015. (b) Thirteen deutan lines DA, DC, DF, DG, DH, DI, DJ, DK, DL, DO, DR, DS, and DU plotted in the CIE 1976 u', v'-chromaticity diagram. The lines pass from the deuteranopic convergence point; u' = 1.2174, v' = 0.7826.

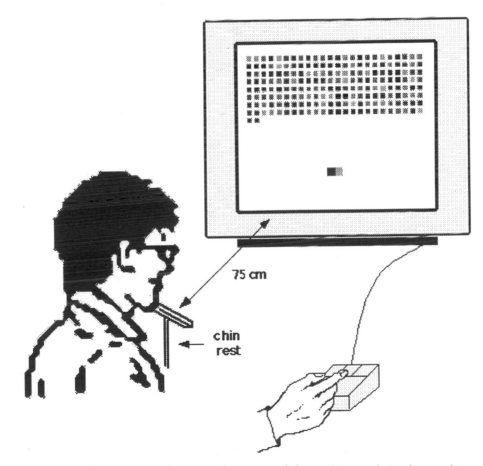

Figure 5.4.7.   The experimental situation for testing of chromaticity confusion by matching.

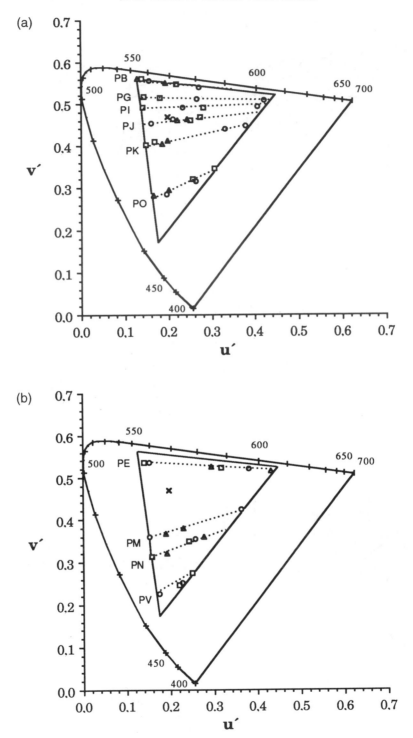

Figure 5.4.8. Matching pairs for the deuteranopic observer plotted in the CIE 1976 u', v'-chromaticity diagram for (a) protan lines PB, PG, PI, PJ, PK, and PO; (b) protan lines PE, PM, PN, and PV; (c) deutan lines DA, DC, DG, DI, DJ, DK and DO; (d) deutan lines DF, DH, DL, DR, DS, and DU. The standard illuminant D white point is indicated by (+). (For parts (c) and (d) see the next page.)

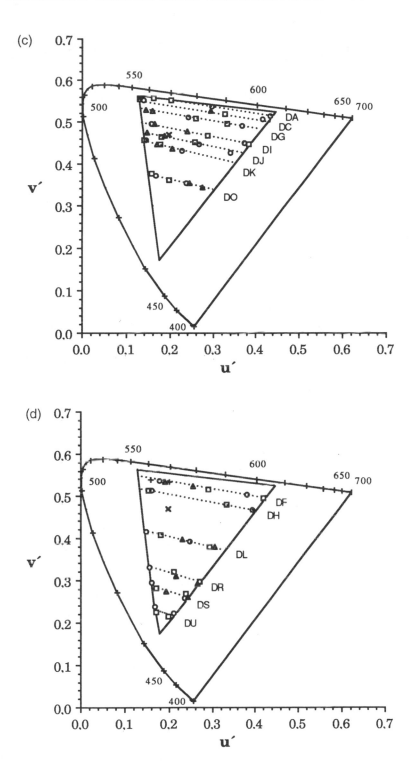

Figure 5.4.8   *continued*

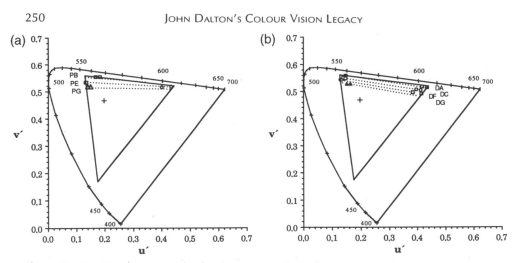

Figure 5.4.9. Matching pairs for the deuteranomalous observer plotted in the CIE 1976 u′, v′-chromaticity diagram for (a) protan lines PB, PE, and PG; (b) deutan lines DA, DC, DF, and DG. The standard illuminant D white point is indicated by (+).

digital R, G, and B (red, green, and blue) combinations can be displayed simultaneously at a resolution of 1280 x 1024. The monitor was a 19-inch 60-Hz non-interlaced Sony Trinitron GDM-1901. Spectrophotometric measurements were made with a Photo Research extended range Spot Spectrascan (PR 713/PC). The CIE 1931 X Y Z tristimulus values were measured for each digital level (0–255) for each phosphor. The CIE 1931 tristimulus values X Y Z of each digital RGB combination displayed on the VDU screen were calculated by the following equations:

$$X = X(R) + X(G) + X(B)$$
$$Y = Y(R) + Y(G) + Y(B)$$
$$Z = Z(R) + Z(G) + Z(B)$$

In these equations X(R) indicates the X tristimulus value at digital level R of the red gun, X(G) the X tristimulus value at digital level G of the green gun, and X(B) the X tristimulus value at digital level B of the blue gun. In the same way Y(R) indicates the Y tristimulus value at digital level R of the red gun, and so on. It was assumed that there were no gun-to-gun interactions. Limitations of data processing necessitated reducing the 16.7 million possible RGB combinations to a colour database of 5000 colour stimuli. The luminance of the 'monitor white' (i.e. RGB = 255, 255, 255, x = 0.2822, y = 0.3425, Y = 153 cdm⁻²) was taken as 100, and the tristimulus values for all other RGB combinations were normalised to this value. The gamut of the colour VDU is shown in Figure 5.4.1. From the colour database, we could select colour stimuli by a colour selection tool (Hedin and Derefeldt, 1990).

5.4.2.2 Procedure

The observer was seated 75 cm in front of the screen with his chin placed on a chin-rest. The observer could freely compare all the different colour stimuli appearing on the screen. For ease of comparison, the observer matched two colour stimuli at a time. These appeared as two reference squares in the lower part of the VDU screen. For a colour stimulus to appear in one of these two lower squares, the subject had only to mark it with a cursor at its place on the VDU screen and then click the mouse. The subject could make it appear in either of the two squares by clicking the mouse: by clicking the right mouse button the colour appeared in the right reference square, by clicking the left mouse button the colour appeared in the left reference square. When two colour stimuli were judged as identical, the subject clicked the middle mouse button, which stored the stimuli in a file. For each line, the subject stored about 10–20 colour matching pairs. The colour stimuli subtended visual angles of 30 min arc and the reference squares visual angles of 1 degree. The colour stimuli were presented against a white background colour.

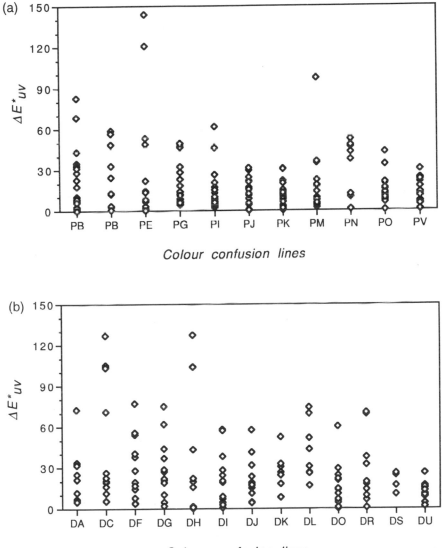

Figure 5.4.10. CIE 1976 E*$_{uv}$ colour differences between matching pairs for the deuteranopic observer for (a) protan lines PB to PV; (b) deutan lines DA to DU.

The fluorescent lighting illuminating the room had correlated colour temperature of 6100 K (Philips TL 40W/55). The room illumination was within the range of normal office lighting. The experimental situation is illustrated in Figure 5.4.7.

5.4.2.3 Subjects

One deuteranope and one deuteranomalous observer took part in the experimental sessions. The two subjects were tested with the Heidelberg anomaloscope and the Farnsworth Panel D-15 test.

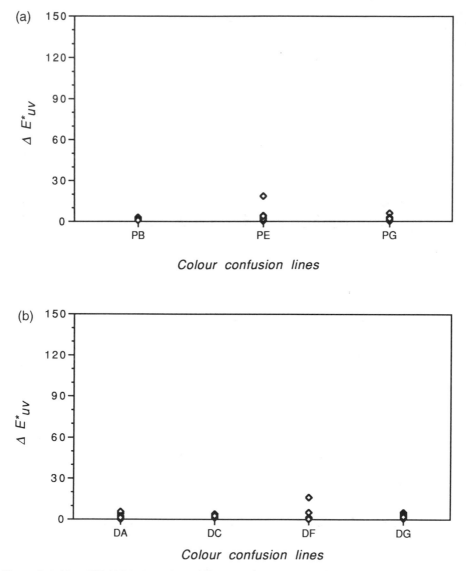

Figure 5.4.11. CIE 1976 E*$_{uv}$ colour differences between matching pairs for the deuteranomalous observer for (a) protan lines PB, PE, and PG; (b) deutan lines DA, DC, DF, DG.

5.4.3   RESULTS

Figures 5.4.8 and 5.4.9 show individual results for the deuteranope and deuteranomalous observers for the different colour confusion lines. Matching pairs are plotted in the CIE 1976 u', v'-chromaticity diagram. To avoid clutter in the figures, we have chosen to illustrate only a few matching pairs for each line. The results show that the deuteranope matched colour stimuli that have large distances on the CIE 1976 u', v'-chromaticity diagram; larger distances than found for the deuteranomalous observers. The results are in line with other data on congenital colour vision deficiencies showing that colour stimuli along chromaticity-confusion lines are difficult to discriminate.

To illustrate the magnitudes of the colour differences, we have also calculated the CIE 1976 E^*_{uv} colour differences between colour matching pairs as illustrated in Figures 5.4.10, and 5.4.11. The ΔE^*_{uv} colour differences of the matching pairs are much larger for the deuteranope than for the deuteranomalous subject. The deuteranomalous subject has much less difficulty in discriminating colours than the deuteranope although his performance does not meet the standards of an observer with normal colour discrimination.

To show how colour stimuli representing the same 'chromaticity-confusion line' may vary in the attributes hue, chroma, and lightness, colour stimuli from two 'chromaticity-confusion lines' are visualised in colour in a CIE 1976 u*, L*-diagram in Figures 5.4.12 and 5.4.13 (see colour section). At each lightness level (L*), the colour differences between the colour samples are equal.

Data on colour confusions illustrated in a CIE 1931 x, y or a CIE 1976 u', v'-chromaticity diagram do not show the differences in luminance or lightness that might exist between the two colour stimuli in a matched pair. Protanopes may perceive isoluminant colours along a chromaticity-confusion line as very unequal in lightness. To illustrate how a deuteranope may match colours with respect to lightness, actual colour matching pairs from six deutan and four protan lines from the deuteranopic observer were plotted in a CIE 1976 u*, L*-diagram. This plot shows that the deuteranope tends to match colour stimuli along deutan lines that are unequal in lightness as indicated by the slope of the lines in Figure 5.4.14.

5.4.4   DISCUSSION AND CONCLUSIONS

The results from this study are in agreement with earlier data showing that protanopic and deuteranopic observers are greatly impaired in their ability to discriminate colour pairs along chromaticity-confusion lines throughout the whole gamut of the VDU compared to both normal and deuteranomalous observers.

The difficulties have been expressed as a distances on a CIE 1976 u', v'-chromaticity diagram and as CIELUV ΔE^*_{uv} distances, and have also been visualised in colour. These results show that the differences between any two colours in a dichromatic colour match can be as large as 127 ΔE^*_{uv}. The CIELUV colour space illustrates to a normal observer the difficulties persons with colour vision deficiencies have in discriminating colours much better than either the CIE 1931 x, y or the 1976 u', v'-chromaticity diagrams. The lightness difference found between the two stimuli in the deuteranopic colour matches will be further studied.

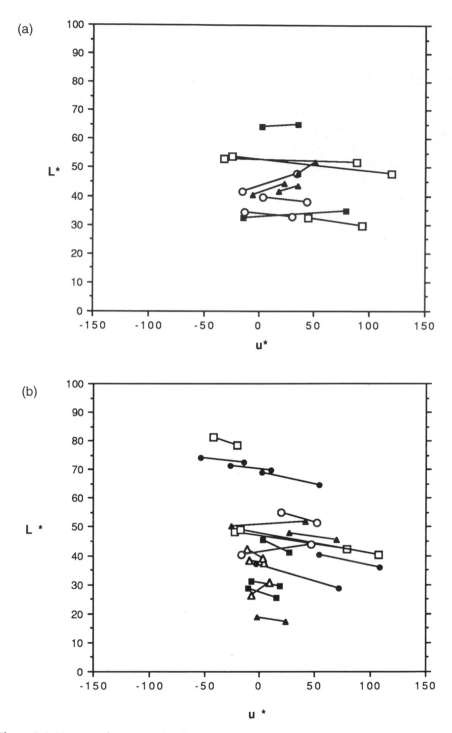

Figure 5.4.14. Matching pairs for the deuteranopic observer plotted in a CIE 1976 u*, L*-diagram. (a) Matching pairs from the protan lines PE (□——□), PM (■——■), PN (○——○), and PV (▲——▲). (b) Matching pairs from the deutan lines DF (●——●), DH (□——□), DL (▲——▲), DR (○——○), DS (■——■), and DU (△——△).

5.4.5   ACKNOWLEDGEMENTS

This study has been mainly supported by a grant from the Swedish Work Environment Fund, contract dnr 86-1410. The authors thank Mr Ulf Berggrund, FOA, for help with the colour plates and Dr Celeste Howard, University of Dayton Research Institute, Armstrong Laboratory (Mesa, Arizona, USA) for help with the manuscript.

5.4.6   REFERENCES

ARDEN, G., GÜNDÜZ, K. & PERRY, S. (1988) Colour vision testing with a computer graphics system: Preliminary results, *Documenta Ophthalmologica*, **69**, 167–174.

BERGMAN, H. & DUIJNHOUWER, F. (1980) Recognition of VDU presented colors by color defective observers. In: *Proceedings of the Human Factors Society*, 24th Annual Meeting, pp. 611–615.

BIRCH, J. & WRIGHT, W. D. (1961) Colour discrimination, *Physics in Medicine and Biology*, **6**, 3–23.

CAVONIUS, C. R., MÜLLER, M. & MOLLON, J. D. (1990) Difficulties faced by color-anomalous observers in interpreting color displays. In: Brill, M. H. (Ed.) *Perceiving, Measuring, and Using Color, SPIE Proceedings Series*, **1250**, 190–195.

CHIORAN, G. M., SELLERS, K. L., BENES, S. C., LUBOW, M., DAIN, S. J. & KING SMITH, P. E. (1985) Color mixture thresholds measured on a color television – a new method for analysis, classification and diagnosis of neuro-ophthalmic disease, *Documenta Ophthalmologica*, **61**, 119–135.

COMMISSION INTERNATIONALE DE L'ÉCLAIRAGE (CIE) (1986) *Colorimetry*, CIE Publication No. 15.2, Vienna: Central Bureau of the CIE.

COLE, B. L. & MACDONALD, W. A. (1988) Defective colour vision can impede information acquisition from redundant colour-coded video displays, *Ophthalmic and Physiological Optics*, **8**, 198–213.

DEREFELDT, G. & HEDIN, C.-E. (1989) Visualization of VDU colours by means of the CIELUV colour space, *Displays*, **10**, 134–146.

DEREFELDT, G., HEDIN, C.-E. & FORSBERG, L. (1989) On the total number of discriminable VDU colours. *AIC, Color 89, Proceedings of the 6th Congress of the Association Internationale de la Couleur*, Buenos Aires, Argentina, 13–17 March, 259–261.

DEREFELDT, G., HEDIN, C.-E., SKOOG, K.-O. & VERRIEST, G. (1991) A VDU colour vision test for congenital colour vision deficiencies. In: Drum, B., Moreland, J. D. & Serra, A. (Eds) *Colour Vision Deficiencies X, Documenta Ophthalmologica Proceedings Series 54*, 95–106, Dordrecht, Boston, London: Kluwer Academic.

DEREFELDT, G., HEDIN, C.-E., SKOOG, K.-O. & SWARTLING, T. (1994) Colour vision deficiencies, Matching and confusion of computer colours, *FOA Report A 50024-5.2, April, National Defence Research Establishment*, 172 90 Sundbyberg, Sweden.

HEDIN, C.-E. & DEREFELDT, G. (1990) Palette – A color selection aid for VDU images. In: Brill, M. H. (Ed.) *Perceiving, Measuring, and Using Color, SPIE Proceedings Series*, **1250**, 165–176.

JUDD, D. B. (1945) Standard response functions for protanopic and deuteranopic vision, *Journal of the Optical Society of America*, **35**, 199–221.

LAKOWSKI, R. (1966) A critical evaluation of colour vision tests, *British Journal of Physiological Optics*, **23**, 186–209.

LAKOWSKI, R. (1969) Theory and practice of colour vision testing: A review. Part 2, *British Journal of Industrial Medicine*, **26**, 265–288.

LAKOWSKI, R. (1971) Calibration, validation and population norms for the Pickford-Nicholson anomaloscope, *British Journal of Physiological Optics*, **26**, 166–182.

MACADAM, D. L., (1942) Visual sensitivities to color differences in daylight, *Journal of the Optical Society of America*, **32**, 247–274.

MIENO, H., TOMIZAWA, G., BAN, Y., TAKAHASHI, K. & TATSUTA, L. (1986) Automatic dyschroma-topsia test. Color blindness test by color graphics display, *The Visual Computer*, **2**, 97–101.

NIMEROFF, I. (1970) Deuteranopic convergence point, *Journal of the Optical Society of America*, **60**, 966–969.

PITT, F. G. H. (1935) Characteristics of dichromatic vision. Medical Research Council, *Report of the Committee on the Physiology of Vision, XIV; Spectral Report Series*, No. 200, London.

PITT, F. G. H. (1944–45) The nature of normal trichromatic and dichromatic vision, *Proceedings of the Royal Society, London, Series B*, **132**, 101–117.

THOMSON, L. C. & WRIGHT, W. D. (1953) The convergence of the tritanopic confusion loci and the derivation of the fundamental response functions, *Journal of the Optical Society of America*, **43**, 890–894.

VERRIEST, G., ANDREW, I. & UVIJLS, A. (1985) Visual performance on a multicolor visual display unit of color-defective and normal trichromatic subjects, *IBM Hursley Technical report TR 12.241*, March, IBM United Kingdom Laboratories Ltd, Hursley Park, Winchester, Hampshire.

VOS, J. J. & WALRAVEN, P. L. (1971) On the derivation of the foveal receptor primaries, *Vision Research*, **11**, 799–818.

Acquired Deficiencies of Colour Vision

A.B. Morland and K.H. Ruddock

5.5.1 INTRODUCTION

Colour vision is defined as the ability to distinguish between light stimuli on the basis of differences in spectral composition, even when all other stimulus parameters, including brightness, are identical. The organisation of primate colour vision has been widely studied by both physiological and psychophysical methods, and the first two sections of this review deal with the results of such studies. Acquired deficiencies of human colour vision are usually described with reference to congenital disorders, the characteristics of which are well established and are summarised in this chapter.

Electrophysiological responses selectively sensitive to the spectral composition or apparent colour of light stimuli are recorded at all levels of the visual pathways, and acquired colour vision deficiencies can be divided into broad categories according to the location of the underlying deficit. We have chosen to differentiate between abnormalities of the peripheral pathways, the retina and optic nerve, and those of cortical origin. There are many conditions which, as a consequence of their effects on the peripheral visual pathways, give rise to abnormalities of colour vision. These have been reviewed by Francois and Verriest (1968), who identified 92 conditions in 1179 patients, and more recent surveys have been given by Krastel and Moreland (1991) and Ruddock (1993). The observed disturbances of colour vision in patients with peripheral disorders can be interpreted reasonably well on the basis of the known spectral responses of retinal and geniculate neurones and we have restricted our consideration of them to a discussion of their general features. In comparison with colour vision deficiencies of peripheral origin, those associated with cortical abnormalities occur at much lower incidence and exhibit much greater variability between individual cases. The present understanding of the cortical mechanisms involved in the processing of colour is incomplete and provides an uncertain basis for the interpretation of central disorders of colour vision. There is a particular difficulty in establishing the full extent of interactions between the different visual cortical areas and, correspondingly, considerable attention has been given to the selective nature of cortical visual disorders, including those involving colour vision. In addition to reviewing published studies on colour vision deficiencies in patients with lesions of the striate cortex or of the fusiform and lingual gyri, we also present the results of studies on three patients, each with a colour vision deficiency associated with abnormal cortical activity.

5.5.2 PHYSIOLOGICAL AND ANATOMICAL MECHANISMS OF COLOUR VISION

The trivariant nature of normal human colour vision is established at photoreceptoral level by the absorption of light in three spectral classes of cone photoreceptors. Their broad-band absorption spectra peak at around 565 nm, 535 nm and 425 nm (Dartnall *et al.*, 1983), which are designated red (R-) sensitive, green (G-) sensitive and blue (B-) sensitive respectively. The reported variability of the absorption spectra within a single spectral class of photoreceptors, which is apparent in the absorption spectra but not in action spectra derived electrophysiologically (Baylor *et al.*, 1987), can be neglected in the context of acquired colour vision deficiencies. The R- and G-sensitive cones cannot be distinguished from each other histologically and estimates of their relative numbers vary, although they are approximately equal. The B-sensitive cones, which are smaller and can be marked selectively by immunohistological staining, constitute an estimated 10–15 per cent of the total and are absent from the central 15 min of the visual field, where colour vision is dichromatic.

Vertebrate photoreceptors hyperpolarise in response to light and this response is transmitted either via sign-conserving synapses to 'off centre' bipolar cells or via sign-inverting synapses to 'on centre' bipolar cells. The responses of post-photoreceptoral neurones in the primate retina are well-established only for ganglion cells, which on anatomical and functional grounds can be divided into at least three groups (Leventhal *et al.*, 1981; Perry and Cowey, 1984; Perry *et al.*, 1984). P-type ganglion cells, identified with the midget cells, constitute about 80 per cent of the 1.5 million ganglion cells, and project to the parvocellular layers of the dorsal lateral geniculate nucleus (dLGN). In the human retina, about 90 per cent of foveal ganglion cells, but only about 40–45 per cent of peripheral ganglion cells are P-type (Dacey, 1993). They have centre-surround antagonistic receptive fields, half of which are 'on'- and the other half 'off'-centre, and are colour opponent, with inputs from R- and G- cones separated into the centre and surround regions of the receptive fields. The spatial distributions of sensitivity to the opponent chromatic inputs are described by Gaussian functions, with the surround input having larger standard deviation and smaller amplitude. The resulting responses have narrow bandwidth spectral characteristics, which contrast markedly with the broad-band spectral characteristics of the photoreceptors. A second class of ganglion cells, which receive their inputs via a specific class of bipolar cells, also project to the parvocellular layers of dLGN, but have larger dendritic fields than the midget cells. Their receptive fields have co-extensive excitatory and inhibitory areas, and are colour coded such that the 'on' response is driven by B-cones, and the 'off' response by combined inputs from R- and G-cones. A small number of cells with the opposite response polarity have been identified electrophysiologically, but not histologically. M-type ganglion cells, which correspond to the parasol cells, constitute 3–5 per cent of parafoveal ganglion cells, and about 20 per cent of those in the peripheral retina. At a given eccentricity, their dendritic receptive fields are larger than those of P-type cells, and correspondingly, their centre surround antagonistic receptive fields are larger. They project mainly to the magnocellular layers of dLGN, but also constitute about 10 per cent of the projection to the superior colliculus. Both the centre and surround of their receptive fields yield achromatic broad-band spectral responses. Other ganglion cells, which project to central areas other than dLGN, including the superior colliculus and the pretectum, appear to generate atypical responses which are also achromatic in nature.

The neuronal responses recorded from the parvo- and magnocellular layers of dLGN correspond to those of the ganglion cells which provide their input signals. In particular, those from the parvocellular layers have colour opponent chromatic responses and low sensitivity to spatial contrast, whereas those from the magnocellular layers have broad-band spectral responses and high sensitivity to spatial contrast. Wiesel and Hubel (1966) identified four spectral classes of neurones in dLGN. Type 1 cells, which constitute 80 per cent of all neurones in the parvocellular layers, have centre-surround antagonistic receptive fields, the vast majority of which are red-green opponent. About one per cent are blue-yellow opponent, and the receptive field centres of these are larger than those of the red-green opponent cells. Type II neurones (about seven per cent of parvocellular cells) also have colour opponent responses, but lack centre-surround spatial organisation, receiving co-extensive inputs of opposite polarities from B- and G-sensitive cones. The remaining neurones of the parvocellular layers have centre surround antagonistic receptive fields, both regions having the same broad-band spectral response, and this Type III response is also recorded from the magnocellular layers. Type IV neurones, found in the magnocellular layers, respond briefly to the onset of a wide range of stimulus wavelengths but generate a sustained inhibitory response to large red stimuli. A few of these cells also exhibit 'red-on, green-off' opponency in response to large stimuli.

These four classes of spectral responses are also observed in recordings from the striate cortex, with colour opponent responses restricted to the columns which, in laminae 2 and 3, are occupied by the 'blobs' revealed by cytochrome oxidase staining. A further class of 'double opponent' responses is also observed, with the receptive field centre receiving two antagonistic spectral inputs (e.g. + R–G) and surround the opposite combination (–R + G). Such cells respond well to chromatic contrast, and there are blue-yellow as well as red-green double opponent responses. They formed a significant proportion of the chromatic responses recorded by Livingstone and Hubel (1984), but only a small fraction of those recorded by T''so and Gilbert (1988). Cells located within the blobs are neither orientation selective nor binocularly driven. Colour opponency is also a feature of neurones located within the thin stripes stained by cytochrome oxidase in visual striate area V2, and together with the V1 blobs, these stripes form a major input pathway for prestriate area V4, neurones of which exhibit sensitivity to stimuli of a given colour appearance rather than spectral composition (Zeki, 1978, 1980).

The evidence reviewed above indicates that chromatic sensitivity is an attribute of the P-projection pathway and of the V1 blob–V2 thin stripe–V4 system of the striate and pre-striate visual areas. It has been demonstrated, however, that magnocellular neurones with non-opponent spectral characteristics can respond to the edge between a pair of equiluminant stimuli, as long as the pair are not tritanopic confusion colours (Kaplan et al., 1991). Thus, chromatic sensitivity is not exclusively an attribute of the P-pathway. Pre-striate areas V2 and V4 receive a sparse, direct input from both magnocellular and parvocellular layers of dLGN, which provides an alternative route for chromatic signals. The relay cells which form this projection survive ablation of the striate cortex and their dendrites are post-synaptic both to retinal fibres and to those from the superior colliculus (Kisvarday et al., 1991). The superior colliculus also projects via the pulvinar to the pre-striate visual cortex, and colour opponent responses have been recorded from the pulvinar (Felsten et al., 1983). These different sources of chromatic signals are all important in the analysis of colour vision deficiencies in patients with cortical lesions.

5.5.3   PSYCHOPHYSICAL MEASUREMENTS OF CHROMATIC RESPONSES IN HUMAN SUBJECTS

Any test colour can be matched by an appropriate mixture of three matching stimuli and values for spectral stimuli published by Wright (1927–28) form a major part of the CIE (1931) standard for a 2 degree colour matching. The trivariant nature of colour matches is determined by the fact that there are three spectral classes of cones and differences between normal colour matches made by different observers are almost entirely attributable to variations in light absorption by the ocular media. The two important contributions are the increase with age in the optical density of the lens (Said and Weale, 1959) and the large variations between individuals in the optical density of the macular pigment (Ruddock, 1963), which is not age related (Ruddock, 1965). Both factors affect the absorption of short wavelength stimuli and cause difficulty in the identification of tritanopic disorders (Moreland, 1994). The spectral sensitivities of the underlying response mechanisms can only be derived from colour matching data with the aid of assumptions about visual function, but they can be investigated directly by the two-colour increment threshold technique, which yields broad-band π-spectral responses closely related to those of photoreceptors (Stiles, 1978). The effective spectral absorption characteristics of the photopigments are only rarely modified by retinal diseases and, except in cases such as those noted in the next section, colour matches and π-spectral response characteristics are normal in patients with acquired colour vision deficiencies.

The overall spectral sensitivity function is influenced both by light absorption in the ocular media, and by variations in the relative contributions of different spectral classes of cone photoreceptors (Rushton and Baker, 1964). Blue sensitive cones make little apparent contribution to the photopic V_λ function, but at mesopic luminance levels both rods and cones influence the spectral sensitivity of the non-foveal retina, with the cone contribution increasing as the luminance level rises, to produce the Purkinje shift from the scotopic V'_λ function to longer wavelengths (Walters and Wright, 1943). In some acquired colour vision deficiencies, rods make an abnormally large contribution to mesopic spectral sensitivity functions. Spectral sensitivity for detection of a monochromatic target presented on a bright, white background is markedly dependent on the nature of the target stimulus. For large targets of long duration, the sensitivity function has prominent maxima and minima, features which are attributed to the contributions of colour opponent mechanisms in the visual detection process (King-Smith and Carden, 1976; Sperling and Harwerth, 1971). In contrast, spectral sensitivity for detection of a target flickering at 25 Hz is broad-band, similar to the V_λ function, and is attributed to detection by a luminance channel, perhaps corresponding to the magnocellular pathway (Lee *et al.*, 1988). This method of investigating the responses of colour opponent, post-receptoral mechanisms has been applied widely in the study of acquired colour vision deficiencies.

Loss of colour discrimination is the defining characteristic of all colour vision deficiencies, and it can be established by several different methods. Wavelength discrimination can be measured only with a specialised monochromator, and care must be taken to ensure that the two fields are maintained at equal brightness. Wright and Pitt (1934) established the essential features of the normal response, but it has been shown subsequently with brighter light sources that the size of the discrimination step at 440-nm is similar to those at 490-nm and 590-nm. If the field size is altered to compensate for the changes in effective field size, the magnitudes of discrimination steps measured at off-axis locations show wavelength dependence similar to those for foveal viewing, but are somewhat larger (van Ensch *et al.*, 1984). Saturation discrimination is measured in terms of the amount of a given spectral light that must be added to a white in order to produce a just noticeable difference in colour. The required stimuli can be generated on a VDU, and the resulting discrimination steps form an ellipse in the chromaticity diagram (e.g. Barbur *et al.*, 1992). Such ellipses are a general feature of discrimination steps measured at other points in the chromaticity diagram (MacAdam, 1942; Wright, 1941). Tests such as the Farnsworth–Munsell (FM) 100 hue test are widely applied in the assessment of discrimination losses in patients with acquired colour vision deficiencies, and the results are analysed in terms of the response patterns associated with the different forms of congenital colour vision deficiencies. It is important to note that responses to such tests, the samples of which have broad-band spectral reflectances, are influenced by light absorption in the ocular media which can, for example, cause apparent loss of blue-green discrimination with increasing age (Ruddock, 1972).

Colour constancy is an important feature of human colour vision, and it is usually examined with Mondrian displays, which consist of multiple coloured elements, in the form of rectangles. Such stimuli eliminate the contribution of cognitive factors to the colour appearance of the samples.

About eight per cent of the normal population has congenital colour vision deficiencies caused by mutations in the genes that code for the cone photopigments (Nathans *et al.*, 1986). There is an extensive literature dealing with the response characteristics of these inherited conditions (see reviews by Ruddock, 1991; Wright, 1946), certain of which form the basis for the classification of acquired deficiencies, even though the latter rarely affect the photopigments. The distinction between congenital and acquired disorders is usually unambiguous, as the former are stable and with very rare exceptions, affect both eyes equally, whereas the latter are often progressive and usually affect the two eyes differently. Further, patients who suffer acquired visual disorders are usually keenly aware of any associated disturbances of colour vision, whereas those with congenital disorders have no perceptual experience of normal colours. A congenital deficit is classified as mono-chromatic, dichromatic or anomalous trichromatic according to the numbers of matching stimuli required for foveal colour matching. These principal categories are divided into sub-groups, each of which corresponds to the involvement of a different set of photopig-ments. There are three classes of dichromacy; protanopia, deuteranopia and tritanopia, which involve loss of the R-, G- and B-sensitive cones respectively. The foveal spectral sensitivities and colour discrimination responses associated with each condition are consistent with activity of the specific cone mechanisms present in the retina, but it should be noted that non-foveal colour vision in many subjects with foveal dichromacy is trichromatic. Formally, the absence of one of the three cone mechanisms implies that the colours with chromaticities on a line passing through a particular point in the chromaticity chart should be indistinguishable from each other. The convergence point, which is different for each form of dichromacy, corresponds to the chromaticity of the missing fundamental response mechanism. This property is exploited in defining responses to tests such as the FM 100 hue in terms of the congenital conditions, and spectral sensitivity functions also provide a basis for comparison between congenital and acquired abnor-malities.

5.5.4 ACQUIRED COLOUR VISION DEFICIENCIES OF PRE-STRIATE ORIGIN

Impairment of colour discrimination in patients with retinal disease usually involves blue-green stimuli, whereas for those with optic nerve disorders, it is observed mainly with red-green stimuli, a dichotomy that was noted by Köllner (1912). There are, however, a number of well-known exceptions of the rule with protanomolous colour matching observed in patients with retinal diseases such as central serous retinopathy and retinitis pigmentosa, and tritan discrimination losses in patients with dominant inherited optic nerve atrophy. Modifications of Köllner's simple classification, which take account of a number of response characteristics, have been suggested. Jaeger and Grützner (1963) divided both the principal groups into two, according to whether or not there was an associated reduction in sensitivity to long wavelength stimuli and Verriest (1963) distinguished three types of acquired vision deficiency. Type I involves red-green discrimination losses and reduction in sensitivity to long wavelength stimuli, with progressive scotopization of the spectral sensitivity function, leading finally to achromatopsia. In Type II, impairment of red-green discrimination is accompanied by less pronounced impairment of blue-green discrimination and Type III involves blue-green discrimination losses accompanied by less prominent losses of red-green discrimination. The last group can be further sub-divided according to whether the Rayleigh colour match is normal or pseudo-protanomalous (Pinckers, 1976; Smith et al., 1978). A different approach to classification was adopted by Marré and Marré (1986), whose scheme is based on the sensitivities of cone spectral response mechanisms measured by two colour increment threshold methods. They take into account the variations with retinal location in the sensitivities of the different spectral response mechanisms, which can be an important factor in disorders involving loss of the central visual field. Unlike the congenital conditions, acquired colour vision deficiencies are frequently progressive in nature, and as they develop, response abnormalities occur for an increasing range of stimulus colours, leading in extreme cases to achromatopsia, the complete absence of colour discrimination. The classification rules are applicable to the early rather than to the later stages in the development of progressive conditions.

The physiological origins of acquired colour vision deficiencies have yet to be explained fully, but some contributory factors have been identified. Observations on patients with central serous retinopathy indicate that the directional Stiles-Crawford effect is abnormal, indicative of mis-alignment of the photoreceptors, which results in a reduction in the effective density of the photopigments. Smith et al., (1978) attribute the pseudo-protanomalous colour matching associated with this condition to photoreceptor misalignment, and propose that a similar mechanism explains the incidence of protanomalous colour matching in other diseases that give rise to impaired blue-green discrimination. There is evidence that protanomalous colour matches established by patients with retinitis pigmentosa may result from low optical density of the cone photopigments (Young and Fishman, 1980). It should be noted, however, that reduction of photopigment density by bleaching always produces a deuteranomalous shift in the normal Rayleigh match (Brindley, 1953; Wright, 1936), a result that is confirmed computationally (Ruddock and Naghshineh, 1974). The appearance of acquired protanomaly in conditions such as choroidopathy must, therefore, involve more than a simple reduction in the density of photopigments. Diabetic patients suffer premature yellowing of the lens and this can give rise to tritan-like responses in colour vision tests (Lütze and Bresnick, 1991).

The tritan nature of colour vision deficiencies caused by retinal diseases suggests that those retinal neurones that form the blue-sensitive pathways are selectively vulnerable to disruption. The incidence of B-cones is much lower than that of the R- and G-cones, thus even if all three were affected equally, there could be a disproportionately large effect on the efficiency of the B-cone pathway. B-cones differ from R- and G-cones in their susceptibility to damage by toxins that cross the outer membrane of cells (de Monasterio et al., 1981) and in their failure to recover after intense bleaching (Harwerth and Sperling, 1975). Light damage to B-cones is observed both as a primary response to repeated, brief exposure to short wavelength light of low luminance and as a secondary effect of continuous exposure to higher luminance levels, for which the primary damage occurs in the pigment epithelium (Ham *et al.*, 1978; Sperling *et al.*, 1980). In the latter case, tritan colour vision deficiencies of several months duration have been observed (Kitahara *et al.*, 1987). Ganglion cells of the blue-sensitive retinal pathway are larger than the midget ganglion cells of the red-green opponent pathway. It has been reported that large ganglion cells are selectively damaged in glaucoma (Quigley *et al.*, 1988), which provides an explanation of the tritan colour vision responses associated with this disease.

The red-green colour discrimination losses that occur in optic nerve diseases imply selective damage of the P-pathway, which comprise optic nerve fibres of small diameter. Pathological examination has shown that tobacco-alcohol amblyopia leads to the loss of small diameter fibres (Rönne, 1910) and demyelination of optic nerve fibres by viral infection has been demonstrated in an animal model (Tansey *et al.*, 1985). Diseases that give rise to red-green discrimination losses also involve reduction of spatial acuity, whereas blue-green discrimination losses are not, at least in the initial stages of disease, accompanied by reduced acuity. This is consistent with the low incidence of B-cones, which prevents their making a significant contribution to spatial resolution (Brindley, 1954).

5.5.5 ACQUIRED DEFICIENCIES OF CENTRAL ORIGIN

Some localised lesions of the pre striate visual cortex produce functional disorders that are expressed only in response to highly specific aspects of the visual stimulus. An example of such a condition is cerebral achromatopsia, in which colour vision is disturbed but most other visual functions remain intact. Lesions of the striate cortex give rise to visual field losses that are homonymous for the two eyes, and are usually absolute and permanent in nature. There are, however, a number of reports that patients with striate lesions are able to respond to certain forms of light stimulation presented within the 'blind' areas of the visual field. Patients who are capable of making such responses are divided between those with 'blindsight', who deny any perceptual experience of the stimulus (Weiskrantz *et al.*, 1974), and those with residual vision who report a 'shadow' or some other primitive percept in response to stimulation (Barbur *et al.*, 1980). Most patients with functional sparing are able to detect and locate transient stimuli presented within the 'blind' field, but in a few cases, other visual functions, including colour discrimination, are also retained. We review briefly the principal features of cerebral achromatopsia and of residual colour discrimination, and we present three case studies that illustrate the response characteristics associated with these conditions.

5.5.6 CEREBRAL ACHROMATOPSIA

There have been several extensive and informative reviews of the literature concerning this condition, including those by Meadows (1974), Zihl and von Cramon (1986), Zeki (1990) and Plant (1991). In extreme cases, achromatopsia involves the complete loss of colour sensations, with visual scenes appearing in shades of grey, white or black. Colour losses in most cases are, however, less severe, the patients perceiving colours as 'washed out', 'dirty' or 'desaturated'. A common characteristic is difficulty in identifying colours, and patients are aware that objects of known colour, such as green grass, elicit the wrong colour sensation. Hue discrimination in tests such as the FM 100-hue test is usually severely impaired, but pseudo-isochromatic plates can often be identified correctly. There have been reports that the condition involves a specific loss of the blue-sensitive response mechanism (Pearlman *et al.*, 1979; Young *et al.*, 1980). In cases of unilateral damage, achromatopsia is restricted to the contralateral visual field. Other aspects of visual function, such as spatial vision, motion perception and stereoscopic function are often essentially normal in achromatopsia, but a majority of patients exhibit losses in the superior visual field, and experience prosopagnosia and topographical agnosia. Some patients, such as MW, whose case is reviewed below, suffer gross impairment of colour vision but retain normal achromatic visual function, including spatial vision. Conversely, patients with apperceptive agnosia are unable to discriminate between any spatial patterns, but retain the ability to identify and discriminate between colours. This double dissociation provides strong evidence of separation between the cortical representation of colour and spatial pattern (Zeki, 1978).

Brain scans and post-mortem pathology establish that achromatopsia is associated with lesions localised to the fusiform and lingual gyri, which in the case of hemi-achromatopsia are restricted to one hemisphere. Positron emission tomographic studies on humans with normal colour vision have shown that this cortical region, which is represented bilaterally, is selectively activated by coloured stimuli. The homology between the colour area in humans and the colour sensitive area V4 in macaque has not been fully established. Lesions of V4 produce small losses of colour discrimination, impairment of colour constancy and significant disruption of spatial vision.

5.5.6.1 Case Study 1 (Kennard *et al.*, 1995)

BL, a 54-year-old male, has highly localised lesions of the lingual and fusiform gyri, which were revealed by an MRI brain scan performed three years ago, after he had suffered an encephalitic illness, believed to be of viral origin. After a period of unconsciousness , he reported that visual scenes appeared dark, without colour, and he had difficulty in recognising faces and finding his way around. Subsequently he has partially recovered, but still exhibits mild prosopagnosia and topographical agnosia. His visual fields are complete, except that the small ($\frac{1}{4}$ mm^2) stationary targets of the Goldmann perimeter are not detected in the upper left quadrants.

We examined a variety of visual functions, in order to determine whether or not non-chromatic responses were affected. BL detects random dot stereograms and experiences binocular rivalry, indicating that his binocular vision is normally organised. His Snellen visual acuity is 6/9 in either eye, and his ST1 spatial frequency response is normal, with a peak at 4 c deg^{-1} (Barbur and Ruddock, 1980). He detects the changes in appearance of a grating stimulus produced by pre-adaptation to another grating of a different orientation or periodicity, and he describes correctly the appearance of illusory spatial images. We conclude that his spatial vision is normally organised, although as already noted, he has mild abnormalities in higher functions such as face recognition. BL's discrimination of velocity for a circular moving target is normal, and he has normal lightness discrimination, measured by asking him to arrange in order 46 grey tiles that formed a reference set for spectrophotometry (Robertson and Wright, 1965). Certain visual discriminations are, therefore, unimpaired.

BL's colour vision has been subject to intensive investigation, the results of which are summarised in Figures 5.5.1–5.5.3. His Rayleigh match of a yellow (590 nm) test against a mixture of red (650 nm) and green (530 nm) matching stimuli is normal, although with larger than average errors. He was unable to establish a blue-green match, but accepted normal matches, made with stimuli chosen to eliminate the effects of variations in density of the macular pigment (Ruddock, 1963). His π_3-spectral sensitivity function is normal (Figure 5.5.1.a), and together with his normal Rayleigh matches this establishes that his cone photoreceptors have normal spectral sensitivities. His threshold sensitivity measured against a white background is similar to that of a normal trichromat with pronounced minima at 590 nm and 490 nm (Figure 5.5.1b), so his post-receptoral colour-opponent response channels also appear to be normal. His wavelength discrimination, however, is impaired, his discrimination steps being some five times greater than normal (Figure 5.5.2a) and his saturation discrimination steps are also larger than those of a normal control (Figure 5.5.2b).

We attempted, particularly, to investigate his colour naming, which is inaccurate, and to examine the effects of change of illumination on his identification of surface colours. Despite the evidence that neuronal responses in area V4 of the macaque are constant under change of illumination (Zeki, 1978, 1980), this aspect of achromatopsia has not been studied. We first determined his verbal identification of 57 colours, generated individually on a VDU screen and placed at the centre of a Mondrian chart. The data (Figure 5.5.3a) show that large areas of the chromaticity chart yield uncertain responses, particularly for blue, green, and grey. No equivalent uncertainty exists for normals, whose well-defined responses are also indicated in Figure 5.5.3a. Although observations were made at two luminance levels, change in luminance had little effect on BL's responses, so the two sets of data were pooled. The categorical divisions of the chromaticity diagram for BL are very similar to those for normal vision, but the areas of uncertainty are much larger. Walsh *et al.* (1992) concluded that macaques with V4 lesions divide the spectrum according to normal colour categories.

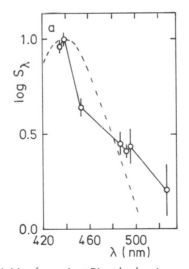

Figure 5.5.1. Spectral sensitivities for patient BL, who has incomplete achromatopsia. (a) The π_3 spectral sensitivity (open circles) recorded by the two-colour increment threshold method. Relative spectral sensitivity, S_λ, is plotted against wavelength, λ. Also shown (broken line) is the standard π_3 response function taken from Wyszecki and Stiles (1982). (b) Relative spectral sensitivity, S_λ, for detection of a target of wavelength λ, presented against a white background (luminance 3 log trolands). Data for BL (open circles) and for a normal control AM (full circles) have been displaced vertically for clarity, and the latter are also plotted as a broken line for purposes of comparison. (For part (b) see next page.)

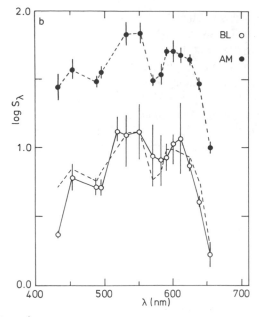

Figure 5.5.1. *continued*

The influence of the illuminant on BL's colour naming was also investigated with the Mondrian display, which was viewed under four illuminants, a white, a red, a green and a blue, and eight test samples were placed sequentially at the centre of the display. BL named each of the samples four times, under each of the four illuminants, and his choice of colour names changed significantly with change of illuminant, as is illustrated in Figure 5.5.3b. If it is assumed that BL has no colour constancy, the apparent colours of the different stimuli under the four illuminants should be defined by the chromaticity co-ordinates, and the colour category with which BL associates those co-ordinates (Figure 5.5.3a). The analysis predicts that under the non-white illuminants, he should make 18 changes of colour name for the 24 test colours (8 samples each viewed under red, green and blue filtered white

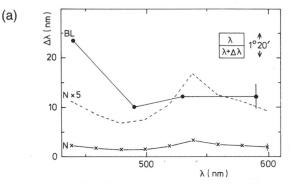

Figure 5.5.2. Discrimination data for patient BL. (a) Wavelength discrimination data for the patient BL (full circles) and for a normal subject (crosses). The normal data are also shown scaled ×5, for comparison purposes. (b) Saturation discrimination for BL (full circles) showing the minimum charge in chromaticity which can be distinguished from the white identified by the central cross. The hatched area shows the corresponding normal values. Data are plotted in the CIE 2° chromaticity diagram, and were determined by the method described by Barbur et al. (1992). (For part (b) see next page.)

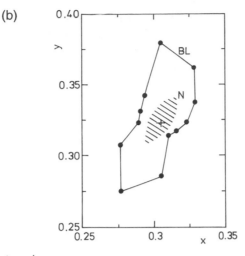

Figure 5.5.2. *continued*

light). In practice he made 16 changes, failing to make three predicted changes and making one which was not predicted. Fifteen of these changes were consistent with the chromaticity shift produced by the source, although only eight correspond to the full shift, others corresponding to a partial displacement (see caption to Figure 5.5.3b). We conclude that BL's colour constancy is at least partially impaired, which prevents his compensating fully for a change in illuminant when naming surface colours. We note that this effect cannot be attributed to reduced colour discrimination, because subjects with congenital red-green colour deficiencies, whose discrimination losses are much more severe than BL's, make many fewer changes of colour naming. This is discussed fully elsewhere (Morland *et al.*, this volume, pp. 463–468).

Our data show that patient BL suffers disturbances of colour vision, with sparing of most other visual functions. Abnormal responses to colour are evident in mildly impaired colour discrimination, erratic naming of colours and failure of colour constancy. These response features are similar to those found in monkeys with V4 ablations (Heywood and Cowey, 1987; Walsh *et al.*, 1993), but BL does not exhibit the major disruption of pattern discrimination associated with such lesions (Heywood and Cowey, 1987; Heywood *et al.*, 1992).

Case Study 2 (Bender and Ruddock, 1974; Hendricks *et al.*, 1981)

MW, a 43-year-old male, has a unique colour vision deficit that has remained unchanged for over 20 years, during which period he has been examined regularly. As far as he is aware, he has throughout his life experienced similar effects when viewing coloured stimuli. Neither ophthalmoscopic examination of his retina nor MRI brain scans reveal any abnormality. His visual responses to achromatic stimuli, including 6/4 Snellen acuity for each eye, are entirely normal. Nonetheless, he exhibits severe visual impairment in response to saturated chromatic stimuli, which inhibit his normal black and white vision not only within the area covered by the coloured stimulus, but also in the surrounding visual field. His chromatic responses are also characterised by highly abnormal increment threshold sensitivity (Figure 5.5.4). Both the spreading inhibition and the disruption of increment threshold sensitivity are particularly severe for red stimuli. Two noteworthy features of the spreading inhibition are its long-term build up, with a correspondingly slow

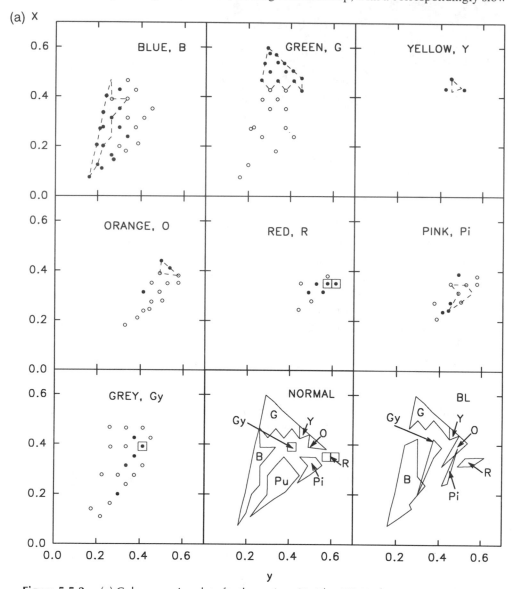

Figure 5.5.3. (a) Colour naming data for the patient BL. The CIE 2° chromaticity co-ordinates of reference samples to which BL gave the different colour names denoted at the top of the panels. Full circles denote identification on three or more of five presentations, open circles to identification on one or two of five presentations. The dotted lines connect the values associated with the different color names by a normal subject (JV), for whom all samples correspond unambiguously to one or other of the colour names. The last two panels summarise the different areas for the normal subject and the patient, BL. Note that the latter did not use the description 'purple' (Pu on the normal panel). Each sample was placed at the centre of a Mondrian (10 degree square) and measured 1.2 degree square.

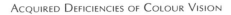

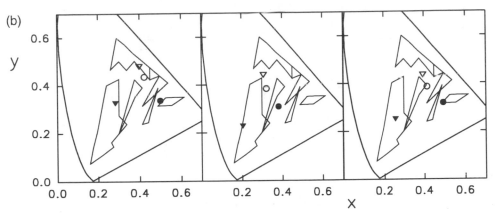

Figure 5.5.3. (b) Colour naming data for the patient BL. The chromaticity co-ordinates of three samples, under white (open circles), red (full circles), green (open triangles) and blue (full triangles) illuminants. Also shown are the colour categories, taken from the bottom right panel of Figure 5.5.3a. For the left hand panel, BL named the samples white, yellow or green (white illuminant), pink (red illuminant), yellow (green illuminant) and blue (blue illuminant), for the central panel green or blue (white illuminant), grey (red illuminant), green, grey or blue (green illuminant) and blue (blue illuminant), and for the right hand panel pink (white illuminant), pink (red illuminant), orange or grey (green illuminant) and blue, green or grey (blue illuminant).

recovery, and its non-uniform effects at different locations in the visual field (Figure 5.5.4b).

Two colour increment threshold measurements isolate the blue-sensitive (π_3^-) and red-sensitive (π_5^-) spectral responses. Although it was not possible to isolate the green-sensitive (π_4^-) spectral mechanism, his responses to yellow are sharply distinguished from those to red, thus he must have a third spectral mechanism, sensitive to long wavelength stimuli. Several features of MW's vision indicate that the spreading inhibition arises cortically. A red filter placed over one eye causes him to become completely blind, he can resolve random dot stereograms viewed through red and green colour separation filters, even though he perceives nothing through the former when the other eye is closed, and his VEPs for an alternating red and black chequerboard are normal, although he fails to perceive the stimulus (Ruddock, 1987).

We have recently examined interactions between MW's responses to colour and those to other stimulus parameters, such as form and motion. We have measured the inhibitory effects of a brief red flash on a second, white stimulus, either in the form of a bar, or a moving post, presented at different latencies relative to the inhibitory stimulus. The results, which are illustrated for the case of the (spatial) line stimulus, show that detection of the latter is influenced by the former, the threshold luminance peaking 200 ms after the white line target (Figure 5.5.5). A similar though temporally less well-defined interaction is also found for a moving white target. These recent measurements have revealed that achromatic moving patterns also generate spreading inhibition, thus this patient displays abnormal responses to colour and movement, while his responses to achromatic, stationary patterns remain intact. The effects of the colour abnormality are particularly severe for red light, and he is effectively blind for monochromatic stimuli of wavelength greater than some 620 nm. The time course of interaction between a briefly presented white target and an inhibitory red light flash demonstrates that interaction is maximum with a significant delay between presentation of the two stimuli. We believe that such measurements will provide a measure

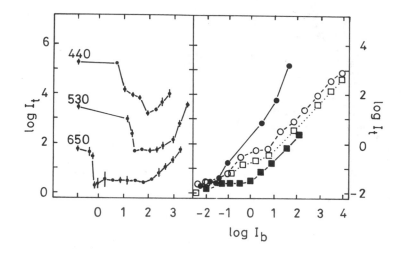

Figure 5.5.4. (a) Data for patient MW, who has a colour vision deficit of central origin. Increment threshold data for detection of a circular target, presented centrally against a circular background. In the left panel, the relative luminance, I_t (log trolands), of the target required for its detection is plotted against the luminance, I_b, of a background stimulus of the same wavelength, as marked in nm on the diagram (target diameter 1.0°, background diameter 7°). The different data sets are displaced arbitrarily along the I_t axis for clarity. The data in the right hand panel refer to a white light target (diameter 3.5°) and a background (diameter 17°) that was either white (open symbols) or of wavelength 636 nm, (full symbols). Both I_t and I_b are expressed in log trolands. Circles refer to MW, and squares to a normal subject IH.

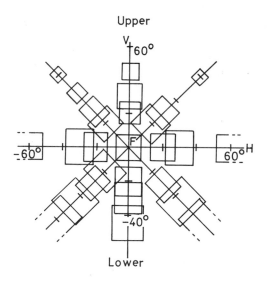

Figure 5.5.4. (b) Data for patient MW who has a colour vision deficit of central origin. The apparent size of a 6.2 degree square red patch (CIE 2° co-ordinates x = 0.505; y = 0.284; Y = 23), as sketched by MW at different points in the visual field, relative to the fixation (F), and the horizontal (H) and vertical (V) meridians.

of the time delays involved in interactions between signals arising in different pre-striate visual areas.

5.5.7   COLOUR VISION IN THE ABSENCE OF STRIATE CORTICAL SIGNALS

As discussed previously, residual vision in the absence of striate input is characterised by sensitivity to transient stimuli presented within the 'blind' region of the visual field. In a minority of cases, however, discrimination of spatial structure and colour have also been reported. Stoerig (1987) found that six of ten patients were able to discriminate between red and green, and Stoerig and Cowey's (1991) three patients were able to name correctly colours presented to their 'blind' fields, making no errors for blue, very few for red, but a larger number for stimuli of wavelength between 525 nm and 580 nm. In the latter study, evidence of rod and cone input to 'blind' field responses was reported, and evidence of colour-opponent activity was obtained by recording spectral sensitivity for targets presented on a white background. Blythe *et al.* (1987) reported that one of 25 patients with hemianopia or quadrantanopia was able to distinguish red from green stimuli presented within the 'blind' area of the field.

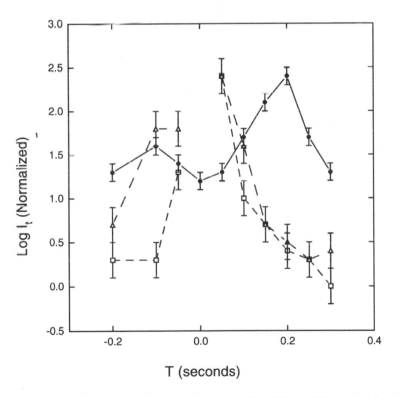

Figure 5.5.5.   Relative luminance, I_t, of a white vertical bar ($6° \times 0.5°$) required for its detection. The bar was presented for 20 ms at a time T relative to the onset of a spatially coincident, red bar (wavelength 665 nm) also presented for 20 ms. Full circles, data for MW; square and triangle, data for two normals, JO and JW respectively. Data for the different subjects have been normalized at the peak value of I_t.

Destriate monkeys can perform red-green colour discriminations (Schilder *et al.*, 1972) and monkeys lacking both striate and prestriate cortical areas can discriminate blues from greens (Keating, 1979). Spectral sensitivity for destriate monkeys is scotopic (Leporé *et al.*, 1975) but the retinal projections to the prestriate cortical areas that survive ablation of the striate cortex receive input signals from cones. Cone activity is observed in recordings from the macaque superior collicus (Kadoya *et al.*, 1971; Marrocco and Li, 1977) and colour-opponent responses have been recorded from pulvinar units (Felsten *et al.*, 1983). The direct projection from the dLGN to the prestriate cortex is influenced by inputs from the superior colliculus, and arises both in P-type and M-type geniculate layers.

5.5.7.1 Case Study 3 (Barbur *et al.*, 1980; Blythe *et al.*, 1986; Brent *et al.*, 1994)

GY, a 36-year-old male, has a hemianopic field loss associated with an extensive lesion of the left striate and pre-striate cortical areas, caused by a traffic accident when he was 8 years old. An MRI scan shows that the left occipital pole and fusiform gyrus are spared, and further details are given in Brent *et al.* (1994) and Wright *et al.* (this volume, pp. 279–286). He has a right hemianopic field loss, with sparing of sensitivity up to 3.5° from fixation, which is consistent with his MRI scans. He is able to respond to a wide range of transient stimuli presented to his 'blind' hemifield, and retains discrimination of brightness and velocity. He cannot, however, discriminate between spatial structures of stimuli that generate his residual vision. Spectral sensitivity measured 30° off axis in the 'blind' hemifield corresponds to the rod V_λ' function, and no Purkinje shift is observed with increased light adaptation. More recent measurements, however, have revealed activity of both the red-(Π_5) and green- (Π_4) sensitive cone mechanisms, and spectral sensitivity measured 10° off axis against a white background is normal. Attempts to isolate the blue- (Π_3) sensitive mechanism were, however, unsuccessful. With large fields, GY is able to identify the colour of monochromatic stimuli drawn from the red-yellow-green region of the spectrum, and he can also distinguish changes in saturation from red to pink to white. Details of these colour responses and a discussion of their physiological substrate are given in this volume by Wright *et al.* (pp. 279–286.)

In summary, GY's residual visual functions permit him to detect transient stimuli presented to the 'blind' hemifield, and to perform limited discriminations between stimuli that differ in velocity and in colour. GY's MRI scans establish that the extensive lesion in his left hemisphere spares both the fusiform gyrus and the pre-striate area associated with sensitivity to movement. A PET scan confirms that areas corresponding to macaque pre-striate V3 and V5 are activated by moving stimuli, although the striate cortex is not (Barbur *et al.*, 1993). Thus those pre-striate cortical regions involved in visual responsiveness to movement and colour are at least partially spared. The retinal projection pathway(s) that provide the input signals responsible for activating these spared central areas have not, however, been identified.

5.5.8   CONCLUSIONS

Human colour vision requires that the spectral composition of the retinal image be encoded in the neuronal signals generated at all levels of the visual pathways. The transduction of light to electrical signals in three spectral classes of cone photoreceptors establishes the trivariant nature of normal colour vision. Post-receptorally, the photoreceptor signals are encoded in colour-opponent responses associated with neurones of the P-projection pathway from the retina, via dLGN to the striate cortex. At cortical level, colour specific responses are observed in the anatomically distinct pathway formed by the blobs in area V1, the thin stripes in area V2 and visual area V4. The complex processing that occurs in this last centre transforms the representation from one defined by the local spectral composition of the stimulus falling within the receptive field of a single neurone to one that takes account of the overall spectral composition of the visual field, that is, colour appearance.

Malfunction at any stage of this chromatic pathway can give rise to an acquired colour vision deficiency, characterised by impairment of colour discriminations. The onset of abnormal colour perception is, in some instances, the first indication of visual disease, although the nature of the colour deficiency rarely, if ever, identifies unambiguously the underlying condition. Certain broad generalisations emerge from studies of acquired colour vision deficiencies in patients with well-defined clinical disorders. In their early stages, most retinal diseases cause impairment of blue-green discriminations, and most optic nerve diseases give rise to abnormal red-green discriminations, but as diseases progress, their associated discrimination losses usually become less specific. Lesions of the fusiform and lingual gyri produce a well-defined condition, known as achromatopsia, in which all colours appear as shades of grey, black or white. Patients with incomplete achromatopsia suffer impaired colour discrimination and make frequent errors in colour identification. Other disturbances of colour vision associated with cortical lesions, such as colour anomia, the mis-naming of colours, do not involve discrimination losses. Some patients with extensive lesions of the striate cortex retain some colour discrimination capacity, although in the case study reviewed previously, GY was able to identify colours only with very large fields.

The principal features of acquired colour vision deficiencies are broadly consistent with the known organisation of chromatic visual pathways. Diseases of the retina and optic nerve are, in most instances, well defined, and associated colour vision dysfunctions can sometimes be interpreted with reference to the histological and physiological properties of single neurones. Modern imaging techniques have improved significantly the accuracy with which cortical lesions can be mapped, but uncertainties regarding cortical functional organisation preclude detailed analysis of visual abnormalities of central origin. Response characteristics of patients with such visual abnormalities do, however, assist in the assessment of electrophysiological and anatomical evidence.

REFERENCES

BARBUR, J.L. & RUDDOCK, K.H. (1980) Spatial characteristics of movement detection mechanisms in human vision. I Achromatic mechanisms, *Biological Cybernetics*, **37**, 77–92.

BARBUR, J.L., RUDDOCK, K.H. & WATERFIELD, V.A. (1980) Human visual responses in the absence of the geniculo-calcarine projection, *Brain*, **103**, 905–928.

BARBUR, J.L., BIRCH, J. & HARLOW, A.J. (1992) Colour vision testing using spatiotemporal luminance masking. Psychophysical and pupillometric methods. In: Drum, B. (Ed.) *Colour Vision Deficiencies XI*, Dordrecht: Kluwer, pp. 417–426.

BARBUR, J.L., WATSON, J.D.G., FRACKOWIAK R.S.J. & ZEKI, S. (1993) Conscious visual perception without VI, *Brain*, **116**, 1293–1302.

BAYLOR, D.A., NUNN, B.J. & SCHNAPF, J.L. (1987) Spectral sensitivity of cones of the monkey *Macaca fascicularis, Journal of Physiology (London)*, **390** 145–160.

BENDER, B.G. & RUDDOCK, K.H. (1974) The characteristics of a visual defect associated with abnormal responses to both colour and luminance, *Vision Research*, **14**, 383–393.

BLYTHE, I.M., BROMLEY, J.M., KENNARD, C. & RUDDOCK, K.H. (1986) Visual discrimination of target displacement remains after damage to the striate cortex in humans, *Nature*, **320**, 619–621.

BLYTHE, I.M., KENNARD, C. & RUDDOCK, K.H. (1987) Residual vision in patients with retro-geniculate lesions of the visual pathways, *Brain*, **110**, 887–905.

BRENT, P.J., KENNARD, C. & RUDDOCK, K.H. (1994) Residual colour vision in a human hemianope: spectral responses and colour discrimination, *Proceedings of the Royal Society of London*, **B 256**, 219–225.

BRINDLEY, G.S. (1953) The effects on colour vision of adaptation to very bright lights, *Journal of Physiology (London)*, **122**, 332–350.

BRINDLEY, G.S. (1954) The summation areas of human colour-receptive mechanisms at increment threshold, *Journal of Physiology (London)*, **122**, 400–408.

DACEY, D.M. (1993). Physiology, morphology and spatial densities of identified ganglion cell types in primate retina, *Higher Order Processing in the Visual System*, CIBA Foundation **184**.

DARTNALL, H.J.A., BOWMAKER, J.K. & MOLLON, J.D. (1983) Human visual pigments: micro-spectrophotometric results from the eyes of seven persons, *Proceedings of the Royal Society of London*, **B 220**, 115–130.

VAN ENSCH, J.A., VAN KOLDENHOFF, A.J., VAN DOORN, A.J. & KOENDERINK, J.J. (1984) Spectral sensitivity and wavelength discrimination of the human periphal visual field, *Journal of the Optical Society of America*, **A 1**, 443–450.

FELSTEN, G., BENEVENTO, L.A. & BURMAN, D. (1983) Opponent-color responses in macaque extrageniculate visual pathways: the lateral pulvinar, *Brain Research*, **288**, 363–367.

FRANCOIS, J. & VERRIEST, G. (1968) Nouvelles observations de déficiences acquises de la discrimina-tion chromatique, *Annales d'Oculistique*, **201**, 1097–1114.

HAM, W.T.JR., RUFFOLO, J.J. JR., MUELLER, H.A., CLARKE, A.M. & MOON, M.E. (1978) Histo-logical analysis of photochemical lesions produced in rhesus by short-wavelength light, *Investigative Ophthalmology and Vision Science*, **17**, 1029–1035.

HARWERTH, R.S. & SPERLING, H.G. (1975) Effects of intense visible radiation on the increment threshold spectral sensitivity of the rhesus monkey, *Vision Research*, **15**, 1193–1204.

HENDRICKS, I.M., HOLLIDAY, I.E. & RUDDOCK, K.H. (1981) A new class of visual defect: spreading inhibition elicited by chromatic light stimuli, *Brain*, **104**, 813–840.

HEYWOOD, C.A. & COWEY, A. (1987) On the role of cortical area V4 in the discrimination of hue and pattern in macaque monkeys, *Journal of Neuroscience*, **7**, 2601–2617.

HEYWOOD, C.A., GADOTTI, A. & COWEY, A. (1992) Cortical area V4 and its role in the perception of color, *Journal of Neuroscience*, **12**, 4056–4065.

JAEGER, W. & GRÜTZNER, P. (1963) Erworbene Farbensinnstöringen. In: Sautter, H. (Ed.) *Ent-wiklung und Fortschritt in der Augenheilkunde 3rd Fortbildungkurs der Deutchen Op-thalmolgischen Gesellschaft*, Stuttgart: Enke, pp. 591–614.

KADOYA, S., WOLIN, L.R. & MASSOPUST, L.C. (1971) Collicular unit responses to monochromatic stimulation in squirrel monkey, *Brain Research*, **32**, 251–254.

KAPLAN, E., LEE, B.B. & SHAPLEY, R.M. (1991) New views of primate retinal function. In: Osborne, N. & Cohaden, J., (Eds) *Progress in Retinal Research*, Oxford: Pergamon, pp. 271–336.

KEATING, E.G. (1979) Rudimentary color vision in the monkey after removal of striate and preoccipital cortex, *Brain Research*, **179**, 379–384.

KENNARD, C., LAWDEN, M., MORLAND, A.B. & RUDDOCK, K.H. (1995) Colour identification and colour constancy are impaired in a patient with incomplete achromatopsia associated with prestriate cortical lesions, *Proceedings of the Royal Society (London)*, **B 260**, 169–175.

KING-SMITH, P.E. & CARDEN, D. (1976) Luminance and opponent-colour contributions to visual detection and adaptation and to temporal and spatial integration, *Journal of the Optical Society of America*, **66**, 709–717.

KISVARDAY, Z.F., COWEY, A., STOERIG, P. & SOMOGYI, P. (1991) Direct and indirect input into degenerated dorsal lateral geniculate nucleus after striate cortex removal in monkey: implica-tions for residual vision, *Experimental Brain Research*, **86**, 271–292.

KITAHARA, K., TAMAKI, R., HIBINO, H. & OYAMA, T. (1987) A case of blue-yellow defect induced by intense blue light. In: Verriest, G. (Ed.) *Colour Vision Deficiences VIII*, Dordrecht: Junk, pp. 21–29.

KÖLLNER, H. (1912) Die Störungen des Farbensinnes: ihre klinische Bedeutung und ihre Diagnose, Berlin: Karger.

KRASTER, H. & MORELAND, J.D. (1991) Colour vision deficiencies in ophthalmic diseases. In: Foster, D.H. (Ed.) *Vision and Visual Dysfunction 7, Inherited and Acquired Colour Vision Deficiencies*, Basingstoke: Macmillan, pp. 115–172.

LEE, B.B., MARTIN, P.R. & VALBERG, A. (1988) The physiological basis of heterochromatic flicker photometry demonstrated in the ganglion cells of the macaque retina, *Journal of Physiology (London)*, **404**, 323–347.

LEPORÉ, F., CARDU, B., RASMUSSEN, T. & MALMO, R.B. (1975) Rod and cone sensitivity in destriate monkeys, *Brain Research*, **93**, 203–221.

EVENTHAL, A.G., RODIECK, R.W. & DREHER, B. (1981), Retinal ganglion cell classes in old world monkey: morphology and central projections, *Science*, **213**, 1139–1142.

LIVINGSTONE, M.S. & HUBEL, D.H. (1984) Anatomy and physiology of a color system in the primate visual cortex, *Journal of Neuroscience*, **4**, 309–356.

LÜTZE, P. & BRESNICK, G.H. (1991) Lenses of diabetic patients 'yellow' at an accelerated rate similar to older normals, *Investigative Opthalmology and Vision Science*, **32**, 194–199.

MACADAM, D.L. (1942) Visual sensitivities to color difference in daylight, *Journal of the Optical Society of America*, **32**, 247–274.

MARRÉ, M. & MARRÉ, E. (1986) *Erworbene Störungen des Farbensehens*, Leipzig: Thieme.

MARROCCO, R.T. & LI, R.H. (1977) Monkey superior colliculus: properties of single cells and their afferent inputs, *Journal of Neurophysiology*, **40**, 844–860.

MEADOWS, J.C. (1974) Disturbed perception of colours associated with localized cerebral lesions, *Brain*, **97**, 615–632.

DE MONASTERIO, F.M., SCHEIN, S.J. & MCCRANE, E.P. (1981) Staining of blue-sensitive cones of the macaque retina by a fluorescent dye, *Science*, **213**, 1278–1281.

NATHANS, J., PIANTANIDA, T.P., EDDY, R.L., SHOWS, T.B. & HOGNESS, D.S. (1986) Molecular genetics of inherited variation in human colour vision, *Science*, **232**, 803–806.

PEARLMAN, A.L., BIRCH, J. & MEADOWS, J.C. (1979) Cerebral color blindness: an acquired defect in hue discrimination, *Annals of Neurology*, **5**, 253–261.

PERRY, V.H. & COWEY, A. (1984) Retinal ganglion cells that project to the superior colliculus and pretectum in the macaque monkey, *Neuroscience*, **12**, 1125–1137.

PERRY, V.H., OEHLER, R. & COWEY, A. (1984) Retinal ganglion cells that project to the dorsal lateral geniculate nucleus in the macaque monkey, *Neuroscience*, **12**, 1101–1123.

PINCKERS, A. (1976) Analysis of acquired disorders of color vision with a view to a distinction from hereditary ocular anomalies, *Ophthalmologia*, **173**, 221–226.

PLANT, G.T. (1991) Disorders of colour vision in diseases of the nervous system. In: Foster, D.H. (Ed.) *Vision and Visual Dysfunction 7, Inherited and Acquired Colour Vision Deficiencies*, Basingstoke: Macmillan, pp. 173–198.

QUIGLEY, H.A., DUNKELBERGER, G.R. & GREEN, W.R. (1988) Chronic human glaucoma causing selectively greater loss of large optic nerve fibres, *Ophthalmology*, **95**, 357–363.

ROBERTSON, A.R. & WRIGHT, W.D. (1965). International comparison of working standards for colorimetry, *Journal of the Optical Society of America*, **55**, 694–706.

RÖNNE, H. (1910) Pathologisch-anatomische Untersuchungen über alcoholishe Intoxikationsamblyopie, *Albrecht v. Graefes Ophthal. Arch. Augenheilk*, **77**, 1–95.

RUDDOCK, K.H. (1963) Evidence for macular pigmentation from colour matching data, *Vision Research*, **3**, 417–429.

RUDDOCK, K.H. (1965) The effect of age upon colour vision. II Changes with age in light transmission of the ocular media, *Vision Research*, **5**, 47–58.

RUDDOCK, K.H. (1972) Light transmission through the ocular media and macular pigment and its significance for psychophysical investigation. In: Jameson, D. & Hurvich, L.M. (Eds) *Handbook of Sensory Physiology* **VIII/4**, *Visual Psychophysics*, Heidelberg: Springer, pp. 455–469.

RUDDOCK, K.H. (1987) Psychophysical testing of normal and abnormal visual function. In: Kennard, C. and Rose, F.C. (Eds) *Physiological Aspects of Clinical Neuro-Ophthalmology*, London: Chapman Hall, pp. 27–55.

RUDDOCK, K.H. (1991) Psychophysics of inherited colour vision deficiencies. In: Foster, D.H. (Ed.) *Vision and Visual Dysfunction 7, Inherited and Acquired Colour Vision Deficiences*, Basingstoke: Macmillan, pp. 4–37.

RUDDOCK, K.H. (1993) Acquired deficiences of human colour vision. In Kennard C (Ed.) *Bailliere's Clinical Neurology: II Visual Perceptual Defects*, London: Bailliere Tindall, pp. 287–337.

RUDDOCK, K.H. & NAGHSHINEH, S. (1974) Mechanisms of red-green anomalous trichromacy: hypothesis and analysis, *Modern Problems in Ophthalmology*, **13**, 210–214.

RUSHTON, W.A.H. & BAKER, H.D. (1964) Red/green sensitivity in normal vision, *Vision Research*, **4**, 75–85.

SAID, F.S. & WEALE, R.A. (1959) The variations with age of the spectral transmissivity of the living crystalline lens, *Gerontologia (Basel)*, **3**, 213–231.

SCHILDER, P., PASIK, P. & PASIK, T. (1972) Extrageniculostriate vision in the monkey. III 'Circle vs triangle' and 'red vs green' discrimination, *Experimental Brain Research*, **14**, 436–448.

SMITH, V.S., POKORNY, J. & DIDDIE, K.R. (1978) Colour matching and Stiles-Crawford effect in central serous choroidopathy, *Modern Problems in Ophthalmology*, **19**, 284–295.

SPERLING, H.G. & HARWERTH, R.S. (1971) Red-green cone interactions in the increment threshold spectral sensitivity of primates, *Science*, **172**, 180–184.

SPERLING, H.G., JOHNSON, C. & HARWERTH, R.S. (1980) Differential spectral photic damage to primate cones, *Vision Research*, **20**, 1117–1125.

STILES, W.S. (1978) *Mechanisms of Colour Vision*, London: Academic Press.

STOERIG, P. (1987) Chromaticity and achromaticity. Evidence for a functional differentiation in visual field defects, *Brain*, **110**, 869–886.

STOERIG, P. & COWEY, A. (1991). Increment threshold spectral sensitivity in blindsight: evidence for colour opponency, *Brain*, **114**, 1487–1512.

TANSEY, E.M., PESSOA, V.F., FLEMING, S, LONDON, D.N. & IKEDA, H. (1985) Pattern and extent of demyelination in the optic nerves of mice infected with Semliki Forest virus and the possibility of axonal sprouting, *Brain*, **108**, 29–41.

TS'O, D.Y. & GILBERT, C.D. (1988) The organisation of chromatic and spatial interactions in the primate striate cortex, *Journal of Neuroscience*, **8**, 1712–1727.

VERRIEST, G. (1963). Further studies on acquired deficiency of color discrimination, *Journal of the Optical Society of America*, **53**, 185–195.

WALSH, V., KULIKOWSKI, J.J., BUTLER, S.R. & CARDEN, D. (1992) The effects of lesions of area V4 on the visual abilities of macaques: colour categorization, *Behavioural Brain Research*, **52**, 81–89.

WALSH, V., CARDEN, D., BUTLER, S.R. & KULIKOWSKI, J.J. (1993) The effects of V4 lesions on the visual abilities of macaques: hue discrimination and colour constancy, *Behavioural Brain Research*, **53**, 51–62.

WALTERS, H.V. & WRIGHT, W.D. (1943) The spectral sensitivity of the fovea and extra-fovea in the Purkinje range. *Proceedings of the Royal Society of London, B*, **131**, 340–361.

WEISKRANTZ, L., WARRINGTON, E.K., SANDERS, M.D. & MARSHALL, J. (1974) Visual capacity in the hemianopic field following a restricted occipital ablation, *Brain*, **97**, 709–728.

WIESEL, T.N. & HUBEL, D.H. (1966) Spatial and chromatic interactions in the lateral geniculate body of the rhesus monkey, *Journal of Neurophysiology*, **29**, 1115–1156.

WRIGHT, W.D. (1927–28) A re-determination of the trichromatic coefficients of the spectra colours, *Transcripts of the Optical Society*, **30**, 141–164.

WRIGHT, W.D. (1936) The breakdown of a colour match with high intensities of adaptation, *Journal of Physiology (London)*, **87**, 23–33.

WRIGHT, W.D. (1941) The sensitivity of the eye to small colour differences, *Proceedings of the Physical Society (London)*, **53**, 93–112.

WRIGHT, W.D. (1946) *Researches on Normal and Defective Colour Vision*, London: Kimpton.

WRIGHT, W.D. & PITT, F.H.G. (1934) Hue-discrimination in normal colour-vision, *Proceedings of the Physical Society (London)*, **46**, 459–473.

WYSZECKI, G. & STILES, W.S. (1982) *Color Science: Concepts and Methods, Quantitative Data and Formulae*, 2nd edn. New York: Wiley.

YOUNG, R.S.L. & FISHMAN, G.A. (1980) Color matches of patients with retinitis pigmentosa, *Investigative Ophthalmology and Vision Science*, **19**, 967–972.

YOUNG, R.S.L., FISHMAN, G.A. & CHEN, F. (1980) Traumatically acquired color vision defect, *Investigative Ophthalmology and Vision Science*, **19**, 545–549.

ZEKI, S. (1978) Uniformity and diversity of structure and function in rhesus monkey prestriate cortex, *Journal of Physiology (London)*, **272**, 273–290.

ZEKI, S. (1980) The representation of colours in the cerebral cortex. *Nature*, **284**, 412–418.

ZEKI, S. (1990) A century of achromatopsia, *Brain*, **113**, 1721–1777.

ZIHL, J. & VON CRAMON, D. (1986) Störungen des Farbensehens, *Zerebrale Sehstörungen*, Stuttgart: Kohlhammer, pp. 66–78.

Colour Discrimination Without Pattern Discrimination in a Human Hemianope

J.R. Wright, P.J. Brent, J.A. Ogilvie and K.H. Ruddock

5.6.1   INTRODUCTION

Lesions of the human striate cortex usually give rise to that loss of sensitivity in those areas of the visual field which project to the damaged cortex. A number of studies have, however, demonstrated that some patients are capable of responding to certain classes of light stimuli presented within the 'blind' areas of the visual field. Such patients can detect and localise transient (flashed and moving) stimuli presented to the 'blind' field, and speed discrimination has also been observed (Ruddock, 1991). Discrimination of spatial structure is rarely found, and only a few patients have been able to make discriminations on the basis of spectral composition (Blythe *et al.*, 1987; Brent *et al.*, 1994; Stoerig, 1987). In some instances, the patient exhibits 'blindsight', in which there is no sensation in response to the light stimulus, and visual discriminations are performed only under 'forced choice' conditions (Weiskrantz *et al.*, 1974). Other patients, however, report that transient light stimuli generate the percept of a 'dark shadow', located within the 'blind' region of the field, and this response mode is designated 'residual vision' (Barbur *et al.*, 1980; Blythe *et al.*, 1986). In this chapter, we examine visual responses in a patient GY, who has suffered hemianopic visual field losses associated with extensive lesions affecting both the striate area V1 and the pre-striate visual areas. We show that GY has residual colour vision without spatial discrimination.

5.6.2   METHODS

The data presented in this paper are concerned primarily with verbal identification of coloured stimuli in the form of a uniform circular field, or a one-dimensional, periodic structure (a grating with square waveform luminance profile). Colour naming was also investigated for stimuli consisting of two different spectral components, of equal luminance, either in the form of alternating bars of different colours (e.g. red and green), or of differently coloured concentric areas. These stimuli were presented for 100 ms and in each experiment, three or four different stimuli were alternated in random sequence, until 20 responses were recorded for each. The 'normal' hemifield was illuminated with white light (luminance 3.0 log troland), in order to suppress sensitivity to intra-ocular stray light from the coloured stimulus. We also examined threshold sensitivity for detection of a target, the luminance of which was selected by a double interleaved staircase method (Cornsweet, 1962), threshold responses corresponding to eight successive reversals of a 'seen', 'not seen' response, set to an accuracy of 0.03 log units. The subject responded to each target presentation by pressing one of two buttons, to denote either target 'seen' or 'not seen'.

5.6.2.1 Equipment

Light stimuli were generated by a three-beam Maxwellian-view optical system, which has been described in detail elsewhere (Barbur and Ruddock, 1980).

5.6.2.2 Procedures

The subject was dark adapted for 15 minutes at the start of each experimental session, and the laboratory remained dark throughout the measurements. Thresholds were determined by a double staircase method, and coloured stimuli were presented in random sequence, for verbal identification. The subject was instructed to fixate on a small, red, circular spot (diameter 1º) that was continuously visible, and the test stimuli were located at selected points in the visual field. Measurements were made with the right eye, for which the 'blind' field falls on the nasal retina. In the initial experiments on colour identification with simple circular fields (data shown in Figure 5.6.2), GY was allowed to examine the stimuli under foveal fixation, so was aware of the composition of the stimulus set. In the experiments with the compound stimuli (data of Figures 5.6.3 and 5.6.4), GY did not perform an initial foveal examination.

5.6.2.3 Observer

GY, a 36-year-old male, has hemianopic fields, homonymous for the two eyes, associated with damage to the left striate and pre-striate cortical areas, incurred 28 years ago in a traffic accident. An MRI scan, similar to that published by Barbur et al. (1993), showed involvement of the lingual gyrus, the striate and pre-striate cortex below the calcarine fissure to within about 1cm of the occipital pole. The medial aspects of the cuneus extending anteriorly to the sulcus parieto-occipitalis, a small strip of the posterior aspect of the pre-cuneus in the parietal lobe and the caudal extremity of the parahippocampal gyrus are also involved. The fusiform gyrus is, however, spared. A less extreme lesion on the right side involves the cortex of the right side of the supra-marginal gyrus, mainly the inferior parietal lobule, and juxta-cortical white matter of the adjacent part of the superior parietal lobule. Much of the geniculo-calcarine fissure on the left, but not that on the right side, is also damaged. No abnormal visual functions were found in testing the left visual field; colour vision responses are normal, and although Hess and Pointer (1989) reported a loss of contrast sensitivity in GY's normal hemifield, increment threshold sensitivity does not differ significantly from that of normal vision (Figure 7b of Barbur et al., 1980). A detailed visual field plot with stationary stimuli shows a right hemianopic loss, with sparing of sensitivity extending up to 3.5º to the right of the fixation point (Barbur et al., 1980). GY can, however, localise and detect transient light stimuli presented to the 'blind' right hemifield. Sensitivity for the detection of a stationary, flashed target is low, but increases linearly with increase in target area, and flicker sensitivity saturates at a low frequency (Barbur et al., 1980).

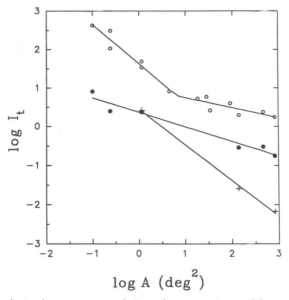

$$\log A \ (\text{deg}^2)$$

Figure 5.6.1. The relative luminance, I_t, of a circular target required for its detection by GY, plotted against the target area, A. Circles refer to a 612 nm target presented for 100 msec 10° off-axis along the horizontal meridian against a white background (luminance 0.9 log troland; diameter 20°); open symbols for the blind hemifield and full symbols for the normal hemifield. Crosses refer to a white target on the same background, presented to the blind hemifield.

Sensitivity for detection of a moving target increases with an increase of the target velocity, and speed discrimination is normal, whereas directional discrimination is impaired (Barbur *et al.*, 1980; Blythe *et al.*, 1987). Spatial resolution for detection of apparent motion is near normal (Blythe *et al.*, 1986), but GY is unable to discriminate shape or any other spatial attribute of stimuli located entirely within the blind hemifield. Although earlier measurements on GY's residual vision revealed neither cone activity (Barbur *et al.*, 1980) nor colour discrimination (Blythe *et al.*, 1987), both have been demonstrated in a recent study (Brent *et al.*, 1994). Positron emission tomography shows that moving stimuli generate activity in pre-striate areas analogous to monkey V3 and V5, both of which are associated with sensitivity to movement, whereas the damaged striate area, V1, remains inactive (Barbur *et al.*, 1993).

5.6.3   RESULTS

The luminance of a circular target required for its detection by GY, measured under conditions that elicit a cone response function (Brent *et al.*, 1994), is plotted as a function of target area in Figure 5.6.1. Also shown are equivalent values measured for white light stimuli, and it should be noted that the change in slope for the data plot for the spectral stimuli is absent in this case. GY's data for colour identification, plotted as the probability of naming correctly the colour of stimuli presented to his 'blind' hemifield, are given for nine sets of stimulus colours (Figure 5.6.2, taken from Brent *et al.*, 1994). The data of Figure 5.6.2 refer to colour naming for spatially uniform coloured fields (see inset to Figure 5.6.2 for the precise configuration). The white hemifield (luminance 1.5 log troland), and the fixation spot, F, were constantly visible, and the target hemifield, with its vertical boundary located 17° from F along the horizontal meridian, was presented for 500 ms. The three target colours in a given experiment were presented 10 times each, in random sequence, and all were of luminance 2.1 log troland. The stimuli were R, 'red', 665 nm; G, 'green', 535 nm; B, 'blue', 440 nm; O, 'orange', 615 nm; Y, 'yellow', 584 nm; P, 'purple', 455 nm; Pi, 'pink', white added in equal photometric proportions to 665 nm; pG, 'pale green', white added in equal photometric proportions to 535 nm; pB, 'pale blue', white added in equal photometric proportions to 440 nm. Experiment (h) was as (a), but with the test half-field reduced to 10° in diameter.

The probabilities for correct identification of the colours and of the spatial disposition of the coloured components for spatially structured fields are shown in Figures 5.6.3 and 5.6.4. Stimuli were presented for 100 ms to GY's blind hemifield. Each stimulus in a set was presented 20 times in random sequence. Labels (a), (b) and (c) refer to rectangular stimuli (18° vertical by 14° horizontal) that were uniformly coloured, or, for the colour pairs, divided vertically (a) or horizontally (b and c). For (d), the stimuli were in a circular configuration, as illustrated. The histogram values denoted 'Pos' show the probability of GY correctly identifying the relative positions of the component colours. It is clear that for large, rectangular elements, GY can detect the presence of red and green components, but

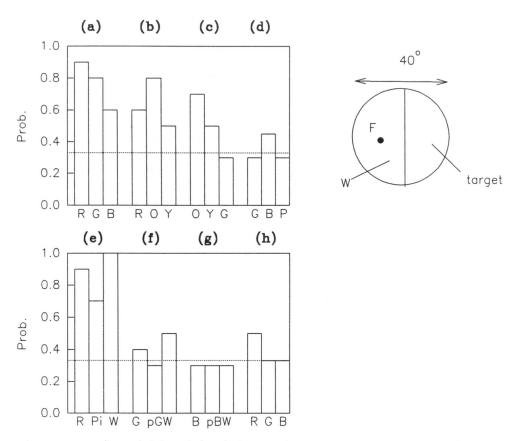

Figure 5.6.2. The probability of identifying correctly the colour of the target hemifield for sets of three stimuli as indicated along the abscissa. The broken lines denote the probability level at chance. Data for GY.

performs poorly in identifying their relative positions (Figure 5.6.3a). Further, he frequently confuses yellow with the red/green mixed fields (Figure 5.6.3b). With the concentric stimuli (Figure 5.6.3d) and the finer rectangular elements (Figure 5.6.4), he is unable to identify the presence of red and green components and adding the outline of the stimulus pattern in the equivalent position of the contralateral field does not improve his performance. He also has difficulty in detecting the presence of blue and yellow components, even with a field consisting of two large rectangular bars (Figure 5.6.3c).

5.6.4   DISCUSSION

Brent *et al.* (1994) demonstrated the activity of the π_5- (red-sensitive) and π_4- (green-sensitive) cone spectral response mechanisms in GY's blind hemifield. They were unable to isolate the blue-sensitive π_3-spectral response and noted that for GY's blind hemifield, rod responses were obtained under several experimental conditions in which cone responses are observed in normal vision. Absence of a Purkinje shift in spectral responses recorded 30° off-axis in GY's 'blind' hemifield had been reported previously by Barbur *et al.* (1980). In addition to recording π-spectral responses, Brent *et al.* also showed that relative spectral sensitivity for a monochromatic target presented on a white background is normal for GY's blind hemifield. They concluded that the post-receptoral response channels that generate this spectral response are normal, although the data provide only weak evidence of those response features that are attributed to the activity of colour opponent mechanisms (Sperling and Harwerth, 1971; King-Smith and Carden, 1976).

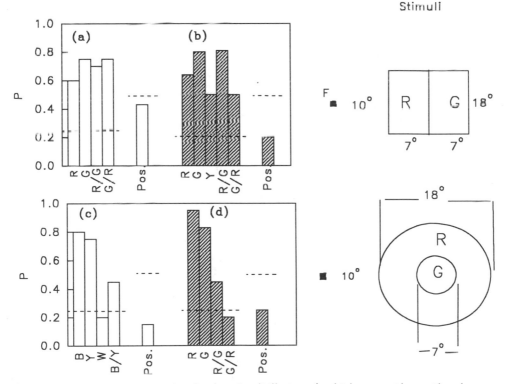

Figure 5.6.3.   As Figure 5.6.2, but for the stimuli illustrated, which were either uniformly coloured, or divided into two equiluminant components (3 log troland) as illustrated.

Stoerig and Cowey (1989, 1991) have reported similar spectral responses for two of three hemianopic patients. The colour naming data (Figure 5.6.2) establish that GY can distinguish stimulus colour in his 'blind' hemifield, and with long wavelength stimuli he discriminates relatively small wavelength steps, e.g. 615 nm from 665 nm (Figure 5.6.2b) or from 585 nm (Figure 5.6.2c) and differences in saturation (Figure 5.6.2f). His performance is less robust for short wavelength stimuli, even for large wavelength differences, which may well be associated with the strong influence of rods evident in his spectral responses. An important feature of GY's discrimination data is his inability to achieve significant discrimination for long wavelength stimuli when the diameter of the field is reduced from 20° to 10° (Figure 5.6.2h).

The observations with the coarse spatial patterns (Figure 5.6.3) show that he can distinguish the rectangular red-green elements from simple red or green patterns of the same area (Figure 5.6.3a,b), but he fails to identify their spatial arrangement. Indeed, on about 25 per cent of presentations, he confused the possible orientations of the boundary between the two rectangles (vertical in Figure 5.6.3a and horizontal in Figure 5.6.3b). When a yellow was included in the stimulus set (Figure 5.6.3b), he identified it as a compound red-green pattern on 50 per cent of presentations, and conversely, he identified a compound grating as yellow on 25 per cent of their presentations. Similarly, with the blue-yellow stimulus set, he performs badly in identifying both white and the mixed yellow-blue fields, making frequent confusion between them (Figure 5.6.3c). We conclude that GY's

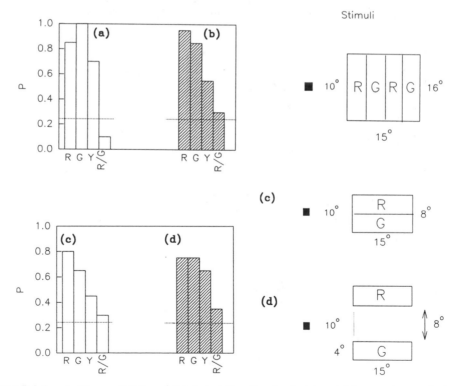

Figure 5.6.4. As Figures 5.6.2 and 5.6.3, but the stimulus in (a) and (b) was a rectangle (16° vertical by 15° horizontal) divided into four equal bars, vertically (a) or horizontally (b), and in (b), an identical black and white pattern was added in the mirror image position of the normal hemifield. The stimulus configurations for (c) and (d) were as illustrated.

apparent ability to resolve coarse patterns, evident in Figure 5.6.3a, is, in reality, based on a change in the perceived colour, the mixture of two components, red and green or yellow and blue, appearing as yellow or white respectively. This is confirmed by the data of Figure 5.6.4, which show that the finer gratings are never resolved at above chance level, and by far the most common confusion was between yellow and the compound colours. Similarly, the pair of colours arranged concentrically were not identified at above chance level (Figure 5.6.3d) but, in this case, the mixture was virtually always identified by the colour of the larger, outer zone. This last stimulus set did not include yellow, although GY was not informed of that fact (see procedures). We conclude that like patients with visual form agnosia caused by carbon monoxide poisoning (Table 11.1 of Ruddock, 1991), GY retains the ability to discriminate colour, but has lost entirely his capacity for spatial discrimination.

GY can, despite his lack of spatial discrimination, localise targets within his 'blind' hemifield (Blythe et al., 1986) and has near normal spatial resolution for apparent motion (Blythe et al., 1987). Threshold detection for white light involves a response mechanism with very extensive spatial summation (Barbur et al., 1980), but the new measurements shown in Figure 5.6.1 establish that under conditions that isolate cone-driven responses, spatial summation is restricted to circular fields of diameter less than some $2.0°$. Thus there appear to be at least two response mechanisms active in GY's residual vision, one with very large receptive fields and the other with much more restricted fields. Barbur et al, (1994), using different methods, also found evidence for two spatial response mechanisms, one with a very large receptive field, and the other with a spatial frequency response which peaks at about 1 c deg^{-1}, similar to the ST2 spatial response described by Holliday and Ruddock (1983). This latter has a centre-surround antagonistic spatial organisation, the central region of which has a diameter of about $1°$, similar to the summation area for the cone thresholds illustrated in Figure 5.6.2. The ST2 mechanism has transient response characteristics, consistent with the fact that GY's residual vision is entirely transient in nature. It should be noted that it was not possible to elicit responses associated with the ST1 mechanism in previous studies of GY's 'blind' hemifield (Barbur et al., 1980).

The principal features of GY's residual vision are consistent with activity in the retino-collicular pathway, and colour-opponent responses capable of providing colour discrimination have been recorded from neurones in the pulvinar (Felsten et al., 1983). It has been demonstrated, however, that monkeys with lesions involving all layers of dLGN are unable to make saccades to locate near threshold stimuli presented within the visual field areas that project to the damaged geniculate area (Schiller et al., 1990). It appears, therefore, that the collicular-pulvinar projection cannot support saccadic localisation in the absence of geniculate input, and suggests that the collicular-geniculate pathway is essential for this function. The residual vision observed in patients such as the one described in this paper is, therefore, likely to involve direct inputs to pre-striate cortex from both retino-geniculate and retino-colliculo-geniculate routes.

5.6.5 REFERENCES

Barbur, J.L. & Ruddock, K.H. (1980) Spatial characteristics of movement detection mechanisms in human vision. I. Achromatic vision, *Biological Cybernetics*, **37**, 77–92.

Barbur, J.L., Ruddock, K.H. & Waterfield, V.A. (1980) Human visual responses in the absence of the geniculo-calcarine projection, *Brain*, **103**, 905–928.

Barbur, J.L., Watson, J.D.G., Frackowiak, R.S.J. & Zeki, S. (1993) Conscious visual perception without V1, *Brain*, **116**, 1293–1302.

BARBUR, J.L., HARLOW, A.J. & WEISKRANTZ, L. (1994) Spatial and temporal response properties of residual vision in a case of hemianopia, *Philosophical Transactions of the Royal Society of London*, **B 343**, 157–166.

BLYTHE, I.M., BROMLEY, J.M., KENNARD, C. & RUDDOCK, K.H. (1986) Visual discrimination of target displacement remains after damage to the striate cortex in humans, *Nature*, **320**, 619–621.

BLYTHE, I.M., KENNARD, C. & RUDDOCK, K.H. (1987) Residual vision in patients with retrogeniculate lesions of the visual pathways, *Brain*, **110**, 887–905.

BRENT, P.J., KENNARD, C. & RUDDOCK, K.H. (1994) Residual colour vision in a human hemianope: spectral responses and colour discrimination, *Proceedings of the Royal Society of London*, **B 256**, 219–225.

CORNSWEET, T.N. (1962) The staircase method in psychophysics, *American Journal of Psychology*, **75**, 485–491.

FELSTEN, G., BENEVENTO, L.A. & BURMAN, D. (1983) Opponent-color responses in macaque extrageniculate visual pathways: the lateral pulvinar, *Brain Research*, **288**, 363–367.

HESS, R.F. & POINTER, J.S. (1989) Spatial and temporal contrast sensitivity in hemianopia. A comparative study of the sighted and blind hemifields, *Brain*, **112**, 871–894.

HOLLIDAY. I.E. & RUDDOCK, K.H (1983) Two spatio-temporal filters in human vision 1. Temporal and spatial frequency response characteristics, *Biological Cybernetics*, **47**, 173–190.

KING-SMITH, P.E. & CARDEN, D. (1976) Luminance and opponent colour contributions to visual detection and adaptation and to temporal and spatial integration, *Journal of the Optical Society of America*, **66**, 709–717.

RUDDOCK, K.H. (1991) Spatial vision after cortical lesions. In: Regan, D.M. (Ed.) *Spatial Vision, Vision and Visual Dysfunction, vol. 10*, London, Macmillan, pp. 4–37

SCHILLER, P.H., LOGOTHETIS, N. & CHARLES, E.R. (1990) Role of colour-opponent and broad-band channels in vision, *Visual Neuroscience*, **5**, 321–346.

SPERLING, H.G. & HARWERTH, R.S. (1971) Red-green cone interactions in the increment threshold spectral sensitivity of primates, *Science*, **172**, 180–184.

STOERIG, P. (1987) Chromaticity and achromaticity: evidence for a functional differentiation in visual field defects, *Brain*, **110**, 869–886.

STOERIG, P. & COWEY, A. (1989) Wavelength sensitivity in blindsight, *Nature*, **342**, 916–918.

STOERIG, P. & COWEY, A. (1991) Increment-threshold spectral sensitivity in blindsight: evidence for colour opponency, *Brain*, **114**, 1487–1512.

WEISKRANTZ, L., WARRINGTON, E.K., SANDERS, M.D. & MARSHALL, J. (1974) Visual capacity in the hemianopic field following a restricted occipital ablation, *Brain*, **97**, 709–728.

Rates of Age-related Declines of Chromatic Discriminations are the Same for Equiluminant Stimuli Lying on Tritan and Constant S-cone Axes

Keizo Shinomori, Brooke E. Schefrin and John S. Werner

5.7.1 INTRODUCTION

Results of colour matching (Gilbert, 1957; Lakowski, 1962; Ohta and Kato, 1975) and hue discrimination (Knoblauch *et al.*, 1987; Smith *et al.*, 1985; Verriest, 1963) tests indicate age-related losses in discrimination. The magnitudes of these losses appear to be greater for discriminations that are mediated by short-wave sensitive S-cones than medium-wave M- and long-wave L-cones. The underlying cause(s) for this tritan-like behaviour associated with age has been a matter of debate. Studies have shown that decreases in retinal illuminance lead to tritan-like behaviour as measured by the Moreland equation and the FM-100 hue test (Gilbert, 1957; Moreland, 1993). These findings suggest that age-related increases in the density of the ocular media, rather than alterations of receptoral or post-receptoral mechanisms, can account for the loss of chromatic discrimination between stimuli composed, in part or entirely, of short-wavelength light. However, models applied to increment threshold data (Schefrin, 1992) suggest that age-related losses in sensitivity of an S-cone pathway are in part due to neuronal changes. Perhaps neuronal changes are also partly responsible for age-related declines in colour discriminations (Knoblauch *et al.*, 1987).

Standard tests of colour vision do not allow the effects of age-related changes in ocular media density to be separated from the effects of senescent neural changes. Because the chromatic differences between caps of the FM-100 hue test along tritan axes are smaller than along the deutan and protan directions (Birch, 1993), age-related tritan-like behaviour obtained with that test may not reflect a physiologically-based selective loss of sensitivity of S-cone pathways. Furthermore, standard tests are influenced by senescent changes in the ocular media and pupil. The luminance levels of the test stimuli are held constant for all observers, so the retinal illuminance of these test stimuli will be lower, on average, for older than younger observers. It has been shown that error scores on arrangement and plate tests will increase with the reduction of intensity level of the illuminant (van Everdingen *et al.*, 1991; Knoblauch *et al.*, 1987; Kudo *et al.*, 1993, Smith *et al.*, 1991).

Our experiment was designed to determine whether age-related losses in chromatic discrimination can simply be explained by senescent changes in the ocular media, or not, when stimuli (unlike lights used in the Moreland equation or caps in the FM-100 hue test) are equated for retinal illuminance for individual younger and older observers. In addition, we also investigated whether rates of age-related losses in chromatic discriminations are greater along a tritan axis than a constant S-cone axis when retinal illuminance is controlled.

5.7.2 METHODS

5.7.2.1 Observers

Data were obtained with 30 observers (15 males, 15 females) ranging from 22.0 to 76.7 years of age. All observers had normal colour vision without a history of ocular disease, surgery, or medications that interfere with ocular or neurological functioning. Colour vision was tested with the Farnsworth Panel D-15 test, the F-2 plate, and the American Optical HRR pseudoisochromatic plates. Each observer possessed a best corrected Snellen acuity of 20/40 or better in the tested eye.

5.7.2.2 Apparatus

The stimuli were presented in Maxwellian-view, using a conventional five-channel system. The 420 nm and 650 nm lights were produced by interference filters (Ealing; bandpass at half power was 8 nm for the 420 nm filters and 12 nm for the 630 nm filters). Other monochromatic lights were produced by three monochromators (Instruments S-A Model H20; 5 nm bandpass at half power). The light intensity of each channel was controlled by neutral density wedges and filters. Two lights for heterochromatic flicker photometry (HFP) measurement were alternated by a sectored mirror placed at the common focal point of each channel. A Powell achromatising lens (Powell, 1981) was used after the final Maxwellian lens and the light was focused onto the plane of the observer's pupil. The final Maxwellian view image, determined by an aperture, was 2 mm in diameter.

Positioning of observers was accomplished using an adjustable chair and a bite-bar assembly with movements in three orthogonal directions. A pupil viewer was used to align the observer's pupil with respect to the final Maxwellian image.

5.7.2.3 Calibrations

Relative radiometric measurements of spectral lights and calibrations of neutral density wedges and filters were made with a silicon photodiode and linear readout system (United Detector Technology 81 Optometer). Photometric calibrations by the method of Westheimer (1966) were made at 570 nm with a Minolta LS-100 photometer. The monochromators were calibrated with a He–Ne laser, and the bandwidths of the monochromators and interference filters were measured with a scanning spectroradiometer (PhotoResearch, model PR-703 A/PC).

5.7.2.4 Procedures

Chromatic discriminations along a tritan axis were measured using individual tritan pairs consisting of a 420 nm and an empirically-determined middle wavelength monochromatic light. The variable wavelength member of the tritan pair, ranging from 525 to 542 nm, was one that produced a metameric match with a 420 nm monochromatic light (2.08 log td) in a 2° bipartite field superimposed on a 3.9° adaptation field (420 nm, 2.08 log td) after observers had adapted to a 420 nm, 2.60 log td, 3.9° adaptation field for five minutes. The spectral composition and intensity of the test light were controlled by the experimenter and the observer, respectively. Discriminations along a constant S-cone axis were measured using a pair of 560 and 630 nm lights.

The retinal illuminance of each pair of test lights was equated by heterochromatic flicker photometry under standard conditions (25 Hz, square-wave flicker of a 2° field). Because there are negligible changes in lens density as a function of age for middle-wavelength lights, the middle-wavelength member of the observer's tritan pair (2 log td) and a 560 nm light (2.08 log td) served as the standard for HFP measurements. Therefore, the retinal illuminance of the 420 nm and 650 nm lights were equated across all observers.

Cone excitation (S-cone or L-cone trolands) was computed following the method of Boynton and Kambe (1980). Chromatic discrimination thresholds along a tritan axis were measured for five S-cone excitation values (1.0, 2.0, 2.5, 3.0 and 3.5 log S td). Thresholds, ΔS, were measured using a temporal two-alternative forced-choice method combined with a 3-down, 1-up staircase procedure. The stimuli consisted of a 2° bipartite field (2.08 log td), divided horizontally by a dark gap (about 10 min arc). The two halves of the field were metameric at the onset of the trial and then in one of two intervals the colour of the lower half field was changed gradually in the direction $\Delta S > 0$ and then back to the original colour. In another interval, both bipartite fields were presented for the same duration, with no change in the appearance of the lower half field. Observers pressed a button to signal the interval in which the appearance of the test light was changed. During a single test session the subject continuously viewed the stimulus and trial onset was signalled by a tone. Because the intensities of two monochromatic lights in the test mixture were changed by small, repetitive asynchronous movements of two neutral density wedges, the colour of the test field could be changed without altering its overall retinal illuminance. The step size for the staircase in terms of S-cone trolands was initially 0.3 log unit and then was reduced to 0.1 log unit following the second reversal. Chromatic discrimination thresholds for each test condition were based on the geometric mean of the last four of six reversals. With this staircase procedure, ΔS was defined by the 79.4 per cent-point of the psychometric function (Levitt, 1970).

The same procedure was used to determine chromatic discriminations mediated by an L/M-cone pathway. Thresholds, ΔL, were measured at two log L values (1.9031 and 2.0154 td) along the constant S-cone axis. The step size for the staircase in terms of L-cone trolands was initially 0.2 log unit and then was reduced to 0.07 log unit following the second reversal.

5.7.3   RESULTS

Figure 5.7.1 shows the relative luminous sensitivity change measured by HFP at 420 nm and 630 nm as a function of age. There is a significant correlation between age and loss of relative luminous sensitivity at 420 nm ($p < 0.05$) but not at 630 nm ($p > 0.05$). The fact that this sensitivity loss with age occurred only at 420 nm suggests that it is caused by an increase in the ocular media density, especially of the lens, but not by receptoral and/or post-receptoral change of the luminance channel, which should decrease the absolute sensitivity at both wavelengths and keep these relative sensitivity values constant with age.

Figure 5.7.2(a) shows log ΔS plotted as a function of log S td. Individual S-cone discrimination functions followed a typical threshold versus radiance (tvr) template. Separate regression analyses were performed for each level of log S. There were significant correlations between age and log ΔS only at the two lowest levels of S-cone stimulation, log $S = 1.0$ ($p < 0.05$) and 2.0 ($p < 0.05$) S-cone td.

In order to compare the data over the tested age range, subjects were divided into three age groups, young (22.0–30.3 years), middle (39.1–54.5 years), and old (59.1–76.7 years). In Figure 5.7.2(b) the averaged data in each age group are shown. The error bars denote ± 1 standard error of the mean. The solid and dashed curves associated with each set of average discrimination thresholds are the best fitting functions to each set of data using Boynton and Kambe's (1980) equation described below. On average, S-cone discrimination thresholds at the plateau of the fitted functions were elevated by 0.66 log units for older observers (mean = 69.5 years) compared with younger observers (mean = 25.8 years). However, in the Weber region, the functions converged for the two groups of observers. Thus, age-

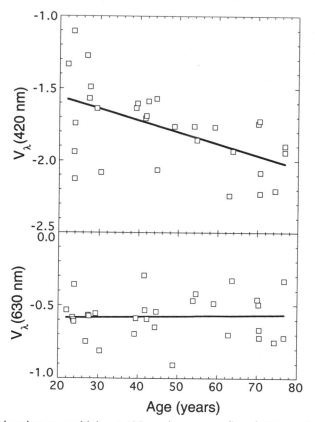

Figure 5.7.1 Luminous sensitivity at 420 nm (upper panel) and 630 nm (lower panel) as a function of age. Squares represent relative luminous sensitivity when luminous sensitivity of the middle-wavelength member of the observer's tritan pair (upper panel) or luminous sensitivity of 560 nm were normalised to the values of Judd's modified V_λ function (Vos, 1978). Regression lines were fitted to each data set using a least-squares criterion.

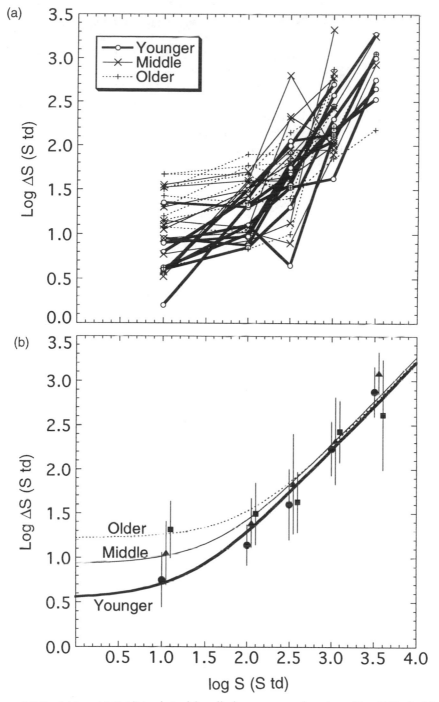

Figure 5.7.2 (a) Log ΔS (S td) is plotted for all observers as a function of log S (S td). (b) Geometric means of these S-cone mediated chromatic discriminations for younger (circles), middle (triangles), and older age-groups (squares) as a function of S-cone stimulation. Error bars represent ±1 SD. Curves show the best fitting functions for each data set calculated from equation (2).

related differences in colour discrimination thresholds along individual tritan axes become smaller as the level of S-cone stimulation increases.

In Figure 5.7.3(a), log ΔL td is plotted as a function of log L td. There was a significant correlation between age and log ΔL only at the lowest level of L-cone stimulation, log $L = 1.903$ ($p < 0.05$) L-cone td. Observers were divided into the same three age groups as in Figure 5.7.2. Figure 5.7.3(b) shows averages of discrimination thresholds for each age group. Results of discrimination tests for an L/M-cone pathway revealed an elevation in threshold for older observers of 0.40 log unit compared with younger observers at log $L = 1.903$ L-cone td, but the averaged data converged for the two groups of observers at log $L = 2.028$ L-cone td.

5.7.4   DISCUSSION

In our experiment, retinal illuminances of the stimuli were equated by individual HFP functions and presented in Maxwellian view in order to compensate for age-related differences of the ocular media density and changes in pupil size. Our results show that even for stimuli equated in terms of retinal illuminance, there is an increase in chromatic discrimination thresholds with age. These age-related losses in chromatic discrimination cannot be explained by senescent changes in the ocular media. Age-related changes at the receptoral and/or post-receptoral levels are required to explain losses in chromatic discrimination along both tritan and constant S-cone axes when the levels of S- and L-cone stimulation are relatively low. We conclude that, while age-related changes in the ocular media contribute to losses in chromatic discrimination under natural viewing conditions, receptoral and/or post-receptoral changes must also be involved.

The age-related loss of chromatic discrimination caused by the neural changes in chromatic pathways has two interesting characteristics. First, the magnitude of the loss depends upon the level of S- and L-cone stimulation. Second, the increase in chromatic discrimination thresholds at relatively low levels of log S- and L-cone excitation is linear with age after approximately 22 years old, as shown in Figure 5.7.4.

5.7.4.1 Comparison of age-related sensitivity loss along different axes

The pattern of age-related losses in chromatic discrimination along a constant S-cone axis is similar to that observed for age-related losses along individual tritan axes. As the level of L-cone stimulation increased, chromatic discrimination thresholds, on average, converge for all three age groups. Figure 5.7.5 shows the ratio between thresholds for each individual at similar cone-excitation levels (log S = 2.0 S td and at log L = 1.9031 L td) plotted as a function of age. The correlation between this ratio and age is not statistically significant ($p > 0.05$). This result supports the tentative conclusion that at levels of cone excitation where age-related changes in chromatic discrimination are evident, the ratio of the losses in discrimination along tritan and constant S-cone axes remain constant with age.

5.7.4.2 Model of chromatic discrimination by S-cone pathway

To investigate the nature of hypothesised age-related receptoral and/or post-receptoral neural changes in an S-cone pathway responsible for mediating tritan discriminations, we

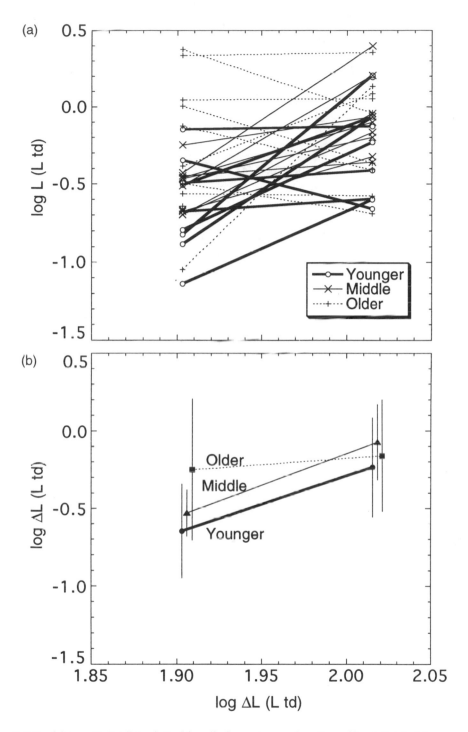

Figure 5.7.3   (a) Log ΔL (L td) is plotted for all observers as a function of log L (L td). (b) Geometric means of these chromatic discriminations along a constant S-cone axis for younger (circles), middle (triangles), and older age-groups (squares) as a function of L-cone stimulation. Error bars represent ±1 SD.

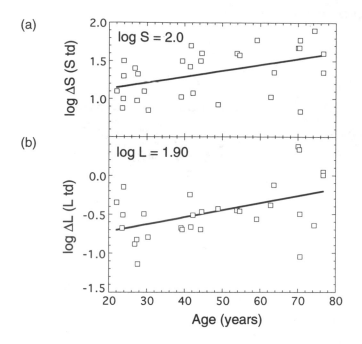

Figure 5.7.4 (a) Chromatic discrimination thresholds along a tritan axis (log ΔS at log S = 2.0; specified in S td) are plotted as a function of age. (b) Chromatic discrimination thresholds along an axis of constant S-cone stimulation (log ΔL at log L = 1.9; specified in L td) are plotted as a function of age. Regression lines in each panel were fitted to each data set using a least-squares criterion.

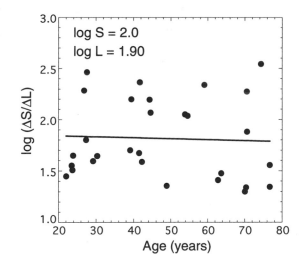

Figure 5.7.5 Log ratio of chromatic discrimination thresholds along tritan axes (ΔS) at log S = 2.0 S-cone td to discrimination thresholds along a constant S-cone axis (ΔL) at log L = 1.903 L-cone td as a function of age. Regression lines were fitted to each data set using a least-squares criterion.

used Boynton and Kambe's (1980) model of chromatic discrimination. The model describes the relation between discrimination thresholds along a tritan axis as a function of S-cone stimulation as:

$$\Delta S/(S + k*S_0) = W \tag{1}$$

ΔS is the chromatic discrimination threshold when the level of S-cone excitation corresponds to S. S_0 is the spontaneous noise (*eigengrau*) occurring prior to sites of light adaptation within an S-cone pathway. These three variables are specified in S-cone td. W is the limiting Weber fraction and k is a multiplicative scalar of the spontaneous noise between observers. We applied this model to the averaged sets of data for the youngest, middle, and oldest groups of observers. As shown in Figure 5.7.2(b), the best-fitting functions to each data set calculated by equation (1) can predict the data well.

Two theoretical explanations can account for the age-related sensitivity losses along a tritan axis. First, the response of the S-cone pathway was reduced with age (i.e. S and ΔS, are reduced to αS and $\alpha\Delta S$ ($\alpha < 1$) in the model). Multiplicative attenuation of S-cone responses and/or post-receptoral changes that reduce the input of S-cone signals are represented by the parameter α in Boynton-Kambe's equation. Second, the spontaneous noise of the chromatic pathway increased with age. This means that the spontaneous noise level, S_0, was raised to βS_0 ($\beta > 1$). Equation (1) is modified by taking account of these two changes.

$$(\alpha*\Delta S)/[\alpha*S + k*(\beta*S_0] = W$$

then,

$$\Delta S/[S + (\beta/\alpha)*k*S_0] = W \tag{2}$$

k and β both scale the noise level and can be reduced to a single constant; they are shown here to emphasise that in addition to the scaling for individual differences (k) proposed by Boynton and Kambe, an age-related scaling (β) is also required. As (β/α) can be replaced by a single parameter that is larger than one, equation (2) indicates that reduction of S-cone response and/or increase of the noise level will have the same effect on chromatic discrimination thresholds. The plateau region of the discrimination curve is elevated by these senescent changes because the constant in the denominator increases. However, discrimination functions in the log ΔS versus log S coordinates for younger and older observers converge in the Weber region of the functions because the Weber fraction is not changed. As shown in equation (2), we cannot distinguish the effects of spontaneous noise within an S-cone pathway from effects caused by reduction of S-cone response within the same visual pathway, either qualitatively or quantitatively, with the results of this study.

5.7.4.3 Comparison between S-cone mediated detection and discrimination

We also wanted to compare age-related changes in chromatic discrimination with age-related losses in sensitivity of increment thresholds mediated by an S-cone pathway. In a previous study (Schefrin *et al.*, 1992), increment thresholds were measured for nine older (mean age, 71 years) and six younger (mean age, 24 years) observers. The stimuli consisted of a 250 ms, 1.03° diameter, 440 nm foveally-viewed test light presented on 470 nm adapting fields and on a 570 nm auxiliary field. In that study, intensities of stimuli were not equated by individual HFP functions, though the lens density of each observer was measured. These lens densities allowed us to compute an HFP function (based on Kraft and Werner, 1994) for the purposes of specifying cone trolands for each age group.

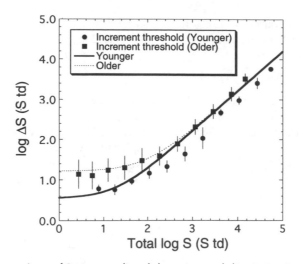

Figure 5.7.6   Comparison of S-cone mediated detection and discrimination. Log ΔS (S td) is plotted as a function of total log S (S td) for increment threshold measurements for younger (circles) and older observers (squares). Curves showing best fitting functions for chromatic discrimination thresholds along a tritan axis are calculated from equation (2).

Figure 5.7.6 shows tvr functions for increment thresholds (circles for younger observers, squares for older observers) and the chromatic discrimination functions along a tritan axis presented in Figure 5.7.3(b). Note that for the increment threshold data, the tvr functions do not converge even at higher S-cone stimulation levels. The tvr function and chromatic discrimination function match well for older observers' data but not for the younger observers' data. Two reasons might account for this discrepancy between S-cone mediated detection and discrimination. First, the observers participating in the two studies are not the same and individual differences may invalidate the comparison. Second in the increment threshold measurements, the stimuli produced not only an S-cone excitation change but also an illuminance change with the presentation of the test stimuli. While the tvr data are clearly mediated by an S-cone pathway, the gain control in this pathway is believed to be influenced by both the rate of photon capture in the S-cones themselves and by the net imbalance at a post-receptoral site of cone antagonism between S-cones and combined signals from M- and L-cones (Pugh and Mollon, 1979). It is possible that signals at the latter (second) site of adaptation were strong enough to shift the tvr function selectively in younger observers relative to older observers.

5.7.5   ACKNOWLEDGEMENT

This research was supported by the National Institute on Aging (Grant AG04058).

5.7.6   REFERENCES

BIRCH, J. (1993) *Diagnosis of Defective Colour Vision*, New York: Oxford University Press.
BOYNTON, R. M. & KAMBE, N. (1980) Chromatic difference steps of moderate size measured along theoretically critical axes, *Color Research and Applications*, **5**, 13–23.

VAN EVERDINGEN, J. A. M., SMITH, V. C. & POKORNY, J. (1991) Sensitivity of tritan screening tests as evaluated in normals at reduced levels of illumination, In: Drum, B., Moreland, J. D. & Serra, A. (Eds) *Colour Vision Deficiencies X*, Dordrecht: Kluwer Academic, pp. 167–175.

GILBERT, J. G. (1957) Age changes in color matching, *Journal of Gerontology*, **12**, 210–215.

KNOBLAUCH, K., SAUNDERS, F., KUSUDA, M., HYNES, R., PODOR, M., HIGGINS, K. E. & DE MONASTERIO, F. M. (1987) Age and illuminance effects in the Farnsworth-Munsell 100-hue test, *Applied Optics*, **26**, 1441–1448.

KRAFT, J. M. & WERNER, J. S. (1994) Spectral efficiency across the life span: flicker photometry and brightness matching, *Journal of the Optical Society of America*, **A 11**, 1213–1221.

KUDO, H., SMITH, V. C. & POKORNY, J. (1993) Sensitivity of five screening tests for tritan discrimination as evaluated in normals at reduced levels of illumination. In: Drum, B. (Ed.) *Colour Vision Deficiencies XI*, Dordrecht: Kluwer Academic, pp. 119–127.

LAKOWSKI, R. (1962) Is the deterioration of colour discrimination with age due to lens or retinal changes, *Die Farbe*, **11**, 69–86.

LEVITT, H. (1970) Transformed up-down methods in psychoacoustics, *Journal of the Acoustical Society of America*, **49**, 467–477.

MORELAND, J. D. (1993) Matching range and age in a blue-green equation. In: Drum, B. (Ed.) *Colour Vision Deficiencies XI*, Dordrecht, Kluwer Academic, pp. 129–134.

OHTA, Y. & KATO, H. (1976) Colour perception changes with age. *Modern Problems in Ophthalmology*, **17**, 345–352.

POWELL, I. (1981) Lenses for correcting chromatic aberration of the eye, *Applied Optics*, **20**, 4152–4155.

PUGH, JR, E. N. & MOLLON, J. D. (1979) A theory of the π_1 and π_3 color mechanisms of Stiles, *Vision Research*, **19**, 293–312.

SCHEFRIN, B. E., WERNER, J. S., PLACH, M., UTLAUT, N. & SWITKES, E. (1992) Sites of age-related sensitivity loss in a short-wave cone pathway, *Journal of the Optical Society of America*, **A 9**, 355–363.

SMITH, V. C., POKORNY, J. & PASS, A. S. (1985) Color-axis determination on the Farnsworth-Munsell 100-hue test, *American Journal of Ophthalmology*, **100**, 176–182.

SMITH, V. C., VAN EVERDINGEN, J. A. M. & POKORNY, J. (1991) Sensitivity of arrangement tests at reduced levels of illumination. In: Drum, B., Moreland, J. D. & Serra, A. (Eds) *Colour Vision Deficiencies X*, Dordrecht: Kluwer Academic, pp. 177–185.

VERRIEST, G. (1963) Further studies on acquired deficiency of color discrimination, *Journal of the Optical Society of America*, **53**, 185–195.

VOS, J. J. (1978) Tabulated characteristics of a proposed 2° fundamental observer, Institute for Perception TNO, Soesterberg, The Netherlands.

WESTHEIMER, G. (1966) The Maxwellian view, *Vision Research*, **6**, 669–682.

Section 6 – Techniques in Colour Vision Testing

Developments in Anomaloscopy

J.D. Moreland

6.1.1 INTRODUCTION

Both Dalton and Rayleigh had a personal interest in colour vision. While Dalton's concern was with his own, Rayleigh's was with his in-laws, the Balfours. In 1881, Rayleigh read his classic paper 'Experiments with colour' before the British Association and published it in *Nature*. In that paper Rayleigh described two new classes of red-green colour vision deficiency (protanomaly and deuteranomaly: the Balfour brothers being in the latter category) distinct from dichromacy and thus laid the foundations of anomaloscopy as a colour vision testing procedure.

However, it was not until 1907 that Nagel, who coined the term *anomaloscope*, published details of a commercial instrument incorporating Rayleigh's equation and reported its use in the differential diagnosis of red-green colour vision deficits.

6.1.2 ANOMALOSCOPY OF RED-GREEN COLOUR VISION DEFICITS

The Rayleigh equation, red + green = yellow, describes a colour match made between a mixture of red and green spectral lights (primaries) and a yellow spectral test light. In Nagel's anomaloscope the match is achieved using only two controls: a primaries ratio control for matching hue and a test radiance control for matching brightness. A third control for saturation is not required because the near-colinearity of the three Rayleigh stimuli in a chromaticity diagram ensures that the saturations of the test and comparison are acceptably matched when hue and brightness have been matched. This colinearity extends to the protanopic and deuteranopic convergence points and so Rayleigh's stimuli lie in the red-green confusion zone common to both dichromacies.

Modern practice with Rayleigh's equation generates three important parameters: matching range (the range of acceptable primary ratios), brightness matches appropriate to the ends of the matching range, and the mid-match point. These three measures respectively can support inferences regarding hue discrimination, spectral sensitivity and, if the matching range is small, photopigment spectra.

Rayleigh's equation is superbly efficient, diagnosing differentially between four X-linked red-green deficiencies: two dichromacies and two anomalous trichromacies. Prota-nopes and deuteranopes have full matching ranges but are readily distinguished by their yellow (brightness) settings, which reflect marked differences in spectral sensitivity. The red- and green-shifted matches of protanomalous and deuteranomalous trichromats respec-tively are due to spectrally shifted photopigments (Piantanida, 1974; Pokorny et al., 1973). Acquired defects may mimic these two anomalies (Pokorny and Smith, 1990). Thus, reduced cone photopigment concentration, due to a strong light bleach or due to a pathologic disorientation of cones, manifests as pseudoprotanomaly while the increase in lens absorbance with age gives rise to pseudodeuteranomaly. In both instances, however, the match point shifts are generally not as large as in X-linked deficiencies.

Recent developments, stimulated by discoveries of new genotypes, particularly those whose photopigments are determined by the alanine/serine amino acid substitution at position 180, show that careful or modified anomaloscope procedures can distinguish successfully between corresponding phenotypes; either by using a dual Rayleigh match technique for normals (He and Shevell, 1994; Sanocki et al., 1994) or by careful brightness matching over the dichromatic matching range (Sharpe et al., 1994)

While the Nagel anomaloscope (and its modern commercial equivalents) is regarded as definitive for diagnosis, it suffers from a design defect, long overlooked. Clinically, a dichromat is defined by a full matching range, meaning that both of the comparisons red-versus-yellow and green-versus-yellow are accepted as matches but these are separate comparisons. Nagel's anomaloscope design precludes the possibility of displaying the doubly 'full' dichromatic comparison red-versus-green. Consequently, a Nagel diagnosis of dichromacy may include a very extreme form of anomalous trichromacy and, indeed, such cases have been detected (Moreland, 1993; Moreland and Bradshaw, 1994). The potential misclassification does have an important bearing on attempts to relate phenotypes with genotypes and on the occurrence of large-field trichromacy in classical 'dichromats', but for vocational purposes the distinction is not important.

Nagel was himself a deuteranope, but he was aware that he could discriminate between a ship's red and green navigation lights when spread by reflections in the water over a larger field of view but not when observed directly (Nagel, 1905). Consequently, he restricted the field of view of his anomaloscope to 2° to ensure a clear clinical distinction between dichromacy and anomalous trichromacy for foveal vision. It has now been established that the anomalous matches that many classical dichromats make with large fields are lumi-nance dependent. The matches are influenced by rod intrusion at modest luminance (Smith and Pokorny, 1977) and by anomalous cones at high luminances (Breton and Cowan, 1981; Jaeger and Krastel, 1984). The greatest change for large fields is shown by deuteranopes who switch from a red- to a green-shifted match as luminance increases.

6.1.3   ANOMALOSCOPY OF BLUE-GREEN[1] COLOUR VISION DEFECTS

The stimuli of the Rayleigh equation are well placed for assessing long- and middle-wavelength sensitive cone function but not for short-wave cones. Indeed, the tritanope's match is normal since the Rayleigh stimuli lie outside the effective response range of the short-wave cone. A number of blue-green equations for assessing short-wave cone function have been proposed from time to time, beginning with Nagel's own in 1907 and these have been discussed in detail elsewhere (Moreland, 1990). The stimuli for such an equation should be sited in the short-middle wavelength region of the spectrum and diagnostic efficiency requires them to be tritanopic isochromes. There are two major problems associated with the wavelength requirement:

1. As the spectrum locus is curved in this region a mixture of short- and middle-wavelength primaries would always be less saturated than any intermediate spectral cyan test that it aims to match. A desaturant must be added to the test for a satisfactory match but this introduces the need for a clinically unergonomic third control.
2. The effect of population variance in macular and lens pigment spectral absorption is much more pronounced for short-wavelength stimuli than in Rayleigh's equation. This results in a wide population distribution of mid-match points and, consequently, a high false-positive rate in diagnosis for some of the proposed equations (Moreland, 1984, 1990).

Both of these issues have been successfully addressed in the Moreland equation. This is a match between indigo and green primaries and a desaturated cyan. While the original motivation was to nullify the effect of macular pigment variance, a systematic study yielded primaries for which the combined effect of macular and lens pigment variances was minimised (Moreland, 1990; Moreland and Kerr, 1979; Zaidi et al., 1982). This study showed that some latitude could be allowed in the spectral location of primaries: 439 and 499 nm (Moreland & Kerr, 1979), 430 and 500 nm (Pokorny et al., 1981) and 436 and 500 nm (Roth, 1984). In a later study additional factors were considered (the interaction of primary wavelength and matching range and the pairing of tritanopic isochromes), which resulted in a fine-tuning of primaries to 436 and 490 nm (Moreland, 1984). Subsequent field trials confirmed the anticipated small but significant improvement in diagnostic precision (Moreland and Roth, 1987).

Particular attention was paid to the desaturation of the test stimulus (Moreland and Young, 1974). The cyan test (480 nm) and yellow desaturant (579 nm) wavelengths were chosen having regard to the curvature of constant hue loci in colour space so that the hue of the test field was unaffected by changes in the ratio cyan/yellow in the region of the normal match. This was done in the interests of clinical viability so that, by locking the saturation control at a mean position for normal matches, matching could be performed using only two controls: effectively those for hue and brightness. Now, when the saturation control is fixed, the cyan/yellow ratio at the receptoral level is determined by inert ocular pigments. We demonstrated that bias due to that cause was avoided by our stratagem (Moreland and Kerr, 1979) and indeed that untrained subjects were able to make satisfactory matches in the presence of small but representative saturation differences. These findings have been confirmed independently (Zaidi et al., 1989).

Moreland matches are sensitive to short-wave cone function (Pokorny and Smith, 1984), but are significantly affected by changes in the ageing lens so a base-line correction for age (Moreland, 1978) is necessary, the effect being some four times larger than in Rayleigh matches (Moreland et al., 1991). Conveniently, just as tritanopes make normal Rayleigh matches, so all X-linked (red-green) colour defectives make normal Moreland matches (Pokorny and Smith, 1990).

6.1.4   TWO-EQUATION ANOMALOSCOPY

The advent of a blue-green equation with a diagnostic precision comparable to Rayleigh's red-green equation has created a demand for an anomaloscope incorporating both. Such an instrument permits the investigation of long-, middle- and short-wavelength cone function and the two-equation method of anomaloscopy is proving to be a powerful analytical and diagnostic tool (Hermès *et al.*, 1989; Pelizzone *et al.*, 1991; Pokorny and Smith, 1990; Roth, 1990; Roth *et al.*, 1987, 1989a,b).

6.1.5   THE OPERATING CONDITIONS REQUIRED IN ANOMALOSCOPY

6.1.5.1 Luminance

The provision of high field luminance in an anomaloscope would facilitate the detection of anomalous extrafoveal cones in classical dichromats, the assessment of residual cone activity in cone degenerations and the availability of retinal luminance compensation for age-related lens changes and miosis. A target luminance to avoid rod intrusion in colour matching and for revealing anomalous cones is about 40–60 cdm^{-2} (Breton and Cowan, 1981).

6.1.5.2 Field size

Now that the luminance dependence of large field colour matching in classical dichromats is understood more clearly than in Nagel's time, the ability to choose different field sizes has a number of benefits. The detection of the switch from dichromacy to anomalous trichromacy has already been mentioned. The genetic implications of anomalous cones in families of classical dichromats is receiving attention by Jaeger *et al.*, (1991) who used field sizes in the range 2–30°. The Rayleigh equation field size effect is a valuable sign, sensitive to disturbances in retinal architecture in the early stage of macular disease (Pokorny *et al.* 1979, 1980; Smith *et al.*, 1978, 1988). A large field size offers the possibility of assessing residual cone activity in cone dystrophies and, indeed, when maculopathy presents with a central scotoma, a large field may provide the only means of performing anomaloscopy (Moreland *et al.*, 1978).

6.1.5.3 Exposure time

Matching range, as a measure of hue discrimination loss, is particularly significant in assessing acquired deficiencies and it is often measured under the two adaptation conditions: *Neutralstimmung* and *Umstimmung* (Krastel and Moreland, 1991). In the former, observation alternates between the matching field (3 s or less) and a large white adaptation field, to maintain a neutral state of adaptation. In the latter, observation of the matching field continues for at least 15 s to maintain a state of chromatic or tuned adaptation. Pelizzone *et al.* (1993) have reported computer-controlled modifications of this procedure. Working with trained normal subjects, they found that matching ranges were narrowest for an exposure time of 1 s in both Rayleigh and Moreland equations. However, since the minima were very shallow, a time of 2–3 s was recommended for use with patients.

6.1.6   SOME ERGONOMIC CONSIDERATIONS

6.1.6.1 The 'brightness' match

Good practice dictates that the patient should decide on equality of brightness between the test and comparison fields before making a hue judgment. Such direct comparison matches are notoriously variable for normals *outside* their Rayleigh matching range, where lumi-nance additivity laws are often not obeyed (Schmidt, 1974). Pelizzone *et al.* (1993) confirmed this but reported much less difficulty with the Moreland equation. The problem of subject inconsistency could be avoided and precision greatly improved by incorporating a simple photometric procedure to establish the relative luminances of the stimuli. Flicker photometry would serve this purpose, being quite rapid, well suited to untrained subjects and, moreover, obeying luminance additivity. It could be used to establish an individual's luminance matches over the whole primary mixture range with the expectation that, within the matching range itself and for some little way beyond, these would also be the correct 'brightness' matches (Pelizzone *et al.*, 1993; Schmidt, 1974). Such a procedure would be particularly relevant to the management of a computer controlled examination protocol.

6.1.6.2 Computer control

Computerised examination protocols have been developed for electronically controlled anomaloscopes (Pelizzone *et al.*, 1991, 1993; Pokorny *et al.*, 1989) and for a mechanically controlled anomaloscope (Pokorny, personal communication). Computerisation offers a number of advantages such as standardised clinical procedure, error-free data acquisition and storage, improved precision in matching range measurement, and reduced examination time.

Computer control allows great flexibility in data presentation. The display could be numerical, giving the matching range, mid-match point and test field luminance in any unit of choice as well as the relevant statistical scores. The power of graphical analysis has been eloquently espoused by Pokorny and Smith (1984, 1990) and a display plot of test luminance versus matching range together with diagnostic limits for dichromacies, normal and anomalous trichromacies and/or other conditions of interest would be very useful in clinical work. A valuable move in this direction is evinced in the novel liquid crystal display of the Heidelberg-Oculus anomaloscope (Krastel *et al.*, 1991) and some other features have been incorporated in the software of the Spectrum 712-Interzeag instru-ment.

6.1.7 NOTE

1 Blue-green is used here to describe a colour confusion that typifies tritanopia (much as red-green typifies both protanopia and deuteranopia). The term blue-yellow, which appears in the literature, is incorrect for tritanopia because yellow is confused with violet.

6.1.8 REFERENCES

Breton, M.E. & Cowan, W.B. (1981) Deuteranomalous color matching in the deuteranopic eye, *Journal of the Optical Society of America*, **71**, 1220–1223.

He, J-C. & Shevell, S.H. (1994) Individual differences in cone pigments of normal trichromats measured by dual Rayleigh-type color matches, *Vision Research*, **34**, 367–376.

Hermès, D., Roth, A. & Borot, N. (1989) The two equation method, II: Results in retinal and optic nerve disorders, *Documenta Ophthalmologica Proceedings Series*, **52**, 325–337.

Jaeger, W. & Krastel, H. (1984) Dichromatic and anomalous trichromatic vision examined with small and large fields by means of the projection anomaloscope, *Documenta Ophthalmologica Proceedings Series*, **39**, 147–154.

JAEGER, W., KRASTEL, H. & MARAT, G. (1991) Large field spectral matches in dichromats, *Documenta Ophthalmologica Proceedings Series*, **54**, 13–19.

KRASTEL, H. & MORELAND, J.D. (1991) Colour vision deficiencies in ophthalmic diseases. In: Foster, D.H. (Ed.) *Inherited and Acquired Colour Vision Deficiencies*, London: Macmillan, pp. 115–172.

KRASTEL, H., GEHRUNG, H., DAX, K. & ROHRSCHNEIDER, K. (1991) Clinical application of the Heidelberg anomaloscope, *Documenta Ophthalmologica Proceedings Series*, **54**, 135–149.

LORD RAYLEIGH (1881) Experiments on colour, *Nature*, **25**, 64–66.

MORELAND, J.D. (1978) Temporal variations in anomaloscope equations, *Modern Problems in Ophthalmology*, **19**, 167–172.

MORELAND, J.D. (1984) Analysis of variance in anomaloscope equations, *Documenta Ophthalmologica Proceedings Series*, **39**, 111–119.

MORELAND, J.D. (1990) The clinical utility of anomaloscopy. In: Ohta, Y. (Ed.) *Color Vision Deficiencies*, Amsterdam: Kugler & Ghedini, pp. 125–143.

MORELAND, J.D. (1993) Design criteria for a clinical anomaloscope, *Documenta Ophthalmologica Proceedings Series*, **56**, 335–344.

MORELAND, J.D. & BRADSHAW, C. (1994) A new class of red-green colour vision deficiency, *Perception*, **23**, 94.

MORELAND, J.D. & KERR, J. (1979) Optimization of a Rayleigh-type equation for the detection of tritanomaly, *Vision Research*, **19**, 1369–1375.

MORELAND, J.D. & ROTH, A. (1987) Validation trials on an optimum blue-green equation, *Documenta Ophthalmologica Proceedings Series*, **46**, 233–236.

MORELAND, J.D. & YOUNG, W.B. (1974) A new anomaloscope employing interference filters, *Modern Problems in Ophthalmology*, **13**, 47–55.

MORELAND, J.D., TORCZYNSKI, E. & TRIPATHI, R.C. (1991) Rayleigh and Moreland matches in the ageing eye, *Documenta Ophthalmologica Proceedings Series*, **54**, 347–352.

MORELAND, J.D., MAIONE, M., CARTA, F. & SCOCCIANTI, L. (1978) Acquired 'tritan' deficiencies in macular pathology, *Modern Problems in Ophthalmology*, **19**, 270–275.

NAGEL, W.A. (1905) Dichromatische Fovea, trichromatische Peripherie, *Z. Psychol. Physiol. Sinnesorg.*, **39**, 83–101.

NAGEL, W.A. (1907) Zwei Apparate für die augenärzliche Funktionsprüfung: Adaptometer und kleines Spektralphotometer (Anomaloskop), *Zeitschr. Augenheilkd.*, **17**, 201–208.

PIANTANIDA, T.P. (1974) A replacement model of X-linked recessive color vision defects, *Annals of Human Genetics*, **37**, 393–404.

PELIZZONE, M., SOMMERHALDER, J., ROTH, A. & HERMÈS, D., (1991) Automated Rayleigh and Moreland matches on a computer-controlled anomaloscope, *Documenta Ophthalmologica Proceedings Series*, **54**, 151–159.

PELIZZONE, M., SOMMERHALDER, J., ROTH, A. & HERMÈS, D. (1993) Automated Rayleigh and Moreland matches: Optimization of stimulus parameters for normal observers, *Documenta Ophthalmologica Proceedings Series*, **56**, 345–355.

POKORNY, J. & SMITH, V.C. (1984) Metameric matches relevant for the assessment of color vision, I: Theoretical considerations, *Documenta Ophthalmologica Proceedings Series*, **39**, 83–94.

POKORNY, J. & SMITH, V.C. (1990) Color matching as a clinical tool: Theory of modification by disease. In: Ohta, Y. (Ed.) *Color Vision Deficiencies*, Amsterdam: Kugler & Ghedini, pp. 255–267.

POKORNY, J., SMITH, V.C. & ERNEST, J.T. (1980) Macular color vision defects: Specialized psychophysical testing in acquired and hereditary chorioretinal diseases, *International Ophthalmological Clinics*, **20**, 53–81.

POKORNY, J., SMITH, V.C. & JOHNSTON, P. (1979) Photoreceptor misalignment accompanying a fibrous scar, *Archives of Ophthalmology*, **97**, 867–869.

POKORNY, J., SMITH, V.C. & KATZ, I. (1973) Derivation of the photopigment absorption spectra in anomalous trichromats, *Journal of the Optical Society of America*, **63**, 232–237.

POKORNY, J., SMITH, V.C. & LUTZE, M. (1989) A computer-controlled briefcase anomaloscope, *Documenta Ophthalmologica Proceedings Series*, **54**, 135–149.

POKORNY, J. SMITH, V.C. & WENT, L. (1981) Color matching in autosomal dominant tritan defect, *Journal of the Optical Society of America*, **71**, 1327–1334.

ROTH, A. (1984) Metameric matches relevant for the assessment of color vision, II. Practical aspects, *Documenta Ophthalmologica Proceedings Series*, **39**, 95–109.

ROTH, A. (1990) The power of metameric color equations in testing color vision. In: Ohta, Y. (Ed.) *Color Vision Deficiencies*, Amsterdam: Kugler & Ghedini, pp. 181–190.

ROTH, A., HERMÈS, D. & PELIZZONE, M. (1987) The diagnosis of acquired colour vision deficiencies by means of metameric matches (using the Besançon anomalometer), *Documenta Ophthalmologica Proceedings Series*, **46**, 203–215.

ROTH, A., PELIZZONE, M. & HERMÈS, D. (1989a) The two-equation method, I. Results in normal colour vision, *Documenta Ophthalmologica Proceedings Series*, **52**, 317–323.

ROTH, A., PELIZZONE, M., HERMÈS, D. & SOMMERHALDER, J. (1989b) Neuere Überlegungen und Entwicklungen zur klinischen Untersuchung des Farbensehens: Die Zwei-Gleichungsmethode, *Fortschr. Ophthalmol.*, **86**, 374–379.

SANOCKI, E., SHEVELL, S.K. & WINDERICKX, J. (1994) Serine/alanine amino acid polymorphism of the L-cone photopigment assessed by dual Rayleigh-type color matches, *Vision Research*, **34**, 377–382.

SCHMIDT, I. (1974) Brightness matches on the Nagel anomaloscope, *Modern Problems in Ophthalmology*, **13**, 19–25.

SHARPE, L.T., NATHANS, J., KLAUSEN, G. & REITNER, A. (1994) Phenotypes and genotypes of red and red-green hybrid pigments, *Perception*, **23**, 86.

SMITH, V.C. & POKORNY, J. (1977) Large field trichromacy in protanopes and deuteranopes, *Journal of the Optical Society of America*, **67**, 213–220.

SMITH, V.C., POKORNY, J., ERNEST, J.T. & STARR, S.J. (1978) Visual function in acute posterior multifocal placoid pigment epitheliopathy, *American Journal of Ophthalmology*, **85**, 192–199.

SMITH, V.C., POKORNY, J. & DIDDIE, K.R. (1988) Color matching and the Stiles-Crawford effect in observers with early age-related macular changes, *Journal of the Optical Society of America*, **A 5**, 2113–2121.

ZAIDI, Q., POKORNY, J. & SMITH, V.C. (1982) Sources of variation in blue-green equations, *Journal of the Optical Society of America*, **72**, 1727A.

ZAIDI, Q., POKORNY, J. & SMITH, V.C. (1989) Sources of individual differences in anomaloscope equations for tritan defects, *Clinical Visual Science*, **4**, 89–94.

A New Panel Test for Tritan Colour Deficiency

Jennifer Birch and Caroline Burden

6.2.1 INTRODUCTION

The Farnsworth D15 test is designed to identify people with 'significant' colour deficiency (Farnsworth, 1943). About five per cent of men fail the test compared with the known prevalence of eight per cent red-green colour deficiency. The test divides, or dichotomises, the population into two groups: people with normal colour vision and slight colour deficiency who pass and people with moderate or severe colour deficiency who fail. The test consists of 16 Munsell colour samples, in matt finish, held in movable circular caps that subtend one and a half degrees at the test distance of 50 cms. The hues are selected from an incomplete hue circle with Munsell value 5 and chroma 4. The x, y co-ordinates of the hues are available from published data and can be represented in the CIE chromaticity diagram 1931 (Birch 1993; Stiles and Wyszecki, 1967). Typical isochromatic colour confusions of protans, deutans and tritans are also represented in the CIE system and this provides the framework for designing colour vision tests utilising Munsell samples. In the D15 test, the subject is required to arrange 15 caps in what he perceives to be a natural colour order beginning from the sixteenth or reference cap. Isochromatic colour confusions are demonstrated when hues from opposite sides of the hue circle are mingled in the arrangement (Figure 6.2.1). The hues are selected to have equal value and chroma so that perceived luminance contrast or saturation differences cannot assist colour deficient subjects to obtain the correct result. The D15 test demonstrates significant protan and deutan colour deficiency effectively but the selection of hues provides less scope for demonstrating tritan defects. Tritan isochromatic colour confusions are limited to four hues, caps 7 and 8 (yellow-green) and caps 14 and 15 (violet). The remaining hues, caps 1–6 and caps 9–13, are within two broad tritan isochromatic colour zones. The colour differences between these caps are small and mis-arrangement can occur in poor overall hue discrimination as well as in tritan colour deficiency. An error score based on the sum of the colour differences in a typical arrangement for tritanopes also demonstrates the limitations on the D15 for tritans. Tritanopes obtain approximately half the error score obtained by protanopes and deuteranopes (Bowman, 1982).

A desaturated version of the D15 test (the Adams test) is in general use (Birch, 1993). The Adams test has the same hues as the standard D15 test. Munsell value 5 is retained but chroma is reduced by two steps (chroma 2). The test has a different pass/fail level and is

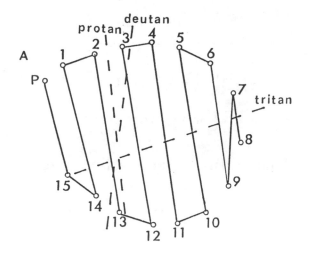

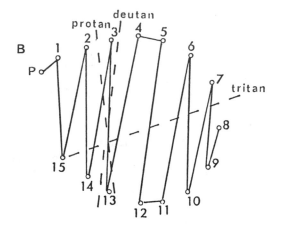

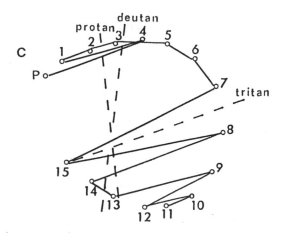

Figure 6.2.1. Isochromatic colour confusions made by dichromats on the Farnsworth D15 test. (a) Protanopia; (b) deuteranopia; (c) tritanopia.

failed by a higher proportion of colour deficient subjects. The test is used to establish an intermediate grade of colour deficiency. However, the classification of dichromats with the Adams test is not as accurate as with the D15 (Dain and Adams, 1990). A panel test containing more saturated hues, the H16 test, may also be included in test batteries. This test does not have the same hues as the D15 test and does not have the capacity to identify tritan defects (Paulson, 1973). The hues have value 5 and chroma 6, 8 and 10.

Two panel tests are often used together in a test battery to grade the severity of colour deficiency. If the D15 test is passed, the Adams test is given, if the D15 test is failed, the H16 test is given. A combination of the D15 and the Adams test is particularly useful in the study of acquired colour deficiency (Adams and Rodic, 1982; Birch, 1989). Most acquired colour vision defects are tritan in type and a panel test that gives more scope for demonstrating and differentiating this type of colour deficiency would be very useful.

We have designed a prototype panel test, the T16 test, which contains more isochromatic tritan hues than the D15 test. Munsell value is kept constant (value 5) but chroma varies as in the H16 test. Results are presented for a representative group of subjects with congenital colour deficiency for a standard and desaturated version of the T16 test.

6.2.2 METHODS

Reference charts of the x, y co-ordinates of Munsell samples (published by Stiles and Wyszecki, 1967) for standard source C were inspected for suitable hues to include in the panel test. Seventeen hues were selected. These form a complete circle in the CIE chromaticity diagram (Table 6.2.1). The hues all have Munsell value 5 but chroma varies between 4, 6 and 8. Chroma is reduced by two for each hue in the desaturated version of the test so that in the desaturated T16 test chroma varies between 2, 4 and 6. The matt finished hues were mounted in D15 caps and illuminated by the MacBeth Easel lamp (Standard source C) giving 400 lux. Both tests were completed by five colour deficient observers who were representative of different types of congenital colour deficiency. There were three

Table 6.2.1. Munsell notations of the T16 test

Cap number		Munsell notation	
Pilot	5	RP	5/8
1	2.5	RP	5/6
2	7.5	P	5/6
3	5	P	5/6
4	10	PB	5/6
5	5	PB	5/4
6	5	B	5/4
7	10	BG	5/6
8	2.5	BG	5/6
9	2.5	G	5/6
10	7.5	GY	5/6
11	2.5	GY	5/4
12	5	Y	5/4
13	10	YR	5/4
14	5	YR	5/6
15	10	R	5/6
16	5	R	5/8

dichromats (a protanope, a deuteranope and a tritanope) and two anomalous trichromats (a protanomalous and a deuteranomalous). Diagnosis of the type of red-green colour deficiency was made with the Nagel Anomaloscope. The diagnosis of tritanopia was made from the colour matches between violet wavelengths shorter than 450 nm and green-yellow wavelengths longer than 500 nm.

The tests were conducted in the same way as the D15 test. Each subject arranged the colour caps in what was perceived as a natural colour order, beginning from the reference cap. A review of the arrangement was allowed after all the 16 moveable caps had been placed in sequence. The cap sequence was then recorded on the results diagram.

6.2.3   RESULTS

The results obtained for the five subjects on both the standard and desaturated T16 tests are shown in Figures 6.2.2, 6.2.3 and 6.2.4. The resulting diagrams show the relative position of the hues in the CIE chromaticity diagram 1931 together with the mean isochromatic line through the neutral point (equivalent to N5) for protans, deutans and tritans. The lines joining the hues as arranged by the subject represent isochromatic confusions. If the test is correctly realised, the results pattern for protans in Figure 6.2.2, deutans in Figure 6.2.3 and for the tritanope in Figure 6.2.4 should have lines parallel to the relevant isochromatic direction.

The three dichromatic observers fail both the saturated and desaturated versions of the test and the results diagrams show the correct classification of the type of colour deficiency.

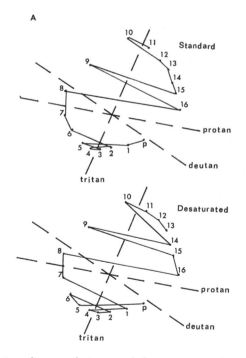

Figure 6.2.2. Isochromatic colour confusions made by protans on the saturated and desaturated T16 test. (a) Protanopia; and (b) protanomalous trichromatism (Nagel matching range 50–55 scale units, normal match 44 SD 2 scale units).

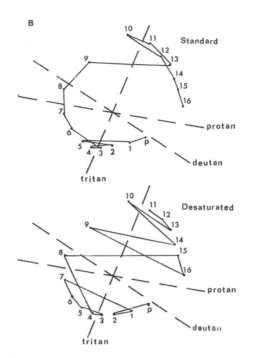

Figure 6.2.2. *continued*

The tritanope makes all the isochromatic colour confusions available in the standard version and is classified correctly as tritan. However, fewer isochromatic errors are made on the desaturated test.

Both the protanomalous and deuteranomalous trichromats (Figures 6.2.2b and 6.2.3b) made more errors on the desaturated version of the test. The classification of the type of colour deficiency was correct in both cases.

It is noted that, as the T16 test contains hues from a complete hue circle, the arrangement may begin either with the cap labelled 1 or the cap labelled 16. People with normal colour vision may obtain the correct result by arranging the colours either in sequence from 1 to 16 or in reverse order from 16 to 1.

6.2.4   DISCUSSION

It is only possible to design a panel test that gives more isochromatic hues for tritans than are available in the D15 test if the selected hues vary in value and chroma. We have adopted a design similar to the H16 test in which the Munsell value is kept constant, at value 5, and only chroma is varied. Perceived variations in saturation occur therefore, but our results show that these do not assist colour deficient observers to obtain the correct result. The anticipated isochromatic confusions are made by protans, deutans and tritans. As expected, anomalous trichromats make more errors on the desaturated version of the test than on the standard test. Although the tritanopic observer made fewer errors on the desaturated T16 test, the desaturated test is not normally given if the standard test is failed. A 'step up' to a more saturated test would be the normal procedure. In view of this, we constructed a test having the same hues as the T16 test but with chroma increased by two to give chroma of

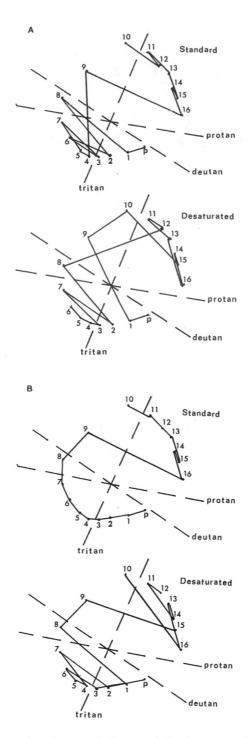

Figure 6.2.3. Isochromatic colour confusions made by deutans on the saturated and desaturated T16 test. (a) Deuteranopia; (b) deuteranomalous trichromatism (Nagel matching range 16–28 scale units, normal match 44 SD 2 scale units).

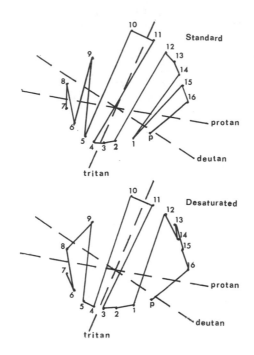

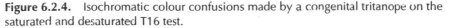

Figure 6.2.4. Isochromatic colour confusions made by a congenital tritanope on the saturated and desaturated T16 test.

6, 8, or 10 throughout the test. The tritanope made the full range of isochromatic colour confusions on this more saturated version of the test. He attributed the result obtained with the desaturated test to the fact that he could not see very many different colours and arranged the colour sequence more or less by chance. Similar results for dichromats on desaturated panel tests have been reported by Dain and Adams (1990).

We consider that the T16 test has a considerable advantage over the D15 test for the examination of acquired colour deficiency because of the increased potential for demonstrating tritan colour deficiency. Acquired type 3 (tritan) defects occur in a number of eye diseases and it is possible that the T16 test will be better able to differentiate poor overall hue discrimination and acquired tritan defects than the conventional D15. This would be helpful for monitoring glaucoma and diabetic retinopathy and for assessing the effect of treatment.

6.2.5   REFERENCES

ADAMS, A.J. & RODIC R. (1982) Use of saturated and desaturated versions on the D15 test in glaucoma and glaucoma suspect patients, *Documenta Ophthalmologica Proceedings Series*, **33**, 419–424.

BIRCH, J. (1989) Farnsworth tests in the study of acquired colour vision defects in diabetic retinopathy, *Documenta Ophthalmologica Proceedings Series*, **52**, 433–440.

BIRCH, J. (1993) *Diagnosis of Defective Colour Vision*, Oxford: Oxford University Press, pp. 85–88.

BOWMAN, K.J. (1982) A method for quantitatively scoring the Farnsworth panel D15, *Acta Ophthalmologica (Kbh)*, **60**, 907–916.

DAIN, S.J. & ADAMS, A.J. (1990) Comparison of the Standard and Adams desaturated D15 tests with congenital colour vision deficiencies, *Ophthalmic and Physiological Optics*, **10**, 40–45.

FARNSWORTH, D. (1943) The Farnsworth-Munsell 100 Hue and dichotomous test for colour vision, *Journal of the Optical Society of America*, **33**, 568–578.

PAULSON, H.M. (1973) Comparison of color vision tests used in the Armed Forces. In: *Colour Vision*, Washington DC: National Academy of Sciences, pp. 34–64.

STILES, W.S. & WYSZECKI, G. (1967) *Colour Science*, New York: John Wiley.

New Method for Investigation of Colour Sensitivity

A.M. Shamshinova, S.N. Endrichovsky, L.I. Nesteruk
and A.A. Yacovlev

6.3.1 INTRODUCTION

The use of reaction time reflects the character and dynamics of psychological and physiological processes. Reaction times include a number of components of the nervous activity from the sensory reaction, to the activity of the motorneuron, but technical difficulties in the organisation of the experiment restrict their practical use. In spite of this, reaction time is used in modern investigations of colour contrast sensitivity and perimetry. The use of the personal computer offers new possibilities in the development of experimental means of psychophysical investigation of the luminance and colour channels of the visual system at each point in the visual field, in order to determine changes that could be an early indication of disease.

6.3.2 METHODS

The possibility of using the reaction time in investigations of the functional state of the cone system of the retina has been conducted with the computer program 'OCULAR'. This program permits us to register the reaction times to the visual stimuli appearing on the display (monitor) screen. The program was realised for IBM-PC DOS 3.1 or higher, with VGA monitor card; it includes stimulus production, and registration, collection, storage, processing and graphical representation of the data. The program enables the operator to change stimulus parameters: size (from 1 to 9mm), brightness (from 0 to 63 units of monitor brightness), the colour of the test ($64 \times 64 \times 64$ combinations of three primary colours: red, green and blue), the position of the stimulus, the number of stimuli (from 1 to 9), the brightness and the colour of the background ($64 \times 64 \times 64$ combinations of the primary colours).

The test, with the necessary intensities and colours, and the scheme of presentation can be set up on the display screen. Investigations were made monocularly. Standards for the investigation of colour vision, and modern data on the foundations of colour vision and perception were taken into account during this work. The time interval between the stimuli changed randomly from 500 to 1500 ms. The reaction time was registered from the time of the appearance of the stimulus to the time of pressing the response key. The stimulus was removed after 1500 ms if no response had occurred in that time. The total dynamic range of the VGA display is 64 arbitrary units, and the precision of step-wise brightness modification was equal to 1 arbitrary unit.

In contrast to the traditional methods of equating colour stimuli by their subjective intensity in the central field of vision, we suggest that the higher reaction time can be used as a criterion of minimum brightness difference. This became the basis of our method of colour campimetry.

Initially, the test and background were different in colour and brightness. The background remained unchanged in colour and brightness in each particular case. The colour of the test stimulus was also constant, but its brightness was modified from more to less bright than the background. In this wide range of variation of the test stimulus brightness, there is an intensity level when the test and background are equal in brightness. Under these conditions the test and background differ only in colour. Because their brightness contrast (which is the most important for detection of the test) was eliminated, the reaction time increased from that measured when they differed both in colour and brightness.

Colour and brightness sensitivity are different in the central and peripheral fields due to the distribution of cones. With the method of colour campimetry, the colour visual sensitivity was investigated in 28 normal subjects and 320 patients with hereditary and acquired colour defects; amblyopia, albinism, glaucoma and Stargardt's dystrophy. The data of the colour campimetry of all patients were compared with the data of electrophysiological investigation and static perimetry (not reported here).

6.3.3   RESULTS AND DISCUSSION

The result of these experiments showed maximum sensitivity in the central visual field for the red and green stimulus and the subsequent decrease in sensitivity to these stimuli in the periphery. The maximum sensitivity to the blue stimulus was 3–7° from the fovea. This conforms with the topography of the distribution of the colour receptors in the retina and the well-known properties of photoreceptors.

Figure 6.3.1 presents the relationship between reaction time and the position of the blue stimulus against the black background. The minimum reaction time was 5–15° from the centre, with a brightness of 0.08–0.24 cdm^{-2}. Both increasing and decreasing the test brightness relative to the background dramatically influences the reaction time. The maximum of the reaction time is achieved when test and background brightness are equal and detection depends on the colour difference. When the test and background are equal both in brightness and colour, the test stimulus is not detected at all, and the reaction time approaches infinity (Figure 6.3.2).

The reaction time for three different levels of background brightness when the test stimuli and backgrounds (blue, green and red) are equated for brightness at a point 5° from the fovea is illustrated in Figure 6.3.3 for six different colour combinations. The general effect of increased background brightness is seen as a reduction in the range between maximum and minimum (irreducible) reaction times. The reaction time is increased for small-sized test stimuli (1–3 mm) and background brightnesses below 10 cdm^{-2}. The intensity of the test stimulus that was needed to match the background brightness as a function of the distance from the fixation point is illustrated in Figure 6.3.4 for three different background brightness levels. For extra-foveal fixation points, the reaction time for equal test-background brightness increases. However, the test stimulus that is equal to the background in the centre of the visual field is not equal to the same background in the periphery. It is necessary to increase the intensity of the extra-foveal stimulus if using the red test stimulus against the blue or green background, or the green against the blue background. But for the blue test colour against the red or green background, and for the green test colour against the red background, the test stimulus must be decreased in intensity.

These results suggest that it is necessary to locally equate the brightness of chromatic stimuli in different parts of the visual field to eliminate effectively the contribution of the brightness channel.

The reaction times for equal brightness of the green stimulus against the purple background, in normals and in patients with various diseases of the eyes, are shown in Figure 6.3.5. The results of the investigation of normals and patients with visual pathology showed a slight increase in reaction time at the point of equal brightness for the normals, but some significant increases of reaction time in pathological conditions. For example, a deuteranopic patient who does not detect the green stimulus against the purple background has a very long reaction time (more than 1500 ms). The same reaction time is recorded not just at the point of equal brightness of the test and background, but also at other closely-adjacent values. A non-symmetric decrease of the light sensitivity is recorded in patients with glaucoma; that is, an increase in the reaction time when the brightness of the test stimulus is lower than the background brightness.

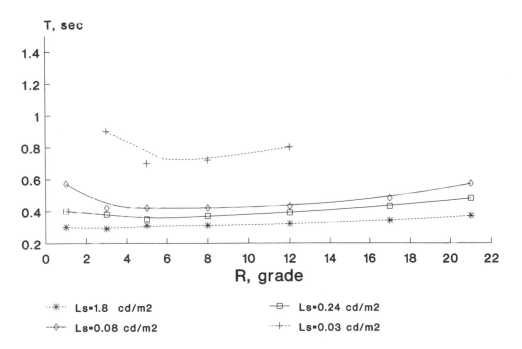

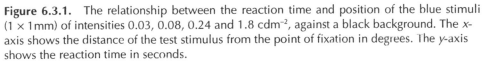

Figure 6.3.1. The relationship between the reaction time and position of the blue stimuli (1 × 1mm) of intensities 0.03, 0.08, 0.24 and 1.8 cdm⁻², against a black background. The x-axis shows the distance of the test stimulus from the point of fixation in degrees. The y-axis shows the reaction time in seconds.

Thus the method of brightness equalisation of the test stimulus and background allows us to measure the reaction time for the different colour test stimuli against different colour backgrounds, at different points in the visual field.

These methods open new possibilities in the research of the light and colour sensitivity in the early diagnosis of pathological processes in the retina and optic nerve. It is evident that the technique requires further elaboration because it is based on the use of the display

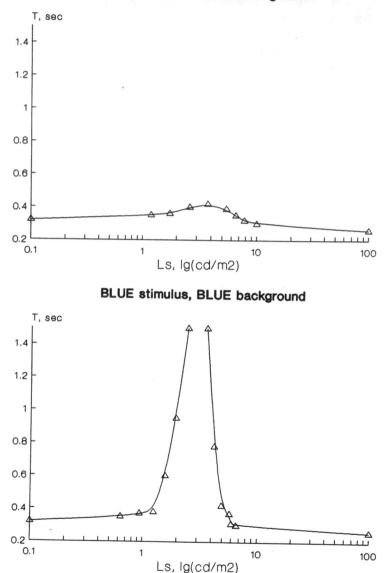

Figure 6.3.2. This shows the reaction time under conditions of equal test and background brightness. The top graph shows the results for the green stimulus against the blue background (3 cdm^{-2}), whilst the bottom plot is for the blue stimulus against the blue background. The x-axis shows the intensity of the stimulus in cdm^{-2}, whilst the y-axis shows the reaction time in seconds.

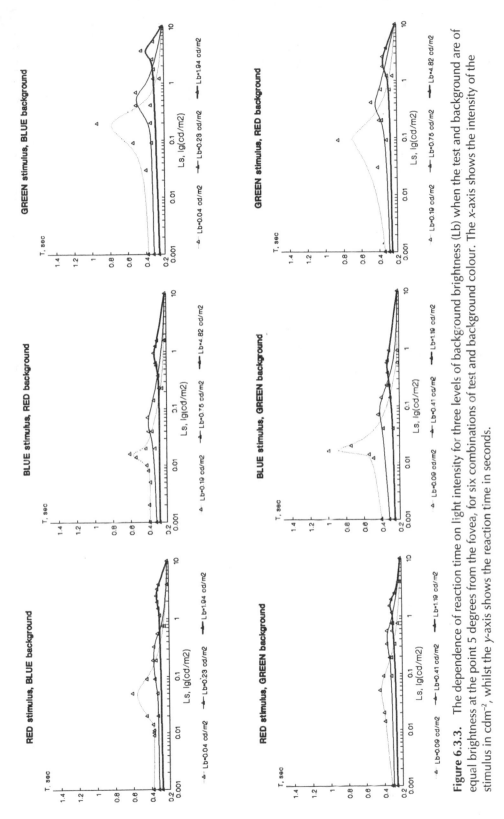

Figure 6.3.3. The dependence of reaction time on light intensity for three levels of background brightness (Lb) when the test and background are of equal brightness at the point 5 degrees from the fovea, for six combinations of test and background colour. The x-axis shows the intensity of the stimulus in cdm^{-2}, whilst the y-axis shows the reaction time in seconds.

Figure 6.3.4. The intensity of the test stimuli needed for equalisation of test (Ls) and background (Lb) brightness (three basic values, given under relevant plot) as a function of the distance from the fixation point. The x-axis shows the distance of the test stimulus from the point of fixation in degrees. The y-axis shows the intensity of the stimulus in cdm⁻².

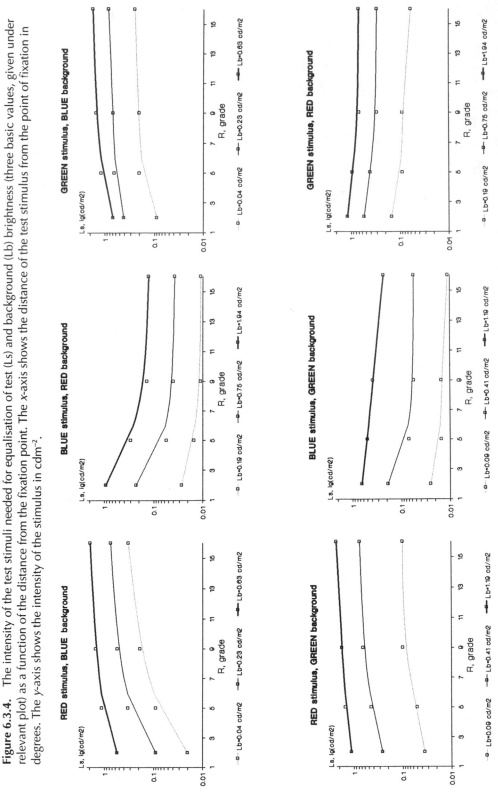

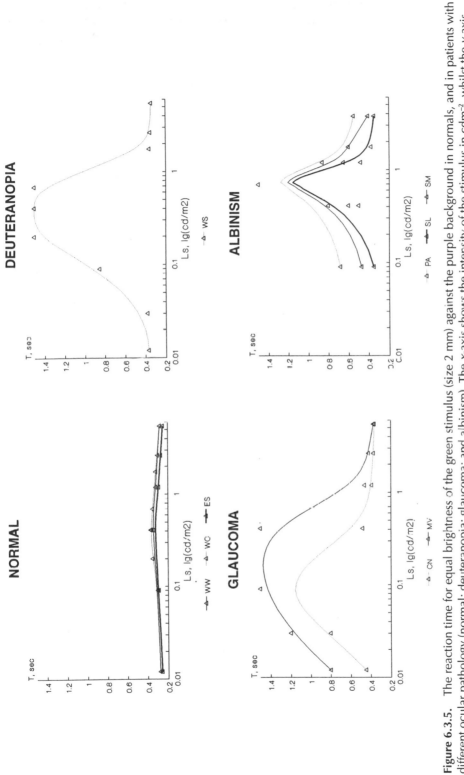

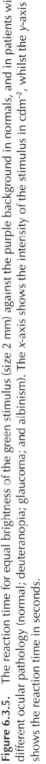

Figure 6.3.5. The reaction time for equal brightness of the green stimulus (size 2 mm) against the purple background in normals, and in patients with different ocular pathology (normal; deuteranopia; glaucoma; and albinism). The x-axis shows the intensity of the stimulus in cdm^{-2}, whilst the y-axis shows the reaction time in seconds.

on the personal computer monitor where the ideal conditions for colour vision investigation cannot be achieved. However, the method of using reaction time to reveal the real differences that exist between normal and those with ocular pathology, allow us to recommend the method of colour campimetry for ophthalmological and psychological studies of the colour sensitivity of the human visual system.

Electrophysiological Correlates of Colour Vision Defects

T. Meigen, M. Bach, J. Gerling and S. Schmid

6.4.1 INTRODUCTION

Since John Dalton studied his own abnormal colour perception (Emery, 1988), the development of basic concepts of colour perception has been closely related to the diagnosis of colour vision deficiencies ('Daltonism'). König and Dieterici (1893) derived three fundamental sensitivity curves (*König fundamentals*) from the confusion lines of dichromats. Later König (1903) found two distinct response systems in dichromats that corresponded in relative spectral sensitivity to two of the three response systems in normal observers. These findings confirmed both the trichromatic nature of colour vision as well as the idea of dichromatism as a reduced form of normal colour vision (Boynton, 1984; Wyszecki and Stiles, 1982). Since then the lack of one cone type in conjunction with the presence of two normal cone types in dichromats induced many paradigms that refined our knowledge of colour vision (Hurvich and Jameson, 1955; Rushton *et al.*, 1973; Smith and Pokorny, 1975; Vos and Walraven, 1971).

Usually colour vision deficiencies are classified psychophysically by means of colour discrimination (pseudo-isochromatic plates) or colour matches (Nagel anomaloscope). For congenital red/green colour vision deficiencies, the abnormal spectral sensitivity of the corresponding cone pigments could be attributed to X-linked genetic abnormalities (Merbs and Nathans, 1992). This may allow an objective classification of colour vision defects.

The aim of this study was to develop a fast, objective colour vision test with electrophysiological methods for the clinical routine. Previous works have looked at the early receptor potential of the ERG, the photopic b-wave, the rapid off-response and ERG flicker photometry in congenital colour vision deficiencies for differentiation (Copenhaver and Gunkel, 1959; Dodt *et al.*, 1958; Jacobs and Neitz, 1991; Kawasaki, 1987; Kawasaki *et al.*, 1984; Yokoyama *et al.*, 1973; Yonemura and Kawasaki, 1979). In an earlier study we used red-green checkerboard patterns with varying intensity ratios $t = I_R (I_R + I_G)$ of the red and green fields (Bach and Gerling 1992; Gerling *et al.*, 1994). We defined the ratio t_0 which evoked minimal flicker ERG responses as an objective measure of red/green colour vision and found a close correlation of t_0 and the subjective equiluminance point. For dichromats, t_0 occurred at different ratios compared to normals. The shift was maximal for protanopic subjects, while an overlap of t_0 values was found for normal and deuteranopic subjects.

Furthermore we could predict the t_0-position from estimating the perceived luminance of the red and green fields by summing the signals of the L- and M-cones after Smith-Pokorny transformation of the stimulus colours (Gerling *et al.*, 1994).

In this study we present an electrophysiological paradigm that uses *cone isolating stimuli* to detect red/green colour vision defects. As the spectral sensitivity functions of the three cone types overlap considerably it is impossible to selectively stimulate only one cone type as long as chromatic adaptation (Krauskopf, 1973; White *et al.*, 1977) is not involved. In this respect the broad-band phosphors of computer monitors are suited just as well as monochromatic colours. Both colour types can be used in the 'silent substitution' technique in which two different colours are chosen that are metameric for two cone types, but lead to a different activation in the remaining third cone type. The term 'silent substitution' was introduced by Donner and Rushton (1959) and reflects a property of visual receptors that Rushton and co-workers have called *the principle of univariance* (Estévez and Spekreijse, 1982; Rushton *et al.*, 1973).

6.4.2   METHODS

Twenty visually normal subjects, 12 protanopes, 4 protanomalous, 11 deuteranopes and 10 deuteranomalous subjects participated in the study. Their acuity was ≥ 1.0, age ranged from 17 to 54 years. Colour vision was assessed using Ishihara plates and the Nagel anomaloscope.

Stimuli were presented on a visual colour display unit (EIZO Flexscan, T660i) controlled by a colour graphics board (Cambridge Research Systems, VSG2, resolution 14 bits per gun). The monitor screen subtended 26' × 34' at a distance of 57 cm (Figure 6.4.1). The stimulus field consisted of a homogeneous, circular area with a diameter of 20° that alternated in colour between red and green at 62.8 reversals per second (i.e. 31.4 Hz). The colour of the yellow mask that surrounded the stimulus field matched the colour mixture of the red and green stimulus colour. The experiment comprised two cone isolating stimuli in which the intensities of the red and green guns temporally modulated one cone type (L or M) and led to 'silent substitution' for the other one. The contribution of the S-cones was negligible in these stimuli. Rod contribution was suppressed by the high stimulus frequency (> 20 Hz). Cone isolating conditions were achieved through several steps:

6.4.2.1 Calibration and gamma correction

The spectral radiant power density of the three monitor phosphors was measured with a spectroradiometer (SpectraScan). This allowed a calculation of the CIE 1964 tristimulus values X, Y, Z and respective chromaticity coordinates x, y, z of the phosphors:

$$\text{Red gun}: \begin{pmatrix} X_R \\ Y_R \\ Z_R \end{pmatrix} = I_R \bullet \begin{pmatrix} 1.76 \\ 1.00 \\ 0.12 \end{pmatrix} \Rightarrow \begin{pmatrix} x_R \\ y_R \\ z_R \end{pmatrix} = \begin{pmatrix} 0.611 \\ 0.346 \\ 0.043 \end{pmatrix} \quad \text{Green gun}: \begin{pmatrix} X_G \\ Y_G \\ Z_G \end{pmatrix} = I_G \bullet \begin{pmatrix} 0.51 \\ 1.00 \\ 0.18 \end{pmatrix} \Rightarrow \begin{pmatrix} x_G \\ y_G \\ z_G \end{pmatrix} = \begin{pmatrix} 0.303 \\ 0.591 \\ 0.106 \end{pmatrix}$$

where I_R and I_G denote gun intensities, measured in cdm^{-2}. A calibration of different intensities and thus a gamma correction was performed with a photodiode (BPW 27).

6.4.2.2 Evaluating relative cone responses

For each gun the relative cone activations L and M were calculated from Smith-Pokorny transformation of the respective tristimulus values X, Y, Z (Wyszecki and Stiles, 1982):

$$\text{Red gun:} \begin{pmatrix} L_R \\ M_R \end{pmatrix} = I_R \bullet \begin{pmatrix} 0.813 \\ 0.187 \end{pmatrix} \quad \text{Green gun:} \begin{pmatrix} L_G \\ M_G \end{pmatrix} = I_G \bullet \begin{pmatrix} 0.617 \\ 0.383 \end{pmatrix} \tag{1}$$

6.4.2.3 Adjusting the intensities I_R and I_G

The temporal modulation of both cone types is given by

$$\text{L}-\text{cones:} \ \Delta L = / L_R - L_G \, | \quad \text{M}-\text{cones:} \ \Delta M = / M_R - M_G \, | \tag{2}$$

L-cone isolation is achieved if silent substitution for the M-cones ($\Delta M = 0$) is adjusted. The appropriate intensity ratio of I_R and I_G can be derived from equations (1) and (2). Likewise M-cone isolation occurs for $\Delta L = 0$. The intensities were chosen to achieve an identical absolute cone modulation in both conditions, i.e. ΔL for L-cone isolation was identical to ΔM for M-cone isolation. The actual intensities and respective cone activations are listed in Table 6.4.1.

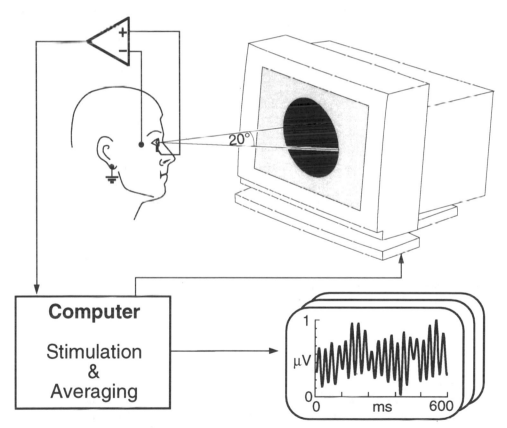

Figure 6.4.1. Experimental setup. Cone isolating colour flicker stimuli (31.4 Hz) were presented within a circular mask on a visual colour display unit. We recorded flicker ERGs from both eyes. The amplified signals were digitised and averaged by a computer that simultaneously generated the visual stimuli.

Both stimuli were presented in an interleaved block design to avoid trend artefacts during a session. ERG responses were recorded separately for both eyes with DTL electrodes (Dawson *et al.*, 1979) above the margin of the lower lid, referenced to the outer canthus. Signals were amplified, filtered and digitised at a sampling interval of 2.65 ms with a small laboratory computer (386 AT-compatible). The sweep time was 637 ms and contained exactly 20 flicker cycles. The computer averaged the sweeps if their amplitude did not exceed ± 100 µV while simultaneously generating the stimuli (Figure 6.4.1). For each stimulus, a total of 160 sweeps were averaged for each condition. These responses were subjected to Fourier analysis and the magnitude at the flicker frequency of 31.4 Hz was used for further analysis.

6.4.3   RESULTS

For each subject and each eye we obtained two ERG responses, one L-cone response and one M-cone response. Figure 6.4.2 shows the averaged ERG responses and respective Fourier spectra for the left eye of one protanopic and one deuteranopic subject. The arrows point to the relevant Fourier component at the flicker frequency of 31.4 Hz (bold arrow: large response; thin arrow: small response). For the protanopic subject the L-cone isolating stimulus evokes no significant ERG response (0.08 µV), while a large response occurs in the M-cone isolating condition (0.43 µV). In the deuteranopic subject this pattern is reversed: a large ERG for L-cone stimulation (0.53 µV) is accompanied by a near-noise response for M-cone stimulation (0.08 µV).

In Figure 6.4.3 the M-cone response is plotted against the L-cone response for all 57 subjects. The overlap between the protan (circles) and deutan (squares) responses was negligible. Protanopic and protanomalous subjects had significant M-cone responses and small L-cone responses. Deuteranopic and deuteranomalous subjects had significant L-cone responses and small M-cone responses. The responses of anomalous and dichromatic subjects in the protan as well as in the deutan group overlapped significantly. For normal subjects (crosses) we found surprisingly low ERG responses in both conditions: no L-cone response was above 0.34 µV, and no M-cone response was above 0.12 µV. Thus the responses of the normal subjects show no overlap with the protan responses, but have magnitudes in the range of low deutan responses.

6.4.4   DISCUSSION

We attempted to develop an electrophysiological colour vision test based on ERG recordings to L- or M-cone isolating colour flicker stimuli (31 Hz). Colour isolating conditions were achieved by alternating red and green fields that temporally modulated one cone type (L or M) and led to silent substitution for the other one. Stimulus conditions were chosen to suppress any contributions of S-cones and rods.

If the M-cone responses are plotted against the L-cone responses, protan and deutan responses are grouped in different clusters with negligible overlap. Thus this test is suitable for a coarse classification of red-green colour vision defects. In dichromatic subjects, one of the two stimuli leads to silent substitution for the remaining cone type. Thus the low ERG response corresponds to the absence of flicker perception in these subjects. However, a further discrimination of protanopia from protanomaly and of deuteranopia from deuteranomaly is not yet possible because these groups overlap considerably. This may be due to the large stimulus field that was necessary to obtain significant ERG responses. It is known

Table 6.4.1. Cone isolating stimuli with silent substitution. The intensities of the red and green monitor guns were chosen to lead to silent substitution either for the M-cones ($\Delta M = 0$) or for the L-cones ($\Delta L = 0$). This corresponds to an isolated modulation of either L- or M-cones. Cone activations were calculated from Smith-Pokorny transformations of the tristimulus values. Though the absolute modulation of the isolated cones was identical in both stimulus conditions (6.9 cdm⁻²) the relative modulation of the luminance channel $Y = M + L$ was reduced in normal subjects compared to both deutan and protan subjects.

Monitor gun	Intensity (cdm⁻²)	Tristimulus values (X, Y, Z)	Cone activation			Modulation			Temporal luminance modulation		
			L	M	Y = L+M	ΔL	ΔM	ΔY	L (deutan)	M (protan)	Y (normal)
L-cone isolation											
R$_L$	13.5	(23.8, 13.5, 1.7)	11.0	2.54	13.54	6.9	0	6.9	46%	0%	34%
G$_L$	6.6	(3.4, 6.6, 1.2)	4.1	2.54	6.64						
M-cone isolation											
R$_M$	21.7	(38.3, 21.7, 2.7)	17.6	4.1	21.7	0	6.9	6.9	0%	46%	14%
G$_M$	28.6	(14.7, 28.6, 5.15)	17.6	11.0	28.6						

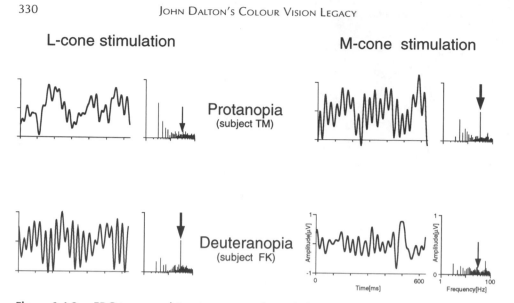

Figure 6.4.2. ERG traces and Fourier spectra of two dichromats. For each subject ERG responses to an L-cone isolating and an M-cone isolating stimulus were recorded. Each ERG trace is the average of 160 sweeps. The Fourier component at the flicker frequency of 31.4 Hz was used for further analysis and is emphasized by arrows (bold arrow: large response; thin arrow: small response). The L-isolating stimulus produced a near-noise response in the protanopic subject and a large response in the deuteranopic subject, with a reversed pattern for the M-isolating stimulus. In both dichromatic subjects, one of the two stimuli leads to a silent substitution for the remaining cone type.

from psychophysical experiments that dichromats behave like anomalous trichromats in conditions with large field stimulation (Pokorny and Smith, 1982).

The responses of normal subjects were significantly different from those of protanopic and protanomalous subjects, but overlapped with those of deuteranopic and deuteranomalous subjects. This result seems related to the findings of Judd (1943) and is in agreement with our study concerning the shift of the equiluminance point in protanopes and deuteranopes obtained with flicker VEP and PERG (Gerling *et al.*, 1994). As we could predict the equiluminance shift by analysing the relative cone activations of L- and M-cones, this derivation might contain a possible explanation for this dissimilarity of protanopia and deuteranopia. L-cones are more sensitive than M-cones, thus the lack of L-cones in protanopia should be easier to detect than the lack of M-cones in deuteranopia.

The small responses of normal subjects in both L- and M-cone isolating conditions (Figure 6.4.3) was the most surprising result in this study. Normals possess both cone types and we would predict a significant response to both stimuli. However, only few responses were above noise in this group. It seems as if the presence of the second cone type, although activated tonically, reduces the response of the modulated cone type. One might postulate an inhibitory interaction between L and M cones. However, a coupling of neighbouring cones could only be found between cones with identical spectral sensitivity (Walraven *et al.*, 1990).

We suggest the following hypothesis to explain the small ERG responses in normal subjects. If L- and M-cones have no direct coupling then the inhibitory interaction might occur beyond the receptor stage where the signals of both cone types are further processed. To quantify the temporal modulation of these processes we revisited our stimulus conditions (Table 6.4.1). Our stimuli were designed to yield identical absolute cone modulations

$\Delta L = \Delta M = 6.9 \ cdm^{-2}$. The stimulus frequency of 31.4 Hz was well above the colour flicker fusion frequency. Thus, the recorded ERG originates from the luminance channel Y = L + M whose absolute modulation was $\Delta Y = 6.9 \ cdm^{-2}$. According to Weber's law increment thresholds are proportional to the background luminance. Thus, the luminance modulations should be divided by the mean luminance to yield a contrast measure as a relevant stimulus parameter. Table 6.4.1 shows the Michelson contrasts for the luminance channel Y. In protanopic subjects this corresponds to the temporal contrast for M-cones as Y = M, in deuteranopic subjects to the temporal contrast for L-cones as Y = L. In normal subjects the silent cone type introduces a tonic luminance pedestal in both stimulus conditions. Compared to dichromats this leads to an increased mean luminance, but also to a reduced contrast. If we assume a monotonic relation between the luminance contrast and the evoked ERG responses, this model predicts a reduction of L-cone and M-cone responses of normals, compared with the responses of dichromats (inset in Figure 6.4.3). The contrast reduction is larger for M-cone isolation than for L-cone isolation (Table 6.4.1). Thus normal responses are shifted towards deutan responses.

Our objective colour vision test is able to discriminate between extreme colour vision defects such as protanopia and deuteranopia. However, a more subtle discrimination of anomalous dichromatic defects and of deutan defects from normal colour vision is currently not possible due to experimental constraints, resulting from the large stimulus field in ERG recordings and the contrast reduction in normal subjects. At this point it is unclear whether this approach can yield data that are precise enough to contribute to the problem of the ratio of L- to M-cones in the human retina.

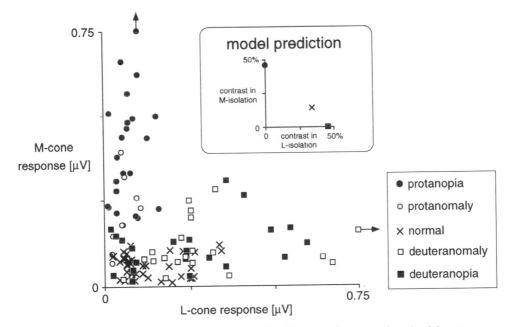

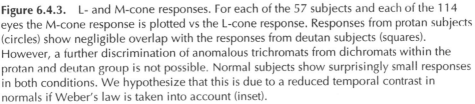

Figure 6.4.3. L- and M-cone responses. For each of the 57 subjects and each of the 114 eyes the M-cone response is plotted vs the L-cone response. Responses from protan subjects (circles) show negligible overlap with the responses from deutan subjects (squares). However, a further discrimination of anomalous trichromats from dichromats within the protan and deutan group is not possible. Normal subjects show surprisingly small responses in both conditions. We hypothesize that this is due to a reduced temporal contrast in normals if Weber's law is taken into account (inset).

6.4.5   REFERENCES

Bach, M. & Gerling, J. (1992) Retinal and cortical activity in human subjects during color flicker fusion, *Vision Research*, **32**, 1219–1223.

Boynton, R. M. (1984) Visual pigments and sensitivity. In: Bartleson, C. J. & Grum, F. (Eds) *Visual Measurements*, vol 5, Optical Radiation Measurements series, Dordrecht: Kluwer Academic.

Copenhaver, R. M. & Gunkel, R. D. (1959) The spectral sensitivity of color defective subjects determined by electroretinography, *Archives of Ophthalmology*, **62**, 55–68.

Dawson, W. W., Trick, G. L. & Litzkow, C. A. (1979) Improved electrode for electroretinography, *Investigative Ophthalmology and Visual Science*, **18**, 988–991.

Dodt, E., Copenhaver, R. M. & Gunkel, R. D. (1958) Photopischer Dominator und Farbkomponenten im menschlichen Elektroretinogramm, *Arch. ges. Physiol.*, **267**, 497–507.

Donner, K. O. & Rushton, W. A. H. (1959) Retinal stimulation by light substitution, *Journal of Physiology*, **149**, 288–302.

Emery, A. E. (1988) John Dalton (1766–1844), *Journal of Medical Genetics*, **25**, 422–426.

Estevez, O. & Spekreijse, H. (1982) The 'silent substitution' method in visual research, *Vision Research*, **22**, 681–691.

Gerling, J., Bach, M. & Meigen, T. (1994) Diagnosis of protan and deutan color vision deficiencies with pattern-ERG and VEP. In: Drum, B. (Ed.) *Colour Vision Deficiencies XII*, Dordrecht: Kluwer Academic, pp. 375–380.

Hurvich, L. M., & Jameson, D. (1955) Some quantitative aspects of an opponent-colors theory. II. Brightness, saturation and hue in normal and dichromatic vision, *Journal of the Optical Society of America*, **45**, 602.

Jacobs, G. H. & Neitz, J. (1991) Deuteranope spectral sensitivity measured with ERG flicker photometry. In: Drum, B., Moreland, J. D. & Serra, A. (Eds) *Colour Vision Deficiencies X*, Dordrecht: Kluwer Academic, pp. 405–411.

Judd, D. B. (1943) Facts about color blindness, *Journal of the Optical Society of America*, **33**, 294–307.

Kawasaki, K. (1987) Electrodiagnosis of red-green colour deficiency, *Japanese Journal of Ophthalmology*, **31**, 50–60.

Kawasaki, K., Yonemure, D. & Nakasato, H. (1984) Empirical detection of congenital dyschromatopsia by electroretinography, *Ophthalmology Research*, **16**, 329–333.

König, A. (1903) *Gesammelte Abhandlungen*, Leipzig: Barth-Verlag.

König, A. & Dieterici, C. (1893) Die Grünempfindungen in normalen und anomalen Farensystemen und ihre Intensitätsverteilung im Spektrum, *Z. Psychol. Physiol. Sinnesorgane*, **4**, 241–347.

Krauskopf, J. (1973) Contributions of the primary chromatic mechanisms to the generation of visual evoked potentials, *Vision Research*, **13**, 2289–2298.

Merbs, S. L. & Nathans, J. (1992) Absorption spectra of the hybrid pigments responsible for anomalous color vision, *Science*, **258**, 464–466.

Pokorny, J. & Smith, V. C. (1982) New observations concerning red-green color defects, *Color Research Applications*, **7**, 159–164.

Rushton, W. A. H., Spitzer Powell, D. & White, K. D. (1973) Exchange thresholds in dichromats, *Vision Research*, **13**, 1993–2002.

Smith, V. C. & Pokorny, J. (1975) Spectral sensitivity of the foveal cone photopigments between 400 and 500 nm, *Vision Research*, **15**, 161–171.

Vos, J.J. & Walraven, P.L. (1971) On the derivation of the foveal receptor primaries, *Vision Research*, **11**, 799–818.

Walraven, J., Enroth-Cugell, C., Hood, D.C., MacLeod, D.I.A. & Schnapf, J.L. (1990) The control of visual sensitivity. In: Spillmann, L. & Werner, J.S. (Eds) *Visual Perception: The Neurophysiological Foundation*, San Diego: Academic Press, pp. 53–101.

White, C.T., Katoaka, R.W. & Martin, J.I. (1977) Colour evoked potentials. In: Desmedt, J.E. (Ed.) *Visual Evoked Potentials in Man: New Developments*, Oxford: Clarendon.

WYSZECKI, G. & STILES, W. S. (1982) *Color science: Concepts and Methods, Quantitative Data and Formulae*, New York: John Wiley & Sons.

YOKOYAMA, M., YOSHIDA, T. & UI, K. (1973) Spectral responses in the human electroretinogram and their clinical significance, *Japanese Journal of Ophthalmology*, **17**, 113–24.

YONEMURA, D. & KAWASAKI, K. (1979) New approaches to ophthalmic electrodiagnosis by retinal oscillatory potential, drug induced responses from retinal epithelium and cone potentials, *Documenta Ophthalmologica*, **48**, 163–222.

An Analysis of VEPs Using Non-linear Identification Analysis Method

Keiko Momose, Akinori Ogawa, Takehiro Ito
and Akihiko Uchiyama

6.5.1 INTRODUCTION

Visual evoked potentials (VEPs) have been analysed to investigate visual systems (Regan, 1970; Regan and Regan, 1988; Sebro and Wright, 1980; Spekreijse and Oosting, 1970; Trimble and Phillips, 1978; Yamanaka et al., 1972). As VEPs can be measured non-invasively and objectively, they have been examined with regard to their possible application to a quantitative description of the human colour system (Regan, 1970; Yamanaka et al., 1973) and testing for colour blindness (Regan and Spekreijse, 1974). It has been reported that the luminosity and chromatic responses found in VEPs are similar to those estimated by psychophysical methods (Regan, 1970; Yamanaka et al., 1973).

As VEPs have non-linear properties, non-linear system identification methods (Marmarelis and Marmarelis, 1978; Schetzen, 1980) have played an important role in describing the relationship between stimulus and VEPs. Often only one wavelength of luminance-modulated stimulus has been used to measure VEPs in the human visual system (Regan and Regan, 1988; Sebro, 1992; Sebro and Wright, 1980; Spekreijse and Oosting, 1970; Sutter, 1987, 1992; Trimble and Phillips, 1978). It is important to study the properties of VEPs at various wavelengths, which could also be useful for detecting colour blindness.

In this study, in order to investigate the non-linearity of VEPs and characteristics of their non-linear parameters to the wavelength of light stimuli, the kernel method using an m-sequence as the input was applied to VEPs in human, because this method is powerful in describing non-linear system characteristics.

6.5.1.1 Theory

Causal and time invariant non-linear systems can be described by their binary expansions so long as the input is in a binary (-1 or +1) sequence,

$$y(t) = b_0 + \sum_{n=1}^{R+1} \sum_{\tau_1=0}^{R} \sum_{\tau_2=\tau_1+1}^{R} \cdots \sum_{\tau_n=\tau_{n-1}+1}^{R} b_n(\tau_1, \ldots, \tau_n) \; x(t-\tau_1) \ldots x(t-\tau_n) \tag{1}$$

335

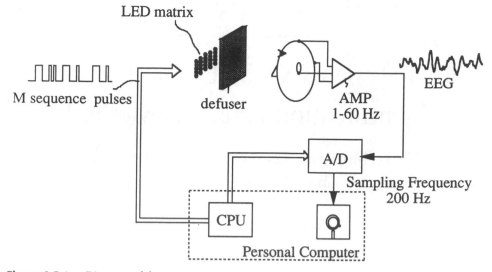

Figure 6.5.1. Diagram of the system.

where x(t) is the input, y(t) is the output, t_n is a time delay, $b_n(t_1, \ldots t_n)$ is the nth-order binary kernel and R is system memory length. Identification of the nonlinear system means to identify its binary kernels. These sliced kernels of all orders are lined up along the first-order cross-correlation cycle between the m-sequence [x(t)] and the corresponding system response [y(t)]. This is because the element-by-element product of relatively shifted versions of a binary m-sequence is still the same sequence except for a known shift (Sutter, 1987, 1992).

6.5.2   METHODS

Figure 6.5.1 shows a diagram of the system used in this study. The stimulus was luminance modulated by a temporal m-sequence whose field was unpatterned. The modulation depth was 100 per cent. Subjects viewed the stimulus binocularly with a visual angle of 5 degrees. The m-sequence used in this study was generated by a 14-bit shift register. The shift register transitions were paced by a clock interval at 5 ms so that the m-sequence period was 81.915 s [$= (2^{14}-1) \times 5$ ms]. Its spectrum was flat from near 0 to 66.6 Hz, covering the range of human VEP flicker response. This sequence output was used to drive 25 LEDs (Stanley products).

The EEG signal was recorded as a bipolar recording between Oz and Cz (the 10–20 electrode system) with grounding at both ears, and was amplified and band-filtered (1–60 Hz) through a bio-amplifier. The amplified signal was applied to an A/D converter in which the sampling frequency was 200 Hz. The stimulus was repeated three times, responses were averaged, and the VEPs were extracted.

Eight stimuli (470, 555, 570, 580, 605, 630, 670 and 700 nm) were used. The time-averaged luminance of these stimuli was constant (10 cdm^{-2}). VEPs for each stimulus were recorded from three colour-normal subjects. Kernel slices were estimated by calculating the first-order cross-correlation function between the m-sequence and the corresponding measured VEP.

6.5.3   RESULTS AND DISCUSSION

Up to third-order kernels were recognised in the cross-correlation functions between VEPs and the m-sequence used as the stimulus (Momose *et al.*, 1994). The first-, second- and third-order kernels obtained from one subject's VEPs are shown in Figure 6.5.2. Figure 6.5.2 (top) shows first-order kernels [$b_1(\tau)$], lines 2–5 show second-order sliced kernels [$b_2(\tau, \tau + \sigma)$, $\sigma = 5$, 15, 35 and 50 ms] and (bottom) shows third-order sliced kernels [$b_3(\tau, \tau + \sigma_1, \tau + \sigma_2)$, $\sigma_1 = 5$ ms, $\sigma_2 = 10$ ms]. The second- and third-order kernels were sliced from three- and four-dimensional data respectively. Two kernels obtained from VEPs in two individual recordings are overlaid. As shown in the figure, the kernels were so reproducible that they could be used as reasonable parameters for describing VEPs. Kernels higher than the fourth order were almost flat. This suggests that the VEP-luminance modulation system can be described in terms of non-linearities up to the third order. In fact, the difference in MSE (mean squared error) between the measured VEPs and the output of the model with estimated kernels up to the third order was minimal (data not shown). This is in agreement with previous studies (Regan and Regan, 1988; Sebro, 1992).

As shown in Figure 6.5.2, the waveforms of first- and second-order kernels depend on the wavelength of the stimulus. The first-order kernel from 150 to 300 ms for the blue stimulus (470 nm) was quite different from those for other stimuli, while the latency of maximum amplitude was almost the same. Furthermore, second-order kernels from 150 to 250 ms were also different. However, the differences among third-order kernels for the four colour stimuli were slight and their amplitudes were smaller than those of the first- and second-order kernels. These results suggest that the first- and second-order kernels include the responses to the colour stimuli. In fact, as shown in Figure 6.5.3, the waveforms of first-order kernels are changed continuously as the wavelength of the light stimuli increase.

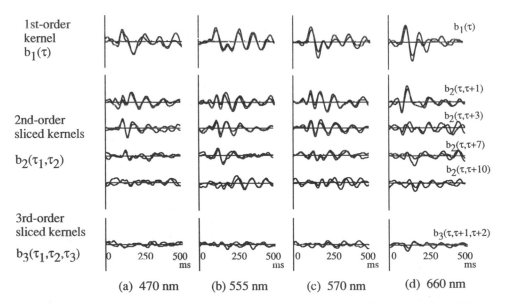

Figure 6.5.2.   Kernels obtained from one subject's VEPs elicited by (a) blue stimulus (470 nm), (b) green stimulus (555 nm), (c) yellow stimulus (570 nm) and (d) red stimulus (660 nm).

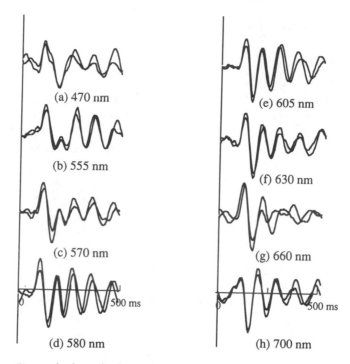

Figure 6.5.3. First-order kernels obtained from one subject's VEPs elicited by eight stimuli. ((a) 470 nm, (b) 555 nm, (c) 570 nm, (d) 580 nm, (e) 605 nm, (f) 630 nm, (g) 660 nm and (h) 700 nm).

It was suggested that first-order kernels included the opponent responses, because they correspond to the impulse responses of the linear system; further it was reported that transient VEPs include the opponent responses (Yamanaka *et al.*, 1973). To examine this suggestion, the principal component analysis (PCA) method, which was used by Yamanaka *et al.* (1973), was applied to evaluate the components included in first-order kernels.

The results from one subject are shown in Figures 6.5.4 and 6.5.5. Figure 6.5.4 shows the first, second and third component vectors $a_i(t)$ ($i = 1, 2, 3, t = 1, \ldots, 100$), which correspond to the time responses. Each vector $a_i(t)$ ($i = 1, 2, 3$) is normalised to be $|a_i(t)| = 1$. Figure 6.5.5 shows the weighting coefficients, $z_i(\lambda)$ ($i = 1, 2, 3$). As shown in Figure 6.5.5, the curves of $z_1(\lambda)$ and $z_2(\lambda)$ are typical curves, while that of $z_3(\lambda)$ is almost flat. The contribution ratios (Table 6.5.1) of the first and second components are higher than those of the third and fourth components. These results show that two components [$a_1(t)$ and $a_2(t)$] are in the first-order kernel.

The curve of $z_1(\lambda)$, shown in Figure 6.5.5(a), is similar to the Y-B chromatic responses found in opponent colour theory (Jameson and Hurvich, 1955). The curve of $Z_2(\lambda)$ is similar to the R-G chromatic responses. This suggests that first-order kernels obtained from VEPs are related to opponent colour responses, a result that is in agreement with Yamanaka *et al.* (1973).

As shown in Figure 6.5.2, the waveforms of first- and second-order kernels for the same colour are almost the same. This implies that colour-opponent responses may be found in second-order kernels. However, the second-order kernel is a non-linear parameter, so it must be considered with regard to the non-linearity of human colour vision.

6.5.4   CONCLUSION

In this study, non-linear properties of human VEPs were investigated by the kernel method using the m-sequence as input. The results showed that a non-linear system can be expressed by the binary kernel up to the third order. Furthermore, it was shown that the waveforms of first- and second-order kernels were dependent on the wavelength of the stimulus, and that first-order kernels include opponent colour responses.

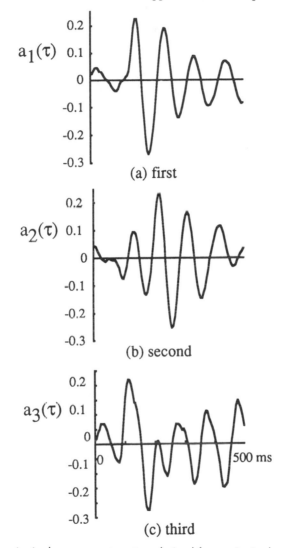

Figure 6.5.4.   The principal component vectors derived from principal component analysis of VEPs.

6.5.5   ACKNOWLEDGEMENTS

The authors would like to thank Dr Masami Miyazaki of Waseda University for the use of his equipment. The authors also thank undergraduate and graduate students of Waseda University who acted as subjects.

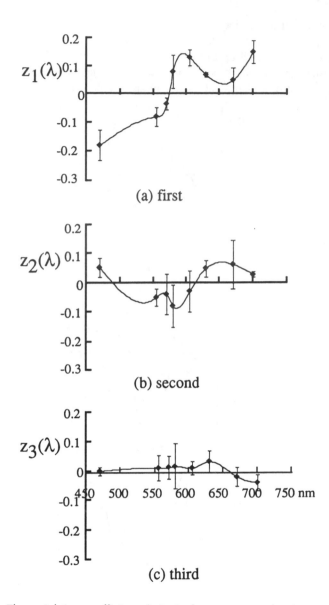

Figure 6.5.5.   The weighting coefficients (principal component values).

Table 6.5.1.   Contribution ratios of three subjects (as %).

	AO	KM	KY
First	51.5	37.0	35.1
Second	23.6	25.9	26.7
Third	6.8	11.3	14.7
Fourth	4.6	6.7	6.3

6.5.6   REFERENCES

JAMESON, D. & HURVICH, L. M. (1955) Some quantitative aspects of an opponent-colour theory I, chromatic responses and spectral saturation, *Journal of Optical Society of America*, **54**, 1031–1040.

MARMARELIS, P. D. & MARMARELIS, V. Z. (1978) *Analysis of Physiological Systems*, New York: Plenum Press.

MOMOSE, K., OGAWA, A. & UCHIYAMA, A. (1994) An analysis of visual evoked potentials elicited by luminance modulated stimulation. In: Ohzu, H. & Komatsu, S. (Eds) *Optical Methods in Biomedical and Environmental Sciences – Optics Within Life Sciences III*, Amsterdam: Elsevier Science.

REGAN, D. (1970) Objective method of measuring the relative spectral luminosity curve in man, *Journal of Optical Society of America*, **60**, 856–859.

REGAN, D. & SPEKREIJSE, H. (1974) Evoked potential indications of colour blindness, *Vision Research*, **14**, 89–95.

REGAN, M. P. & REGAN, D. (1988) A frequency domain technique for characterizing nonlinearities in biological systems, *Journal of Theoretical Biology*, **133**, 293–317.

SCHETZEN, M. (1980) *The Volterra and Wiener Theories of Nonlinear Systems*, New York: Wiley.

SEBRO, R. (1992) An analysis of the VEP to luminance modulation and of its nonlinearity, *Vision Research*, **32**, 1395–1404.

SEBRO, R. & WRIGHT, W. W. (1980) Visually evoked potentials to pseudorandom binary sequence stimulation, *Archives of Ophthalmology*, **98**, 196–198.

SPEKREIJSE, H. & OOSTING, H. (1970) Linearlizing: A method for analysing and synthesizing nonlinear systems, *Kybernetik*, **7**, 22–31.

SUTTER, E. E. (1987) A practical nonstochastic approach to nonlinear time-domain analysis. In: Marmarelis, V.Z. (Ed.) *Advanced Methods of Physiological System Modeling*, Los Angeles: University of Southern California, pp. 303–315.

SUTTER, E. E. (1992) A deterministic approach to nonlinear system analysis. In: Pinter, R. B. & Nabet, B. (Eds) *Nonlinear Vision*, CRC Press, pp. 171–220.

TRIMBLE, J. & PHILLIPS, G. (1978) Nonlinear analysis of the human visual evoked response, *Biological Cybernetics*, **30**, 55–61.

YAMANAKA, T., SOBAGAKI, H. & NAYATANI, Y. (1973) Opponent-colours responses in the visually evoked potential in man, *Vision Research*, **13**, 1319–1333.

Chromatic Thresholds in Visual Disorders

P. Ewen King-Smith, Sara L. Alvarez, Gilbert E. Pierce and Michael J. Earley

Thresholds measured with coloured test targets can be applied in various ways to the study of visual disorders. For example, a comparison between thresholds for, say, red and green test spots can be used to study the relative amounts of scotopic and photopic loss in diseases such as retinitis pigmentosa (Massof and Finkelstein, 1979). More commonly, measurements of chromatic thresholds have been used to study colour vision losses and they have a number of advantages compared with more standard clinical colour tests such as plate and arrangement tests. For example, chromatic thresholds can be used to study localised losses whereas plate and arrangement tests are not typically localised in the visual field; thus, chromatic test spots are becoming popular in static perimetry (e.g. Johnson *et al.*, 1993). An important advantage of using chromatic threshold measurements is that they provide a direct measure of the loss in colour sensitivity compared with normal; for example, a patient's loss of sensitivity may be expressed directly in log units relative to normal, whereas an error score for a plate or an arrangement test does not give this information. Expressing loss of chromatic sensitivity in log units facilitates comparison with other types of visual threshold measurement, e.g. with thresholds for an achromatic test spot (including perimetry), or for sinusoidal gratings or flicker (King-Smith, 1991).

In this review, a comparison is made between different methods for studying colour vision losses in visual disorders based on thresholds for chromatic targets. A major distinction can be made between methods designed to isolate responses from individual cone types and those that attempt to isolate post-receptoral processes; in both cases, two main types of method will be discussed. The discussion will emphasise acquired colour defects, rather than the congenital colour defects sometimes associated with Dalton's name; references will be limited to representative examples.

6.6.1 ISOLATION OF RESPONSES FROM INDIVIDUAL CONE TYPES

A popular method of attempting to isolate responses from an individual class of cones is the two-colour threshold technique of Stiles (1978), Wald (1964) and Marré (1973). Thresholds for a test spot of one colour are measured on a background of another colour. This background is typically chosen to reduce the response of two types of cone so that the remaining type becomes more sensitive; for example, a bright yellow background reduces the sensitivity of both medium (M) and long (L) wavelength cones so that the S cones become more sensitive than the other cones. Magenta and blue backgrounds can likewise be used to help isolate M and L cones respectively. One application of the two-colour technique is to measure a spectral sensitivity curve superimposed on one of these three coloured backgrounds (e.g. Marré, 1973) – this yields a 'spectral test sensitivity' curve that typically provides fairly good isolation of the corresponding cone type in one region of the spectrum.

In addition to specifying the background colour, the test spot colour may be chosen to favor the cone type to be isolated – e.g. on a yellow background, a blue-violet test light could be used to favour S cone responses because, in comparison with the other cone types, S cones are relatively sensitive to this colour. For M and L cones, corresponding combinations might be green on magenta and red on blue backgrounds, respectively. The 'isolation' obtained is typically not perfect – e.g. there may be a small M cone contribution in conditions designed to isolate the L cones; isolation of S cones is typically better than for M and L cones. Common applications of the two-colour technique with fixed test and background colours include perimetry (e.g. Johnson et al., 1993) and threshold versus background intensity studies (e.g. Kalloniatis et al., 1993).

Information from L, M and S cones is recoded into achromatic, red-green and blue-yellow signals at least by the stage of the ganglion cells and probably also in bipolar cells (Gouras, 1991). Thus it might seem that the two-colour threshold technique, which is designed to isolate cone responses, is less suitable for studying post-receptoral function and losses; however, there are at least three situations where the two-colour technique can be usefully applied to post-receptoral losses. First, it should be noted that S cones send their output almost exclusively through blue-yellow processes (Krauskopf et al., 1982); therefore, a loss of blue-yellow vision can be tested by using an S cone-isolating stimulus and this helps to justify the use of blue-on-yellow perimetry in evaluating glaucoma (Johnson et al., 1993), which is thought to be a largely post-receptoral disorder. A second use of the two-colour technique is in demonstrating that a red-green loss in a suspected acquired colour defect is not due to a concurrent congenital colour defect. In both dichromats and anomalous trichromats, spectral sensitivity curves measured on, say, magenta and blue backgrounds have almost identical shapes (see Boynton and Wagner, 1961); this typically is not the case for red-green colour losses caused by post-receptoral defects (e.g. King-Smith et al., 1980) so comparison of spectral sensitivity on blue and magenta background provides a valuable test for a concurrent congenital colour defect. A final application of the two-colour technique is as an indicator of selective loss of the red-green process relative to the achromatic process. It may be shown that contributions from red-green opponency tend to move the peak wavelengths of spectral sensitivities on blue and magenta backgrounds away from each other, while contributions of the black-white process have the opposite effect; thus, a selective loss of red-green sensitivity, relative to achromatic sensitivity, may cause the peak wavelengths on blue and magenta backgrounds to move towards each other (King-Smith, 1991).

A second method of isolating responses of individual cone types is the '(cone) silent substitution' method. In this method a test stimulus is generated by a combination of incremental and decremental stimuli so that only one of the three cone types is stimulated; such combinations of incremental and decremental stimuli are readily generated on a colour video display. For example, a certain combination of a red increment and a green decrement can be used to generate a test spot that stimulates L cones without stimulating S and M cones; a different combination (with a weaker green decrement) stimulates M cones, but not S and L cones. As expected, thresholds for the corresponding dichromat (e.g. protanope thresholds for an L cone-isolating stimulus) are large or infinite (Sellers *et al.*, 1986). It may be noted that the cone-isolation achieved by this method can be theoretically perfect (assuming that the spectral sensitivities of the subject's cones are known exactly, and do not vary throughout the extent of the test target); however, in practice, the isolation achieved by the two-colour technique may be better, particularly the excellent isolation of S cones, which can be obtained by blue on yellow.

Application of this method to acquired colour defects is subject to some of the same considerations as the two-colour technique. Thus, in a disorder affecting post-receptoral processes, an S cone-isolation stimulus is suitable for isolating the blue-yellow process. As discussed previously, isolation of M and L cones is probably less informative in post-receptoral disorders, because information from these cones is transmitted along both chromatic and achromatic processes. Thus, for example, whereas Yu *et al.* (1991) have developed a promising screening test for glaucoma using stimuli on protan, deutan and tritan axes, the tritan stimulus is preferable to the others on theoretical grounds, if glaucoma is mainly a post-receptoral disorder.

6.6.2 ISOLATION OF RESPONSES FROM POST-RECEPTORAL PROCESSES

The first method of isolating post-receptoral processes is based on Sperling and Harwerth's (1971) observation that spectral sensitivity for a relatively large, long duration, foveal test spot on a bright white background shows three peaks near 440, 520 and 600 nm, which seem to correspond to blue-yellow (440 nm) and red-green (520 and 600 nm) opponent processes; thus, for example, the spectral sensitivity at long wavelengths (above about 580 nm) can be modelled by a difference between L and M cone sensitivity as might be expected for a red-green opponent process. As expected, the threshold for colour recognition of these spots is very close to the detection threshold (King-Smith and Carden, 1976); also, these spectral peaks correspond closely to those of the 'spectral valence' curves of Hering's chromatic processes (Hurvich and Jameson, 1957). It seems that the third Hering process – the black-white process, which would be expected to contribute a peak near 555 nm – contributes little to the spectral sensitivity in these conditions because it is relatively insensitive; it has been argued that the relatively large size (e.g. 1°) and long duration (e.g. 0.2 s) of the test spots, as well as the bright white background, all tend to favour the chromatic opponent processes rather than the black-white process (King-Smith and Carden, 1976). Using the same equipment, it is possible to test for black-white function by asking the subject to detect high frequency (25 Hz) flicker in the spectral test spot; this gives rise to a spectral sensitivity curve that is very similar to the photopic luminosity curve, with a peak sensitivity near 555 nm (King-Smith *et al.*, 1976).

It follows that a selective loss of post-receptoral chromatic processes, relative to the black-white process, might change the three-peaked curve to a curve with a single peak near 555 nm; this predicted change is clearly evident in hereditary optic atrophies (King-Smith *et al.* 1980). Flicker recognition thresholds may be more elevated than thresholds for long duration test flashes in some disorders (e.g. retrobulbar neuritis, Zisman *et al.*, 1978) suggesting that the black-white process is more affected than the chromatic processes; however, loss of flicker sensitivity might be caused by a change in temporal processing characteristics (see Trautzettel-Klosinski and Aulhorn, 1987) rather than by a general loss of black-white sensitivity.

A second method of isolating post-receptoral processes is similar to the 'cone silent substitution' method for isolating photoreceptors discussed previously; however, in this case the combination of incremental and decremental stimuli should stimulate one of the three post-receptoral detection processes (red-green, blue-yellow and black-white) but not the other two, and so could be described as 'post-receptoral silent substitution'. For example, a certain combination of a red increment and green decrement can be used to stimulate the red-green opponent process without stimulating blue-yellow or black-white processes; the proportions of red and green are intermediate between those for isolating the L and M cones. Another example would be a test spot that stimulates S cones but not L and M cones (one of the 'cone silent substitution' stimuli); because S cones contribute little or nothing to red-green and black-white detection mechanisms (Krauskopf et al., 1982), this stimulus will stimulate only the blue-yellow process. By definition, both the preceding stimuli are 'equiluminous', in that they do not stimulate the black-white process. Finally, a white spot on a white background appears colourless, and so presumably stimulates the black-white process but not the two chromatic processes. The three stimuli discussed above define 'cardinal' axes in colour space (Krauskopf et al., 1982).

The most direct way of applying these ideas is to measure thresholds along the three cardinal axes, possibly including both positive and negative directions along each axis, i.e. equiluminous red and green or blue and yellow, and light and dark test spots (e.g. Fallowfield and Krauskopf, 1984). Our own approach has been to measure thresholds along a number of directions within two planes in colour space, one defined by the red and green phosphors of our video monitor and the other defined by the blue phosphor and a yellow that corresponds to equal contrasts (Weber fractions) of the red and green phosphors. Thresholds are plotted in these colour planes, e.g. the contrast of the green component is plotted as a function of the contrast of the red component; increments and decrements are represented by positive and negative contrasts respectively. Ellipses, typically centred at the origin, are fitted to the data. A selective enlargement of the ellipse along an axis of negative slope (corresponding to a combination of, say, red increment and green decrement, thus yielding a chromatic stimulus) indicates a selective loss of chromatic sensitivity. This occurs, for example, in anomalous trichromacy where the major axis of the ellipse is considerably elongated and has a negative slope, corresponding to the relatively high red-green chromatic threshold (Sellers et al., 1986). Our method automatically takes account of differences in spectral sensitivity between observers; for example protanomals and deuteranomals can be studied using the same set of red-green stimuli, and their sensitivity difference is indicated by a change in the direction of the major axis of the ellipse (Sellers et al., 1986). Some acquired colour deficiencies (particularly hereditary optic atrophies, Grigsby et al., 1991) also show a selective elongation along an axis of negative slope, which may occur for both red-green and blue-yellow mixtures, indicating a selective loss of the corresponding chromatic process relative to the black-white process. A selective enlargement along an axis of positive slope (e.g. both blue and yellow increments) would indicate a selective increase in black-white thresholds; this type of enlargement is sometimes seen for blue-yellow mixtures (e.g. King-Smith et al., 1989) but does not seem to occur for red-green mixtures (presumably because a disorder that generates a severe black-white loss also causes a red-green loss of at least comparable magnitude).

Various advantages and disadvantages of our method may be noted. One advantage is that red-green mixture thresholds are more sensitive than the spectral sensitivity on white method in detecting selective loss of the red-green process (Chioran et al., 1985). As already noted, our method allows for differences in spectral sensitivity (e.g. between protan and deutan) without having to perform flicker photometry to determine the relative luminances of the three phosphors. Because the results are expressed in terms of the physical stimulus from the monitor (i.e. contrast of each phosphor), the plot is not dependent on any assumptions about spectral sensitivities of the post-receptoral detection processes. Our experience is that clinicians can readily interpret the data, i.e. it seems easier to appreciate that a certain shape of ellipse implies a selective chromatic or achromatic loss, than to deduce this from, say, a bar chart of chromatic and achromatic thresholds. A limitation of our method is that our equiluminous blue and yellow differ somewhat from the tritan confusion axis (Grigsby et al., 1991), which may be the optimum axis for isolating the blue-yellow detection process (Krauskopf et al., 1982). Also, our red-green mixtures do not include a strictly achromatic stimulus, although calculations indicate that the black-white process is more sensitive to yellow (equal contrasts of red and green) than the blue-yellow process in nearly all subjects; thus, red-green and black-white losses can be compared using the red-green mixture thresholds.

In choosing a technique for studying post-receptoral losses in acquired colour defects, one needs to take into account how well any method isolates one of the three post-receptoral detection processes as well as the sensitivity of that method in detecting loss of that process. For the blue-yellow process, the two-colour technique (e.g. blue on yellow) provides excellent isolation and may also be more sensitive than other methods (Kalloniatis et al., 1993). For the red-green process, the last method discussed ('post-receptoral silent substitution'), provides better isolation than measuring spectral sensitivity on a white background (Chioran et al., 1985).

6.6.3 REFERENCES

BOYNTON, R.M. & WAGNER, M. (1961) Two-color threshold as test of color vision, *Journal of the Optical Society of America*, **51**, 429–440.

CHIORAN, G.M., SELLERS, K.L., BENES, S.C., LUBOW, M., DAIN, S.J. & KING-SMITH, P.E. (1985) A new method for analysis, classification and diagnosis of neuro-ophthalmic disease, *Documenta Ophthalmologica*, **61**, 119–135.

FALLOWFIELD, L. & KRAUSKOPF, J. (1984) Selective loss of chromatic sensitivity in demyelinating disease, *Investigative Ophthalmology and Visual Science*, **25**, 771–773.

GOURAS, P. (1991) Precortical physiology of colour vision. In: Gouras, P. (Ed.) *The Perception of Colour*, London: MacMillan, pp. 163–178.

GRIGSBY, S.S., VINGRYS, A.J., BENES, S.C. & KING-SMITH, P.E. (1991) Correlation of chromatic, spatial and temporal sensitivity in optic nerve disease, *Investigative Ophthalmology and Visual Science*, **32**, 3252–3262.

HURVICH, L.M. & JAMESON, D. (1957) An opponent process theory of color vision, *Psychological Reviews*, **64**, 384–404.

JOHNSON, C.A., ADAMS, A.J., CASSON, E.J. & BRANDT, J.D. (1993) Progression of visual field loss as detected by blue-on-yellow and standard white-on-white automated perimetry, *Archives of Ophthalmology*, **111**, 651–656.

KALLONIATIS, M., HARWERTH, R.S., SMITH, E.L. & DeSANTIS, L. (1993) Color vision anomalies following experimental glaucoma in monkeys, *Ophthalmic and Physiological Optics*, **13**, 56–67.

KING-SMITH, P.E. (1991) Psychophysical methods for the investigation of acquired colour vision deficiencies. In: Foster, D.H. (Ed.) *Inherited and Acquired Colour Vision Deficiencies*, London: MacMillan, pp. 38–55.

KING-SMITH, P.E. & CARDEN, D. (1976) Luminance and opponent color contributions to visual detection and adaptation and to temporal and spatial integration, *Journal of the Optical Society of America*, **66**, 709–717.

KING-SMITH, P.E., KRANDA, K. & WOOD, I.C.J. (1976) An acquired color defect of the opponent color system, *Investigative Ophthalmology*, **15**, 584–587.

KING-SMITH, P.E., ROSTEN, J.G., ALVAREZ, S.L. & BHARGAVA, S.K. (1980) Human vision without tonic ganglion cells? In: Verriest G. (Ed.) *Colour Vision Deficiencies V*, Bristol: Adam Hilger, pp. 99–105.

KING-SMITH, P.E., VINGRYS, A.J., BENES, S.C., GRIGSBY, S.S. & BILLOCK, V.A. (1989) Detection of light and dark, red and green, blue and yellow. In: Kulikowski, J.J., Dickinson, C.M. and Murray, I.J. (Eds) *Seeing Contour and Colour*, Oxford: Pergamon Press, pp. 381–391.

KRAUSKOPF, J., WILLIAMS, D.R. & HEELEY, D.W. (1982) Cardinal directions in color space, *Vision Research*, **22**, 1123–1131.

MARRÉ, M. (1973) The investigation of acquired colour deficiencies. In: *Colour 73*, London: Adam Hilger, pp. 99–135.

MASSOF, R.W. & FINKELSTEIN, D. (1979) Rod sensitivity relative to cone sensitivity in retinitis pigmentosa, *Investigative Ophthalmology and Visual Science*, **18**, 263–272.

SELLERS, K.L., CHIORAN, G.M., DAIN, S.J., BENES, S.C., LUBOW, M., RAMMOHAN, K. & KING-SMITH, P.E. (1986) Red-green mixture thresholds in congenital and acquired color defects, *Vision Research*, **26**, 1083–1097.

SPERLING, H.G. & HARWERTH, R.S. (1971) Red-green cone interactions in the increment threshold spectral sensitivity of primates, *Science*, **172**, 180–184.

STILES, W.S. (1978) *Mechanisms of Colour Vision*, New York: Academic Press.

TRAUTZETTEL-KLOSINSKI, S. & AULHORN E. (1987) Measurement of brightness sensation caused by flickering light. A simple and highly specific test for assessing the florid stage of optic neuritis, *Clinical Vision Sciences*, **2**, 63–82.

WALD, G. (1964) The receptors of human color vision, *Science*, **145**, 1007–1017.

YU, T.C., FALCAO-REIS, F., SPILEERS W. & ARDEN, G.B. (1991) Peripheral color contrast: a new screening test for preglaucomatous visual loss, *Investigative Ophthalmology and Visual Science*, **32**, 2779–2789.

ZISMAN, F., KING-SMITH, P.E. & BHARGAVA, S.K. (1978) Spectral sensitivities of acquired color defects analyzed in terms of color opponent theory, *Modern Problems in Ophthalmology*, **19**, 254–257.

Electrophysiological Investigation of Adult and Infant Colour Vision Deficiencies.

N.R.A. Parry and I.J. Murray

6.7.1 INTRODUCTION

In previous studies, we have shown that occipital Visual Evoked Potentials (VEPs) can best reflect the integrity of red-green opponency when isoluminant gratings are presented in on-off mode (e.g. Murray *et al.*, 1987). The negative going waveform seen at isoluminance reverts to a positive-going 'achromatic' response at non-isoluminant red-green ratios. Furthermore, the symmetry between responses to onset and to offset of achromatic gratings indicates that these stimuli favour transient neural mechanisms, while the asymmetric chromatic responses show the presence of a substantial sustained component (Kulikowski and Parry, 1987). The chromatic-achromatic differences are best revealed when low contrast is used, as might be expected from primate studies. Macaque studies using chromatic or achromatic stimuli of low contrast and low spatial frequency showed relatively selective activation of parvocellular and magnocellular streams (Tootell *et al.*, 1988). In this chapter, we describe some of our adult and infant studies of normal and defective colour vision.

6.7.1.1 Inherited colour vision deficiencies

Individuals with inherited colour vision deficiencies can be classified as dichromats or anomalous trichromats. The former appear to have a 'missing' cone mechanism, either red (protanopes) or green (deuteranopes), whereas in the protanomals and deuteranomals both red and green cones appear to be present, but the function of one or other is abnormal. Dichromats do not generally show red-green opponency in their central visual field (Romeskie and Yager, 1978), while this is to some extent preserved in anomalous trichromats (Romeskie, 1978). Therefore, a VEP that reflects the activity of colour opponent mechanisms might be expected to distinguish between these two groups.

Abnormalities of colour vision have been revealed when coloured stimuli are used to generate VEPs. Regan and Spekreijse (1974) showed that onset of red-green checkerboards elicited a response in colour-normals, but not in a deuteranope. Murray *et al.* (1987) produced similar findings in their study of responses to chromatic and achromatic gratings. In the present study we consider the extent to which the evoked potential can discriminate dichromats from anomalous trichromats. The VEP might be expected to exhibit different properties when the red-green ratio is varied for subjects with qualitatively different forms of colour vision deficiency.

6.7.1.2 Development of chromatic vision in infants

There is some doubt as to when trichromatic vision is fully established in infants. The foveae of infants are very immature at birth, there is a relatively large rod-free area and the outer segments of the foveal cones are short (Yuodelis and Hendrickson, 1986). Anatomical studies (Hickey, 1977) suggest that the parvocellular pathway, which mediates colour vision, remains immature until around 12 months postnatal. There is, however, a wealth of behavioural and electrophysiological studies showing that some form of chromatic vision is established much earlier. Brown and Teller (1989) were able to demonstrate a notch in the spectral sensitivity function of three-month-old infants at around 580 nm indicating the presence of red-green opponent mechanisms. Allen *et al.* (1993) used rapid contrast reversal stimuli to generate VEPs and suggested that apparent delays in development of colour vision can be attributed simply to a generalised lack of visual sensitivity. Morrone *et al.* (1993), again using reversal stimuli, claimed that chromatic and achromatic vision develop at different rates with chromatic responses being evident at 8–10 weeks postnatal, whilst achromatic responses were present from birth. For a review of these issues see Brown (1990) and Teller's chapter in this volume (pp. 217–224).

In the adult studies reported here we concentrate on the differences between anomalous trichromats and dichromats. We also report preliminary observations on the development of chromatic on-off VEPs in colour normal infants and those with a family history of inherited colour vision deficiency.

6.7.2   METHODS

6.7.2.1 Stimulus

Sinusoidal gratings were generated using a 12-bit Millipede VR1000 grating generator in an Opus PCV microcomputer, and displayed on a Barco Calibrator high-resolution colour monitor with a frame refresh rate of 100Hz. Red and green gratings were superimposed in antiphase and their mean luminances (R and G respectively) adjusted to give a range of red-green ratios $(R/(R+G))$ between 0 (green only) and 1 (red only). Contrast was defined using the Michelson equation $(C = (Lmax - Lmin)/(Lmax + Lmin)$, where Lmax and Lmin are the grating's maximum and minimum luminance). Chromatic contrast can be operationally defined as the Michelson contrast of the constituent gratings (Regan, 1973). Because of the overlap of the spectral characteristics of TV phosphors, we normally apply a correction factor of 0.25 log units, which gives a maximum chromatic contrast of 0.56 when red-green ratio is 0.5 (Murray *et al.*, 1987). However, because both contrast and red-green ratio are manipulated in the present study, we refer throughout this paper to the achromatic contrast of the red and green components, which were always equal. At maximum contrast (component contrast = 1), the constituent gratings had unity luminance contrast, and one spatial cycle of the displayed pattern changed from 'pure' red to 'pure' green. Temporal presentation was on-off: gratings were presented for 270 ms then replaced for 270 ms with a plain field, with no change in space-averaged hue or luminance (30 cdm^{-2}). Other conditions differed in the two studies; these are described in the relevant sections.

6.7.2.2 VEP recording

Visual evoked potentials were recorded monopolarly from a Ag/AgCl electrode mounted on the occipital scalp at position Oz (on the midline, at a distance above the inion corresponding to 10 per cent of the inion-nasion distance; this is usually about 3.5 cm in adults and 2.5 cm in infants). Reference was provided by linked ear electrodes (adults) or a right mastoid electrode (infants). The earth electrode was placed on either the forehead (adults) or the left mastoid (infants). Electrode impedance was kept below 2kΩ. Signals were amplified and averaged using a Medelec Sensor system (bandwidth 0.3–30 Hz). The VR1000 grating generator card was modified by the manufacturers to provide a trigger impulse that could be gated by the monitor's vertical synchronisation pulse. Consequently the averager trigger always occurred at the beginning of a video frame. Each sweep was triggered by grating onset and each VEP waveform was the average of 128 sweeps.

6.7.3   EXPERIMENT 1: DIFFERENTIATING DICHROMACY FROM ANOMALOUS TRICHROMACY

Spatial frequency was 2c/deg. Viewing distance was 162cm. A centrally fixated circular field, 3º in diameter, was used. Each subject set isoluminance using heterochromatic flicker photometry, determining the red-green ratio (RGR) giving the minimum percept of flicker when the gratings were phase-reversing at 12.5Hz. In this chapter the use of the term 'isoluminant' refers simply to the RGR giving minimum flicker, and is not intended to carry any implications about chromatic stimulation for a given subject.

One colour-normal subject (NRAP) and four colour defectives participated in this study. Subjects were classified using a Nagel Model I anomaloscope (Schmidt and Haensch). Two were classified as dichromats as they matched yellow to all combinations of red and green; one was a protanope and one a deuteranope. The other two were anomalous trichromats with anomalous quotients (AQ) of 3.81 (protanomal) and 0.39 (deuteranomal). NRAP's AQ was 1.12. All three had narrow matching ranges, and all five subjects had corrected visual acuity of at least 6/6.

6.7.3.1 Results and comments

In this experiment, VEPs were recorded in all five subjects for gratings with a range of red-green ratios (RGR) and component contrast of 0.2. Where possible, extra recordings were made around each subject's isoluminant point.

In Figure 6.7.1, the normal results (NRAP, column A) confirm the effect described by our earlier papers (e.g. Carden *et al.*, 1985; Murray *et al.*, 1987). At extremes of the RGR, when the grating was achromatic (luminance-modulated red or green), the onset response was characterised by a major positivity with a time-to-peak (latency) of 130ms. Also noteworthy is the similarity between green-only and red-only VEPs. Given the fact that they are both achromatic, their temporal modulation would be expected to activate the same neural mechanism. There is a marked similarity between the responses to achromatic onset and offset. Stimulus offset is an event that activates principally transient mechanisms,

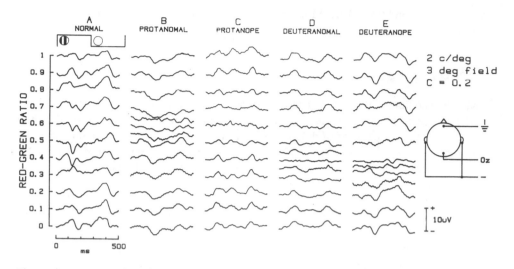

Figure 6.7.1. Visual evoked potentials generated by one normal and four colour deficient observers. Red and green sinusoidal gratings were superimposed in antiphase and their relative mean luminances (R and G) varied to produce red-green ratios (R/(R + G)) from 0 (green only) to 1 (red only). Timing: 270ms on, 270ms off. Mean luminance 30 cdm⁻². Isoluminant red-green ratios: A = 0.5, B = 0.64, C = 0.58, D = 0.39 and E = 0.37.

eliciting VEPs related to the transient change in contrast. It is thus considered to be equivalent to contrast reversal (Estevez and Spekreijse, 1974; Kulikowski, 1977; Kriss and Halliday, 1978). Onset can activate both sustained and transient mechanisms, although in what proportion depends on the other stimulus characteristics (Kulikowski, 1977). Thus, when on and off times are equal, a major difference between on and off responses is indicative of the presence of a sustained mechanism; by implication, their similarity suggests a principally transient mechanism.

NRAP's isoluminant RGR was 0.5. As RGR approached this value, there was a marked transition in the shape of the onset response, which became principally negative-going, with the same latency (130ms) as the achromatic positivity. The offset response did not undergo any substantial transition, remaining positive-going at all RGRs. The resultant marked distinction between chromatic on and off responses reflects the sustained nature of the chromatic onset response, as demonstrated by Kulikowski and Parry (1987).

One feature common to all the colour defective data (Figure 6.7.1, columns B–E) was that there was a range of RGRs where the VEP was barely discernable from noise. In each case this coincided approximately with the isoluminant RGR (see caption). Nulling of the VEP has been used in previous studies as evidence of a red-green colour vision deficiency (Allen *et al.*, 1990; Berninger *et al.*, 1989; Murray *et al.*, 1987; Parry *et al.*, 1987; Regan and Spekreijse, 1974). Certainly, a null response would be expected in the dichromatic VEP data. As already discussed, these subjects are unlikely to show an opponent-type response to red-green stimulation. There are, however, fundamental differences between dichromats and trichromats and it is surprising that these are not reflected more fully in the red-green ratio data. As a degree of red-green opponency is likely to be present in the anomalous trichromatic central visual field (e.g. Romeskie, 1978), we would expect to see some form of 'chromatic' VEP near their isoluminant point. One possible explanation for the absence of such a response is that the chromatic contrast used here was insufficient to modulate their anomalous colour opponent mechanism.

If the chromaticities of the red and green phosphors of a colour TV are plotted on the CIE chromaticity diagram, they can be seen to lie along both protanopic and deuteranopic confusion lines (Pitt, 1935). Reducing the contrast of a red-green grating decreases the separation of the chromaticities of the red and green bars. The nature of these confusion lines suggests that these colours will be confused by a dichromat, whatever the contrast. If the colour confusions of the anomalous trichromats were plotted on the same physical colour space, the result is likely to be a compromise between dichromatic confusion lines and the small ellipses that describe normal colour vision (MacAdam, 1942), appearing as enlarged zones of confusion (Birch, 1973). It would then follow that, if the contrast of a red-green grating is increased sufficiently for its chromaticities to fall outside an anomalous trichromat's confusion zone, then a measurable VEP should be obtained at isoluminance. This response should reflect sustained neural characteristics. No such transition should occur in dichromats. To test this, VEPs were recorded from the same five subjects as before. Six levels of component contrast were employed, between 0.1 and 1.0. For each subject, the RGR that gave minimum flicker was used. Finally, VEPs were recorded at maximum contrast as RGR was varied. Other conditions were the same as in experiment 1.

Figure 6.7.2 shows the effect of increasing chromatic contrast in the colour normal and the four classes of colour defect. Note that their isoluminant red-green ratio was unaffected by this increase in contrast. In each case, the lowermost waveform was generated by an achromatic high contrast pattern, taken from the extreme point of the high-contrast red-green ratio run (broken lines). Together, this waveform and the highest contrast isoluminant VEP are representative of the full range of red-green ratio data, which are therefore not reproduced here. The figure shows that, at higher contrasts, VEPs were obtained to chromatic stimulation contrast in all four colour defective subjects, as well as the normal. There were, however, qualitative differences between the responses generated by the dichromats and the anomalous trichromats.

Both anomalous trichromats (B and D) had isoluminant onset responses which differed from the offset; indeed, an offset response was barely recordable even at the highest contrast. As we have already described, this suggests that the overall responses were

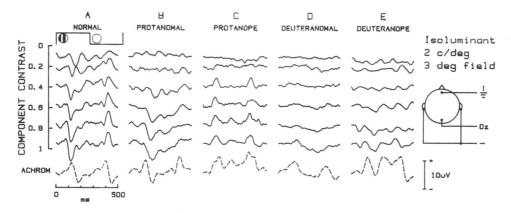

Figure 6.7.2. Solid lines: isoluminant VEPs as a function of contrast. Subjects and other conditions as in Figure 6.7.1. Broken lines: responses to high contrast gratings with red-green ratio = 1.

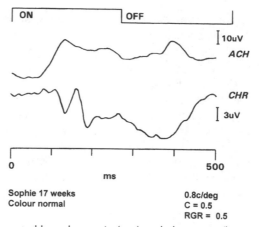

ON   OFF   10uV

ACH

CHR

3uV

0   500

ms

Sophie 17 weeks   0.8c/deg
Colour normal   C = 0.5
RGR = 0.5

Figure 6.7.3. VEPs generated by achromatic (top) and chromatic (botttom) sinusoidal gratings in a 17-week-old baby girl with no family history of colour vision abnormalities. The chromatic negativity was maximal when RGR was 0.5 (lower trace); the achromatic response was elicited by the equivalent yellow/dark-yellow grating. Timing: 270ms on, 270ms off. Spatial frequency: 0.8c/deg. Contrast: 0.5. Mean luminance: 50 cdm^{-2}.

dominated by contributions from sustained mechanisms (see the achromatic data, where onsets were similar to offsets). The VEPs of the dichromats (C and E) behaved in a different fashion. Once contrast was sufficient to elicit a measurable response, they showed little difference between on and off, even at the highest possible contrast. Furthermore, the high contrast 'chromatic' and 'achromatic' responses were similar.

There are major differences in the temporal response characteristics of these dichromats and anomalous trichromats when red-green stimuli are used. Dichromats exhibit only a luminance response that has transient characteristics, manifest in the VEP in the form of similar responses to onset and offset. Anomalous trichromats, who have residual colour opponency, may generate a response similar to that obtained from normals, but only when high contrast is used.

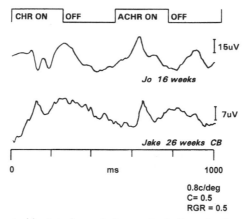

Figure 6.7.4. VEP generated by interleaved chromatic (left) and achromatic (right) sinusoidal gratings in a 16-week-old boy with a 50 per cent chance of inheriting protanomaly (Jo, top trace) and a 26-week-old protanomalous boy (Jake, lower trace). Jo's chromatic negativity was maximal when RGR was 0.5; Jake's responses did not change throughout the range of RGRs. Other conditions as in Figure 6.7.3.

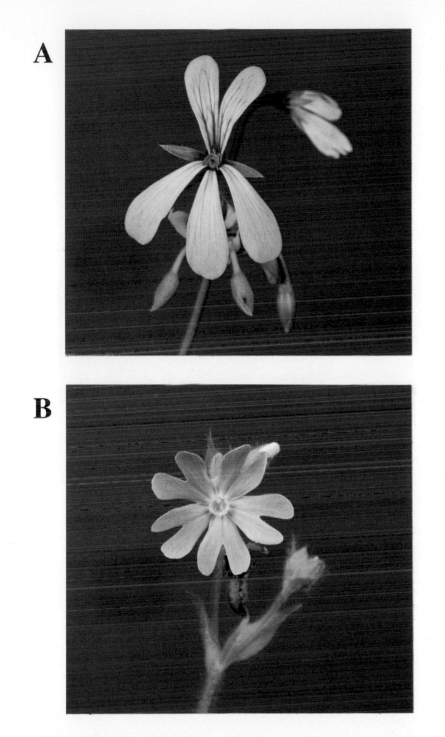

Figure 1.3.1 (a) is *Pelargonium zonale* and (b) is red campion, *Lychnis dioica*.

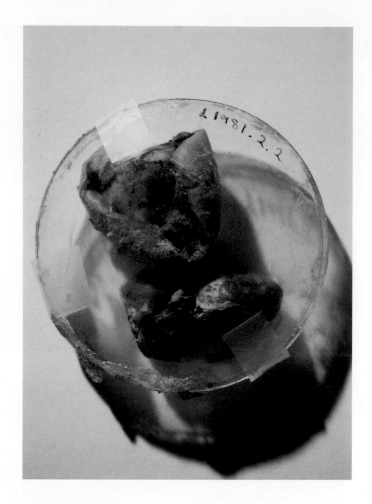

Figure 1.3.2 John Dalton's eye tissue.

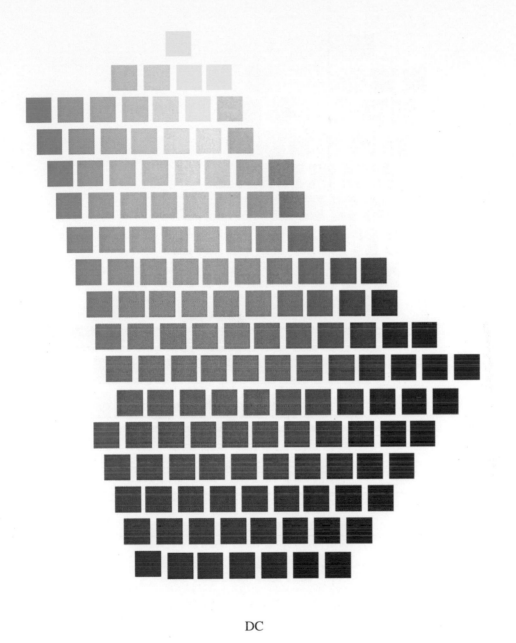

DC

Figure 5.4.12 Colour stimuli representing colours from the deutan line, DC, are visualised in a CIE 1976 u*, L*-diagram.

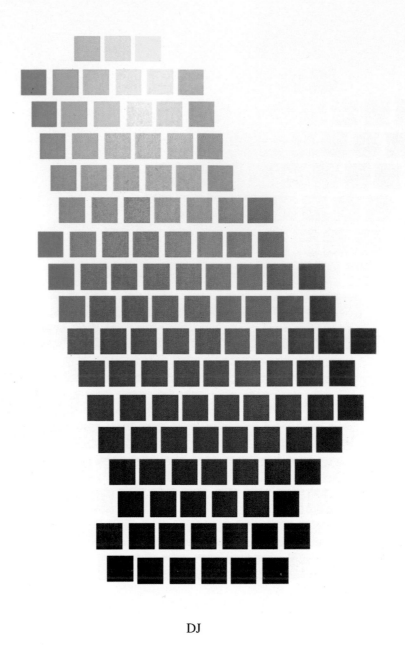

DJ

Figure 5.4.13 Colour stimuli representing colours from the deutan line, DJ, are visualised in a CIE 1976 u*, L*-diagram.

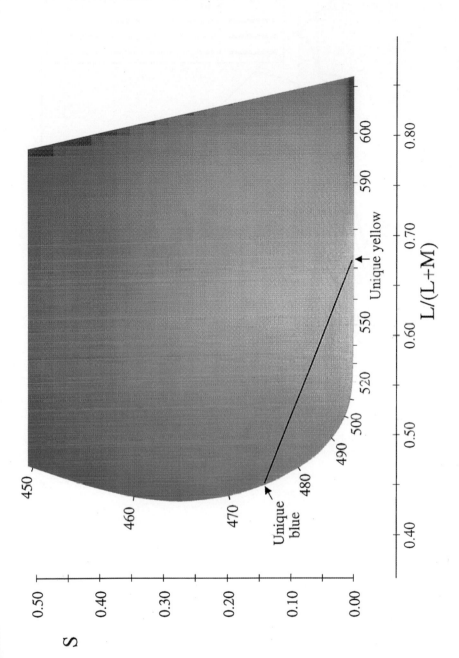

Figure 7.1.1 MacLeod and Boynton chromaticity diagram. The two ordinates of the diagram correspond to the two chromatic channels that have been identified in the early visual system. In this space the line running from unique-yellow to unique-blue is not vertical but oblique. (We are grateful to Ben Regan for preparation of the original colour figure.)

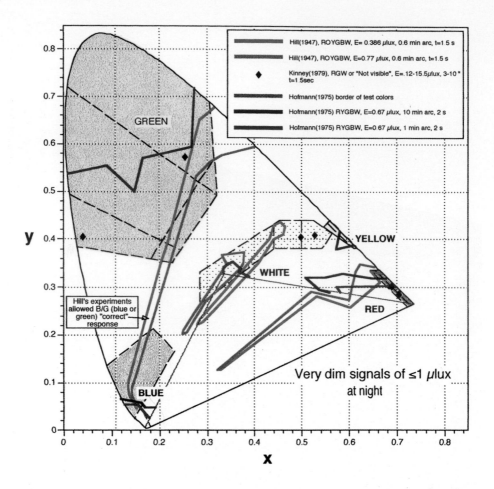

Figure 10.2.1 The 1931 CIE chromaticity diagram showing the 90 per cent probability of recognition contours for very dim signals. The 1975 CIE recommended colour domains are shown by dashed lines.

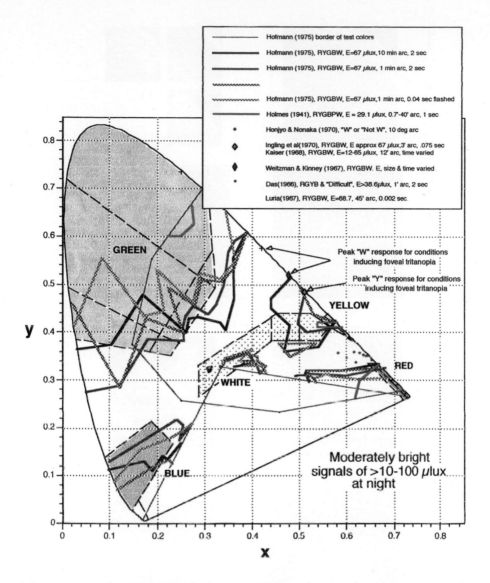

Figure 10.2.2 The 1931 CIE chromaticity diagram showing the 90 per cent probability of recognition contours for moderately bright signals. The 1975 CIE recommended colour domains are shown by dashed lines.

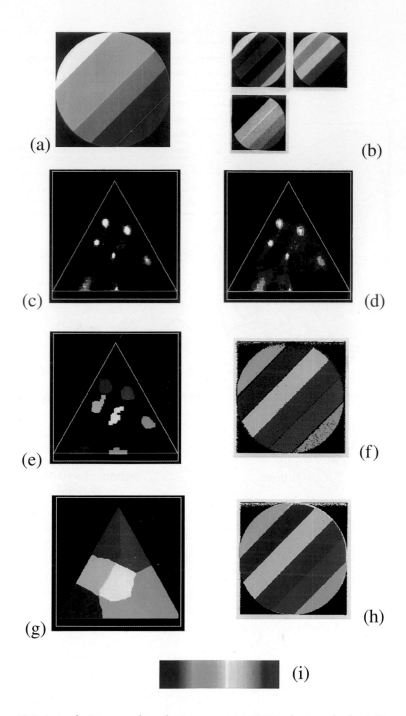

Figure 10.5.4 Analysing a multi-colour pattern. (a) Original artwork. (b) RGB colour separations. (c) Colour scattergram. (d) Pseudo-colour display of the colour scattergram. (e) Processed colour scattergram. (f) PCF output when trained on image (e). (g) Application of colour generalisation. (h) PCF output when trained on image. (i) Pseudo-colour display of an intensity wedge, black on the left and white on the right.

6.7.4 EXPERIMENT 2: DEVELOPMENT OF THE CHROMATIC VEP IN NORMAL AND COLOUR DEFICIENT INFANTS

In this study the stimulus conditions were modified to encourage fixation. A cartoon was displayed on a black and white video monitor, which was placed at right angles to the display screen with a sheet of glass interposed at 45º, thus allowing the two image planes to be superimposed. Although the sound track was played at all times, with the loudspeaker in front of the baby, the two images were not displayed simultaneously. Periodically the gratings were switched off and the video switched on to help the babies attend. Recordings were only made when the baby was watching the gratings. The rest of the room was mesopically illuminated to minimise distraction. To take account of variabilities in the infants' attention, chromatic and achromatic stimuli were interleaved in a single session. Thus each sweep of the VEP was elicited by the following stimulus cycle: chromatic on (270ms); chromatic off 270ms; achromatic on (270ms); achromatic off (270ms).

6.7.4.1 Results and comments

Here we present data from three babies with different likelihoods of inheriting colour vision deficiency. In Figure 6.7.3 it can be seen that a clear chromatic negativity was recorded in a 17-week-old girl with no family history of colour blindness. In all, 14 presumably colour-normal babies were included in this study. In this group, there was no evidence of a chromatic negativity before 14 weeks, despite investigating a range of contrasts and red-green ratios around normal isoluminance. Red-green onset either produced no measurable response, or a small positivity that was similar to the achromatic response. Reversal presentation over a range of red-green ratios produced similar results to other studies (e.g. Allen et al., 1993; Morrone et al., 1993) in that the major effect was a reduction in amplitude. Figure 6.7.4 shows data from a 16-week-old baby boy whose mother was a known carrier of protanomaly. From the clear chromatic negativity we can assume that he had not inherited this. The negativity was maximal at a red-green ratio of 0.5. Also in Figure 6.7.4 are the responses of a 26-week-old boy whose mother was protanomalous and who could therefore be assumed to be similarly affected. At no red-green ratio did his results differ from those shown here; there was no difference between responses to onset of chromatic and achromatic gratings.

6.7.5 DISCUSSION

We have shown that occipital potentials can be used to selectively monitor the activity of parvocellular and magnocellular pathways in the human visual system. In primates, these pathways have different physiological characteristics. Only one mediates chromatic vision and they have different temporal frequency characteristics. Hence the underlying physiology dictates that it is desirable to consider not only the chromaticity of the stimulus but also the difference between onset, offset and reversal responses (Kulikowski and Parry, 1987). It is evident that, in adult dichromats, varying red-green ratio does not change the predominantly transient nature of the responses, whereas anomalous trichromats may show sustained activity (presumably parvo-mediated) if chromatic contrast is sufficiently high.

The precise nature of post-receptoral processing in dichromats is not well understood. Although the molecular genetics of cone pigment abnormalities are being unravelled (see, for example, Jacobs and Calderone's chapter in this volume), the impact this has on the anatomical and physiological characteristics of retinal ganglion cells and parvo and magno cellular pathways remains unclear. Our current experiments on the temporal characteristics of anomalous colour vision are expected to shed further light on these issues.

Our adult studies demonstrate that VEPs to the onset rather than the reversal of isoluminant gratings gives a recordable response that is specific to chromatic processing. One of the cornerstones of this approach is that chromatic processing is sluggish and demands the use of low temporal frequencies. Fast reversal can be used to reveal chromatic processing in the sense that a zero response is obtained at isoluminance (Kulikowski and Russell, 1989; Kulikowski *et al.*, 1991). This might explain some of the controversy surrounding the presumed onset of adult-like colour vision in early infancy (Allen *et al.*, 1993; Morrone *et al.*, 1993) as these studies used reversing stimuli. We have observed that the chromatic onset negativity seen in adults is not recorded before about 14 weeks of age. This would suggest that before then the chromatic visual system is immature. What remains uncertain is the relative rates of maturation of the chromatic and achromatic pathways (Allen *et al.*, 1993). The on-off studies illustrated in this chapter complement the use of contrast reversal in that they monitor *directly* the activity of the parvocellular pathway.

6.7.6   ACKNOWLEDGEMENTS

We are grateful for the help and cooperation of our subjects and the families whose babies volunteered so willingly. Our infant studies were supported by the Medical Research Council.

6.7.7   REFERENCES

ALLEN, D., BANKS, M.S., NORCIA, A.M. & SHANNON, L. (1990) Human infants' VEP responses to isoluminant stimuli, *Investigative Ophthalmology and Visual Science*, **31**, 10.

ALLEN, D., BANKS, M.S. & NORCIA, A.M. (1993) Does chromatic sensitivity develop more slowly than luminance sensitivity? *Vision Research*, **33**, 2553–2562.

BERNINGER, T.A., ARDEN, G.B., HOGG, C.R. & FRUMKES, T. (1989), Separable evoked retinal and cortical potentials from each major visual pathway: preliminary results, *British Journal of Ophthalmology*, **73**, 502–511.

BIRCH, J. (1973) Dichromatic convergence points obtained by subtractive colour matching, *Vision Research*, **13**, 1755–1765.

BROWN, A. (1990) Development of visual sensitivity to light and colour vision in human infants: A critical review, *Vision Research*, **30**, 1159–1188.

BROWN, A. & TELLER, D.Y. (1989) Chromatic opponency in 3-month-old human infants, *Vision Research*, **29**, 37–46.

CARDEN, D., KULIKOWSKI, J.J., MURRAY, I.J. & PARRY, N.R.A. (1985) Human occipital potentials evoked by the onset of equiluminant chromatic gratings, *Journal of Physiology*, **369**, 44P.

ESTEVEZ, O. & SPEKREIJSE, H. (1974) Relationship between pattern appearance-disappearance and pattern reversal responses, *Experimental Brain Research*, **19**, 233–235.

HICKEY, T.L. (1977) Postnatal development of human lateral geniculate nucleus: Relationship to a critical period for the visual system, *Science*, **198**, 836–838.

KRISS, A. & HALLIDAY, A.M. (1978) A comparison of occipital potentials evoked by pattern onset, offset and reversal by movement. In: Barber, C. (Ed.) *Evoked Potentials I*, Lancaster: MTP.

KULIKOWSKI, J.J. (1977) Separation of occipital potentials related to the detection of pattern and movement. In: Desmedt, J.E. (Ed.) *Visual Evoked Potentials in Man: New Developments*, Oxford: Clarendon.

KULIKOWSKI, J.J. & PARRY, N.R.A. (1987) Human occipital potentials evoked by achromatic or chromatic checkerboards and gratings, *Journal of Physiology*, **388**, 45P.

KULIKOWSKI, J.J. & RUSSELL, M.H.A. (1989) Electroretinograms and visual evoked potentials elicited by chromatic and achromatic gratings. In: Kulikowski, J.J., Dickinson, C.M. & Murray, I.J. (Eds) *Seeing Contour and Colour*, Oxford: Pergamon Press.

KULIKOWSKI, J.J., MURRAY, I.J. & RUSSELL, M.H.A. (1991) Effect of stimulus size on chromatic and achromatic VEPs. In: Drum, B., Moreland, J.D. & Serra, A. (Eds) *Colour Vision Deficiencies X*, Dordrecht: Kluwer.

MACADAM, D.L. (1942) Visual sensitivities to color difference in daylight, *Journal of the Optical Society of America*, **32**, 247–274.

MORRONE M.C., BURR, D.C. & FIORENTINI, A. (1993) Development of infant contrast sensitivity to chromatic stimuli, *Vision Research*, **33**, 2535–2552.

MURRAY, I.J., PARRY, N.R.A., CARDEN, D. & KULIKOWSKI, J.J. (1987) Human visual evoked potentials to chromatic and achromatic gratings, *Clinical Vision Science*, **1**, 231–244.

PARRY, N.R.A., MURRAY, I.J. & KULIKOWSKI, J.J. (1987) VEPs to chromatic stimulation: comparison of normals and colour defectives, *Electroencephalography and Clinical Neurophysiology*, **67**, 75P.

PITT, F.H.G. (1935) Characteristics of dichromatic vision with an appendix on anomalous trichromatic vision, *Special Report Series No. 200*, Medical Research Council, London: HMSO.

REGAN, D. (1973) Evoked potentials specific to spatial patterns of luminance and colour, *Vision Research*, **13**, 2381–2402.

REGAN, D. & SPEKREIJSE, H. (1974) Evoked potential indications of colour blindness, *Vision Research*, **14**, 89–95.

ROMESKIE, M (1978) Chromatic opponent-response functions of anomalous trichromats, *Vision Research*, **18**, 1521–1532.

ROMESKIE, M. & YAGER, D. (1978) Psychophysical measures and theoretical analysis of dichromatic opponent-response functions, *Modern Problems in Ophthalmology*, **19**, 212–217.

TOOTELL, R.B.H., HAMILTON, S.L. & SWITKES, E. (1988) Functional anatomy of macaque striate cortex. IV. Contrast and magno-parvo streams, *Journal of Neuroscience*, **8**, 1594–1609.

YUODELIS, C. & HENDRICKSON, A. (1986) A qualitative and quantitative analysis of the human fovea during development, *Vision Research*, **26**, 847–855.

Clinical Applications of an Automated Test of Chromatic Discrimination

S.J. Tregear, L.G. Ripley, P.J. Knowles, V. Tanner,
D.V. de Alwis, J.P. Reffin, S.V. Vickers, A.G. Casswell
and R.T. Gilday

6.8.1 INTRODUCTION

We have developed an automated cathode ray tube (CRT) based chromatic discrimination test that has been specifically designed to be used in a clinical environment (de Alwis, 1993; de Alwis *et al.*, 1993; Reffin, 1992; Tregear *et al.*, 1993; Tregear *et al.*, 1994). The system enables us to measure chromatic discrimination along any chromatic axis in colour space bounded by the gamut of the CRT. We have found that a constant R/G-cone (tritan) axis and a constant S-cone (red-green) axis, which pass through white, are most useful (Figure 6.8.1). These chromatic axes correspond to the cardinal axes in CIE colour space that were originally proposed by Krauskopf *et al.* (1982).

Chromatic stimuli are presented in the form of a static, isoluminant, sinusoidal, low spatial frequency (0.66 cpd) grating on a high resolution CRT (luminance: 20 cdm^{-2}). Test subjects are positioned 2m from the CRT so that the stimuli subtend a central visual angle of 4° and are then instructed to press a hand-held button if they see stripes on the screen following an auditory warning tone. They are instructed not to press the button if stripes are not seen or if they are unsure. To ensure that the subject understands the procedure, a short practice routine is performed binocularly. The test proper is then carried out monocularly on one or both of the subject's eyes with the eye not being tested occluded.

The chromaticity of the gratings is modulated about the white point along either the red-green or tritan axis. The chromatic amplitudes at which the subject can just distinguish gratings are determined using a double staircase reversal algorithm (Cornsweet, 1962). These are taken to be measures of the red-green and tritan discrimination thresholds respectively.

A complete test session, which involves giving instructions to the subject, a practice routine, and measurement of red-green and tritan discrimination in both eyes, takes an average of 15 minutes. All procedures are carried out under automated software control with the user interface being an easy-to-operate Microsoft Windows based system.

In this chapter we present some of the work that we have carried out at the Sussex Eye Hospital where we have assessed the usefulness of automated chromatic discrimination testing in a clinical environment.

6.8.2 CHROMATIC DISCRIMINATION AND DIABETIC RETINOPATHY

Diabetic retinopathy is the most common cause of blindness amongst the working age group in the western world (Grey *et al.*, 1989; Herman *et al.*, 1983; Jerneld, 1987; National Diabetes Data Group, 1985; Sjølie and Green, 1987; Sorsby, 1972). This should not be the case in that most forms of retinopathy can be treated effectively using laser photocoagulation. Unfortunately, many diabetics who have retinopathy are not picked up in the early

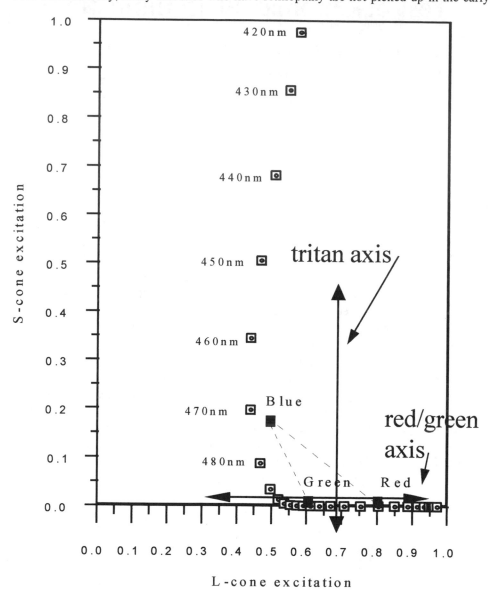

Figure 6.8.1. The position of the constant R/G-cone (tritan) and the constant S-cone (red-green) axis in constant luminance cone excitation space as proposed by MacLeod and Boynton (1979, 1980). Both axes pass through the white point with CIE co-ordinates 0.33, 0.33 (on conversion to CIE colour space). The solid boxes labeled Red, Green and Blue represent the position of the three CRT phosphors used.

stages of the disease when laser treatment would be most effective. Great efforts are now being made to improve the ways in which diabetics are screened in an attempt to decrease the number of blind registrations due to diabetic retinopathy. Ideally, all diabetics would be examined once a year by an ophthalmologist. This is, however, not practical and, as a result, different methods of screening the diabetic population for severe diabetic retinopathy need to be developed that are not only sensitive, but cost effective. Automated chromatic discrimination testing is a candidate for such a role.

We have measured red-green and tritan discrimination thresholds in 358 eyes of 358 diabetic patients. Each diabetic eye was graded into one of five categories depending on its retinopathy status as determined by an ophthalmologist using an ophthalmoscope and a 78 D lens through dilated pupils. The five categories were: no retinopathy; background retinopathy; maculopathy; ischaemic (pre-proliferative) retinopathy; and proliferative retinopathy. Those patients classified as being in the maculopathy, ischaemic retinopathy or proliferative retinopathy sub-groups were classified as having severe diabetic retinopathy, which is potentially sight threatening. Exclusion criteria included history of other eye disease, presence of a diabetic cataract, and previous laser treatment. Patients taking prescribed drugs other than those related to diabetes were deliberately not excluded because it is common for diabetics to be taking other medication.

We have found that tritan discrimination thresholds were increased more than red-green discrimination thresholds in all diabetic sub-groups (Figure 6.8.2). Furthermore, we have found that it was possible to use the tritan discrimination threshold obtained to screen for severe diabetic retinopathy. When compared to normal age-matched tritan discrimination threshold data obtained from 150 normal controls, it was found that 97 per cent of diabetics with maculopathy, 67 per cent of diabetics with ischaemic (pre-proliferative) retinopathy, and 93 per cent of diabetics with proliferative retinopathy had abnormal tritan discrimination thresholds. However, 18 per cent of diabetics with no retinopathy and 30 per cent of diabetics with background retinopathy also had abnormal tritan discrimination thresholds. Thus it can be seen that although tritan discrimination is very sensitive, it is not very specific. A good screening technique needs to flag effectively those patients who have severe diabetic retinopathy (high sensitivity) but it should not flag those patients with non-severe diabetic retinopathy (high specificity).

As a result we decided to investigate the possibility that the abnormal tritan discrimination thresholds seen in the diabetics with non-severe diabetic retinopathy were preceding a deterioration in retinopathy status to severe diabetic retinopathy. To this end we have recalled those patients who were originally categorised as having non-severe diabetic retinopathy 18 months after the initial test. Each was re-examined by an experienced ophthalmologist (PJK) to establish whether a deterioration in retinopathy status had occured. To date, 87 such patients have been re-examined. It turned out that 12 of the 19 (63 per cent) of the diabetics originally classified as having background retinopathy and who showed abnormal tritan discrimination deteriorated to a more severe form of retinopathy. However, only 6 of the 68 (9 per cent) diabetics originally classified as having background retinopathy and who had normal triton discrimination showed such a deterioration. These findings show that those patients with non-severe diabetic retinopathy and abnormal tritan discrimination are significantly more at risk of developing severe diabetic retinopathy within the next 18 months than are those with normal tritan discrimination (χ^2 $p < 0.0001$).

The results obtained to date lead us to conclude that automated tritan discrimination testing provides us with a clinically viable tool with which we can not only detect those diabetics who have severe diabetic retinopathy but those diabetics who are most at risk of developing it within a relatively short space of time.

6.8.3   CHROMATIC DISCRIMINATION AND THYROID EYE DISEASE

Approximately 90 per cent of patients suffering from Graves' hyperthyroidism will develop the related complication of thyroid eye disease (Weetman, 1991). Of these, 5–10 per cent will develop sight-threatening optic nerve compression (Trobe *et al.*, 1978).

Orbital decompression can be carried out via orbital radiotherapy, steroids, or surgical intervention. As with other disease processes, early intervention is desirable and the early

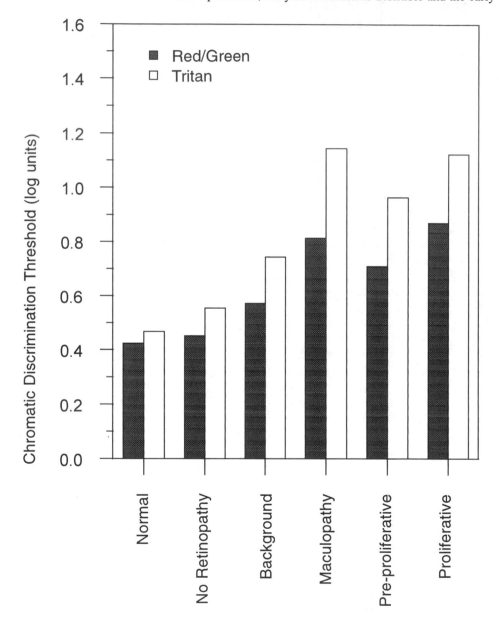

Figure 6.8.2.   The increases in tritan discrimination thresholds and red-green discrimination thresholds, showing the greater increase in the former in all diabetic retinopathy categories.

recognition of optic nerve compression is becoming increasingly important. Unfortunately, the diagnosis of optic nerve compression is often difficult due to its insidious nature.

Traditionally, the methods by which optic nerve compression is assessed include measurement of Snellen visual acuity, observing the presence of a relative afferent pupillary defect (RAPD), examination of the optic disc, and screening for a red-green colour deficit as with the Ishihara plates. Unfortunately the aforementioned indicators are not always present in the early stages of optic nerve compression. It has been demonstrated that up to 50 per cent of patients who have optic nerve compression have normal optic discs and that performance on the Ishihara plates is only significantly decreased if visual acuity is below 20/40 (Trobe *et al.*, 1978).

The Ishihara plates are commonly used in ophthalmic out-patient departments in an attempt to determine early colour-vision deterioration. However, the results of such tests are theoretically flawed as the plates were originally designed as a test of congenital colour deficiency rather than acquired deficiency. Therefore, we feel that the Ishihara test score may not adequately reflect the degree of optic nerve compression present in Dysthyroid Optic Neuropathy (DON). There are other colour vision tests available such as the American Optical (HRR) plates and the Farnsworth-Munsell 100 hue test (FM 100 hue test). However, these require strict testing conditions, and in the case of the FM 100 hue test, a lot of time to administer.

A report already exists that demonstrates that decreased colour sensitivity, as measured with Arden's automated chromatic contrast system, is associated with optic nerve compression (Potts *et al.*, 1990). Encouraged by this we have assessed the viability of automated chromatic discrimination sensitivity as a possible test for the early diagnosis of optic nerve compression using 39 eyes from 39 volunteer thyroid patients.

One eye from each patient was randomly chosen and the automated chromatic discrimination test was then carried out as described earlier. Following this, each patient was assessed by an experienced ophthalmologist using a standard clinical format that included Snellen visual acuity, corneal and conjunctival appearance, lid retraction, exophthalmometer reading, an orthoptic assessment, red-green colour vision using the Ishihara plates, and observing for the presence of a RAPD. Based on the clinical assessment, each patient was then graded using the NOSPECS classification system as originally described by Werner (1969). The NOSPECS classification system is summarised in Table 6.8.1. Patients classified as NOSPECS grade 6 were considered as having clinically significant optic nerve compression.

We found a consistent decrease in chromatic discrimination sensitivity in all cases of

Table 6.8.1.   The NOSPECS classification as described by Werner (1969). This is the classification system used to classify clinically the patients with thyroid eye disease in this paper.

Grade	Description
Grade 0	No ocular symptoms
Grade 1	Only signs, no symptoms: signs limited to upper lid retraction with or without lid lag and mild proptosis.
Grade 2	Soft tissue involvement: oedema of conjunctivae or lids, extrusion of orbital fat.
Grade 3	Proptosis: mild 21–23 mm: moderate 24–27 mm: marked >28 mm.
Grade 4	Extrinsic muscle involvement.
Grade 5	Corneal involvement: minimal, corneal stippling: moderate, ulceration: marked, necrosis and perforation.
Grade 6	Sight loss secondary to optic nerve involvement.

optic nerve compression (NOSPECS grade 6). This decrease was also found in three patients who were classified as non-compressive (NOSPECS grade 5). No other non-compressive patients showed a decrease in chromatic discrimination sensitivity. The greatest decrease in chromatic discrimination seen in the patients with reduced colour vision occurred on the tritan axis. All three of the patients who were classified as grade 5 and who had reduced colour vision subsequently developed clinically significant optic nerve compression within a few months of the original classification.

We believe that monitoring chromatic discrimination, especially along a tritan confusion axis, provides the ophthalmologist with a sensitive tool that will help in the early diagnosis of optic nerve compression in patients suffering from thyroid eye disease.

6.8.4 CHROMATIC DISCRIMINATION AND OPTIC NEURITIS RECOVERY

Several studies have investigated colour discrimination sensitivity in patients with chronic deficits (Alvarez et al., 1982; Fallowfield and Krauskopf, 1984; Ménage et al., 1993; Mullen and Plant, 1987). Most of these investigations have examined a number of selected patients with chronic optic neuritis (ON) who have continued to complain of visual symptoms after the ON attack had long since subsided. The time since the attack has rarely been considered and, in general, patients were considered stable or chronic if more than two months had passed since the attack. For this study it was hypothesised that a better understanding of the relationship between colour vision and optic neuritis could be gained by studying the dynamics of the recovery process rather than looking for patterns of residual deficit in chronic patients.

All patients presenting over a six-year period at the Sussex Eye Hospital Accident and Emergency Department with optic neuritis symptoms were considered for this study. Patients who showed evidence of having had a previous attack or who had a history of any other ocular complaints were rejected. Not all suitable patients were recruited. This was mainly due to the impracticalities of their repeated attendance at the hospital. Ten out of the 47 patients originally recruited do not appear in the results. This was due to non-attendance in five cases and a change in diagnosis in a further five cases. Most of the patients in the study received no treatment. However, two patients were given a three-day course of intravenous steroids (methyl-prednisolone) in the first week of the attack. The recovery curves of these two patients did not differ from those who were untreated and their results are included in this study.

On a number of occasions following initial presentation, each patient's chromatic discrimination sensitivities were measured using the automated chromatic discrimination test. Ideally the patients were tested on a weekly basis. However, the frequency of visits depended to a very large degree on the patients' cooperation. As a result, weekly visits were not always possible.

Figure 6.8.3 shows a typical set of serial chromatic discrimination sensitivity results obtained from one of our patients (AK) as central vision recovered. A method of analysing such results was devised that allowed comparisons between subjects and between stimuli conditions. First, the date on which the recovery commenced was determined. This was done by establishing from the patients and from their medical records the date when vision subjectively began to improve. Chromatic discrimination sensitivity data were then translated into recovery curves by subtracting the age-matched normal threshold for each stimulus condition from the measured threshold. Figures 6.8.4a, b, c, and d show examples of typical recovery curves produced using the above method for four different patients.

It can be seen that all the recovery curves show a strong resemblance. In almost all cases, chromatic discrimination recovered in a smooth, continuous and predictable manner being rapid at first and then tailing off with time. It turned out that the recovery curves can be described by using a simple exponential model that encapsulates the observed recovery behaviour using just two coefficients for each patient. The first represents the size of the deficit reached before recovery commences and the second describes its rate of decay. The larger the decay constant, the faster the rate of recovery. The coefficients can be estimated by making straight-line fits to log-transformed data. The intercept of the line with the ordinate axis gives an estimate of the size of the initial deficit and the slope gives an estimate of the decay constant. An extrapolation of the straight line allows a prediction of the time at which the deficit will have decayed to such an extent that vision may be considered normal.

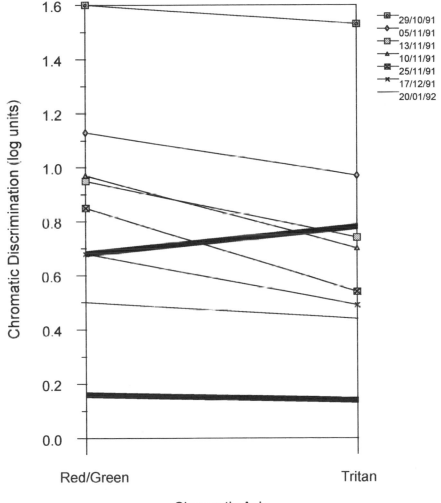

Figure 6.8.3.   A typical set of chromatic discrimination data obtained from a patient (AK) as optic neuritis recovery occurred. The thick solid lines represent the upper and lower limits of normal chromatic discrimination for this patient's age group.

Thus if the deficit is described as:

$$y = A\exp(-Bt)$$

then,

$$\ln(y) = \ln(A) - Bt$$

and recovery time is given by

$$t_r = [\ln(A) - \ln(T)]/B$$

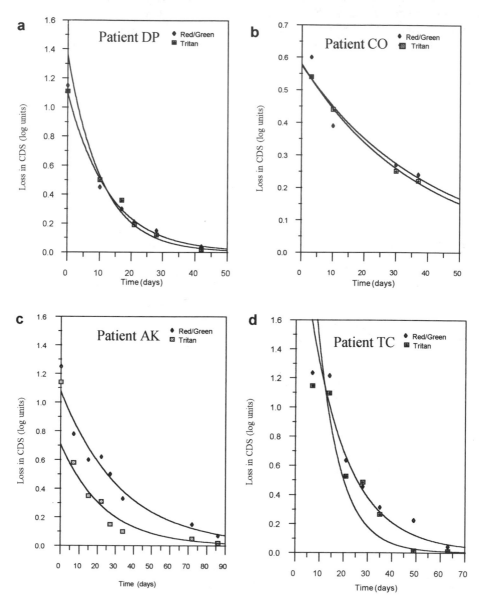

Figure 6.8.4. The recovery in chromatic discrimination of four patients (DP, AK, TC and CO), who suffered unilateral optic neuritis. (Note how well the exponential curves fit the data in all four cases.)

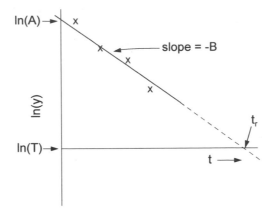

Figure 6.8.5.   Straight-line fit of log-transformed data allows prediction of recovery.

if T is the criterion of normality. We have taken this to be two standard deviations of the age-matched normal threshold. This model is illustrated in Figure 6.8.5.

On analysis of the data using the exponential decay model, it was found that only two patients deviated significantly from that predicted by the model. Both seem to have suffered a second 'clinically silent' attack while recovering from the initial attack. It is not uncommon for further attacks to follow within a week of the primary attack and it is not unusual for these attacks to go unnoticed by the patient. Nuclear magnetic resonance (NMR) studies have demonstrated dramatically that a large number of demyelinating lesions can occur in multiple sclerosis without giving rise to noticeable signs or symptoms (Omerod *et al.*, 1987).

In order that we might understand more about the mechanisms of the recovery process it would be useful to correlate recovery patterns of chromatic discrimination sensitivity with NMR images that can detect changes in optic nerve appearance during recovery. Better understanding of the changes in optic nerve performance during recovery could also be achieved by correlating more closely visual evoked potential data with chromatic discrimination data, particularly using small field evoked potentials from chromatic stimuli (Russell *et al.*, 1991).

Our work on chromatic discrimination and optic nerve recovery following an optic neuritis attack demonstrates how automated chromatic discrimination sensitivity techniques can be used to monitor the progress of recovery following an optic neuritis attack. The exponential recovery model can also be used to predict recovery times for the component sub-systems of central vision at an early stage in the recovery process. This offers significant advantages in the management of optic neuritis patients who are very disturbed by the uncertainty surrounding the prognosis for recovery of vision. Furthermore, the decay model may offer a simple way of looking at the effect of demyelinating lesions and their subsequent recovery elsewhere in the central nervous system.

6.8.5   SUMMARY

Using the automated chromatic discrimination system we have investigated acquired colour vision deficits in patients with diabetes, thyroid eye disease, and optic neuritis. We have shown that tritan discrimination losses can be used to screen for severe diabetic retinopathy and also to predict those who are likely to develop it within 18 months. We have also confirmed that acquired tritan discrimination losses are a very useful indicator of optic-nerve compression in thyroid eye disease. Finally, we have found that colour-vision losses in optic neuritis patients allow us to track recovery of visual function.

The work presented in this chapter is being continued, and further work into other areas is being carried out where we are investigating the effects of other eye diseases on chromatic discrimination in order that we might identify other possible clinical applications for the test. Some of these areas include the investigation of colour vision in asymptomatic and symptomatic HIV patients, colour vision in pseudophakes, and the effects of low-dose radiotherapy used in treatment of thyroid eye disease.

6.8.6   ACKNOWLEDGEMENTS

This work has been supported by grants from the Sir Halley Stewart Trust.

We would like to thank the consultants and the business manager of the Sussex Eye Hospital who have supported this work over the past years: Mr A. F. Harden, Mr A. C. Casswell, Mr D. V. Ingram, Mr G. P. Britain, and Mr J. Basket. We would also like to thank all those who have volunteered to be subjects in this study.

6.8.7   REFERENCES

ALVAREZ, S. *et al.* (1982) Luminance and colour dysfunction in retrobulbar neuritis, *Docum. Ophthal. Proc. Ser.*, **33**, 441.

CORNSWEET, T. N. (1962) The staircase method in psychophysics, *American Journal of Psychology*, **75**, 485–491.

DE ALWIS, D. V., REFFIN, J. P., TREGEAR, S. J., RIPLEY, L.G. & CASSWELL, A.G. (1993) Should management of diabetic retinopathy be based upon measurements of visual function rather than observations of retinal morphology, *Investigative Ophthalmology and Visual Science*, **34**, 719.

DE ALWIS, D. V. (1993) The role of automated chromatic contrast sensitivity tests in the management of diabetic retinopathy, MPhil Thesis, University of Sussex, Falmer, Brighton, UK.

FALLOWFIELD, L. & KRAUSKOPF, J. (1984) Selective loss of chromatic sensitivity in demyelinating disease, *Investigative Ophthalmology and Visual Science*, **25**, 771.

GREY, R. H. B., BURNS-COX, C. J. & HUGHES, A. (1989) Blind and partial sight registration in Avon, *British Journal of Ophthalmology*, **73**, 88–94.

HERMAN, W. H., TEUTSCH, S. M. & SEPO, S. J. (1983) An approach to the prevention of blindness in diabetes, *Diabetes Care*, **6**, 608–613.

JERNELD, B. (1987) Prevalence of diabetic retinopathy: A population study from the Swedish island of Gotland, DPhil Thesis. Department of Ophthalmology, Karolinski Institute, Stockholm, Sweden.

KRAUSKOPF, J., WILLIAMS, D.R. & HEELY, D.N. (1982) The cardinal directions of colour space, *Vision Research*, **22**, 1123– 1131.

MACLEOD, D. I. & BOYNTON, R. M. (1979) Chromaticity diagram showing cone excitation by stimuli of equal luminance, *Journal of the Optical Society of America*, **69**, 1183–1186.

MACLEOD, D. I. & BOYNTON, R. M. (1980) Rectangular chromaticity diagram showing cone excitations at constant luminance, In: Verriest, G. (Ed.) *Colour Deficiencies* V, Bristol: Adam Hilger, 65–68.

MÉNAGE, M. J., PAPAKOSTOPOULOS, D., DEAN-HART, J. C., PAPAKOSTOPOULOS, S. & GOGOLITSYN, YU (1993) The Farnsworth-Munsell 100 hue test in the first episode of demyelinating optic neuritis, *British Journal of Ophthalmology*, **77**, 68.

MULLEN, K. T. & PLANT, G. T. (1987) Anomalies in the appearance of colour and of hue discrimination in optic neuritis, *Clinical Vision Sciences*, **4**, 303.

NATIONAL DIABETES DATA GROUP (1985) Diabetes in America: Diabetes data compiled in 1984, Public Health Services, NIH publication number 85, Bethesda MD: US Department of Health and Human Services, pp. 1468.

OMEROD, I. E. C., MILLER, D.H., MCDONALD, W.I., DU BOULAY, E.P., RUDGE, P., KENDALL, B.E., MOSLEY, I.F., JOHNSON, G., TOFTS, P. & HALLIDAY, A.M. (1987) The role of NMR imaging in the assessment of multiple sclerosis and isolated neurological lesions, *Brain*, **110**, 1579–1616.

POTTS, M. J., FELLS, P., FALCAO-REIS, F., BUCETTI, S. & ARDEN, G. B. (1990) Colour contrast sensitivity, pattern ERGs and cortical evoked potentials in dysthyroid optic neuropathy, *Investigative Ophthalmology and Visual Science*, **31**, 189.

REFFIN, J. P. (1992) The design and clinical application of tests of colour vision, DPhil Thesis, University of Sussex, Falmer, Brighton, UK.

RUSSELL, M.H.A., MURRAY, I.J., METCALFE, R. & KULIKOWSK, J.J. (1991) Visual evoked potentials and psychophysical investigation of chromatic and achromatic visual function in humans: application in the investigation of MS and optic neuritis, *Brain*, **114**, 2419–2435.

SJØLIE, A. K. & GREEN. A. (1987) Blindness in insulin treated diabetic patients with age onset < 30 years, *Journal of Chronic Diseases*, **40**, 215–220.

SORSBY, A. (1972) The incidence and causes of blindness in England and Wales 1963–1968. Report on public health and medical subjects number 128, London: HMSO, pp. 33–51.

TREGEAR, S. J., KNOWLES, P. J., RIPLEY, L. G. & CASSWELL, A. G. (1993) Colour vision deficits predict the development of severe diabetic retinopathy in diabetic subjects with background retinopathy, *Investigative Ophthalmology and Visual Science*, **34**, 719.

TREGEAR, S. J., RIPLEY, L. G., KNOWLES, P. J., GILDAY, R. T., DE ALWIS, D. V. & REFFIN, J. P. (1994) Automated Tritan Discrimination: A new clinical technique for the effective screening of severe diabetic retinopathy, *International Journal of Psychophysics*, **16**, 191–198.

TROBE, J. D., GLASER, J. S. & LAFLAMME, P. (1978) Dysthyroid optic neuropathy: Clinical profile and rationale for management, *Archives of Ophthalmology*, **96**, 1199–1209.

WEETMAN, A. P. (1991) Thyroid-associated eye disease: Pathophysiology, *The Lancet*, **338**, 25–28.

WERNER, S. C. (1969) Classification of the eye changes of Graves' disease, *Journal of Clinical and Endocrinological Metabolism*, **29**, 782.

First Experiences with the Trafford Anomaloscope

L.G. Ripley, F. Dean, R.T. Gilday, C. Kon and S.J. Tregear

6.9.1 INTRODUCTION

The use of the Rayleigh match in the assessment of colour vision is well known (Birch, 1993). Normal subjects are able to make a precise colour match between a monochromatic spectral yellow and a suitable mixture of monochromatic red and monochromatic green. Abnormal subjects can be categorised according to how they fail to make a normal match.

The Rayleigh match is often measured with the Nagel anomaloscope or its derivatives which are relatively complicated and expensive optical instruments and which suffer from various shortcomings (Jordan and Mollon, 1993). The current availability of efficient solid-state sources of monochromatic light (light emitting diodes) makes it feasible to manufacture an electronic anomaloscope that, in principle, ought to be cheap and robust. A first attempt at this led to various lessons being learned so that the second machine which was produced appeared to be suitable for routine use. Three copies of this were made and independently tested and it was discovered that the protocol of operation is a very important parameter.

6.9.2 DESIGN AND CONSTRUCTION

From the beginning it was understood that there was a wide variety of possible solutions to the problem of using light emitting diodes (LEDs) in an anomaloscope. For instance, diodes are now available that emit blue light and modern electronics would allow the incorporation of a lot of computational power even into small, portable apparatus. However, it was decided to begin at the beginning to make the simplest possible red-green machine. Tritan testing and microprocessor control will feature in later systems, which are currently under development. The first aim was to make a screener that could replace the Ishihara plates in terms of reliability, cost and ease of operation.

Figure 6.9.1 shows the prototype device and Figure 6.9.2 is a cross-section of it. The body is made from plastic pipe sprayed with a matt black finish and the eye piece, which

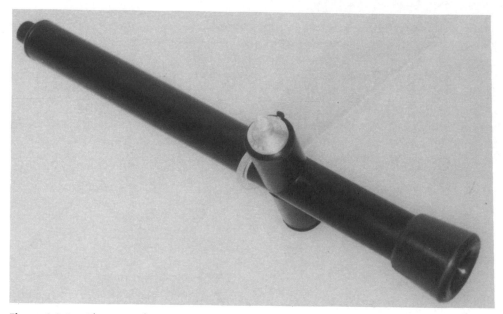

Figure 6.9.1.   The anomaloscope prototype.

supports the lens, was moulded in the laboratory from silicone rubber. The iris was required to cut down glare and reflection from the inside of the pipe to an acceptable level.

The circuitry runs off about 3 volts which is provided by two standard AA cells in a conventional holder (RS 507-545) that allows them to be changed very easily when necessary. More volts would allow for the use of a regulator that would give more protection against the effects of the cells running down. However, the holder used was the only one available that would fit into the pipe which had been chosen.

The circuit is required to provide non-interacting adjustments of the brightness of a yellow light emitting diode and the proportions of red and green in a constant-luminance

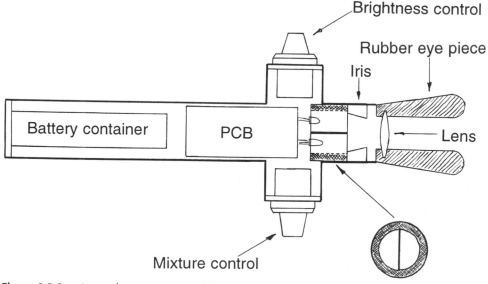

Figure 6.9.2.   Anomaloscope construction.

mixture. The first function is easily achieved by using a variable series resistance, VR_4. A fixed series resistance is used for safety to limit the maximum current through the diode and hence determines the maximum brightness. Given the non-linearities otherwise involved, the only feasible technique to control the red-green mixture easily is switching two LEDs in antiphase with a variable mark-space ratio. This is shown in Figure 6.9.3. The op-amp has been configured as a modified Smitt oscillator so that, because of diodes D_1 and D_2, there are different time constants for the rising and falling relaxations that depend on R_A and R_B respectively. However, as $R_A + R_B = VR_1$ which is constant, then adjustment of the slider of VR_1 does not alter the overall frequency of oscillation, which can be set to about 10 kHz so that there is no chance of any flicker being perceived.

Transistors TR_1 and TR_2 are used as switches to turn on the red and green light emitting diodes respectively during each part of the cycle of oscillation. There are series resistances that can be used to adjust the brightness of each diode and, by temporarily increasing C_1 by a factor of about one hundred, flicker photometry can be used to achieve an equiluminant match while the mark-space ratio is set to 50 per cent. This calibration will avoid problems due to spreads in component values and diode efficiencies.

The light emitting diodes that were used were primarily chosen for their low price and

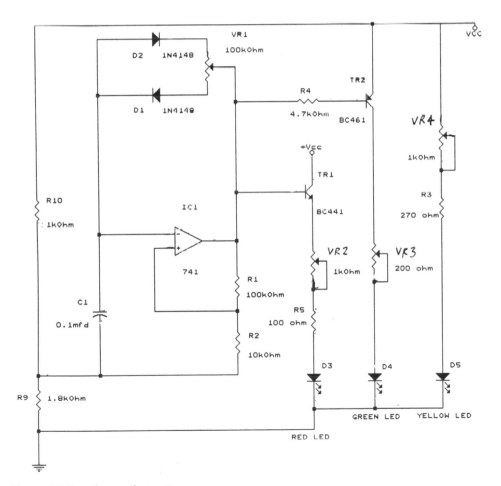

Figure 6.9.3. Electrical circuit.

easy availability. The yellow source is an ultrabright LED (RS 578-238) with an output peaking at 590 nm. The red and green sources are an ultrabright tricolour LED (RS 564-166) with peaks at 660 nm and 567 nm respectively. This device has the two diodes in one package and is called 'tricolour' because it is intended to be an indicator lamp that can glow red, green or yellow according to whether either or both diodes are turned on.

The outputs from the LEDs are plotted on the CIE diagram as points R, Y and G as shown in Figure 6.9.4. These points do not lie exactly on the spectral locus because of the finite bandwidth of the LEDs, but they do lie on a straight line, which indicates that a good match should be possible, as indeed it is. For comparison, r, y and g indicate the ideal locations of the Nagel sources (whose bandwidths are not known). These Nagel sources were presumably chosen not so much for any profound physiological reason but because sodium lamps and so on were easily available in the pre-LED age. The colours of the two sets of sources are not very different.

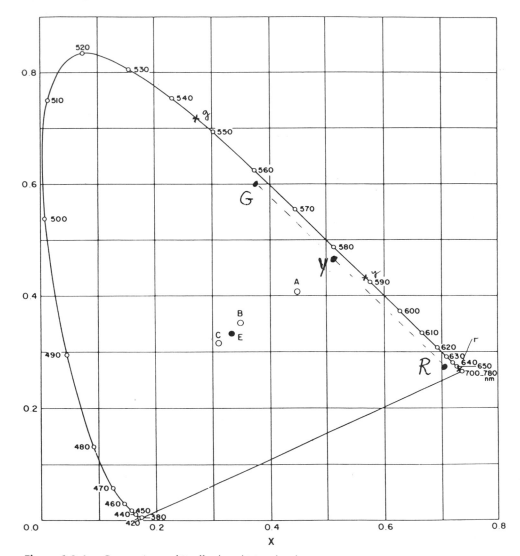

Figure 6.9.4. Comparison of Trafford and Nagel colour sources

A very important aspect of the instrument is how the yellow light and the red-green mixture are presented for comparison. By dint of much experimentation we have realised a bipartite field by potting the LEDs in a translucent resin which evens out variations of brightness while not attenuating the light too much.

The brightness control, VR_4, is a single-turn potentiometer with a scale marked 0–100 in arbitrary units. The mixture control, VR_1, is a ten-turn potentiometer with a scale marked 0 to 100, which corresponds almost exactly to the percentage of red light being displayed. Thus, for example, a low setting produces a very green light and is the result that could be expected from testing a deuteranomolous subject.

6.9.3 EXPERIMENTS

A prototype machine was tried out on some of the faculty and research students in the School of Engineering of the University of Sussex with immediate success. Two subjects with known colour-vision deficiencies were very obviously different from the rest of their colleagues and a bimodal distribution of the results led to the hypothesis of a bimorphism, which, unknown to the inventor, had been previously discovered elsewhere (Mollon, 1992).

It was with great optimism that three more machines were made. These were tried out by the authors on themselves and it was confirmed that they all behaved very similarly so that they ought to produce comparable results with no need for any normalisation or re-calibration.

Each machine was then used independently on three different populations with no evidence of ocular pathology. A test protocol was initially agreed but the operators were given freedom to vary this in the light of experience in that, at this stage, it was just as important to learn how to operate the device most effectively as it was to obtain experimental data. However, it was obviously desirable to see whether viable data could be collected to be compared with those of other workers with other machines.

In essence, each subject was twice asked to set the machine so that the two halves of the field were identical. This required some degree of coaching from the researchers in some cases and, even so, four subjects professed themselves incapable of operating the machine. The Ishihara plates were administered to all subjects in the normal way and their visual acuity was assessed with a Snellen chart.

6.9.4 RESULTS

Data were obtained from 237 out of 241 subjects. All of these had a corrected VA of 6/6 or better and none of them, even those who could not operate the machine, failed the Ishihara test. This latter finding was a great surprise for 91 of the subjects were male and several of them would have been expected to show some congenital colour-vision deficiency.

Figure 6.9.5 is a histogram of the average mixture setting and is much as expected with most of the subjects in the range 50 ± 10, i.e. with anomaloquotients between 0.67 and 1.5. Apparently no protanomalous subjects were tested and although there appears to be a deuteranomolous tail, none of these did fail the Ishihara test. This was also surprising in that we had expected this to happen when mixtures were set outside the range of about 25–75.

As intimated earlier, the researchers were aware of considerable differences among subjects. There was a wide range of confidence and precision in performing the test. Figure

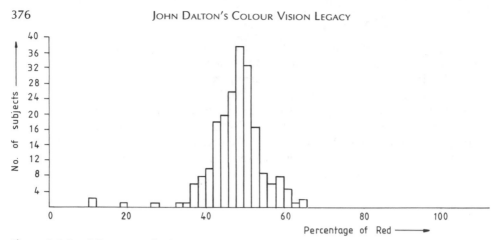

Figure 6.9.5.   Histogram of mixture settings.

6.9.6 is a histogram of the set/reset spread. This shows that whereas Figure 6.9.5 looks quite respectable, some of the data must be highly suspect if, to take one extreme instance, a figure of 43 is derived from averaging 14 and 72.

It is tempting to deduce from Figure 6.9.6 that meaningful data have been obtained only from a sub-group who have repeated the mixture settings with a spread of no more than about seven. However, a histogram of the 'best half' of the mixture settings which were averages of figures with a spread of 3 or less, does not look significantly different from Figure 6.9.5.

Further analysis of the data in terms of brightness setting, age, male/female performance and so on has failed to reveal any significant trend.

6.9.5   CONCLUSIONS

It is clear that, before we go any further, we need to review the ergonomics of the machine to see if there is any way in which we can improve the subjects' experience. Without doubt, the most important thing we have to do is to devise a better test protocol. This will have to involve a significant amount of instruction for it is clear that the general public is far less

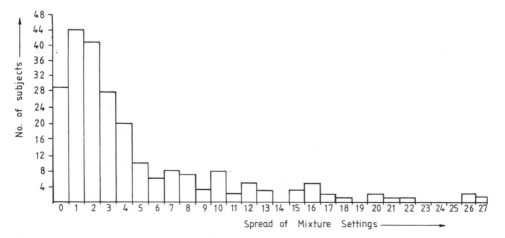

Figure 6.9.6.   Histogram of spread of mixture settings.

able to learn how to operate a new device than are the members of a university engineering group.

6.9.6   ACKNOWLEDGEMENTS

The Trafford Anomaloscope has been named for the late Lord Trafford, who did so much to foster medical research at The University of Sussex, and for his widow, Lady Helen Trafford, who inspires us all with her enthusiasm and her unflagging fundraising, without which we would not be able to carry on so successfully.

The Trafford Anomaloscope would still be a heap of pieces on the bench if Brian Stothard had not put them together.

6.9.7   REFERENCES

BIRCH, J. (1993) *Diagnosis of Defective Colour Vision*, Oxford: Oxford University Press.
JORDAN, G. & MOLLON, J.D. (1993) The Nagel anomaloscope and seasonal variation of colour vision, *Nature*, **363**, 546–549.
MOLLON, J. (1992) Worlds of difference, *Nature*, **356**, 378–379.

Section 7 – Colour Categories

On the Nature of Unique Hues

J. D. Mollon and Gabriele Jordan

7.1.1 INTRODUCTION

There exist four colours, the *Urfarben* of Hering, that appear phenomenologically un-mixed. The special status of these 'unique hues' remains one of the central mysteries of colour science. In Hering's Opponent Colour Theory, unique red and green are the colours seen when the yellow-blue process is in equilibrium and when the red-green process is polarised in one direction or the other. Similarly unique yellow and blue are seen when the red-green process is in equilibrium and when the yellow-blue process is polarised in one direction or the other. Most observers judge that other hues, such as orange or cyan, partake of the qualities of two of the *Urfarben*. Under normal viewing conditions, however, we never experience mixtures of the two components of an opponent pair, that is, we do not experience reddish greens or yellowish blues (Hering, 1878).

These observations are paradigmatic examples of what Brindley (1960) called Class B observations: the subject is asked to describe the quality of his private sensations. They differ from Class A observations, in which the subject is required only to report the identity or non-identity of the sensations evoked by different stimuli. We may add that they also differ from the performance measures (latency; frequency of error; magnitude of error) that treat the subject as an information-processing system and have been increasingly used in visual science since 1960. Sensory observations of Class A can be interpreted if one allows merely the hypothesis that physiologically indistinguishable signals sent from the sense organs to the brain cause indistinguishable sensations. But to this day we have no secure way of interpreting Class B observations, no way of knowing what weight to place on them. Some might suppose that there exist specific cortical cells (or structures or processes) that give rise to – secrete – sensations of redness and other units that secrete sensations of blueness, and so on; and that mixed hues are seen when two types of cortical cell are concurrently secreting their proper sensations. Psychophysical linking hypotheses of this kind are not often made so unashamedly explicit, but it is a good idea to make them so. For all we really know is that in a given state of adaptation some chromaticities map on to hue sensations that typical observers describe as pure, whereas other chromaticities map on to mixed sensations.

7.1.2 THE CHROMATIC CHANNELS OF THE VISUAL PATHWAY

When chromatically antagonistic signals were first recorded in the retinae of fish (Svae-tichin and MacNichol, 1958) and in the lateral geniculate nucleus of macaques (De Valois *et al.*, 1966), it was widely assumed that Hering had been vindicated and that the neural channels of the primate LGN corresponded to the red-green and yellow-blue processes of Opponent Colours Theory. The standard zone model of the 1960s had a receptoral 'Helmholtz' stage and a second 'Hering' stage (Walraven, 1962). Such a view still survives in psychology textbooks and other secondary sources. Today, however, most colour scientists are agreed that the chromatically opponent cells of the early visual system (the 'second stage' of models of colour vision) do not correspond colorimetrically to red-green and yellow-blue processes. Two main types of neural channel have consistently been reported in Old World primates: a phylogenetically recent channel in which the signal of the long-wave cones is opposed to that of the middle-wave cones and a phylogenetically older channel in which the signal of the short-wave cones is opposed to some combination of the signals of the L and M cones (Derrington *et al.*, 1984; Gouras, 1968; Mollon and Jordan, 1988). Figure 7.1.1 (see colour section) shows the chromaticity diagram of MacLeod and Boynton (1979), the axes of which correspond to the two chromatic channels of the early visual system. In such a diagram, a line that runs from unique yellow (c. 572 nm) to unique blue (c. 475 nm) is oblique, and not vertical as it should be if it represented a fixed, equilibrium, ratio of the quantum catches of the M and L cones. Indeed, unique blue is close to the wavelength (460 nm) that maximises the ratio M/L (Mollon and Estévez, 1988).

Recognising this discrepancy, the authors of recent models of colour vision have usually postulated a 'third stage', in which the second-stage signals are re-transformed to give channels that do correspond to those of Hering (De Valois and De Valois, 1993; Guth, 1991). It may be that a third stage of this kind does exist, but electrophysiological recording has not yet revealed it. Lennie *et al.* (1990) recording from neurons in the striate cortex of *Macaca fascicularis*, found that there was a large variation between cells in their preferred direction in colour space, with some bias towards the 'second stage' axes; only a few cells behaved as would be expected of the putative 'red-green' and 'yellow-blue' mechanisms of Hering. In the prestriate region V4, Zeki (1980) reported cells with narrow spectral sensitivities, but the wavelengths of peak sensitivity were distributed through the spectrum, with some avoidance of the yellow region; and extraspectral purples were well represented. Komatsu *et al.* (1992) examined the colour selectivity of neurons in the inferior temporal cortex and found that the population of cells together covered most of the chromaticity diagram. There were, for example, cells that gave their most vigorous response to a desaturated pink.

Lennie *et al.* (1990) speak of the 'red-green and yellow-blue mechanisms whose existence is so firmly established by psychophysics'. Yet what is this psychophysical evidence? The psychophysical experiments most commonly invoked to support a third stage are the chromatic cancellation measurements of Jameson and Hurvich (1955; see also Werner and Wooten, 1979): in these experiments the strength of, say, the green chromatic response was established by finding at each wavelength the amount of a fixed, reddish, wavelength that needed to be added to yield a light that looked neither reddish nor greenish. These measurements are certainly quantitative, but they too are Class B observations and they are in effect only an extension of the basic determination of the unique hues. This is clear when one considers that it is not necessary to perform the measurements as cancellations. It is completely equivalent to ask the subject to identify directly the sets of non-spectral chromaticities that are neither reddish nor greenish or are neither bluish nor yellowish: in a chromaticity diagram these sets form (often curved) loci that connect the wavelengths of the unique hues to the white point (Burns *et al.*, 1984). Conventional colorimetry will then allow the reconstruction of cancellation curves in the form presented by Jameson and Hurvich.

So the cancellation experiments amount to the extended determination of unique hues. They show us that the topology of chromaticity space is preserved in our phenomenological colour space, but they remain Class B observations and, as evidence for a third stage, they add nothing to the original observation that some hues are unique and some are phenomenal mixtures.

7.1.3   DOCTRINE OF COINCIDENT CATEGORIES

In the hypothesis that each unique hue represents the activity of a discrete class of cortical cell, we can recognise a modern form of Müller's Doctrine of Specific Nerve Energies. And in judging this hypothesis we should place it in its broader context: one of the chief unsolved questions of brain science is that of whether the elements of perception and thought are represented by the activities of individual cells (Barlow, 1972, 1995).

It may be useful to identify a more general form of the hypothesis, in which we replace 'cell' by a term that can refer to any discrete 'structure' or 'process' or 'neural signal'. Let us speak of 'neural primitives'. It may also be useful to make explicit the distinct question of whether these neural primitives always map exactly on to our phenomenological categories. In the case of colour, then, we can ask: does the existence of unique and non-unique hues tell us that the neural representation of colour is discontinuous, and do the phenomenally unique hues correspond to the discrete primitives of this neural representation whereas mixed hues correspond to more than one kind of neural primitive? We might use the term *Doctrine of Coincident Categories* for the idea that phenomenological categories correspond to neural primitives in the above way.

Suppose that the Doctrine of Coincident Categories were wrong in the following sense. Suppose that colours were represented centrally only by neural primitives that corresponded to the axes of the MacLeod-Boynton space, i.e. primitives that did not correspond to redness, greenness, yellowness and blueness. This would imply that the transformation between the two categorical organisations (the transformation from the second to the third stage in current theories) arose in the relationship between the neural representation and the phenomenological, whatever that relationship might be. But now we are on radical ground. For it is easy for the normal trichromat to base his behaviour, verbal or otherwise, on the categories red, green, yellow and blue — much more easily than he can base his behaviour on the categories of the MacLeod-Boynton space. We should thus be allowing that strictly phenomenological categories can influence behaviour.

It is clear that if we understood the status of unique hues we should probably understand something useful about the general question of neural representation and its relationship to conscious experience. For the present, the nature of the unique hues remains mysterious and we do not know whether they tell us anything about the neural organisation of the visual system. In asking what they are, it may be instructive to adopt a Gibsonian view and to look outside the observer as well as within the fixed wiring of his visual system. Either in phylogeny or in ontogeny, is there some property of the external environment that sets the chromaticities that appear unique?

7.1.4   INDIVIDUAL DIFFERENCES IN UNIQUE YELLOW

One traditional approach to unique hues has been to study the undoubted differences that exist amongst colour-normal observers in the exact wavelength of each equilibrium colour. Let us consider two different hypotheses that have been advanced to explain the variation in unique yellow.

7.1.4.1 Cone ratios

An example of a model that seeks the variation within the fixed wiring of the visual system is that of Cicerone (1990). She proposes that the wavelength of unique yellow depends on the relative proportions of long- and middle-wave cones: the greater the proportion of long-wave cones, the shorter the wavelength of unique yellow. We have carried out two tests of this hypothesis.

A traditional index of L and M cone ratios is offered by the relative flicker-photometric sensitivity at middle and long wavelengths (De Vries, 1947). A measure closely related to flicker photometry is that given by the OSCAR test, in which the subject is asked to minimise apparent flicker by adjusting the relative depths of modulation of a long-wave light and of a middle-wave light, which are modulated in counterphase (Estévez et al., 1983). Negative values on the OSCAR test indicate low sensitivity to long wavelengths. In the course of a recent study in collaboration with Emma-Louise Dormand we had occasion to obtain OSCAR settings and estimates of unique yellow from 50 young men. To measure unique yellow, we used a Maxwellian-view optical system that incorporates a computer-controlled monochromator with integral stepping motor. This system allows us to determine unique hues by a procedure in which four staircases are randomly interleaved (Jordan and Mollon, 1995). Sternberg has estimated that an adaptive method of this kind gives a stimulus sequence that is as random as that of the Method of Constant Stimuli (Sternberg et al., 1982), while it avoids the chief disadvantage of the Method of Constant Stimuli – the tendency of subjects to give equal numbers of responses of the two types and thus to yield a setting in the middle of the fixed range of stimuli. In the present experiment, the background was dark, the stimuli were circular and subtended one degree, and the stimulus duration was one second. Instead of the negative correlation predicted by Cicerone's hypothesis, we found no significant relationship between the OSCAR setting and the wavelength of unique yellow ($r = 0.066$).

A second and particularly interesting test of Cicerone's hypothesis is offered by women who are heterozygous for the common forms of dichromacy. Although such women usually exhibit Rayleigh matches that are within the normal range (Jordan and Mollon, 1993), their retinae almost certainly contain abnormal proportions of L and M cones, owing to the process of X-chromosome inactivation or Lyonisation. Although a woman inherits two X-chromosomes, one from each parent, only one of the two is actually expressed in any individual cell of her body (Gartler and Riggs, 1983; Lyon, 1972). In the retina of a heterozygote, a subset of cones will express the abnormal opsin array that she has inherited from one parent and which will lead to dichromacy if she passes it on to a son. Thus, carriers of protanopia are thought to have reduced numbers of functional long-wave cones, whereas carriers of deuteranopia have reduced numbers of middle-wave cones. It is well established that most carriers of protanopia show a reduced sensitivity to long wavelengths but exhibit a normal Rayleigh match (Schmidt, 1934). This is the behaviour expected if the normal photopigments are present but the long-wave cones are reduced in number (Rushton and Baker, 1964).

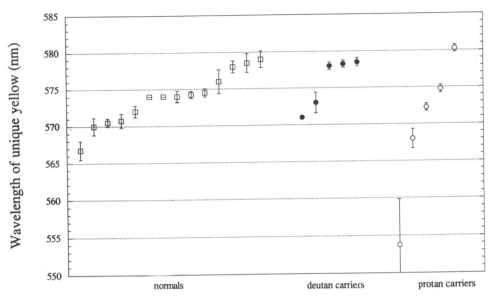

Classification

Figure 7.1.2. The wavelength set as unique yellow is plotted for individual normal observers (open squares), carriers of deuteranopia (filled circles) and carriers of protanopia (open circles). There is no significant difference between these groups of observers. Note that one carrier of protanopia exhibits a very short value of unique yellow.

We have collected in Cambridge a panel of obligate heterozygotes whose sons' phenotypes have been established in detail (Jordan and Mollon, 1993). We have determined unique yellow for members of this panel and for normal controls. Results from this experiment are shown in Figure 7.1.2. As groups, neither protanopic nor deuteranopic carriers differ significantly from the normals. One carrier of protanopia sets unique yellow at a very short wavelength (and has a very large standard deviation), but her setting is displaced in the direction opposite to that predicted by Cicerone. In sum, by testing populations who have extreme ratios of L and M cones, we find no evidence for Cicerone's hypothesis.

From the same population of heterozygotes we did concurrently obtain OSCAR settings, as a direct measure of relative sensitivity to middle and long wavelengths. On this test, most individual protan carriers reveal themselves by a clearly depressed sensitivity to long wavelengths, a finding consistent with the hypothesis that they have reduced numbers of long-wave cones. As a population, deutan carriers show a lower relative sensitivity to middle wavelengths than do normals, although in this case the normal and heterozygote distributions overlap substantially. We found that the wavelength of unique yellow showed a non-significant positive correlation with OSCAR setting ($r = 0.32$), a relationship opposite in direction to that expected from Cicerone's hypothesis (Figure 7.1.3).

7.1.4.2 Cone sensitivities

The hypothesis of Pokorny and Smith (1977) is one that relates unique yellow to properties of both the observer and the environment. It supposes that unique yellow is that wavelength that produces in the L and M cones the same ratio of quantum catches as does the average illumination of the observer's environment. A view of this kind was also adopted by Mollon (1982). A neural adjustment with a relatively long time constant would control the channel that differences the L and M cone signals and would ensure that the equilibrium point of the channel corresponded to the average stimulus.[1] Departures from the equilibrium point would be represented by neural signals of opposite sign and (here a psychophysical hypothesis enters) by sensations of opposite quality.

Pokorny and Smith developed their hypothesis to account for the spectral position of unique yellow in protanomaly and in deuteranomaly, and they treated the normal observer as a single phenotype. But it is natural to extend such a hypothesis to account for the variation in unique yellow between normal subjects. We now know that the long- and middle-wavelength photopigments are polymorphic; that is to say, there exist individual variations in the amino-acid sequence of the opsins. Some of these variations produce spectral displacements in the absorbance spectrum of the photopigment: most notably the substitution of alanine for serine at site 180 shifts the peak sensitivity to shorter wavelengths, but there are small, non-additive effects of other sites in the amino acid sequence (Asenjo et al., 1994; Merbs and Nathans, 1992).

These genetic polymorphisms account for a significant part of the variance in Rayleigh matches (Winderickx et al., 1992). Now, in hypotheses of the type advanced by Pokorny and Smith, unique yellow is a kind of a colour match: it is a tritanopic match between a monochromatic yellow and a remembered broad-band white. So we might expect some correlation between a subject's Rayleigh match and his unique yellow, a correlation that reflects underlying variations in the spectral positions of the L and M pigments. In fact, a

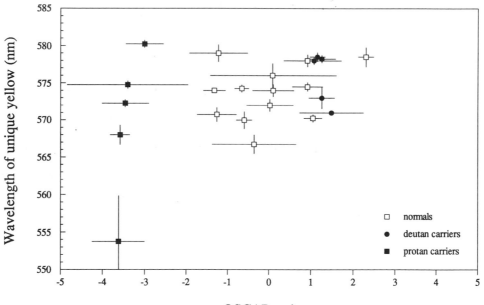

OSCAR units

Figure 7.1.3. The wavelength set as unique yellow is plotted as a function of the observer's OSCAR setting for normal observers (open squares), carriers of deuteranopia (filled circles) and carriers of protanopia (filled squares). There is no significant correlation between the two variables. The error bars indicate the standard deviations of five settings on the OSCAR and four estimates of unique yellow (drawn from four interleaved staircases). However, unlike the settings of unique yellow, the OSCAR settings separate well the deutan and protan carriers.

correlation was reported by Donders (1884) for a sample of colour-normal observers: the more red a subject required in the Rayleigh match, the shorter the wavelength of unique yellow. We have plotted in Figure 7.1.4 the data that Donders gives in the tables on pages 536–537 of his paper. However, a study by Hailwood and Roaf (1937) found no correlation at all between Rayleigh matches and unique yellow. This was also the case for our recent sample of 50 young colour-normal males: the value of r was 0.01, giving no hint at all of a relationship. So this test offers no support for the extended Pokorny-Smith hypothesis.

There is a second test of the extended Pokorny-Smith hypothesis that we can employ. Suppose we supply a reference white during the experiment. It is plausible that this will supplant the stored white. So, in a chromaticity diagram, the subject's unique yellow ought to lie on the projection of a line that passes through the tritanopic copunctal point and the (supplied) white. For such a line represents a set of chromaticities that produce a constant ratio of quantum catches in the L and M cones, i.e. a set of lights that would be confused by an observer who lacked the short-wave cones.

To test this prediction, we have recently measured the wavelength of unique yellow for one-degree targets presented within a 10-degree steady white annulus. Three different chromaticities, lying close to illuminants A, C and E, were chosen for the annulus. Unique yellow was estimated by means of the four-staircase method described above. The results, shown in Figure 7.1.5, make it clear that unique yellow does not lie on a tritan line passing through the reference white: the hypothesis is not supported. The lines pass much closer to the spectral region of unique blue. There is thus an interesting discrepancy between (1) the wavelength of supra-threshold unique yellow in the presence of a white annulus and (2) the wavelength of Sloan's notch for increment thresholds measured on a white background. In

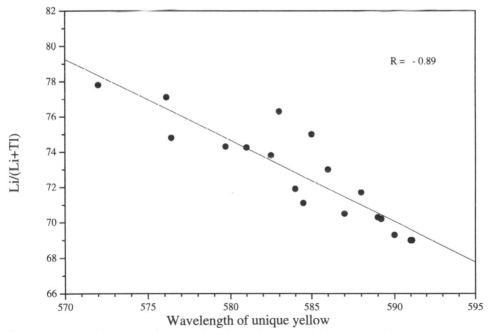

Figure 7.1.4. Rayleigh matches are plotted as a function of the wavelength seen as unique yellow. The data are taken from tables published by Donders in 1884. Li and Tl denote the Fraunhofer lines for spectral red and green. The higher the amount of red in the red-green mixture needed to match the standard yellow (Na), the shorter the wavelength set as unique yellow. This relationship was later termed *Donder's law* by Westphal (1910).

the latter case, the wavelength of minimal sensitivity does lie closely on a tritan line passing through the chromaticity of the background white (Fach and Mollon, 1987).

In summary then, our own investigations have failed to relate unique yellow to either the relative numbers or the spectral sensitivities of the long- and middle-wave cones. Nor does unique yellow prove to be a tritan metamer of a white reference supplied in the experiment. Let us turn to unique green, a case where we have found one correlate of individual differences.

7.1.5   INDIVIDUAL VARIATIONS IN UNIQUE GREEN

Unique green has traditionally been found to vary more than does unique yellow or unique blue. There have been recurrent suggestions that the distribution is bimodal (Richards,

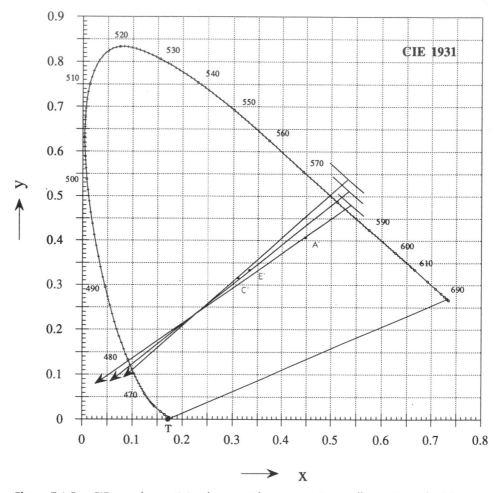

Figure 7.1.5.   CIE x, y chromaticity diagram. The mean unique yellow settings for 19 observers are plotted as a function of three different white backgrounds. The short bars parallel to the spectrum locus indicate standard deviations. Lines connect each mean unique yellow with its associated reference white point (A, E, C respectively). Note that these lines do not pass through the tritanopic copunctal point (T).

1967; Rubin, 1961), and indeed some have held that the two phenotypes correspond to two phenotypes revealed by Rayleigh matches (Waaler, 1967). Hurvich *et al.* (1968) suggested that the apparent bimodalities arose from differential chromatic adaptation. Using our randomised staircase procedure to avoid systematic biases in adaptation, we have obtained estimates of unique green from a sample of 97 male observers (Jordan and Mollon, 1995). The background was dark. The distribution (Figure 7.1.6) was not bimodal, although, as others have found, it was skewed to long wavelengths. There was no correlation at all with the observers' Rayleigh matches. We may relate the increased spread of unique green, and the skew, to the way hue discrimination varies in this part of the spectrum: at wavelengths shorter than the modal value of unique green, most colour-normal observers exhibit very fine wavelength discrimination and subjective hue changes quickly, whereas at wavelengths longer than the modal value discrimination is poorer. We may suppose that subjects can more readily tolerate errors towards longer wavelengths than towards shorter.

Our study did, however, reveal one correlate of unique green. The experimenter rated the lightness of each subject's iris on a three-point scale and a Kruskal-Wallis test showed that there was a significant relationship between these ratings and unique green (H = 13.12, $p < 0.001$): subjects with light irises have unique green settings that lie at shorter wavelengths than do subjects with medium or dark irises.

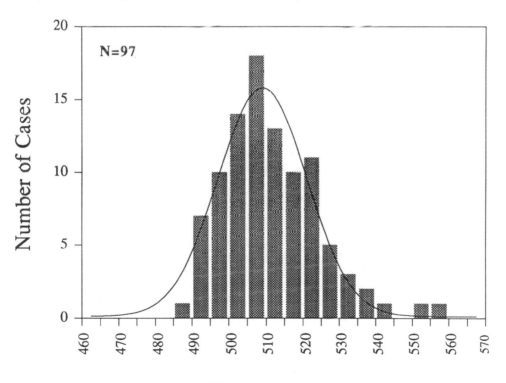

Figure 7.1.6. Distribution of the wavelength set as unique green by 97 normal male observers. The mean value is 511 nm with a standard deviation of 13 nm. The normal distribution with the same mean and standard deviation is shown as a solid line overlaid on the histogram. (The figure is replotted from Jordan and Mollon, *Vision Research*, 1995.)

Is there a clue here as to the nature of unique green? The lightness of the iris is often taken to be an index of the level of pigmentation present in the fundus of the eye, behind and between the photoreceptors. The absorption of light transmitted through the iris and sclera, and of light scattered within the eye, is greatest at short wavelengths, and so will modify the spectral composition of the light actually absorbed in the photoreceptors. However, the stimuli commonly used to establish unique hues are near-monochromatic ones, and ocular pigmentation should not modify the ratios of quantum catches that a given wavelength produces in the different cone types. Yet suppose that the spectral position of unique green does not correspond to a genetically fixed set of cone signals, but instead depends on the observer's interaction with broad-band stimuli in the real world. Consider two observers, one with light pigmentation, one with heavy, but with identical photopigments. Suppose that these observers agree that a certain leaf is neither glaucous nor yellowish. The ratios of quantum catches that the leaf produces in the cones of one observer must differ from the corresponding ratios for the other observer. If these two observers agree on unique green in the real world, then they ought to differ when we bring them into the laboratory and confront them with monochromatic lights. For they will need different monochromatic lights to imitate the cone ratios.

This approach to unique hues makes a clear prediction. The variance between observers should be less when they judge surface colours than when they judge spectral colours. We end by recalling the case of Dr Sulzer, examined by Donders (1884). The Rayleigh match for Dr Sulzer's left eye lay at the protan end of the normal distribution whereas the match for his right eye lay at the deutan end. With his left eye Dr Sulzer chose 577 nm for unique yellow, and with his right eye he chose 587 nm, but there was no difference between his eyes when he was asked to choose the unique yellow in a set of graded papers differing in steps of one j.n.d.

7.1.6   ACKNOWLEDGEMENTS

The experimental work reported here was supported by MRC Grant G911363 and by a Wellcome Research Fellowship to G. Jordan.

7.1.7   NOTES

1. It might seem more accurate to express the hypothesis not in terms of the spectral composition of the average illumination of the observer's world but in terms of the average illumination of the retina. However, the latter stimulus may not correspond to the colour we perceive as neutral, for the average reflectance of surfaces in the observer's world may not correspond to a grey colour but be biased, say to olive green (Brown, 1994). It is the illuminant chromaticity that we judge to be achromatic. This consideration might be taken to suggest that the long-term reference white was neurally incorporated not in the equilibrium points of retinal channels but in a more central process.

7.1.8   REFERENCES

ASENJO, A. B., RIM, J. & OPRIAN, D. D. (1994) Molecular determinants of human red/green color discrimination, *Neuron*, **12**, 1131–1138.

BARLOW, H. B. (1972) Single units and sensation: A neuron doctrine for perceptual psychology? *Perception*, **1**, 371–394.

BARLOW, H. B. (1995) The neuron doctrine in perception. In: Gazzaniga, M. (Ed.) *The Cognitive Neurosciences*, Boston: MIT Press, pp. 415–435.

BRINDLEY, G. S. (1960) *Physiology of the Retina and Visual Pathway*, London: Arnold.

BROWN, R.O. (1994) The world is not grey, *Investigative Ophthalmology and Visual Science*, **35**, 2165.

BURNS, S. A., ELSNER, A. E., POKORNY, J. & SMITH, V. C. (1984) The Abney effect: chromaticity coordinates of unique and other constant hues, *Vision Research*, **24**, 479–489.

CICERONE, C. M. (1990) Color appearance and the cone mosaic in trichromacy and dichromacy. In: Ohta, Y. (Ed.) *Colour Vision Deficiencies. Proceedings of the Symposium of the International Research Group on Color Vision Deficiencies*, Amsterdam: Kugler & Ghedini, pp. 1–12.

DE VALOIS, R.L. & DE VALOIS, K.K. (1993) A multi-stage color model, *Vision Research*, **33**, 1053–1065.

DE VALOIS, R.L., ABRAMOV, I. & JACOBS, G.H. (1966) Analysis of response patterns of LGN cells, *Journal of Optical Society of America*, **56**, 966–977.

DE VRIES, H. (1947) The heredity of the relative numbers of red and green receptors in the human eye, *Genetica*, **24**, 199–212.

DERRINGTON, A.M., KRAUSKOPF, J. & LENNIE, P. (1984) Chromatic mechanisms in lateral geniculate nucleus of macaque, *Journal of Physiology*, **357**, 241–265.

DONDERS, F. C. (1884) Farbengleichungen, *Archiv f. Anat. u. Physiol. Physiol. Abthig.*, 518–552.

ESTÉVEZ, O., SPEKREIJSE, H. VAN DALEN, J. T. W. & VERDUYN LUNEL, H. F. E. (1983) The Oscar color vision test: theory and evaluation (Objective Screening of Color Anomalies and Reductions), *American Journal of Optometry and Physiological Optics*, **60**, 892–901.

FACH, C. & MOLLON, J. D. (1987) Predicting the position of Sloan's notch, *Investigative Ophthalmology and Visual Science*, **28**(3), 213.

GARTLER, S. M. & RIGGS, A. D. (1983) Mammalian X-chromosome inactivation, *Annual Review of Genetics*, **17**, 155–190.

GOURAS, P. (1968) Identification of cone mechanisms in monkey ganglion cells, *Journal of Physiology*, **199**, 535–547.

GUTH, S. L. (1991) Model for color vision and light adaptation, *Journal of the Optical Society of America*, **A 8**, 976.

HAILWOOD, J. G. & ROAF, H. E. (1937) The sensation of yellow and anomalous trichromatism, *Journal of Physiology*, **91**, 36–47.

HERING, E. (1878) *Zur Lehre vom Lichtsinne. Sechs Mittheilungen an die Kaiserliche Akademie der Wissenschaften in Wien*, Wien: Carl Gerlold's Sohn.

HURVICH, L. M., JAMESON, D. & COHEN, J. D. (1968) The experimental determination of unique green in the spectrum, *Perception and Psychophysics*, **4**, 65–68.

JAMESON, D. & HURVICH, L. M. (1955) Some quantitative aspects of an opponent-colors theory. I Chromatic responses and spectral saturation, *Journal of the Optical Society of America*, **45**, 546–552.

JORDAN, G. & MOLLON, J. D. (1993) A study of women heterozygous for colour deficiencies, *Vision Research*, **33**, 1495–1508.

JORDAN, G. & MOLLON, J. D. (1995) Rayleigh matches and unique green, *Vision Research*, **35**, 613–620.

KOMATSU, H., IDEURA, Y., KAJI, S. & SHIGERU, Y. (1992) Color selectivity of neurons in the inferior temporal cortex of the awake macaque monkey, *Journal of Neuroscience*, **12**, 408–424.

LENNIE, P., KRAUSKOPF, J. & SCLAR, G. (1990) Chromatic mechanisms in striate cortex of macaque, *Journal of Neuroscience*, **10**, 649–669.

LYON, M. F. (1972) X-chromosome inactivation and development patterns in mammals, *Biological Reviews*, **47**, 1–35.

MACLEOD, D. I. A. & BOYNTON, R. M. (1979) Chromaticity diagram showing cone excitation by stimuli of equal luminance, *Journal of the Optical Society of America*, **69**, 1183–1186.

MERBS, S. L. & NATHANS, J. (1992) Absorption spectra of human cone pigments, *Nature*, **356**, 433–435.

MOLLON, J. D. (1982) Color vision, *Annual Review of Psychology*, **33**, 41–85.

MOLLON, J. D. & ESTÉVEZ, O. (1988) Tyndall's paradox of hue discrimination, *Journal of the Optical Society of America*, **A5**, 151–159.

MOLLON, J. D. & JORDAN, G. (1988) Eine evolutionäre Interpretation des menschlichen Farbensehens, *Die Farbe*, **35/36**, 139–170.

POKORNY, J. & SMITH, V. C. (1977) Evaluation of single-pigment shift model of anomalous trichromacy, *Journal of the Optical Society of America*, **67**, 1196–1209.

RICHARDS, W. (1967) Differences among color normals: classes I and II, *Journal of the Optical Society of America*, **57**, 1047–1055.

RUBIN, M. L. (1961) Spectral hue loci of normal and anomalous trichromats, *American Journal of Ophthalmology*, **52**, 166.

RUSHTON, W. A. H. & BAKER, H. D. (1964) Red-green sensitivity in normal vision, *Vision Research*, **4**, 75–85.

SCHMIDT, I. (1934) Über manifeste Heterozygotie bei Konduktorinnen für Farbensinnstörungen, *Klinische Monatsblätter für Augenheilkunde*, **92**, 456–467.

STERNBERG, S., KNOLL, R. L. & ZUKOFSKY, P. (1982) Timing by skilled musicians: perception, production, and imitation of time ratios. In: Deutsch, D. (Ed.) *The Psychology of Music*, New York: Academic Press.

SVAETICHIN, G. & MACNICHOL, E. F. (1958) Retinal mechanisms for chromatic and achromatic vision, *Annals of the New York Academy of Sciences*, **74**, 385–404.

WAALER, G. H. M. (1967) Heredity of two types of normal colour vision, *Nature*, **215**, 406.

WALRAVEN, P. L. (1962) *On the Mechanisms of Colour Vision*, The Netherlands: Institute for Perception RVO-TNO.

WERNER, J. S. & WOOTEN, B. R. (1979) Opponent chromatic response functions for an average observer, *Perception and Psychophysics*, **25**, 371–374.

WESTPHAL, H. (1910) Unmittelbare Bestimmungen der Urfarben, *Z. Sinnesphysiologie*, **44**, 182–230.

WINDERICKX, J., LINDSAY, D. T., SANOCKI, E., TELLER, D. Y., MOTULSKY, A. G. & DEEB, S. S. (1992) Polymorphism in red photopigment underlies variation in colour matching, *Nature*, **356**, 431–433.

ZEKI, S. (1980) The representation of colours in the cerebral cortex, *Nature*, **284**, 412–417.

On the Existence of a Fixed Number of Unique Opponent Hues

J. van Brakel and B.A.C Saunders

7.2.1 INTRODUCTION

Many textbook reviews of colour science claim there are two opponent pairs of unique hues: red-green and yellow-blue. What is the basis for this purported fact? Answers must face two further questions:

1. Is there psychophysical and/or neurophysiological support for singling out exactly *two* pairs of opponent and unique hues?
2. Is there any support for a close – perhaps causative – connection between colour categories encoded in ordinary language (English or any other language) and the relevant categories in colour vision research?

The answer to both questions must be a resounding: 'No'.

After a brief historical note on the idea of unique hue and the idea of opponency, we review the relevant evidence from psychophysics, neurophysiology, and anthropology respectively.

7.2.2 HISTORICAL NOTE ON UNIQUE HUES AND OPPONENCY

A unique hue is defined as a 'perceived hue that cannot be further described by the use of hue names other than its own' (CIE, 1987); a definition that goes back to Hering's suggestion that: 'language has long since singled out red, yellow, green, and blue as the principal colors of the multiplicity of chromatic colors'.[1] Although many colour vision scientists will stress non-linguistic evidence for the existence of four unique hues, throughout the colour literature, unique hues are always explained and justified in linguistic terms, as in the CIE definition.[2]

There is a long tradition deriving from Pliny's *Natural History* proposing four colours as 'basic'. Leonardo, for example, in *Trattato della Pittura* associated yellow, green, blue, and red with the four elements: earth, water, air, and fire. Mach, however, correctly disputed the relevance of these earlier views for Hering's proposal of four *Urfarben*: Leonardo's and earlier views were making a point of natural philosophy, not of unique perceptions or experiences.[3]

The concept of polarity used by Hering and revived by Jameson and Hurvich, had already been used by Goethe, who claimed certain colours reciprocally evoke each other. However this idea does not imply *two* pairs of opponent hues. In Goethe's colour circle there are three opponent pairs: red-green, orange-blue, and yellow-purple. Many earlier colour circles showing 'opponency' – ones including black and white – exist. In the nineteenth century, Grassmann might be said to have codified five pairs of opponent hues.[4] So the idea of a fixed number of unique hues and the idea of opponent colours must be kept separate. Evidence for the one is not evidence for the other.

7.2.3   PSYCHOPHYSICAL EVIDENCE FOR TWO OPPONENT PAIRS OF UNIQUE HUES

A considerable range of wavelengths are identified as unique green, blue or yellow. Unique red, not being in the spectrum, moreover, raises questions about the operational meaning of a unique hue. The unique points reported cover the spectral range of these colours, apart from 21 nm of yellow-green. Hence, unique is not that unique. Moreover, there is disagreement about whether brown is unique or not. In addition, metallic colours have been described as a 'group of colors we perceive as unique'.[5] It is true that if one averages the data into a Standard Observer, the unique hues become more constant; that, after all, is what averaging does. But the issue is not whether English speakers roughly agree on what, for example, is unique green or whether brown is, or is not, unique. The issue is whether asking people to point out the unique hues reveals anything more than their command of English colour terms (defined by the average speaker). Therefore, quoting Sternheim and Boynton (1966, or others) as having shown that most English speakers can describe all spectral colours with the four unique-hue names is pointless. Moreover, because of the spread of Western science, education and technological products, this Standard Observer is now found in the greater part of the world. Similarly, therefore, there is no point in quoting, as Pokorny *et al.* (1991) do, experiments that reconfirm for American and Japanese speakers the thesis of eleven Basic Color Terms, first proposed by Berlin and Kay (1969): Japanese colour vocabulary has changed over the past 100 years to conform with modern techno-science and American English in particular.[6]

Although there is conclusive non-linguistic evidence for trichromaticity and some sort of opponent processes, it is less clear what exactly the non-linguistic support is for the two pairs of opponent unique hues. Evidence for just two opponent hue channels with red-green and yellow-blue as poles is thin at best. Discrepancies in the standard model display themselves primarily in the form of non-linearities, which are then attributed to various non-standard interactions between cone types.[7] Consequently there have been many proposals for adjustments and modifications. There is talk of mixtures of opponent and non-opponent channels and of multiple 'red-green' channels; it has been suggested that fixed spectral sensitivity functions should be given up and detection mechanisms are thought to be tuned to a wide variety of hues.[8]

Moreover, most measurement techniques rely on some sort of threshold detection, not representative of ordinary colour vision at suprathreshold levels. Further, most experiments are carried out with spectral lights (as distinct from coloured surfaces), which cannot be thought representative of the chromatic world in which humans live. It is also a matter of controversy whether the chromatically opponent channels suggested by additivity experiments are the same as account for the results of cancellation experiments.[9] Finally, in general introductions to the subject, the Bezold-Brücke phenomenon of invariant hues is often quoted, the same data from Purdy's 1929 dissertation always being reproduced. These invariant hues are then assimilated to the unique hues, as for example Hurvich does (1981, p. 73). However Purdy had already noted that the invariant hues are not the same as the unique hues. Recent technical publications remain as unclear about the issue as they are about other characteristics of the invariant hues.[10]

Without denying psychophysical evidence for opponent mechanisms (the brain somehow taking advantage of the difference between adding and subtracting information), these very general ideas, or motivations for research, are remote from the postulate of exactly two opponent channels of a specified sort. The *instrumental* success of the idea of opponent channels is obvious; *two* chromatic channels may indeed be sufficient to do the job *in some cases.* That is to say, psychophysically distinct channels might well emerge in particular types of well-determined experimental conditions. But these channels do not exist outside the experimental situations. In this sense, psychophysically speaking, there might be *many* opponent channels (of which *one* might be red-green), while neurophysiologically speaking there are none.

7.2.4   NEUROPHYSIOLOGICAL EVIDENCE FOR TWO OPPONENT PAIRS OF UNIQUE HUES

Recent work in neurophysiology provides strong evidence that between retina and cortex, processing of wavelength information is intricately mixed with luminosity, form, texture, movement responses, and other changes in the environment; 'the absence of a distinct 'achromatic' pathway is the most troublesome physiological finding'.[11] Evidence for a blue-yellow neural pathway is exceptionally weak. Most evidence has been reported for a red-green pathway, but, even with identical spatial and temporal stimuli and identical adapting conditions, there can be extreme variation in the neutral points of individual 'red-green' ganglion cells (which allegedly support a red-green pathway).[12] If one averages the results for many cells, the average 'cell' does give opponent signals when stimulated by a red or green light and there are excellent grounds for talking about *opponent* cells. But that is a far cry from there being individual red-green opponent cells. For one thing, whether a cell behaves *as if* responding differently to red and green may depend on characteristics of the stimulus other than being red or green. For another, it leaves unclear what the purpose is of a variety of cells higher up the visual system that seem to duplicate the procedure. Similar unclarities arise with identifying the properties of double-opponent cells and their contribution to a fixed number of modular pathways.[13]

Sometimes the suggestion arises, in the context of neurophysiological research, that words such as 'colour', 'opponent', 'red', etc. have a technical meaning that is independent of the colloquial sense of these words. If that were true, then *we* do not know what colour science is about. Consider the following quotation of Gregory (1994), from a review of Zeki's *A Vision of the Brain*: 'Zeki is rightly renowned for his discovery of specific neurones generating the experiences of colours.' Surely, the word 'colours' here is not a technical term.

The suggestion that there is no neurophysiological evidence for the existence of two pairs of opponent hues is not new. Gouras and Eggers (1984) explicitly deny Hering's opponent colour channels in the primate retinogeniculate pathway. D'Zmura (1991) says 'observers [also] possess chromatic detection mechanisms tuned to intermediate hues such as orange'. Teller (1991, p. 530) suggests: 'The retinal coding scheme requires further recoding if neurons fully worthy of the name red/green and (particularly) yellow/blue are to emerge. Such neurons have not yet been seen in primate visual systems, and no one knows where or whether they will ever be seen.' Similarly, Mollon (1992), in a review of Davidoff (1991), claims the latter's appeal to 'chromatically opponent cells which signal redness and greenness or blueness and yellowness' is 'pseudo-physiology' because the neurons required to substantiate the view are not those that have so far been found electrophysiologically in the visual pathway (see also Mollon, 1987). Of course none of this denies the existence of a variety of opponent types of cells. That is not the issue here. The point is that there is no convincing evidence for exactly *two* well-determined pairs of opponent hues.

7.2.5   CROSS-CULTURAL EVIDENCE FOR A FIXED NUMBER OF BASIC COLOUR CATEGORIES

In 1901, Ladd-Franklin claimed that 'the acute tribe of Eskimo examined by Mr Rivers [1901] have discovered for themselves – that red, yellow, green and blue (and no other colors) are of a unitary character'. Later developments include the claim of Berlin and Kay (1969) that *eleven* basic colour categories exist which appear labelled in the languages of the world according to an evolutionary sequence. If it were true that *four* unique hues or *eleven* basic colour categories were a universal human cognitive grounding, cross-cultural research should lend support to it. That is to say, before deciding that there is *scientific* evidence for four unique hues (or any other number of 'primitive' or 'basic' colours), it is necessary to be sure that one is not simply fitting one's data to the particular idiosyncrasies of, for example, modern English.

As it happens, empirical evidence for a fixed number of perceptuo-linguistic culturally universal colour categories (whether four or any other number), is as phantasmagoric as virtual reality, although empirical research tends to confirm the cross-cultural validity of European categories by simply imposing them on other languages when these are first inscribed or translated. For example, the well-known anthropologist Boas, in decades of work transcribing and codifying the Kwakw'ala language on Vancouver Island, always glossed *lhenxa* as 'green' although Kwakw'ala speakers still describe both a green apple and a yellow lemon as *lhenxa*.[14] Similar problems arise for numerous other languages,[15] including European languages of the past.[16]

7.2.6   CONCLUSION

In the space available we can refer to only a very small portion of the evidence supporting our claims. Nonetheless taking this other evidence into account our main conclusions are as follows:

1. Neither structural nor functional opponency can be denied. But neurophysiology and psychophysics do not support the view that there are only two pairs of opponent unique hues.

2. Both the history of western art and science and a cursory cross-cultural glance reveal that to rely on (macro-) folk perception to establish four primitive hues, eleven basic colour categories, or any other perceptual categorisation of colour held to be universal because of salience, innateness, or whatever, is an unreliable procedure. There is no convincing evidence that particular colour primitives exist at any kind of pre-linguistic, phenomenal or biological level.

3. The separation of colour into hue, brightness and saturation might more profitably be viewed as an artefact of technoscience. Thus there is nothing 'natural' about either the

combination or the separation of these three attributes. There is no 'natural' way, in which, say, luminance and brightness could be related by a strict law.

4. No one-to-one correspondence can be shown to exist between physiological pathways and psychophysical channels. Different functional channels are (partly) embodied in the same set (pattern) of anatomic cells and different contexts may require different sets of functional channels. In particular there is no neurophysiological evidence for an autonomous colour pathway, or cells responsible for hue alone. There is no unequivocal cross-cultural evidence for colour as a clear and distinct universal cognitive grounding.

5. There is no evidence (physiologically or phenomenologically) for specific mechanisms corresponding to Hering's four unique hues. In western cultures the four unique hues may have a techno-sociological or historical significance: colour scientists must decide for themselves how relevant they find this.

7.2.7 NOTES

1 CIE 1987, cf. Wyszecki and Stiles 1982; Hering 1964 [1878], p. 48.

2 Hurvich 1981, pp. 1-11, 53; Lennie and D'Zmura 1988, p. 337; Kuehni 1983, p. 39; Quinn et al. 1988; Pokorny et al. 1991.

3 Gage 1993; Richter 1977, p. 137; Mach 1919, p. 54f.

4 Sepper 1988; Dcrefeldt 1991; Sherman 1981.

5 Dimmick and Hubbard 1939, Schefrin and Werner 1990; Hering 1964 [1878], p.58; Bartleson 1976, Fuld et al. 1983, Quinn et al. 1988; Kuehni 1983, p. 42.

6 McNeill 1972; Wierzbicka 1990; Iijima et al. 1982; Johnson and Tomiie 1985; Stanlaw 1987; Boynton and Olson 1987; Uchikawa and Boynton 1987.

7 Ayama and Ikeda 1986, Boynton 1988, Ejima and Takahashi 1984, 1985, Elsner et al. 1987, Elzinga and de Weert 1984, Ikeda and Ayama 1980, 1983, Ingling and Martinez 1985 Suppes et al. 1990, Lec et al. 1989, Lennie and D'Zmura 1988, Schefrin and Werner 1990, Shevell and Humanski 1988, Switkes and De Valois 1983, van Dijk and Spekreijse 1983, van Esch et al. 1983, Yaguchi and Ikeda 1982. See further Gouras 1984, Haegerstrom-Portnoy and Adams 1983, Hess et al. 1989, Rabin and Adams 1992, Shevell 1992, Sperling et al. 1983, Stockman et al. 1991, Stromeyer et al. 1991, Thornton and Pugh 1983, Vos 1982, Wolf and Scheibner 1983.

8 Albright 1991; D'Zmura 1991; Flanagan et al. 1990; Krauskopf et al. 1982, 1986; Lennie et al. 1990; Paulus and Kröger-Paulus 1983; Webster and Mollon 1991.

9 Shevell and Handte 1983; Brown and Teller 1989.

10 Purdy 1931,1937; Ejima and Takahashi 1984, 1985; Elsner et al. 1987; Suppes et al. 1990; Paulus and Kröger-Paulus 1983; Pokorny et al. 1991; Vos 1986; Zrenner 1985.

11 Lennie and D'Zmura 1988, p. 372. See further: Boynton 1988; Derrington et al. 1984; DeValois and De Valois 1975; Estévez and Dijkhuis 1983; Gouras 1984; Gouras and Eggers 1984; Finkelstein 1988; Hood and Finkelstein 1983; Tansley et al. 1983; Zrenner 1983. Also on the interaction with motion detection: Albright 1991; Gouras 1991; Hubel and Livingstone 1990, 1991; Ingling and Grigsby 1990, 1991; Ingling and Martinez 1985; Kooi and De Valois 1992; Krauskopf and Farell 1990; Merrigan 1989; Mollon 1989, 1990; Ohmura 1988; Schiller et al. 1990.

12 Gouras 1984, Zrenner 1983, 1985.

13 Billock 1991, Boynton 1988, Estévez and Dijkhuis 1983, Krüger and Fischer 1983, Lennie and D'Zmura 1988, Lennie et al. 1990, Livingstone and Hubel 1984, 1988, Schein and Desimone 1990, Shapley 1990, Teller 1984, Ts'o and Gilbert 1988, Zeki 1984, 1985.

14 See Boas 1892, 1931, 1934; Boas and Hunt 1905; cf.Curtis 1916. However, Dawson (1887), Grubb (1977) and Lincoln and Rath (1980) gloss it as 'yellow, green'.

15 Ayama and Ikeda 1986, Boynton 1988, Ejima and Takahashi 1984, 1985, Elsner *et al.* 1987, Elzinga and de Weert 1984, Ikeda and Ayama 1980, 1983, Ingling and Martinez 1985, Suppes *et al.* 1990, Lee *et al.* 1989, Lennie and D'Zmura 1988, Schefrin and Werner 1990, Shevell and Humanski 1988, Switkes and De Valois 1983, van Dijk and Spekreijse 1983, van Esch *et al.* 1983, Yaguchi and Ikeda 1982. See further Gouras 1984, Haegerstrom-Portnoy and Adams 1983, Hess *et al.* 1989, Rabin and Adams 1992, Shevell 1992, Sperling *et al.* 1983, Stockman *et al.* 1991, Stromeyer *et al.* 1991, Thornton and Pugh 1983, Vos 1982, Wolf and Scheibner 1983.

16 André 1949; Gage 1993; Mead 1899; Barley 1974; Ardener 1971.

7.2.8 REFERENCES

ALBRIGHT, T.D. (1991) Color and the integration of motion signals, *Trends in Neuroscience*, **14**, 266-69.

ANDRÉ, J. (1949) *Etude sur les termes de couleur dans la langue latine*, Paris: Klincksieck.

ARDENER, E. (ED.) (1971) *Social Anthropology*, London: Tavistock.

AYAMA, M. AND IKEDA, M. (1986) Additivity of yellow chromatic valence, *Vision Research*, **26**, 763–769.

BARLEY, N.F. (1974) Old English colour classification: where do matters stand?, *Anglo-Saxon England*, **3**, 15–28.

BARTLESON, C.J. (1976) Brown, *Color Research and Application*, **1**, 181–191.

BERLIN, B. & KAY, P. (1969) *Basic Color Terms: Their Universality and Evolution*, Berkeley: University of California Press; reprint 1991.

BILLOCK, V.A. (1991) The relationship between simple and double opponent cells, *Vision Research*, **31**, 33–42.

BOAS, F. (1892) Vocabulary of the Kwakiutl language, *Proceedings of the American Philosophical Society*, **30**, 34–82.

BOAS, F. (1931) Notes on the Kwakiutl vocabulary, *International Journal of American Linguistics*, **6**, 163–178.

BOAS, F. (1934) *Geographical Names of the Kwakiutl Indians*, New York: AMS Press.

BOAS, F. & HUNT, G. (1905) *Kwakiutl Texts* (The Jesup North Pacific Expedition, vol. 3; Memoir of the American Museum of Natural History, New York, vol.3; Leiden: Brill, New York: Stechert), New York: AMS Press.

BOYNTON, R.M. (1988) Color vision, *Annual Review of Psychology*, **39**, 69–100.

BOYNTON, R.M. & OLSON, C.X. (1987) Locating basic colors in the OSA space, *Color Research and Application*, **12**, 94–105.

BROWN, A.M. & TELLER, D.Y. (1989) Chromatic opponency in 3-month-old human infants,*Vision Research*, **29**, 37–45.

CIE (1987) *International Lighting Vocabulary*, Publication CIE No. 17.4, Genève: Bureau Central de la Commission Electrotechnique Internationale.

CURTIS, E.S. (1916) *The North American Indian*, vol. 11, New York: Johnson Reprint.

D'ZMURA, M. (1991) Color in visual search, *Vision Research*, **31**, 951–966.

DAVIDOFF, J. (1991) *Cognition Through Color*, Cambridge MA: The MIT Press.

DAWSON, G.M. (1887) *Notes and Observations on the Qwakiool People of the Northern Part of Vancouver Island and Adjacent Coasts, Made During the Summer of 1885*, Fairfield WA: Ye Galleon Press.

DE VALOIS, R. L. & DE VALOIS, K. K. (1975) Neural coding of color. In: Carterette, E.C. & Friedman, M.P. (Eds), *Handbook of Perception*, New York: Academic Press, pp. 117–166.

DEREFELDT, G. (1991) Colour appearance systems. In: Gouras, P. (Ed.) *The Perception of Colour*, London: Macmillan, vol. 6, pp. 218–261.

DERRINGTON, A.M., KRAUSKOPF, J. & LENNIE, P. (1984) Chromatic mechanisms in lateral geniculate nucleus of macaque, *Journal of Physiology*, **357**, 241–265.

DIMMICK, F.L. & HUBBARD, M.R. (1939) The spectral location of psychologically unique yellow, green, and blue, *American Journal of Psychology*, **52**, 242–254.

EJIMA, Y. AND TAKAHASHI, S. (1984) Bezold-Brücke hue shift and nonlinearity in opponent-color processes, *Vision Research*, **24**, 1897–1904.

EJIMA, Y. & TAKAHASHI, S. (1985) Interaction between short- and longer-wavelength cones in hue cancellation codes: Nonlinearities of hue cancellation as a function of stimulus intensity, *Vision Research*, **25**, 1911–1922.

ELSNER, A.E., BURNS, S.A. & POKORNY, J. (1987) Changes in constant-hue loci with spatial frequency, *Color Research and Application*, **12**, 42–50.

ELZINGA, C.H. & DE WEERT, C.M.M. (1984) Spectral sensitivity functions derived from brightness matching: Implications of intensity variance for color-vision models, *Journal of the Optical Society of America*, A **3**, 1173–1181.

ESTÉVEZ, O. & DIJKHUIS, T. (1983) Human pattern evoked potentials and colour coding. In: Mollon, J.D. & Sharpe, L.T. (Eds) *Colour Vision: Physiology and Pyschophysics*, London: Academic Press, pp. 261–268.

FINKELSTEIN, M.A. (1988) Spectral tuning of opponent channels is spatially dependent, *Color Research and Application*, **13**, 106–112.

FLANAGAN, P., CAVANAGH, P. & FAVREAU, O.E. (1990) Independent orientation-selective mechanisms for the cardinal directions of colour space, *Vision Research*, **30**, 769–778.

FULD, K., WERNER, J.S. & WOOTEN, B.R. (1983) The possible elemental nature of brown, *Vision Research*, **23**, 631–637.

GAGE, J. (1993) *Colour and Culture: Practice and Meaning from Antiquity to Abstraction*, London: Thames and Hudson.

GOURAS, P. (1984) Color vision. In: Osborn, N. & Chader, J. (Eds) *Progress In Retinal Research*, **3**, London: Pergamon Press, pp. 227–260.

GOURAS, P. (1991) Precortical physiology of colour vision. In: Gouras, P. (Ed.) *The Perception of Colour*, London: Macmillan, pp. 163–178.

GOURAS, P. & EGGERS, H. (1984) Hering's opponent color channels do not exist in the primate retinogeniculate pathway, *Ophthalmic Research*, **16**, 31–35.

GREGORY, R. (1994) Escape from the obvious, *Times Literary Supplement*, 14 January, p. 5.

GRUBB, D. McC. (1977) *A Practical Writing System and Short Dictionary of Kwakw'ala (Kwakiutl)*, Ethnology Service Paper No. 34, Ottawa: National Museums of Canada.

HAEGERSTROM-PORTNOY, G. & ADAMS, A.J. (1983) Spatial sensitization properties of the blue-sensitive pathways. In: Mollon, J.D. & Sharpe, L.T. (Eds) *Colour Vision: Physiology and Psychophysics*, London: Academic Press, pp. 505–514.

HERING, E. (1964) *Outlines of a Theory of the Light Sense*, transl. Hurvich, L.M. & Jameson, D., Cambridge: Harvard University Press; first German edition 1878, translation of 1920 edition.

HESS, R.F., MULLEN, K.T. & ZRENNER, E. (1989) Human photopic vision with only short wavelength cones: post-receptoral properties, *Journal of Physiology*, **417**, 151–172.

HOOD, D.C. & FINKELSTEIN, M.A. (1983) A case for the revision of textbook models of color vision: the detection and appearance of small brief lights. In: Mollon, J.D. & Sharpe, L.T. (Eds) *Colour Vision: Physiology and Psychophysics*, London: Academic Press, pp. 385–398.

HUBEL, D.H. & LIVINGSTONE, M.S. (1990) Color and contrast sensitivity in the lateral geniculate body and primary visual cortex of the Macaque monkey, *Journal of Neuroscience*, **10**, 2223–2237.

HUBEL, D.H. & LIVINGSTONE, M.S. (1991) Comment on Ingling & Grigsby 1990, *Vision Research*, **31**, 1655–1656.

HURVICH, L.M. (1981) *Color Vision*, Sunderland: Sinauer.

IIJIMA, T., WENNING, W. & ZOLLINGER, H. (1982) Cultural factors of color naming in Japanese: naming tests with Japanese children in Japan and Europe, *Anthropological Linguistics*, **24**, 245–262.

IKEDA, M. & AYAMA, M. (1980) Additivity of opponent chromatic valence, *Vision Research*, **20**, 995–999.

IKEDA, M. & AYAMA, M. (1983) Nonlinear nature of the yellow chromatic valence. In: Mollon, J.D. & Sharpe, L.T. (Eds) *Colour Vision: Physiology and Psychophysics*, London: Academic Press, pp. 345–352.

INGLING, C.R. & MARTINEZ, E. (1985) The spatiotemporal properties of the r-g X-cell channel, *Vision Research*, **25**, 33–38.

INGLING, C.R. & GRIGSBY, S.S. (1990) Perceptual correlates of magnocellular and parvocellular channels: Seeing form and depth in afterimages, *Vision Research*, **30**, 823–828.

INGLING, C.R. & GRIGSBY, S.S. (1991) Perceptual correlates of magnocellular and parvocellular channels: Seeing form and depth in afterimages (reply), *Vision Research*, **31**, 1657–1658.

JOHNSON, E.G. & TOMIIE, T. (1985) The development of colour-naming in four- to seven-year old children: A cross-cultural study, *Psychologia: An International Journal of Psychology in the Orient*, **28**, 216–227.

KOOI, F.J. & DE VALOIS, K.K. (1992) The role of color in the motion system, *Vision Research*, **32**, 657–668.

KRAUSKOPF, J. & FARELL, B. (1990) Influence of colour on the perception of coherent motion, *Nature*, **348**, 328–331.

KRAUSKOPF, J., WILLIAMS, D.R. & HEELEY, D.W. (1982) Cardinal directions in color space, *Vision Research*, **22**, 1123–1131.

KRAUSKOPF, J., WILLIAMS, D.R., MANDLER, M.B. & BROWN, A.M. (1986) Higher order color mechanisms, *Vision Research*, **26**, 23–32.

KRÜGER, J. & FISCHER, B. (1983) Colour columns and colour areas. In: Mollon, J.D. & Sharpe, L.T. (Eds) *Colour Vision: Physiology and Psychophysics*, London: Academic Press, pp. 291–296.

KUEHNI, R.G. (1983) *Color: Essence and Logic*, New York: Van Nostrand.

LADD-FRANKLIN, C. (1901) Color-introspection on the part of the Eskimo, *Psychological Review*, **8**, 396–402.

LEE, B.B., MARTIN, P.R. & VALBERG, A. (1989) Nonlinear summation of M- and L-cone inputs to phasic retinal ganglion cells of the macaque, *The Journal of Neuroscience*, **9**, 1433–1442.

LENNIE, P. & D'ZMURA, M. (1988): Mechanisms of color vision, *Critical Reviews in Neurobiology*, **3**, 333–400.

LENNIE, P., KRAUSKOPF, J. & SCLAR, G. (1990) Chromatic mechanisms in striate cortex of macaque, *Journal of Neuroscience*, **10**, 649–699.

LINCOLN, N.J. & RATH, J.C. (1980) *North Wakashan Comparative Root List*, Canadian Ethnology Service Paper No. 68, Ottawa: National Museums of Canada.

LIVINGSTONE, M.S. & HUBEL, D.H. (1984) Anatomy and physiology of a color system in the primate visual cortex, *Journal of Neuroscience*, **4**, 309–356.

LIVINGSTONE, M.S. & HUBEL, D.H. (1988) Segregation of form, color, movement, and depth: anatomy, physiology, and perception, *Science*, **240**, 740–749.

MACH, E. (1919) *Die Analyse der Empfindungen*, Jena: Fischer.

MCNEILL, N.B. (1972) Colour and colour terminology, *Journal of Linguistics*, **8**, 21–23.

MEAD, W.E. (1899) Color in old English poetry, *Publications of the Modern Language Association of America*, **14** (new series 7(2)), 169–206.

MERIGAN, W.H. (1989) Chromatic and achromatic vision of Macaques: Role of the P pathway, *Journal of Neuroscience*, **9**, 776–783.

MOLLON, J.D. (1987) On the nature of models of colour vision, *Die Farbe*, **34**, 29–46.

MOLLON, J.D. (1989) 'Tho She Kneeld In That Place Where They Grew . . .': The uses and origins of primate colour vision, *Journal of Experimental Biology*, **146**, 21–38.

MOLLON, J.D. (1990) Neurobiology: the club-sandwich mystery, *Nature*, **343**, 16–17.

MOLLON, J.D. (1992) Review of Davidoff 1991, *Trends in Neuroscience*, **15**, 194.

OHMURA, H. (1988) Disparities of shape and color in determining the type of apparent movement, *Japanese Psychological Research*, **30**, 1–10.

PAULUS, W. & KRÖGER-PAULUS, A. (1983) A new concept of retinal colour coding, *Vision Research*, **23**, 529–540.

POKORNY, J., SHEVELL, S.K. & SMITH, V.C. (1991) Colour appearance and colour constancy. In: Gouras, P. (Ed.) *The Perception of Colour*, London: Macmillan, vol. 6, pp. 43–61.

PURDY, D. MCL. (1931): Spectral hue as a function of intensity, *American Journal of Psychology*, **43**, 541–559.

PURDY, D. MCL. (1937): The Bezold-Brücke phenomenon and contours for constant hue, *American Journal of Psychology*, **49**, 313–315.

QUINN, P.C., ROSANO, J.L. & WOOTEN, B.R. (1988) Evidence that brown is not an elemental color, *Perception & Psychophysics*, **43**, 156–164.

RABIN, J. & ADAMS, A.J. (1992) Lightness induction in the S-cone pathway, *Vision Research*, **9**, 1771–1774.

RICHTER, I.A. (1977) *Selections from the Notebooks of Leonardo da Vinci*, Oxford: Oxford University Press.

SCHEFRIN, B.E. & WERNER, J.S. (1990) Loci of spectral unique hues throughout the life span, *Journal of the Optical Society of America*, **A 7**, 305–311.

SCHEIN, S.J. & DESIMONE, R. (1990) Spectral properties of V4 neurons in macaque and their relationship to a physiological model of color vision, quoted in D'Zmura (1991).

SCHILLER, P.H., LOGOTHETIS, N.K. & CHARLES, E.R. (1990) Functions of the colour-opponent and broad-band channels of the visual system, *Nature*, **343**, 68–70.

SEPPER, D.L. (1988) *Goethe Contra Newton*, Cambridge: Cambridge University Press.

SHAPLEY, R. (1990) Visual sensitivity and parallel retinocortical channels, *Annual Review of Psychology*, **41**, 635–658.

SHERMAN, P.D. (1981) *Color Vision in the Nineteenth Century*, Bristol: Hilger.

SHEVELL, S.K. (1992) Redness from short-wavelength-sensitive cones does not induce greenness, *Vision Research*, **32**, 1551–1556.

SHEVELL, S.K. & HANDTE, J.P. (1983) Postreceptoral adaptation in suprathreshold color perception. In: Mollon, J.D. & Sharpe, L.T. (Eds) *Colour Vision: Physiology and Psychophysics*, London: Academic Press, pp. 399–407.

SHEVELL, S.K. & HUMANSKI, R.A. (1988) Color perception under chromatic adaptation: Red/green equilibria with adapted short-wavelength cones, *Vision Research*, **28**, 1345 1356.

SPERLING, H.G., VIANCOUR, T., MATHENY, J. & MEHARG, L. (1983) Blue and green increment thresholds on a sine-wave varying yellow. In: Mollon, J.D. & Sharpe, L.T. (Eds) *Colour Vision: Physiology and Psychophysics*, London: Academic Press, pp. 527–534.

STANLAW, J.M (1987) *Color, Culture, and Contact: English Loanwords and Problems of Color Nomenclature in Modern Japanese*, PhD Thesis, University of Illinois at Urbana-Champaign.

STERNHEIM, C.E. & BOYNTON, R.M. (1966) Uniqueness of perceived hues investigated with a continuous judgmental technique, *Journal of Experimental Psychology*, **72**, 770–776.

STOCKMAN, A., MACLEOD, D.I.A. & DEPRIEST, D.D. (1991) The temporal properties of the human short-wave photoreceptors and their associated pathways, *Vision Research*, **31**, 189–208.

STROMEYER, C.F., ESKEW, R.T., KRONAUER, R.E. & SPILLMANN, L. (1991) Temporal phase response of the short-wave cone signal for color and luminance, *Vision Research*, **31**, 787–803.

SUPPES, P., KRANTZ, D.M., LUCE, R.D. & TVERSKY, A. (1990) *Foundations of Measurement*, New York: Academic Press, vol. 2, chapter 15.

SWITKES, E. & DE VALOIS, K.K. (1983) Luminance and chromaticity interactions in spatial vision. In: Mollon, J.D. & Sharpe, L.T. (Eds) *Colour Vision: Physiology and Psychophysics*, London: Academic Press, pp. 465–470.

TANSLEY, B.W., ROBERTSON, A.W. & MAUGHAN, K.E. (1983) Chromatic and achromatic border perception. In: Mollon, J.D. & Sharpe, L.T. (Eds) *Colour Vision: Physiology and Psychophysics*, London: Academic Press, pp. 445–454.

TELLER, D.Y. (1984) Linking propositions, *Vision Research*, **24**, 1233–1246.

TELLER, D.Y. (1991) Simpler arguments might work better, *Philosophical Psychology*, **4**, 51–60.

THORNTON, J.E. & PUGH JR, E.N. (1983) Relationship of opponent colours cancellation measures to cone-antagonistic signals deduced from increment threshold data. In: Mollon, J.D. & Sharpe,

L.T. (Eds) *Colour Vision: Physiology and Psychophysics*, London: Academic Press, pp. 361–374.

Ts'o, D.Y. & GILBERT, C.D. (1988) The organisation of chromatics and spatial interaction in the primate striate cortex, *Journal of Neuroscience*, **8**, 1712–1727.

UCHIKAWA, K. & BOYNTON, R.M. (1987) Categorical color perception of Japanese observers: Comparison with that of Americans, *Vision Research*, **27**, 1825–1833.

VAN DIJK, B.W. & SPEKREIJSE, H. (1983) Nonlinear versus linear opponency in vertebrate retina. In: Mollon, J.D. & Sharpe, L.T. (Eds) *Colour Vision: Physiology and Psychophysics*, London: Academic Press, pp. 173–182.

VAN ESCH, J.A., NOORLANDER, C. & KOENDERINK, J.J. (1983) Sensitivity to spatiotemporal colour contrast. In: Mollon, J.D. & Sharpe, L.T. (Eds) *Colour Vision: Physiology and Psychophysics*, London: Academic Press, pp. 425–432.

VOS, J.J. (1982) On the merits of model making in understanding color vision phenomena, *Color Research and Application*, **7**, 69–77.

VOS, J.J. (1986) Are unique and invariant hues coupled?, *Vision Research*, **26**, 337–342.

WEBSTER, M.A. & MOLLON, J.D. (1991) Changes in colour appearance following post-receptoral adaptation, *Nature*, **349**, 235–238.

WIERZBICKA, A. (1990) The meaning of color terms: Semantics, culture and cognition, *Cognitive Linguistics*, **1**, 99–150.

WOLF, E. & SCHEIBNER, H. (1983) The blue fundamental primary – a revision based on dichromatic alychnes. In: Mollon, J.D. & Sharpe, L.T. (Eds) *Colour Vision: Physiology and Psychophysics*, London: Academic Press, pp. 479–486.

WYSZECKI, G. & STILES, W.S. (1982) *Color Science*, New York: Wiley, 2nd ed.

YAGUCHI, H. & IKEDA, M. (1982) Nonlinear nature of the opponent-color channels, *Color Research and Application*, **7**, 187–190.

ZEKI, S. (1984) The construction of colours by the cerebral cortex, *Proceedings of the Royal Institution of Great Britain*, pp. 231–257.

ZEKI, S. (1985) Colour pathways and hierarchies in the cerebral cortex. In: Ottoson, T. & Zeki, S. (Ed.) *Central and Peripheral Mechanisms of Colour Vision*, New York: Macmillan, pp. 19–44.

ZRENNER, E. (1983) *Neurophysiological Aspects of Color Vision in Primates*, Berlin: Springer.

ZRENNER, E. (1985) The zero signal detector. In: Ottoson, T. & Zeki, S. (Ed.) *Central and Peripheral Mechanisms of Colour Vision*, New York: Macmillan, pp. 165–182.

The Influence of White Light on the Location of Unique Green

Jeffery K. Hovis and Richard Van Arsdel

7.3.1   INTRODUCTION

Unique green is a term used to describe a light that appears green without a yellowish or bluish component. Within opponent colours theory, the spectral location of unique green is important, because it is one light that produces a balance of the excitatory and inhibitory receptor inputs into the blue-yellow opponent channel. (The other lights that produce a balanced input into the blue-yellow mechanism are perceived as white or as unique red.) By altering the viewing conditions the receptor balance can be disturbed, resulting in a shift in the location of unique green and the direction of the unique green shift reflects the relative change in the receptor inputs. For example, decreasing field size, duration, or luminance can shift the unique green location to a longer wavelength (Dagher, *et al.*, 1958; Ingling and Tsou, 1977; Nagy, 1979; Drum, 1989a). The shift to a longer wavelength associated with these changes in viewing conditions suggests that the relative input of the cone mediating the blue signal has increased.

In addition to field size, duration and luminance, receptor inputs into the blue-yellow channel are also affected by the admixture of a white desaturant or a brightness reduction induced by a white surround. Relative to viewing monochromatic lights on a dark background, both of these conditions have been reported to shift unique green to a shorter wavelength (Fuld and Otto, 1985; Guth, 1991; Kurtenback *et al.*, 1984).

Assuming that the simultaneous contrast effects of the white surround would produce the opposite effect of the white desaturant, Fuld and Otto's (1985) report of unique green shifting to a shorter wavelength in the presence of a white surround is unexpected. Furthermore, previous work (Coren and Keith, 1970) has shown that an induced brightness reduction produced hue shifts that, in general, were consistent with hue shifts associated with decreasing luminance. That is, Bezold-Brücke hue shifts can be induced by both a direct and indirect brightness reduction. If the induced brightness reduction by an achromatic surround has the equivalent effect on the receptor inputs into the blue-yellow channel as decreasing luminance, then unique green should have shifted to a longer, not shorter, wavelength.

The discrepancy between the data and the expected direction of the unique green shift in the presence of a white surround does not appear to be related to stray light effects. Stray light from the surround could desaturate the monochromatic light and produce a shift to a shorter wavelength (Guth, 1991; Kurtenback *et al.*, 1984). However, Fuld and Otto (1985) concluded that, based upon stray light calculations, scattered light from an equal brightness surround was negligible. A factor that could explain the discrepancy between the expectation and their results is that the location of unique green was interpolated from colour naming data. Because the wavelength interval used in the colour naming experiment was 20 nm and colour naming functions were often irregular, Fuld and Otto recognised that interpolating hue loci could be subject to considerable error.

The purpose of this short study is to investigate more directly the effect of an induced brightness reduction on the location of unique green. Low photopic levels were selected because the shifts in unique green with varying intensity are more evident at retinal illuminances below 2 log td (Ingling and Tsou, 1977). To minimise the effects of stray light, only an equal-brightness surround was used. In addition, this study reinvestigates the effects of a white desaturant on the location of unique green and examines qualitatively the combined effects of the desaturant and surround on the receptor inputs into the blue-yellow channel by superimposing the spectral lights on a white background.

7.3.2 METHODS

7.3.2.1 Apparatus

Achromatic lenses imaged lights from a Bausch and Lomb monochromator and a tungsten-halogen lamp onto separate diffusing screens. These screens were optically superimposed with a beam splitting cube. The diffusing screens were masked so that the monochromatic light, white desaturant, and inner diameter of the white annulus subtended 1°. The white background and the outer diameter of the annulus subtended 5°. A plus lens located at the subject's spectacle plane imaged the target at optical infinity. Subjects viewed the stimulus monocularly with their natural pupils. Central fixation was maintained without the aid of fixation lights. An electronic shutter flashed the stimuli in both the white and unique green trials for 0.7 second every 10 seconds.

The experimenter maintained constant brightness of the monochromatic lights by adjusting a mirrored-neutral density wedge to predetermined settings during the inter-stimulus interval. These wedge settings were interpolated from the mean values of the four subjects' brightness matching results in 5 nm steps to a 2.5 cdm^{-2} whitish surround.

After adjusting the white light's colour temperature, its luminance (measured by a Tektronix Spot Meter) was set at 2.5 cdm^{-2} for the annulus condition and 1.6 cdm^{-2} for the desaturant and background trials using mirrored-neutral density filters. (Initially, the desaturant and background luminances were set to 2.5 cdm^{-2}, but the subjects reported that the stimuli were too desaturated to make reliable hue judgements.)

7.3.2.2 Determination of white

Prior to each session in which the white light was present, the spectral emittance of the tungsten-halogen lamp was altered with Kodak Colour Correcting Filters so that the white field appeared achromatic to each subject using the following procedure. After 10 min of dark adaptation, the subject viewed 5° whitish lights whose colour temperature varied randomly from 4000K to 7500K. Subjects responded as to whether the light appeared bluish or yellowish. The colour temperature of the achromatic light was determined by interpolating to the colour temperature that corresponded to 50 per cent of the yellowish responses. If the colour temperature was impossible to obtain with the filter set, then the next highest obtainable colour temperature was selected.

7.3.2.3 Unique green determination

Following 10 min of dark adaptation, subjects adjusted the wavelength of the mono-chromator during the dark interstimulus interval until the subsequent coloured stimulus appeared neither bluish nor yellowish. This setting was repeated five times with the starting wavelength chosen randomly by the experimenter to be within 15 nm of the subject's previous setting. The experimenter alternated between starting at a wavelength that was either longer or shorter than the previous setting. The viewing condition was held constant throughout the session. Each condition was evaluated five times using a random block design.

7.3.2.4 Subjects

The four male subjects had normal colour vision as determined by the Ishihara Colour Vision Screening Plates and the Farnsworth Munsell 100 Hue test. Subjects J and R were highly experienced observers in colour naming and colour matching experiments, whereas subjects C and L were inexperienced. All subjects were naive as to their results during the experiment.

7.3.3   RESULTS

Figure 7.3.1 shows each subject's unique green wavelengths for the various test conditions. Each point represents the average of the five session means. The results demonstrate that, relative to a dark background, an equal brightness white annulus shifts unique green to a longer wavelength, whereas a white desaturant shifts unique green to a shorter wavelength. Statistical analyses on the individual subject's results (one-way ANOVA and Tukey's *posthoc* Test) revealed that, except for the annulus condition for subject C, these shifts were significant at the $p \le 0.05$ rejection level. The effect of the white background on the locus of unique green is less certain. For subjects J and L, the white background shifted unique green to a longer wavelength, whereas the location for subjects R and C was unaffected by the background. The shifts for J and L were significant at the $p \le 0.05$ rejection level. Although subject J's unique green location is unusually high, it is consistent with measurements in several previous experiments.

7.3.4   DISCUSSION

The shift of unique green to a shorter wavelength when admixed with a white desaturant confirms previous results that a white desaturant produces a yellowish hue shift for wavelengths near 500 nm (Guth, 1991; Kurtenback *et al.*, 1984). Although the shift of unique green to a longer wavelength in the presence of a white surround is consistent with predictions based upon a contrast induced brightness reduction, this result disagrees with Fuld and Otto's (1985) colour naming data. This inconsistency may be a result of the different procedures used to determine the unique green location. As Fuld and Otto mentioned, interpolating hue locations from irregular functions can be subject to error.

It is unlikely that the conflicting results between the colour naming experiments and our direct measurements are due to a yellowish component in the white annulus inducing blue in the test stimulus, because the colour temperature of the white light was intentionally biased towards a bluish white. In fact, a slightly bluish surround probably reduced the effect of the brightness reduction because a bluish component in the surround would induce yellow in the test field that would counteract the shift of unique green to a longer wavelength.

Although rod influence cannot be discounted at the luminance level used in this study (Aguilar and Stiles, 1954), stimulation of the rods would have also counteracted the shift to a longer wavelength. A blue signal in the surround due to the rods (Stabell *et al.*, 1987; Trezona, 1970) would induce a yellowish component into the test stimulus that would also oppose the shift of unique green to a longer wavelength.

The effect of superimposing a monochromatic light on a slightly dimmer white background on the location of unique green is less certain. The result that the unique green locus remained the same as the dark background for two subjects suggests that the shift due to desaturating the monochromatic light was counteracted by the lateral contrast effects of the surround. However, for the other two subjects, the shift to a longer wavelength suggests

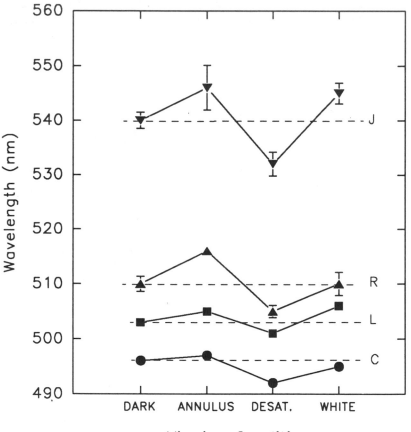

Figure 7.3.1. Spectral location of unique green for the four subjects under the various viewing conditions. The labels on the x-axis are: Dark is the dark background; Annulus is the equal brightness white surround; Desat. is when admixed with a white light; and White is when the spectral lights are superimposed on a white background.

that the induced effects of the surround predominated. Although the number of subjects is limited, these between-subject differences in the unique green shift on a white background are reminiscent of differential adaptation affects reported by others (Hurvich *et al.*, 1968; Ingling and Tsou, 1977; Richards, 1967).

Data from the background condition for subjects J and L are opposite to the shifts predicted from Drum's (1989b) experiment. Results from his study suggest that unique green should shift to a shorter wavelength when superimposed on a dim-to-moderately bright white background. However, in Drum's experiment the luminance of the mono-chromatic light was increased for the white background conditions to maintain a constant increment above threshold, whereas the luminances of the monochromatic lights for the dark and white backgrounds in this experiment were equal. Thus, Drum's stimuli on the white background may have appeared more saturated than the green light in our study and this increased saturation may account for the differences. Of course, inter-subject differences could also be responsible for the apparent conflict.

Theoretical interpretations of the present results are limited because of the narrow range of viewing conditions examined. Nevertheless, the annulus data indicate that the relative receptor inputs into the blue-yellow channel are influenced by a contrast induced brightness reduction, and this effect is equivalent to lowering the test light luminance. Both the direct and indirect brightness reductions shift unique green to a longer wavelength, which implies a relative increase in the response of the receptor mediating the blue signal. Drum (1989a,b) and Ingling (1977; Ingling and Tsou, 1977) propose that the shift in unique green to a longer wavelength reflects a relative increase of the middle-wavelength sensitive (M) cone input into the blue signal.

The mechanism responsible for the shift of unique green to a shorter wavelength when admixed with white has been attributed to the influence of the S-cone on the yellow chromatic signal via either successive or simultaneous contrast affects (Drum, 1989a,b), inhibition of the M-cone by the S-cone (Ingling, 1977; Ingling and Tsou, 1977) or non-linear gain control on all three types of cone input into the blue-yellow channel (Guth, 1991). Although Ingling and Drum's explanations are mostly qualitative, their hypotheses are more attractive because, unlike the Guth model, they also account for the shift in unique green with decreased brightness. Nevertheless, the Guth model can be modified to account for the shifts in unique green with changes in luminance, but these modifications may weaken the other predictions.

7.3.5   ACKNOWLEDGEMENT

We thank S. Lee Guth for his helpful advice and comments.

7.3.6   NOTE

Disclaimer: Opinions expressed in this article are those of the authors and do not reflect the official policy or position of the US Air Force, Department of Defense or the US Government.

7.3.7   REFERENCES

Aguilar, M. & Stiles, W.S. (1954) Saturation of the rod mechanism of the retina at high levels of stimulation, *Optica Acta*, **1**, 59–65.

COREN, S. & KEITH, B. (1970) Bezold-Brüke effect: pigment or neural locus? *Journal of the Optical Society of America*, **60**, 559–562.

DAGHER, M., CRUZ, A. & PLAZA, L. (1958) Colour thresholds with monochromatic stimuli in the spectral region 530–630 nm. In: *Visual Problems of Colour I*, NPL Symp. No. 8, London: HMSO.

DRUM, B. (1989a) Hue signals from short-and middle-wavelength-sensitive cones, *Journal of the Optical Society of America*, **A 6**, 153–157.

DRUM, B. (1989b) Colour scaling of chromatic increments on achromatic backgrounds: Implications for hue signals from individual classes of cones, *Colour Research Applications*, **14**, 293-308.

FULD, K. & OTTO, T.A. (1985) Colours of monochromatic lights that vary in contrast-induced brightness, *Journal of the Optical Society of America*, **A 2**, 76-83.

GUTH, S.L. (1991) Model for colour vision and light adaptation, *Journal of the Optical Society of America*, **A 8**, 976–993.

HURVICH, L., JAMESON, D. & COHEN, J.D. (1968) The experimental determination of unique green in the spectrum, *Perception and Psychophysics*, **4**, 65–68.

INGLING, C.R. (1977) The spectral sensitivity of the opponent-colour channels, *Vision Research*, **17**, 1083–1109.

INGLING, C.R. & TSOU, B.H.P. (1977) Orthogonal combination of the three visual channels, *Vision Research*, **17**, 1075–1082.

KURTENBACK, W., STERNHEIM, C.E. & SPILLMANN, L. (1984) Change in hue of spectral colours by dilution with white light (Abney effect), *Journal of the Optical Society of America*, **A 1**, 365–372.

NAGY, L.A. (1979) Unique hues are not invariant with brief stimulus durations, *Vision Research*, **19**, 1427–1432.

RICHARDS, W.(1967) Differences among colour normals. Classes I and II, *Journal of the Optical Society of America*, **57**, 1047–1055.

STABELL, B., NORDBY, K. & STABELL, U. (1987) Light-adaptation of the human rod system, *Clinical Vision Sciences*, **2**, 83–91.

TREZONA, P.W. (1970) Rod participation in the 'blue' mechanism and its effect on colour matching, *Vision Research*, **10**, 317–332.

Categorical Characteristics of Multiple-colour Memory

K. Uchikawa, H. Ujike and T. Sugiyama

7.4.1 INTRODUCTION

It has been shown that when we remember a colour we tend to confuse it with colours in the same category rather than with those colours that have small colour differences (Boynton *et al.*, 1989; Uchikawa, 1992; Uchikawa and Shinoda, 1990). Some previous studies (Uchikawa, 1993; Uchikawa and Sugiyama, 1993; Uchikawa *et al.*, 1994) measured an ambiguity area of identifying a test colour in memory from a large number of colours. This identification ambiguity area was defined as an area in which colours were judged to match the test colour with a certain criterion.

Uchikawa (1993) and Uchikawa and Sugiyama (1993) developed a new memory colour matching method called cascade colour matching. In cascade colour matching, first, a test colour sample was presented and the subject memorised it; then, some seconds later, he selected colour samples that matched the test colour in his memory from a set of many different colour samples. There were four consecutive stages that corresponded to different memory ambiguity levels of identification. In stage 1, the subject rejected colour samples that appeared definitely different from the test colour in his memory. In stage 2, he examined the colour samples that remained in stage 1, and again rejected colour samples that appeared probably different. In stage 3, the subject selected some colour samples that matched the test colour. He could hardly decide which one was the correct test colour even if they appeared different. In stage 4, the subject was forced to choose a colour sample that most probably matched the test colour. This colour was the final matched colour.

Uchikawa and Sugiyama found that, in a uniform colour space, the ambiguity areas obtained in stages 1 – 3 did not uniformly spread around the test colour, but were restricted to the regions of the eleven basic categorical colours (Berlin and Kay, 1969); red, green, yellow, blue, brown, orange, purple, pink, white, black and grey. Their results suggested that colours were somehow categorically organised in memory.

In this report, we studied multiple-colour memory. Our memory is usually used to remembering many colours, not just a colour presented in a simple experimental procedure. Therefore it is important to see whether there is any interference among multiple colours in memory, and whether multiple colours are memorized categorically as shown in the case of single-colour memory.

7.4.2   METHODS

7.4.2.1 Stimulus

We used the OSA uniform colour scales as stimulus colours. The OSA uniform colour scales consist of 424 colour samples that are arranged in a three-dimensional space. The three axes in the space are j for the yellow-blue direction, g for the green-red direction and L for the lightness direction. All samples in the OSA space are placed in equal colour-difference steps in any direction based on their colour appearance. This is the reason why we used the OSA space as a scale of stimulus colours in our experiments.

We measured the chromaticity and the luminance of all 424 OSA samples under the D65 illuminant, and in the present experiments we simulated these OSA samples on a colour CRT monitor. A stimulus colour was a square subtending $2.4^{\circ} \times 2.4^{\circ}$ of visual angle, surrounded by a $7.1^{\circ} \times 7.1^{\circ}$ grey stimulus ($L = -2$, $j = 0$, $g = 0$) of 10 cdm^{-2}.

7.4.2.2 Procedure

In the preliminary experiment, the subject performed the categorical colour naming for all test stimulus colours. The observer named a test colour sample using only Berlin and Kay's eleven basic colour names. This categorical colour naming was repeated twice for each subject (five times for subject TS). We defined the categorical colour region in the colour space as the positions of colour samples that were named twice (four times for subject TS) with the same basic colour name. Focal colours in the colour categories were also determined by each subject. The focal colour was defined as a colour sample whose colour-appearance best represented the colour category.

In the present study, at first, we carried out a single-colour memory experiment as a control. A test colour was presented on the CRT screen for 5s, then 30s later the subject started the cascade colour matching. In the present experiments, we did not use all stages in the cascade matching but, to save time, used only the stage 2, that is, the subject examined all colour samples to reject the colour samples that appeared probably different from the test colour in his memory.

In the multiple-colour memory experiments, the subject saw three or five test colours, depending on the session, consecutively for 5s each with an ISI of 1s. With a 30s delay the subject started selecting colours that matched the test colours in his memory with the criterion of the stage 2. In the case of five test colours, before, during and after the stimulus presentation the subject made an arithmetic calculation with a loud voice to prevent him using a verbal expression of a test colour. The calculation was a consecutive subtraction of three from a three-digit number.

Three male subjects and two male subjects were used in three-colour memory and five-colour memory experiments, respectively. They were colour normal.

7.4.3   RESULTS AND DISCUSSION

Figures 7.4.1(a) and (b) show examples of selected colours obtained in the three-colour memory and the single-colour memory experiments, respectively. The three focal colours in the blue, purple and orange categories were used as test colours in both experiments. Three groups of the selected colours in the single-colour memory experiment were obtained in different sessions. The solid lines show the categorical regions of blue, purple and orange determined for this subject in the categorical colour naming procedure.

It was found, in the multiple-colour memory, that the selected colours were also restricted in the categorical regions and they distributed in a very similar way to that in the single-colour memory. This indicates that the subject memorises categorically multiple colours as well as a single colour, and there seems no interaction among colours in memory.

Figure 7.4.2 shows other examples of the three-colour memory. In this case, test colours are not focal colours, but chosen from border areas between two categorical regions. Here, again, selected colours spread very similarly between the cases of the multiple-colour memory and the single-colour memory.

Figure 7.4.3 shows the results of the five-colour memory. In this case, focal colours of blue, purple, brown, pink and orange were used as test colours. In this multiple-colour memory, selected colours for blue, purple, brown and pink spread in the same area as those in the single-colour memory. However, selected colours for orange in the multiple-colour memory were found to be totally missing from the area that existed in the single-colour memory.

In Figure 7.4.4, test colours are three focal colours in blue, green and yellow regions and two non-focal colours on the borders of purple-pink and brown-orange. Selected colours for the green, yellow and purple-pink are shown to correspond to those in the single-colour memory, but again no selected colours for the blue were found in the multiple-colour memory.

In Figure 7.4.5 all test colours are non-focal. They locate on the borders between two categorical regions as shown in the left figure. These results seem to show that, in the

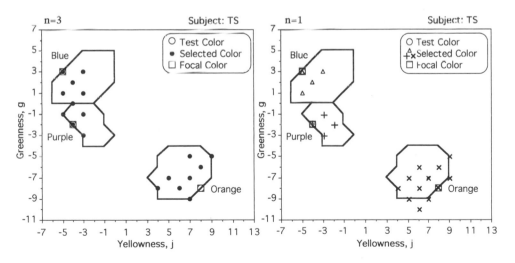

Figure 7.4.1. The distribution of selected colours. Test colours are three focal colours. Solid lines indicate the categorical colour regions. Subject: TS, (a) the multiple-colour memory, selected colours were obtained in an experimental session; (b) the single-colour memory, selected colours shown by the different symbols were obtained in different experimental sessions.

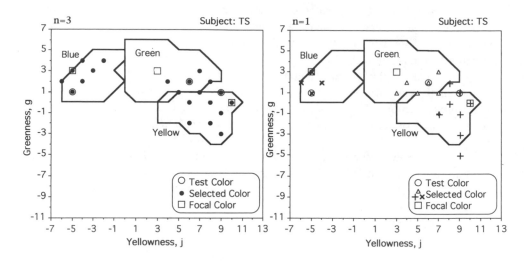

Figure 7.4.2. Same as in Figure 7.4.1, but for three non-focal test colours.

multiple-colour memory experiment, the subject could select colours for the purple-pink and probably the red-orange and the red-brown, but failed to select colours for the blue-green and the yellow-orange. In his memory these test colours seemed to completely disappear.

The results shown in Figure 7.4.1–7.4.5 indicate that there is no clear distinction in memory among focal and non-focal colours. One might have predicted that focal colours may be remembered easier than non-focal colours, but it was not true. This is probably

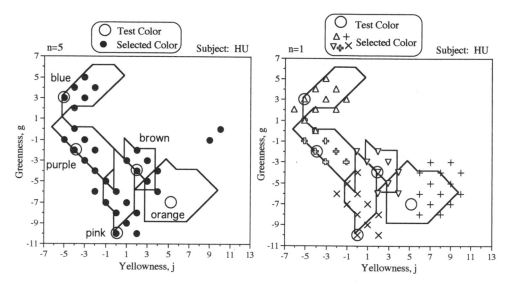

Figure 7.4.3. The distribution of selected colours. Test colours are five focal colours. Solid lines indicate the categorical colour regions. Subject: HU, (a) the multiple-colour memory, selected colours were obtained in an experimental session; (b) the single-colour memory, selected colours shown by the different symbols were obtained in different experimental sessions.

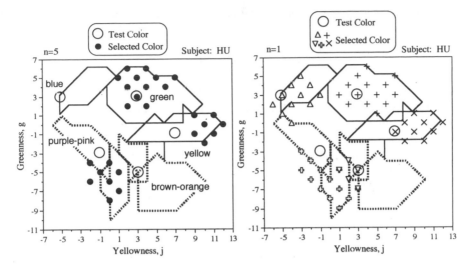

Figure 7.4.4. Same as in Figure 7.4.3, but for three focal and two non-focal test colours. Dashed lines indicate the categorical colour regions for non-focal test colours.

because when we store colours in our memory it might be the case that colours are coded in a categorical way regardless of focal or non-focal colours so that their appearance differences are no more effective in memory.

Komatsu *et al.* (1992) reported some physiological evidence that indicated a categorical processing of colour signals in the cortex. They tested colour selectivity of neurons in the inferior temporal (IT) cortex of awake macaque monkeys. Colour selective cells responded exclusively to some particular regions of a chromaticity diagram. This colour field is of a similar size and, for some cells, a similar shape to the categorical colour regions shown in the present experiments. Although the agreement between our data and the physiological data do not assure us that the IT cells remember categorical colours, it seems that there is

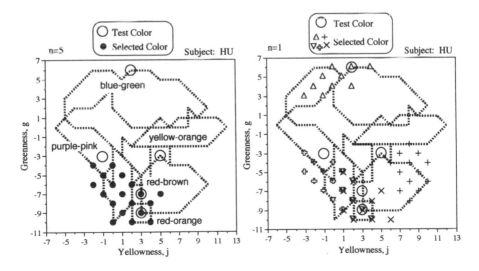

Figure 7.4.5. Same as in Figure 7.4.4, but for five non-focal test colours.

a physiological mechanism for categorical colour perception, which is the base of colour memory.

7.4.4 CONCLUSIONS

1. Selected colours for multiple test colours did not spread uniformly around the test colours, but were restricted within each categorical colour region.
2. The distribution for multiple test colours, if any, was similar to those for corresponding single test colours. In some trials, a distribution for one of multiple test colours was totally missing.
3. These results indicate that colours are hardly changed by other colour in memory, and that they are categorically processed in memory.

7.4.5 REFERENCES

BERLIN, B. & KAY, P. (1969) *Basic Color Terms: Their Universality and Evolution*, Berkeley: University of California Press.

BOYNTON, R. M., FARGO, L., OLSON, C. X. & SMALLMAN, H. S. (1989) Category effects in color memory, *Color Research Applications*, **14**, 229–234.

KOMATSU, H., IDEURA, Y., KAJI, S. & YAMANE, S. (1992) Color selectivity of neurons in the interior temporal cortex of the awake macaque monkey, *Journal of Neuroscience*, **12**, 408–424.

UCHIKAWA, K. (1992) 'Categorical characteristics of color discrimination in memory', presentation at the Advances in Color Vision Topical Meeting, Irvine, January.

UCHIKAWA, K. (1993) 'Categorical nature of color memory', presentation at the OSA Annual Meeting, Toronto, October.

UCHIKAWA, K. & SHINODA, H. (1990) Effects of color memory on color appearance. In: Ohta, Y. (Ed.) *Color Vision Deficiencies* (Proceedings of the Symposium of the International Research Group on Color Vision Deficiencies, Tokyo, Japan, 1990), Amsterdam: Kugler & Ghedini Publications, pp. 35–43.

UCHIKAWA, K. & SUGIYAMA, T. (1993) Effects of eleven basic color categories on color memory, *Investigative Ophthalmology and Visual Science*, **34**, 745.

UCHIKAWA, K., SUGIYAMA, T. & UJIKE, H. (1994) 'Categorical distribution of memory-matched colors in the OSA uniform color space', presentation at the 17th ECVP, Eindhoven, September.

Estimation of Object's Hue Using Maximum-likelihood Principle

Vytautas Petrauskas and Tom Troscianko

7.5.1   INTRODUCTION

There are numerous colour models dealing with colour perception (Buchsbaum and Gottshalk, 1983; DeValois and DeValois, 1993; Guth, 1991; Hunt, 1991; Ingling and Tsou, 1977; Izmailov and Sokolov, 1991; Vaitkevicius *et al.*, 1993) that use different approaches and/or try to model different stages of the visual system and are intended to account for known perceptual phenomena. One feature, however, which is common to all the above cited models is that they assume a given configuration of the visual system and then try to describe the functioning of its different stages.

The aim of this chapter is to present a computational approach of how the visual system might be constructed to compute and transmit visual information about colour available from the visual environment.

It is reasonable to assume that evolution has acquired a visual system with efficient mechanisms for detecting changes in visual stimuli in order to survive the competition with other species. This assumption might apply for detection of colour differences as well. The basic source for a change in the major classic attributes of an object's colour such as hue, saturation and brightness is a change in a spectral distribution of reflected light. Our aim is to propose a method of generating filters whose property is to detect and evaluate shifts in the spectral distribution of light incident on the retina in as efficient a manner as possible. We will relate this shift with the change in the percept of hue.

7.5.2   MODEL

For the sake of simplicity let us assume that we have a Gaussian-like spectral distribution at some point in the retinal image (Figure 7.5.1):

$$I(\lambda) = I_0 \exp\left(-\frac{(\lambda - \lambda_0)}{s^2}\right),$$

$$(1)$$

where I_0 = const, λ denotes wavelength, λ_0 is the mean and s defines the spread of the distribution. The psychophysical meaning for λ_0 is that it gives rise to the perception of hue

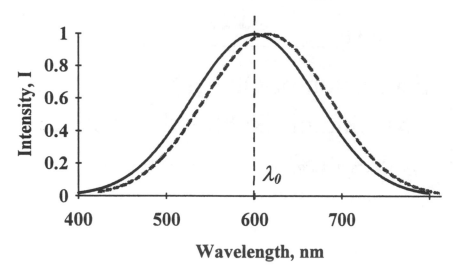

Figure 7.5.1. Gaussian-like spectral distributions demonstrating the shift that is intended to represent the shift in hue perception.

of the colour represented by the spectral distribution in Figure 7.5.1 and the change in λ_0 leads to the change in hue. We will look for a means of representing this value efficiently.

Let us assume that the signal $I(\lambda)$ is sampled by some definite number of sensors distributed uniformly and is transformed to its sampled version $I(\lambda_i)$, where $i = 1 \ldots n$ denote sampling points along the λ axis. At this point we do not make any speculations about the number of the sensors. The sampling might be described as the operation during which the continuous function $I(\lambda)$ is associated to its sampled version $I(\lambda_i)$ by the following expression:

$$I(\lambda_i) = I(\lambda)comb(\lambda/d),$$

where $comb(\lambda/d) = \Sigma\, \delta(\lambda\text{-}i)$. The sampling function consists of an array of δ functions, spaced at intervals of width d in the λ direction. As a next step normally distributed noise is added to conform with the known existence of noise in sampling of real scenes. In this case the sampled signal should be taken for the sum of $I(\lambda_i)$ and noise $N(\lambda_i)$:

$$R(\lambda_i) = kI(\lambda_i) + N(\lambda_i),$$

$$(2)$$

where $R(\lambda_i)$ denotes the response of the i-th sensor and $N(\lambda_i)$ denotes the random noise at the output of $R(\lambda_i)$. We will take the coefficient $k = 1$ (despite the fact that in reality it might have quite a complicated expression), as this coefficient is not important for the demonstration of the approach we wish to present here. To simplify notation we are going to use i instead of (λ_i). Given this we will have the following simplified expressions from now on:

$$R(\lambda_i) \Rightarrow R_i, \quad I(\lambda_i) \Rightarrow I_i, \quad N(\lambda) \Rightarrow N_i$$

Let N_i's be independent and normally distributed random variables with means $\mu = 0$ and variances σ^2, i. e. $N_i(0,\sigma)$. The receptor outputs R_i are also distributed normally with means $\mu_i = I_i$ and variances σ^2.

$$p(r_i, \lambda_0) = (4\pi\sigma) \exp - \frac{(r_i - I_i)^2}{2\sigma^2}),$$

(3)

where r_i stands for a possible realisation of a random variable R_i. The term $p(r_i, \lambda_0)$ stands for the probability density of the i-th photoreceptor having an output signal equal to r_i with the co-ordinate λ_0 serving as parameter. Now we shall use the method of maximum-likelihood estimation to find the estimator for λ_0. First, we shall try to explain briefly the maximum-likelihood method.

Let each R_i have the distribution density $p(r_i, \lambda_0)$. We can estimate the parameter $i\lambda_0$ by a function of $r_i's$, say $\lambda_0(r_i)$. This means that for any realisation of a random variable, r_i, we get different values for λ_0. Therefore, λ_0 (which we shall call an estimator), is itself a random variable with its own probability distribution, mean and variance. The particular value taken by λ_0, based on a particular set of $r_i's$, (that is the realisations of λ_0) is called an estimate. It is intuitively desirable that the distribution of $\lambda_0(r_i)$ should be centred at λ_0, that is

$$E(\lambda_0(r_i)) = \lambda_0.$$

(4)

The estimators possessing this property are called unbiased. The second step is to find a minimum-variance unbiased, or efficient estimator, that is, to find such an estimator that has a high probability of being close to λ_0. The minimum-variance unbiased estimator is unique when it exists. The most commonly used method of estimation that gives the efficient estimator (when it exists) is the method of maximum-likelihood estimation, where λ_0 is estimated by that value of $\lambda_0(r_i)$ which maximises the joint density of the independent observations, L:

$$L = p(r_i, \lambda_0) \, p(r_2, \lambda_0) \, p(r_3, \lambda_0) \ldots p(r_n\lambda_0).$$

(5)

Loosely speaking, we may say we choose λ_0 so as to make observations most likely, a criterion that clearly has an intuitive appeal. We take λ_0 as a solution of the likelihood equation

$$\frac{\delta L}{\delta \lambda_0} = 0.$$

(6)

Substituting equations (3) and (5) into equation (6), then expanding it in a Taylor series up to the first order, and solving it, we get

$$\lambda - \lambda_0 = \frac{\Sigma_i W_1(\lambda_i) I(\lambda_i)}{\Sigma_i W_2(\lambda_i) I(\lambda_i)},$$

(7)

where λ_0 is the point about which the Taylor series is taken, $W_1(\lambda_i) = I'(\lambda_i)$ and $W_2(\lambda_i) = I''(\lambda_i)$ are the first and second derivatives of spectral distribution, $I(\lambda_i)$, respectively. It should be noted that formula (7) is a solution of a maximum-likelihood equation that is valid only for small deviations from λ_0. As can be seen from Figure 7.5.2, one filter is odd- and the other even-symmetric. The ratio of outputs of these filters gives the maximum-likelihood estimation for λ_0 in the spectral distribution shown in Figure 7.5.1.

One interpretation of formula (7) is that estimator λ_0 might be thought of as the orientation of a two-dimensional vector with the components W_1 and W_2 shown in Figure 7.5.2. The other interpretation of the formula might be that λ_0 is some kind of non-linear mean in the spectral distribution.

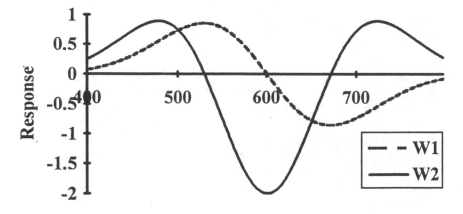

Wavelength, nm

Figure 7.5.2. W_1 and W_2 represent first and second derivatives of the function presented by solid line in Figure 7.5.1.

7.5.3   DISCUSSION

The main assumption for linking this model with perception is that the change in the mean of the spectral distribution leads to the change in hue. As an estimate for the mean a maximum-likelihood estimator is used. The results of modelling show that the most sensitive estimator for the change in the mean of the spectral distribution under study is the ratio of output signals of the odd-and even-symmetric filters. If a non-symmetric spectral distribution was used the above filters would be non-symmetric, however, they would remain opponent-like, i.e. as is the case in the human visual system.

The most important implication of the fact that the form of the filters depends on the spectral distribution is that different species which have more than one photoreceptor type and have habitats in different regions on the Earth, should have different colour filters to allow them to detect differences in spectral distributions of objects as precisely as possible as this might be of primary importance for their survival.

The other implication concerns the minimal number of different colour sensors that are needed to build up opponent-like filters. As can be clearly seen from Figure 7.5.2, only three types of Gaussian-like filters, if summed with different weights, would be enough to construct the above opponent-like filters.

In conclusion, we want to point out that we are not aiming to quantitatively account for known perceptual phenomena but rather have made a first attempt to use a computation approach to try to understand basic principles of how the visual system might be built up. Of course, the model needs to be fitted to real data and known properties of colour perception should be accounted for. On the other hand, however, it is interesting that a very simplified demonstration of the above approach may allow us to understand colour processing in the visual system from the purely theoretical assumptions about the physical correlate of hue and about the nature of its evaluation. This leads to the following conclusions:

1. To precisely and efficiently evaluate shifts in light spectral distribution opponent-like colour mechanisms are needed.
2. To ensure opponent-type processing at least three different types of colour sensor are needed.

7.5.4 ACKNOWLEDGEMENT

The work was aided by support from Lithuanian government grant No 114-92, from a travel grant from Lithuanian Open Fund and DRA Grant D/ER/1/9/4/2034/102. Thanks to Zydrunas Stankevicius for assistance in mathematics.

7.5.5 REFERENCES

BUCHSBAUM, G. & GOTTSHALK, A. (1983) Trichromacy, opponent colours coding and optimum colour information transmission in the retina, *Proceedings of Royal Society, London*, **220**, 89–113.

DEVALOIS, R.L. & DEVALOIS K.K. (1993) A multi-stage color model, *Vision Research*, **33**, 1053–1065.

GUTH, S.L. (1991) Model for color vision and light adaptation, *Journal of the Optical Society of America*, **8**, 976–993.

HUNT, R.W. (1991) A model of colour vision. In: Hunt, R.W. (Ed.) *Measuring Colour*, 2nd edn, London: Ellis Horwood Ltd, pp. 213–258.

INGLING, C.R. & TSOU, B.M. (1977) Orthogonal combination of three visual channels, *Vision Research*, **17**, 1075–1082.

IZMAILOV, CH.A. & SOKOLOV, E.N. (1991) Spherical model of color and brightness discrimination, *Psychological Science*, **2**, 249–259.

VAITKEVICIUS, H.H., STANKEVICIUS, Z. & SOKOLOV, E.N. (1993) Opponent colour functions and colour discriminability, *Sensory Systems*, **7**, 58–66.

Are Colour Categorical Borders Stable Under Various Illuminants?

H. Jordan and J.J. Kulikowski

7.6.1 INTRODUCTION

Following Hering's original studies of colour opponency, psychological experiments have consistently reported that there are at least four basic colour categories: blue, green, yellow and red (Boynton and Gordon, 1965; Boynton and Olson, 1990) and a cross cultural consistency in the use of seven other colour terms (Berlin and Kay, 1969). These findings are consistent with the everyday experience that the chromatic spectrum is divisible into discrete colour categories, and are broadly consistent with the organisation of colour opponent mechanisms R/G and B/Y (see Crook et al., 1987; Derrington et al., 1984; Krauskopf et al., 1982). Hurvich and Jameson (1955) reported five spectral components along two functions, obtained from their hue cancellation method. Four of these components are consistent with the four basic colours of psychological studies. However, at short wavelengths it is necessary to add red to a mixture of hues to balance the sensation of violet. This is consistent with the characteristics of the long-wavelength cones (or 'red' cones), which show a secondary sensitivity peak in the region of 380–400 nm. Thus, the L-cones span the whole range of wavelengths of the visible spectrum. Psychophysical findings would suggest the possibility of a fifth colour category at the shortest wavelengths of the visible spectrum. It is still debatable how to relate the four colour categories of Hering model studies to the five possible categories of strict psychophysical mechanisms (Mullen and Kulikowski, 1990), although the latter have similar spectral properties to visual cortical cells (Vautin and Dow, 1985; see section 7.6.4 Discussion).

Early psychophysical colour categorisation studies utilised a small spot with the intention of stimulating a single cone. Krauskopf (1978) directed a spectral (500–650 nm) spot (1.3 min arc) at the retinal mosaic with the intention of stimulating a single cone. He reported that the observer identified a percentage of the stimuli with a single colour term. Thus, certain pure colours may be identified through the activation of a single cone with an appropriate action spectra. Other responses were interpreted as stimulating two or more 'detectors'. The identification of wavelengths, other than a few 'pure' colours, is a result of the interaction between two or more cones. However, the sensation of colour experienced by the individual should not be interpreted in terms of individual cones acting as trigger units. The cones do not act as trigger feature units; rather, the sensation of colour is a product of cone opponency at post-receptoral stages.

Nearly all spectral spots that are substantially greater than 7 min arc are detected by the cone opponency system. King-Smith and Carden (1976) suggested that it is possible to discriminate a spectral test stimulus from background white at intensities close to the detection threshold. Mullen and Kulikowski (1990) developed a paradigm whereby measuring discrimination rates allowed the identification of colour category borders at threshold. They identified four categorical colour borders at threshold that were approximately 455, 489, 566 and 585 nm, under an illuminant with the colour temperature of 2450 K, outlining the colour categories of violet, blue, green, yellow and orange (red). The location of the category borders suggests that colour categorisation is carried out by mechanisms of the post-receptoral pathways.

Mullen *et al.* (1989) attempted to identify the four neural mechanisms that are associated with the four distinct colour sensations at threshold. The boundaries between the categories correspond closely to the peaks and troughs of the spectral sensitivity function. They proposed that the two longer wavelength categories, 'red' and 'green' are the product of the combined L and M cone opponent channels. They suggested that the short wavelength categories, 'violet' and 'blue' are composed of two mechanisms, although they did not suggest what these may be. They also suggested that the categorical border at 580 nm ('yellow') was a product of the summed output of the L and M channels, although they did not dismiss the possibility of a contribution from the luminance channel. In order to assess the role of the luminance channel to wavelength discrimination it is necessary to reduce the sensitivity of the achromatic system, and measure the performance of the chromatic system alone.

The achromatic mechanisms have higher temporal and spatial resolution limits than the chromatic system. Centrally fixated stimulus spots subtending an angle of up to 7 min arc activate (at threshold) the achromatic system, resulting in low sensitivity to short wavelengths, and a lack of distinct peaks in the middle wavelength range (for review, see Kulikowski and Walsh, 1991). However, Mullen and Kulikowski (1986) reported that a small spot (10') can activate the red-green opponent mechanisms at longer wavelengths (above 500 nm). The achromatic system relies on the mixture of the L,M cone input, in the same way as yellow relies on the $[(L+M)-S]$ input. However, when the experimental conditions are controlled so as to desensitise the achromatic system, full discrimination between yellow and white spots is possible. Thus, it has been shown that under optimised conditions, yellow is a categorical colour in its own right (Sharanjeet-Kaur and Kulikowski, 1992).

If the achromatic system is more sensitive than the chromatic system in certain regions of the spectrum, i.e. in the region of yellow, it is difficult to evaluate the functioning of the cone opponency system for these wavelengths. Wavelength discrimination is affected by certain experimental conditions in just the same way as spectral sensitivity. Sharanjeet-Kaur and Kulikowski (1992) reported conditions under which selectivity of identification of yellow can be improved. The use of an annulus fitted around the stimulus selectively aids discrimination in the region, by masking achromatic contrast detection (Kulikowski and Walsh, 1991) between the spot and the background. (This does not eliminate the contribution of the achromatic system to the detection of temporal transients.) The use of a higher colour temperature will also aid discrimination in the middle wavelength region, as it increases the sensitivity of the yellow branch of the blue-yellow chromatic-opponent system.

On the basis of experimental work on the V4 cortical region of monkeys, Walsh *et al.* (1992) suggested that basic colour categories are formed before colour-constancy processes are completed. They predicted that colour-constancy thresholds will show similar categorical effects to those involving colour memory, i.e. constancy effects will be more robust for wavelengths that are categorical centroids (or typical colours) than for categorical borders. Kulikowski and Walsh (1993) reported that colour constancy observations of human subjects matching Munsell chips under two illuminants (6500 K and 2700 K) did show the predicted categorical effects. Illuminant changes showed a greater effect on border colours than on categorical centroids (see also Kulikowski *et al.*, this volume, pp. 521–531). Additionally, border colours were observed to change category under different illuminants. (However, their 'colour constancy' paradigm minimised the effect of the adaptation of the cones to the background illuminant, whereas in the present study, the subject is fully adapted to the background.)

The first part of this study attempts to explore the effects of changing illuminant on colour categorisation borders at threshold and supra-threshold intensity levels. This effect is examined by first replicating the previous data (Mullen and Kulikowski, 1990) and then introducing the second illuminant. The first illuminant is determined by a background colour temperature close to illuminant A, similar to that used by Mullen and Kulikowski (1990). The second background colour chosen was close to illuminant D. It is supposed that the location of categorical yellow, and its borders with green and red will show the effects of adaptation to the background illuminant, by shifting in the same direction as predicted by the Sloan notch (although the categorical yellow may not be determined by the Sloan notch).

The second part of this study attempts to relate the position of categorical borders and centroids at threshold, to the location of typical colours set at suprathreshold intensity levels. It is expected that while colour constancy of typical colours or centroids (basic perceptual prototypes) is robust (showing little shifts), colour categories expressed in terms of wavelengths should shift accordingly (Zeki, 1983).

7.6.2   PART 1: CATEGORICAL BORDERS AND CENTROIDS AT THRESHOLD

7.6.2.1 Method

A stimulus spot, generated by a monochromator, is presented using a two-channel Maxwellian view system at 500 ms duration. The spot, which subtends an angle of one degree, is presented against a uniform photopic background at 1000 td. An annulus subtending 10 min of arc, is placed around the spot stimulus, obscuring the contour between the stimulus and the background, in order to exert masking upon the achromatic response (Kulikowski and Kranda, 1977). Initially, the surround colour temperature is 2950 K (close to illuminant A). Blue colour-correction filters (Lee) are placed in the background channel to change the surround colour temperature to 6550 K (close to illuminant D65).

A two alternative forced choice (2AFC) procedure is used to simultaneously measure the detection of, and discrimination between, spots of two different wavelengths ($\lambda 1$ and $\lambda 2$). Each trial consists of two time intervals. One of the time intervals is blank and the spot stimulus is added in the other. The interval in which the stimulus is displayed is varied randomly by a microprocessor. The wavelength of the spot stimulus presented is also varied randomly between $\lambda 1$ and $\lambda 2$, under the control of a microprocessor. After each trial the subject is first required to indicate the time interval in which the spot stimulus occurred, and thus determine the detection rate at a particular intensity. The subject is also required to indicate whether the spot stimulus presented was $\lambda 1$ or $\lambda 2$, thus determining the discrimination rate. Within each experiment both wavelengths were presented at least 60 times, at each of four intensities spanning the threshold. The subjects familiarised themselves with the appearance of the two wavelengths before the experiment began.

The detection and discrimination psychometric functions for both of the wavelength pairs were plotted using a probit analysis. The detection threshold was set at the intensity where 90 per cent of the stimulus spots were correctly detected. The rate of discrimination was calculated as the percentage of trials correctly discriminated, when 90 per cent of these trials were correctly detected. The discrimination rate for each of the two wavelengths is averaged to produce a final value for the discrimination rate between the two wavelengths. This rate varied between 50 per cent (random) and 90 per cent (complete) discrimination as good as detection.

A fixed wavelength is chosen, and paired with successively longer wavelengths until complete discrimination is obtained. The initial fixed point was chosen on the basis of the spectral sensitivity function of the observer. The point chosen was around the maximum sensitivity of the broad middle wavelength peak. The wavelength at which 70 per cent discrimination is obtained is considered the categorical border between the fixed and varied wavelength.

7.6.2.2 Results and comments

The results for one subject (HJ), using both illuminants are shown in Figure 7.6.1. The filled circles indicate the fixed wavelengths, and the open circles indicate the wavelengths with which it was paired. The vertical arrows show the positions of the categorical borders (i.e. 70% discrimination at 90% detection) in each case.

Section A of Figure 7.6.1, top, shows the results of pairing 530 nm with successively longer wavelengths. Thus the region of the spectrum, which subjectively appears 'green' to the observer, is traversed. Once the 530 nm is paired with wavelengths of 575 nm or longer, 90 per cent discrimination at 90 per cent detection is achieved. This indicates that discrimination is possible as soon as detection between the two wavelengths. The categorical border, chosen as 70 per cent discrimination was achieved at 565 nm. Thus, arbitrarily, this wavelength is taken as the separation of the spectrum, by the observer, into discrete 'green' and 'yellow' colour categories.

The next fixed point (Figure 7.6.1, top, section B) is selected as falling beyond the first and within the second categorical spectral region. The wavelength of 575 nm is completely distinguishable from wavelengths of 620 nm and longer. Seventy per cent discrimination is achieved at approximately 580 nm, indicating that this is the border between 'yellow' and 'red' chromatic sensations.

Similarly, the borders between the categories in the shorter wavelength regions are determined. A fixed point is chosen which is within the previous spectral region, but beyond any other categorical spectral range. The fixed point is matched with shorter wavelengths to determine the locations of the borders of the short wavelength categories of 'blue' and 'violet'. Thus, colour category borders under illuminant A were established at 455, 490, 565 and 580 nm. These results compare closely with those reported by Mullen and Kulikowski (1990).

The 90 per cent discrimination points can be tentatively taken as close to the 'centroids' of each of the colour categories. The centroids of each of the colour sensations under illuminant A were as follows: violet, below 410 nm (not fully discriminable); blue, 480 nm; green, 530 nm; yellow, 575 nm; red, about 620 nm.

Figure 7.6.1 (bottom) shows the results for the same subject with a background colour temperature of 6550 K (close to illuminant D). The results were collected in the same manner as those under illuminant A. The same initial fixed point was chosen, and the subsequent fixed points were determined, as before, by the discrete spectral ranges identified by the discrimination rates.

Five discrete colour sensations were also perceived under illuminant D. The categorical borders were established at 450, 492, 555 and 585 nm. Thus, a significant shift was found for the borders between 'violet' and 'blue', 'green' and 'yellow', and 'yellow' and 'red'. Only a small shift was experienced for the border between 'blue' and 'green'. The colour 'centroids' were as follows: violet, stayed about 410 nm; green, 530 nm; and red, about 620 nm; the others were shifted, blue, 475 nm; yellow, 568 nm.

Thus, this study confirmed that there are five distinct spectral colour sensations at threshold: violet, blue, green, yellow and red (Mullen and Kulikowski, 1990) forming the basis of early colour categorisation.

The 90 per cent discrimination points are tentatively taken as close to the 'centroids' of each of the colour categories. The shift of the centroid of the yellow category is most conspicuous. There is also a significant shift in the location of the blue centroid, whereas green and red correspond to the broad maxima of the spectral sensitivity function (which are hardly shifted). There are also greater shifts in the borders between the red and yellow

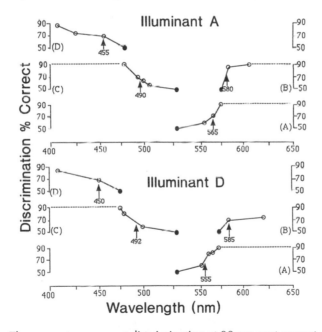

Figure 7.6.1.   The percentage correct discrimination at 90 per cent correct detection, under illuminant A (top) and D (bottom) is plotted for pairs of wavelengths. In a series of 2AFC experiments, one wavelength remains fixed (filled symbol) and matched with a second wavelength stimulus (hollow symbol). The solid lines are fitted by eye. The dashed lines indicate 90 per cent correct discrimination at 90 per cent correct detection (i.e. when discrimination is as good as detection). Vertical arrows indicate the wavelength at which discrimination reaches 70 per cent correct in each series of pairings (categorical borders). Subject HJ.

and green and yellow categories, than with the other borders, as shown in Figure 7.6.2. Thus, these preliminary data suggest that categorical borders at threshold are subject to some shifts due to a change of illuminant.

7.6.3   PART 2: THE LOCATION OF TYPICAL COLOURS AT SUPRATHRESHOLD LEVELS OF INTENSITY

7.6.3.1 Method

A stimulus spot of 1 degree and 500 ms duration was presented on a photopic background of 1000 td. The stimuli was produced by a monochromator, and presented by a two-channel Maxwellian view system. The background colour temperature was varied between 2950 K (close to illuminant A) and 6550 K (close to illuminant D) using Lee colour correction filters in the background channel. An annulus was fitted around the stimulus spot.

Five subjects (mean age 21 years) with normal colour vision were instructed to set the threshold intensity of a spot stimulus at 36 different wavelengths between 401 nm and 652 nm. Three intensities were recorded for each wavelength and the mean intensity plotted,

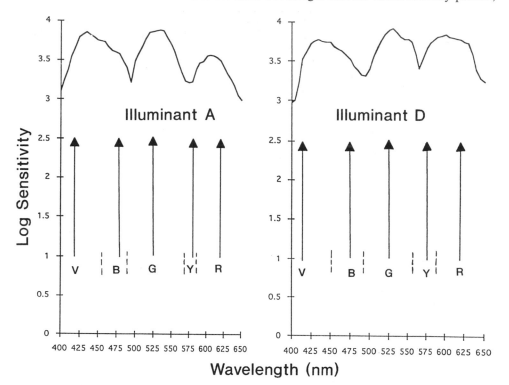

Figure 7.6.2.   Mean spectral sensitivity function to the test stimuli in log units as a function of the wavelength of the stimulus under illuminant A (left) and D (right). Sensitivity is the reciprocal of the intensity of the stimulus at threshold. Arrows indicate the point at which 90 per cent correct discrimination at 90 per cent correct detection occurs between stimuli (ie. centroids), whereas the dashed lines indicate 70 per cent correct discrimination at 90 per cent correct detection, ie. borders (taken from Figure 7.6.1). The spectral regions between the dashed lines correspond to violet, blue, green, yellow and red.

producing the distinctive triple-peak spectral sensitivity function. Each subject was asked to follow this procedure for both illuminants.

The subjects were then asked to select the wavelength that most closely resembled its 'typical colour'. The 'typical' hue, for that category, was not supposed to contain components of the adjacent categories (the procedure was a modified version of that for setting unique hues). The intensity was set at one log unit above the threshold they had set previously for that wavelength read off the spectral sensitivity function. Each subject set a wavelength resembling its 'typical' colour for each of the five categories at least three times. This procedure was repeated for illuminant D.

7.6.3.2 Results

Table 7.6.1 shows the mean wavelength settings for the typical colours of each of the five categorical regions across all five subjects under the two illuminants. The standard deviations are given for each colour to indicate the variation between wavelength setting for each of the colours.

With the exception of yellow, there are large inter-subject variations in the mean wavelength settings of each of the five 'typical' colours under the two illuminants. The change in illuminant, therefore, has no significant effect on the location of these typical colours. However, there is a significant difference ($t = 4.03$, df $= 35, p = 0.001$) between the location of typical yellow under the two different illuminants. The shift at suprathreshold intensity levels is in the same direction as the shift for centroids at threshold intensity levels.

Although the instructions were carefully worded and the settings were repeated several times (there was little intra-subject variation), the subjects continued to display consistent differences in their wavelength settings across all five colours. Apparently, the subjects in this study did not have the same prototypes of the appearance of 'typical' spectral colours (inter-subject variations are considerable, see section 7.6.4).

7.6.4 DISCUSSION

In the present study, we used spectral stimuli, that serve well to characterise both psychophysical and neural mechanisms of colour vision (although natural colours are

Table 7.6.1. Wavelengths of typical colours and centroids (in nm) for the illuminants A and D.

	The mean wavelengths of the typical colours and standard deviations (SD)					
	Illuminant	Violet	Blue	Green	Yellow	Red
Typical						
Mean	A	421	478	525	579	621
SD	A	11.3	9.9	11.2	4.7	8.6
Typical						
Mean	D	419	476	525	570	622
SD	D	8.5	9.1	10.7	4.5	10.5
Centroids	A	<410	480	530	575	~620
	D	~410	475	530	568	~620

usually non-spectral). The centroid spectral colours, obtained here, are those for which threshold detection is practically the same as discrimination. Thus, the pairs of hues that are adjacent centroids are fully distinguishable at detection threshold. Hence the centroids represent optima of elementary colour mechanisms, determined psychophysically. It is, therefore, important to examine whether these elementary (threshold) mechanisms are correlated with known neurophysiological data, on the one hand, and with suprathreshold perception of typical colours, on the other.

Perhaps the closest electrophysiological study is that by Vautin and Dow (1985) which reported cells in the macaque primary visual cortex with spectral maxima grouped around red, yellow and green. Some cells with spectral properties around categorical blue and violet (and non-spectral purple) have also been found. Similarly, tuned cells were also reported in related studies on visually activated areas (V4 – Schein and Desimone, 1984, and in the adjacent temporal cortex – Komatsu et al., 1992).

Perceptually, each subject obviously has a fairly clear idea of the region of the visible spectrum that belongs to a particular 'colour'. This is a typical finding of research that is concerned with categorical perception. Thus, the data broadly support Hering's model of colour vision in that they confirm the presence of four basic colour categories at threshold intensity levels (a better quantitative fit would probably be obtained using multi-stage models, e.g. the simplest linear model of De Valois and De Valois, 1993). The distinct spectral region in the very shortest wavelength portion of the visible spectrum is probably due to L cones responding in this region. The inter-subject variations seem to parallel those reported for unique hues, obtained for spectral colours (but not for broad-band hues, see Mollon and Jordan, this volume, pp. 381–392).

The location of a 'yellow centroid' is very similar to that of the mean typical (or unique) yellow. Moreover, the shifts (with illuminant changes) of both centroid and typical yellow are roughly consistent with the shift of the Sloan notch in the spectral sensitivity characteristics (Figure 7.6.1). The wavelength of this notch is theoretically obtained using the x/y (CIE) co-ordinates: the tritanopic confusion line is drawn from the tritan co-punctal point and through the background illuminant. The Sloan notch determines the wavelength at which red-green opponent mechanisms are not involved (this does not necessarily imply that the yellow-blue opponent response should be maximal there). Under the present conditions the Sloan notch location shifts by about 10 nm from a longer wavelength (approximately 578 nm) under illuminant A to a shorter wavelength (approximately 567 nm) under illuminant D. The shift in the location of centroid yellow at threshold levels was in the same direction, but by a smaller magnitude (A: 575 nm to D: 568 nm); the mean shift of typical yellow was also smaller than indicated by the Sloan notch (A: 579 nm to D: 570 nm).

The locations of the remaining threshold centroids and typical colours under the two illuminants are also similar, but not identical (Figure 7.6.1 and Table 7.6.1). For example, centroids for green are located at longer and red centroids at shorter wavelengths than the corresponding suprathreshold typical colours; these shifts are broadly consistent with the changes of dominant wavelengths as a function of saturation.

Finally it should be stressed that the apparent stability, or wavelength 'constancy' observed here (yellow excepted) for a change in illuminant from A to D is not in conflict with colour constancy, which in turn holds best in the mid-spectral range of colours (yellow and green, see Kulikowski et al., this volume, pp. 521–531, but note that constancy for long-term adaptation is still better).

The typical colours (except for yellow) are relatively stable for at least two reasons:

1. The centroid colours are located on the broad maxima of the spectral sensitivity function, and this may partly account for the stability of these colours.
2. When illuminant changes from D to A and colour constancy holds well, the changes in dominant wavelengths for most typical colours (but not for yellow) happen to be relatively small. For yellow, adaptation most readily desensitise components of the opponency system $[(R + G)/B]$ and accordingly acts to shift the wavelength sensitivity of this mechanism. Thus sensation of yellow is a 'litmus' test of a rule that colour and wavelength constancy cannot generally hold together.

7.6.5   SUMMARY

There are five spectral regions that can be discriminated at threshold, forming the psychophysical basis for threshold colour categories: red, yellow, green, blue and violet. A change in colour temperature of the adapting background (illuminants A and D) shifts mostly the borders of categorical yellow, the remaining categories are relatively insensitive. These results are also correlated with suprathreshold sensation of typical colours.

7.6.6   REFERENCES

BERLIN, B. & KAY, P. (1991) *Basic Color Terms: Their Universality and Evolution*, Berkeley: University of California Press.

BOYNTON, R.M. & GORDON, J. (1965) Bezold-Brücke hue shift measured by color naming technique, *Journal of the Optical Society of America*, **55**, 78–86.

BOYNTON, R.M. & OLSON, C.X. (1990) Salience of chromatic basic terms confirmed by three measures, *Vision Research*, **30**, 1311–1317.

CROOK, J.M., LEE, B.B., TIGWELL, D.A. & VALBERG, A. (1987) Thresholds to chromatic spots of cells in the macaque geniculate nucleus as compared to detection sensitivity in man, *Journal of Physiology*, **392**, 193–211.

DE VALOIS, R.L. & DE VALOIS, K.K. (1993) A multi-stage color model, *Vision Research*, **33**, 1053–1066.

DERRINGTON, A., KRAUSKOPF, J. & LENNIE, P. (1984) Chromatic mechanisms in the LGN of macaque, *Journal of Physiology*, **357**, 241 265.

HURVICH, L.M. & JAMESON, D. (1955) Some quantitative aspects of opponent colours theory, Part 3, *Journal of the Optical Society of America*, **45**, 602.

KING-SMITH, P.E. & CARDEN, D. (1976) Luminance and opponent colour contributions to visual detection and adaption and temporal and spatial integration, *Journal of the Optical Society of America*, **66**, 709–717.

KOMATSU, H., IDEURA, Y., KAJI, S. & YAMANE, S. (1992) Color selectivity of neurons in the inferior temporal cortex of the awake macaque monkey, *Journal of Neuroscience*, **12**, 408–424

KRAUSKOPF J. (1978) On identifying detectors. In: Armington, J.C., Krauskopf, J. & Wooten B.R. (Eds), *Visual Psychophysics and Physiology*, New York: Academic Press, pp. 283–295.

KRAUSKOPF J., WILLIAMS D.R. & HEELEY D.M. (1982) The cardinal directions of colour space, *Vision Research*, **22**, 1123–1131.

KULIKOWSKI, J.J. & KRANDA, K. (1977) Detection of coarse patterns with a minimum contribution from rods, *Vision Research*, **17**, 853–856.

KULIKOWSKI, J.J. & WALSH, V. (1991) On the limits of colour detection and discrimination. In: Kulikowski J.J., Walsh, V. & Murray, I.J. (Eds), *Limits of Vision*, Basingstoke: Macmillan, pp. 202–220.

KULIKOWSKI, J.J. & WALSH, V. (1993) Colour vision: Isolating mechanisms in overlapping streams, *Progress in Brain Research*, **95**, 417-426.

MULLEN, K.T. & KULIKOWSKI, J.J. (1986) The detection and recognition of small and large spots by chromatic mechanisms, *Perception*, **15**, A26–27.

MULLEN, K.T. & KULIKOWSKI, J.J. (1990) Wavelength discrimination at detection threshold, *Journal of the Optical Society of America*, **A 7**, 733–742.

MULLEN, K.T., KULIKOWSKI, J.J. & CARDEN, D. (1989) The identification of spectral colour sensations. In: Kulikowski, J.J., Dickinson, C.M. & Murray, I.J. (Eds), *Seeing Contour and Colour*, Oxford: Pergamon Press, pp. 263–268.

SCHEIN, S. & DESIMONE, R. (1984) Spectral properties of V4 neurons in the macaque, *Journal of Neuroscience*, **10**, 3369–3389.

SHARANJEET-KAUR & KULIKOWSKI, J.J. (1992) Detection and discrimination of categorical yellow, *Perception*, **21**, 77.

VAUTIN, R.G. & DOW, B.M. (1985) Color cell groups in foveal striate cortex of the behaving macaque, *Journal of Neurophysiology*, **54**, 273–292.

WALSH, V., KULIKOWSKI, J.J., BUTLER, S.R. & CARDEN, D. (1992) The effects of V4 lesions on the visual abilities of macaques: Colour categorization, *Behavioral Brain Research*, **52**, 81–89.

ZEKI, S.M. (1983) Colour coding in the cerebral cortex: the reaction of cells in monkey cortex to wavelengths and colours, *Neuroscience*, **9**, 741–765.

The Paucity of Evidence for Cardinal Mechanisms

John Krauskopf

We have been encouraged for some time to believe that, while colour vision begins with the absorption of light in the three different kinds of cones, important events take place within three mechanisms that combine the outputs of the cones algebraicly. This trend started with Hering and was promoted diligently by Hurvich and Jameson in the form of the opponent colours theory in which these second stage mechanisms were associated with unique hues resulting in the red-green, yellow-blue and black white opponent mechanisms (Hering, 1905 [1964]). A number of other suggestions about the nature of the second stage mechanisms have been made. One is embodied in the colour space that Dave Williams, Dave Heeley, Andrew Derrington, Peter Lennie and I have employed, which is illustrated in Figure 7.7.1 (Derrington *et al.*, 1984; Krauskopf *et al.*, 1982).

This is a three-dimensional extension of the chromaticity diagram developed by MacLeod and Boynton (1979). There are a number of labels that have been applied to the

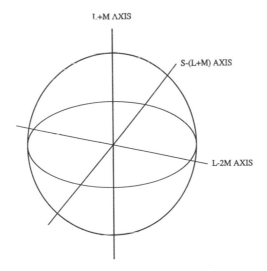

Figure 7.7.1. Colour space.

axes of this space. We prefer to specify the axes in terms of the weights assigned to the cones by mechanisms that would respond uniquely to stimuli modulated along the axes. In this scheme there are two axes in the isoluminant plane labelled L–2M, and S–(L + M) and an axis perpendicular to them at the equal-energy white point, which is labelled L + M. One could alternatively label the axes in terms of the variation of the modulations of the cones along these axes, in which case the labels would be L–M, S and 2L + M + S, respectively.

It is useful to use polar co-ordinates to specify chromatic modulation. The equatorial plane is defined by the L-2M and S-(L + M) axes. The azimuth (ϕ) of a modulation vector is defined by its projection in this plane. The positive (reddish) end of the L–2M axis is assigned an azimuth of 0°. We assign an azimuth of 90° to the positive (purplish) end of the S–(L + M) axis. Elevation (θ) is defined as the angle between the modulation vector and the isoluminant plane with positive elevation signifying increasing luminance.

The specification of other than axial colour directions requires a determination of units for measurement along the axes. It is general practice to use threshold based units.

This kind of space has many uses but I want to concentrate on whether the mechanisms implied or explicitly invoked when using such spaces have the same status as cones would have in a space using cone co-ordinates. The thesis that I will try to promote is that the evidence argues against the existence of three well-defined classes of second stage mechanisms, that is, mechanisms which attach precise weights to the responses of the cones.

The habituation experiments that I did with Dave Williams and Dave Heeley some time ago seemed, at first, to provide evidence for independent mechanisms tuned along the two isoluminant axes and the luminance axis of Figure 7.7.1 (Krauskopf et al., 1982). In those experiments thresholds were measured for modulations away from the equal-energy white point at the centre of the sphere before and after the viewing of fields modulated sinusoidally along some line through the white point. The outstanding result was the selective effect of the direction of modulation of the habituation stimulus on the elevation of the detection thresholds. When the habituation stimulus was modulated along one of the cardinal axes, thresholds for detection along that axis were raised substantially while thresholds along the other cardinal axis were unchanged and thresholds along intermediate axes were somewhat elevated. The effect of habituation along non-cardinal directions was to raise thresholds more generally.

However, there was at least a hint of selectivity in the data for non-axial habituation. When we pursued this quantitatively by applying Fourier analysis to the whole set of data we found clear evidence of selectivity, a finding inconsistent with a simple theory that detection was mediated solely by mechanisms responsive along the cardinal axes. The recent experiments of Webster and Mollon (1991, 1994) on the effects of habituation on colour appearance yielded results of similar form to, and of greater completeness than, ours, which cannot be explained solely by postulating independent detection and desensitisation within cardinal mechanisms.

Zaidi and Shapiro (1993) have suggested that the effects of habituation could be explained by invoking adaptive orthogonalisation among cardinal mechanisms. However, other evidence inconsistent with independent processing of stimuli within cardinal mechanisms comes from experiments which do not involve habituation.

For example, consider chromatic discrimination. Inspired by Craik's classical work on the effect of the level of light adaptation on discrimination thresholds at various luminance levels Karl Gegenfurtner and I measured chromatic discrimination at loci removed from the adaptation point (Krauskopf and Gegenfurtner, 1992). The observer viewed a TV screen, which had a luminance of about 35 cdm^{-2} upon which four disks were displayed for one second. One of the disks was always different in some way from the other three. The observers' task was to identify the odd disk. In one set of experiments, the three test disks were excursions along one of the cardinal directions; the comparison disk was also an excursion along the same axis but different in amplitude by the amount DELTA, which was varied in a staircase procedure to measure the threshold for discrimination. In a complementary set of experiments, the test disks were the same but the DELTA was in the direction of the other cardinal axis.

The results were quite clear-cut as shown in Figure 7.7.2 and Figure 7.7.3. When the test and DELTA lie along the same cardinal axis, the discrimination threshold increases linearly with the amplitude of the test excursion. On the other hand when the DELTA is parallel to the other cardinal axis, thresholds are independent of amplitude. The first result is a nice confirmation of the Craik generalisation that discrimination is best when the stimuli to be discriminated are in the vicinity of the stimuli to which the observer is adapted. The second result provides evidence in favour of the notion that discrimination is performed independently by mechanisms tuned along the cardinal axes.

However, further scrutiny reveals evidence inconsistent with this view. Figure 7.7.4 plots discrimination ellipses around test vectors in 16 directions from the equal-energy white point. The ellipses in the four cardinal directions agree with, and expand on, the results just shown. Briefly, the expectation based on the theory of independent detection is that the major axes of all the ellipses should be parallel to the nearest cardinal axis, except

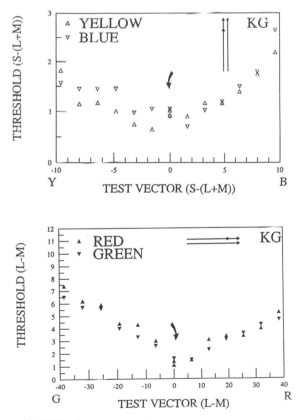

Figure 7.7.2. Test and DELTA along same axis.

for test vectors 45° from the axes, in which case the thresholds should plot on circles. Sometimes the predictions hold convincingly and sometimes they fail convincingly, convincingly because there is a high degree of symmetry in the results.

In a different sort of experiment, Qasim Zaidi, Marc Mandler and I measured simultaneous colour induction with a cancellation procedure (Krauskopf *et al.*, 1986b). The

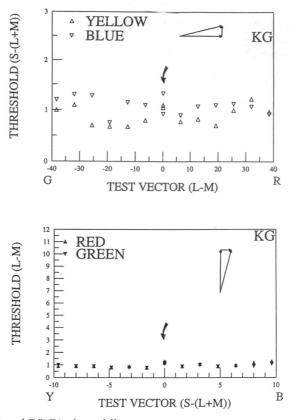

Figure 7.7.3. Test and DELTA along different axes.

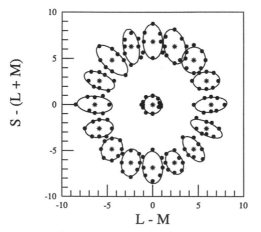

Figure 7.7.4. Discrimination ellipses.

results deviated significantly from the prediction based on independent induction processes within cardinal mechanisms.

Another bit of evidence comes from experiments on discrimination and detection of chromatic pulses (Krauskopf et al., 1986a). In a two interval – two stimulus forced choice procedure observers were required to say in which interval which of two classes of chromatic pulse was presented. In one condition, the pulse was along one of two cardinal axes. In another condition, the pulses were along lines 45° away from the cardinal axes in neighbouring quadrants.

It was hypothesised that there are independent mechanisms that respond to the components along the cardinal axes and that they evoked unique experiences when activated. This might be called in modern language the 'labelled line hypothesis', in older parlance the 'Doctrine of Specific Nerve Energies'. If this hypothesis is correct, all weak, near threshold stimuli actually detected should be correctly identified. When appropriate allowance was made for guessing, this, in fact, was found to be true for all cardinal pairs.

For each 45° stimulus, detection should occur sometimes when one of the neighbouring cardinal mechanisms is activated, sometimes when the other is, and sometimes when both are. This will lead to an ambiguity corrupting the discrimination between such stimuli. Quantitatively the effect is small but would be easily measurable if it occurred. It does not. Pairs of 45° pulses are perfectly discriminable at threshold. Thus, once again, we seem to be required to postulate mechanisms tuned to directions other than cardinal.

The final piece of psychophysical evidence I want to consider concerns the coherence of plaids generated as in the experiments of Adelson and Movshon (1982) by simultaneously presenting pairs of drifting gratings. People tended to see these patterns as a unitary drifting plaid rather than superimposed moving gratings to the degree that the component gratings are similar in contrast and spatial frequency. Bart Farell and I asked whether the similarity rule held with respect to chromatic composition (Krauskopf and Farell, 1990). We found that people reported seeing gratings drifting past one another when the components were modulated along different chromatic axes but appeared coherent when the components were modulated in directions 90° apart but rotated 45° with respect to the cardinal axes.

Recently Hai-jung Wu and I have tried to make precise measurements of the locus of the cardinal axes using plaid patterns. The basic idea is illustrated in Figure 7.7.5 (left), which depicts the isoluminant plane. Test patterns were made up consisting of one drifting grating that was always modulated along one presumed cardinal direction, in this case the L-2M direction, while a second drifting grating was modulated along one of five directions in the vicinity of the S–(L + M) axis. A two-interval forced choice procedure was used. One pairing of fixed and variable gratings was presented in the first 1.0 s interval and after a 0.5 s interval a pair consisting of the fixed grating and a different variable grating was presented for 1.0 s.

As Farell and I had found that grating pairs modulated along different cardinal directions appeared to slip past one another, we asked the observers to decide which one of the pairs seemed less coherent. All 20 possible pairings were presented five times. Figure 7.7.6 plots the frequency with which each pairing was chosen as least coherent against all the other pairings. The form of these data is typical. We wanted to have a measure of the pairing that was least coherent and found it convenient and empirically reasonable to fit the data with a Gaussian and to use the mid-point of the curve as the measure of the least coherent pairing.

We used this method to obtain what appeared to be highly reliable estimates of the loci of the cardinal axes for several observers. Then we turned our attention to what happens

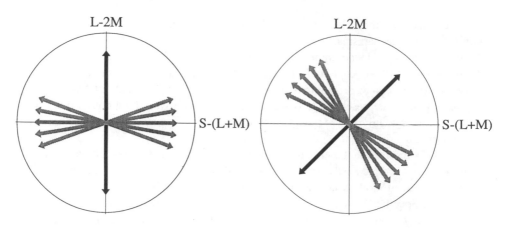

Figure 7.7.5. Paired comparison stimuli.

when the fixed modulation is not along a cardinal axis as illustrated in Figure 7.7.5 (right). My expectation was based on the rule that the greater the similarity between the component gratings the more likely the perception of coherence and this meant that for the pairings on the right the perception of *coherence* should be most likely when the gratings are modulated in directions 90° apart. This was simply wrong. The data for the two cases shown were much the same. The least coherent pair consisted of grating modulated along directions at 45° and 135°.

This seems to be at odds with the results of Krauskopf and Farell (1990). This fortunately is not the case. In that experiment the choice was 'coherent' or 'slipping', but the perceptions are not really binary. A stimulus could be judged as 'coherent' and yet be seen as slipping more than another stimulus.

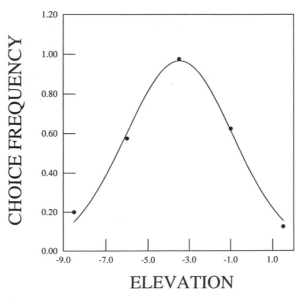

Figure 7.7.6. Paired comparison results.

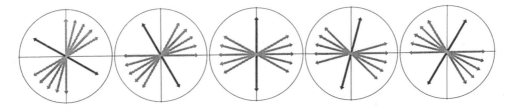

Figure 7.7.7. Paired comparison with fixed stimuli at 15° intervals.

We pursued this further and performed the experiment diagrammed in Figure 7.7.7. We set the fixed grating at different angles in different sessions to sample the whole isoluminant plane. The results of this experiment are given in Figure 7.7.8. The abscissa is the direction of the fixed modulation direction, the ordinate the direction of modulation for the grating that when paired with it produces the minimal impression of coherence. For each modulation direction coherence is minimal when the paired grating is modulated in a direction 90° away. This suggests once again that there are a multiplicity of mechanisms tuned to respond best to modulations in some direction and minimally to modulation 90° away.

To protect Bart Farell's reputation and mine we did one more variation on these experiments illustrated in Figure 7.7.9. We used our paired comparison procedure with pairs of gratings like those shown here again asking the observers to pick the pair that was least coherent. The answer confirming our previous work was that the best pairing was close to 0° and 90°.

The idea that there are three well-defined second stage mechanisms was strongly reinforced by the finding of two classes of cells in the monkey lateral geniculate nucleus that derive their chromatically and spatially opposed inputs in the majority group from the long- and middle-wavelength cones, and in the minority group from the short-wavelength

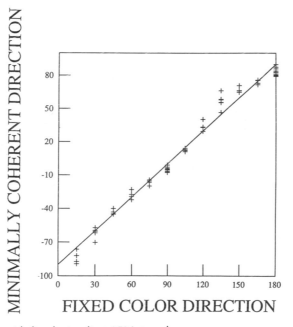

Figure 7.7.8. Results with fixed stimuli at 15° intervals.

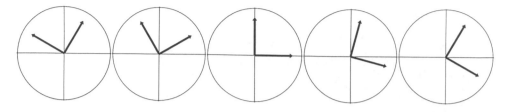

Figure 7.7.9.   Conditions for comparing relative coherence of pairs 90° apart.

cones opposed by both the long- and middle-wavelength cones (DeValois *et al.*, 1966; Wiesel and Hubel, 1966).

We measured the responses of macaque LGN cells to modulations in different directions through the white point of our colour space (Derrington *et al.*, 1984). We fit the data to a linear model, which held that each cell had a preferred direction in colour space to which it responded best and that its responses to other directions were proportional to the cosine of the angle between the modulation direction and the best direction. This model could also

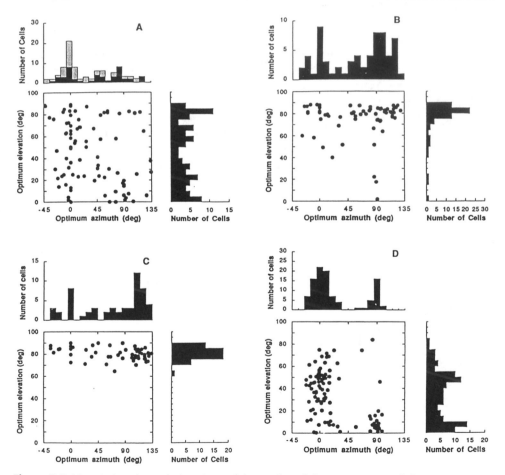

Figure 7.7.10.   Azimuths and elevations of the preferred directions: upper left – non-oriented units in V1; upper right – simple cells in V1; lower left – complex cells in V1; lower right – parvocellular neurones in LGN.

be expressed in terms of the algebraic weights that each cell assigned to the S, L and M cones.

Figure 7.7.10 shows distributions of the best directions of the parvocellular units from those experiments together with results from V1 obtained by Peter Lennie, Gary Sclar and I (Lennie *et al.*, 1990). The LGN data in the lower right corner show clustering into two distinct groups, one whose azimuths cluster about 0°, that is, the L-2M axis, and about 90°, the S–(L + M) axis. While this might be thought to provide a substrate for cardinal mechanisms, at least two facts argue against this interpretation. LGN neurons do not habituate even when maximally stimulated. Their responses are very nearly linear, which means the information they carry is decoded by elements later in the chain.

The lower left panel shows the preferred directions for complex cells. They are really more tightly clustered than this picture, a Mercator projection, suggests because at the North Pole azimuth is of little consequence.

The upper two panels depict the preferences of units without orientation preferences that respond well to low spatial frequencies (left), and simple cells (right). What can be seen is that the distribution of preferred azimuths is broader for these units than for those in the LGN though there remains some residual clustering about the cardinal azimuths. No one knows which of these units are the relevant substrate for the psychophysical phenomena I have discussed but the broad scatter in the distributions of the preferred directions is consonant with the expectations fostered by the psychophysical results discussed here.

7.7.1 ACKNOWLEDGEMENTS

I thank Walter Kropfl of the Center for Neural Science for his work in designing and constructing the expanded ATVistaBoard display system and for his development of the Postq experimental control system, and the various collaborators mentioned above. The work was supported by NIH grant EY 06638.

7.7.2 REFERENCES

ADELSON, E.H. & MOVSHON, J.A. (1982) Phenomenal coherence of moving visual patterns, *Nature*, **300**, 523–525.

DERRINGTON, A.M., KRAUSKOPF, J. & LENNIE, P. (1984) Chromatic mechanisms in lateral geniculate nucleus of macaque, *Journal of Physiology*, **357**, 241–265.

DEVALOIS, R.L., ABRAMOV, I. & JACOBS, G.H. (1966) Analysis of Response Patterns of LGN Cells, *Journal of the Optical Society of America*, **56**, 966–977.

HERING, E. (1905) *Outline of a Theory of the Light Sense* (edited and translated by Hurvich, L. & Jameson, D. (1964)), Cambridge: Harvard University Press.

KRAUSKOPF, J. & FARELL, B. (1990) The influence of chromatic content on the perception of coherent motion, *Nature*, **348**, 328–331.

KRAUSKOPF, J. & GEGENFURTNER, K. (1992) Colour discrimination and adaptation, *Vision Research*, **32**, 2165–2175.

KRAUSKOPF, J., WILLIAMS. D.R. & HEELEY, D.W. (1982) Cardinal Directions of Colour Space, *Vision Research*, **22**, 1123–1131.

KRAUSKOPF, J., WILLIAMS, D.R., MANDLER, M.B. & BROWN, A.M. (1986a) Higher order colour mechanisms, *Vision Research*, **26**, 23–32.

KRAUSKOPF, J., ZAIDI, Q. & MANDLER, M.B. (1986b) Mechanisms of simultaneous colour induction, *Journal of the Optical Society of America*, A **3**, 1752–1757.

LENNIE, P., KRAUSKOPF, J. & SCLAR, G. (1990) Chromatic mechanisms in striate cortex of macaque, *Journal of Neuroscience*, **10**, 649–669.

MacLeod, D.I.A. & Boynton, R.M. (1979) Chromaticity diagram showing cone excitation by stimuli of equal luminance, *Journal of the Optical Society of America*, **69**, 1183–1186.

Webster, M.A. & Mollon, J.D. (1991) Changes in colour appearance following post-receptoral adaptation, *Nature*, **348**, 235–238

Webster, M.A. & Mollon, J.D. (1994) The influence of contrast adaptation on colour appearance, *Vision Research*, **34**, 1993–2020.

Wiesel, T.N. & Hubel, D.H. (1966) Spatial and chromatic interactions in the lateral geniculate body of the rhesus monkey, *Journal of Neurophysiology*, **29**, 1115–1156.

Zaidi, Q & Shapiro, A.G. (1993) Adaptive orthogonalization of opponent-colour signals, *Biological Cybernetics*, **69**, 415–428.

Colour Appearance and the CIE System

C.J. Hawkyard

7.8.1   INTRODUCTION

The internationally accepted method of defining a colour numerically was first formulated by the CIE in 1931. It takes into account the nature of the illuminant or coloured light, as defined by its spectral power distribution, and the colour matching characteristics of the 'standard observer', for a 2° or 10° field of view (Figure 7.8.1). These curves are called colour matching functions.

The standard observer data is the average results of panels of observers who were asked to match monochromatic lights with a mixture of red, green and blue primaries. As the value of one of these is negative at all visible wavelengths, Deane Judd introduced the theoretical stimuli X, Y and Z to enable all the 'tristimulus values' to be positive or zero.

When a surface is observed by reflection a third parameter, namely the reflectance characteristics of the surface, must be introduced. The measured reflectance data may vary, depending on whether the surface is glossy, matt, fluorescent, pearlescent or metallic. It is therefore important to stipulate the geometry, specular content, angle of measurement, etc., when using reflectance data.

7.8.2   SCALING

The tristimulus values of an illuminant are defined as follows:

$$X = k \int P\lambda.\bar{x}\lambda \, d\lambda$$
$$Y = k \int P\lambda.\bar{y}\lambda \, d\lambda \tag{1}$$
$$Z = k \int P\lambda.\bar{z}\lambda \, d\lambda$$
$$k = 100 \int P\lambda.\bar{y}\lambda \, d\lambda$$

The system is therefore relative, not absolute, since it is scaled so that the Y tristimulus value is always 100. As the areas under the $\bar{x},\bar{y},\bar{z}$ curves are equal, the tristimulus values for a light source with equal power at all wavelengths are:

$$X = Y = Z = 100$$

This applies regardless of the absolute power, i.e. the intensity of the light (Figure 7.8.2).

The tristimulus values of a surface viewed by reflection are similarly scaled. Thus:

$$X = k \int P\lambda.\bar{x}\lambda.R\lambda \ d\lambda$$
$$Y = k \int P\lambda.\bar{y}\lambda.R\lambda \ d\lambda \tag{2}$$
$$Z = k \int P\lambda.\bar{z}\lambda.R\lambda \ d\lambda$$

k being defined as above.

The perfect white diffuser, with a reflectance of 100 per cent at all wavelengths, has X = Y = Z = 100 for the equal energy illuminant.

7.8.3   LIGHT SOURCES

Coloured lights and self-luminous displays may be measured with a tristimulus filter instrument or a spectroradiometer. The instruments will usually provide readings for luminance L, often erroneously termed Y. The two are linearly related.

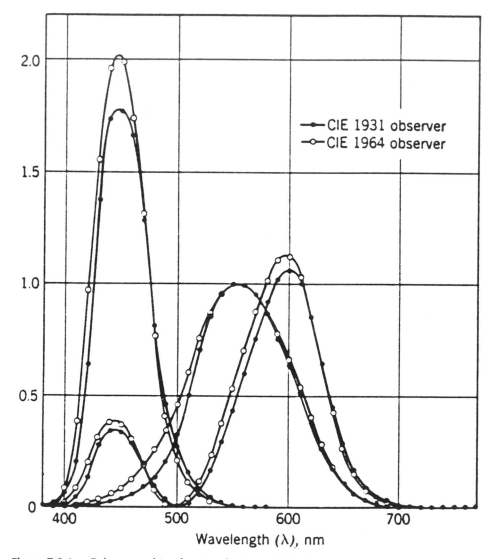

Figure 7.8.1.   Colour matching function for 2° and 10° observers.

Power

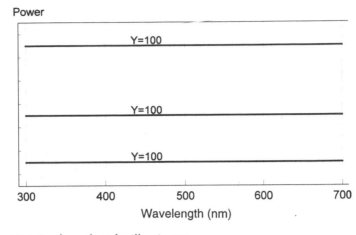

Y=100

Y=100

Y=100

300   400   500   600   700

Wavelength (nm)

Figure 7.8.2. Y tristimulus values for illuminants.

$$L = K.Y \qquad (3)$$

where K is the luminance factor.

As L is also used for lightness, this nomenclature can cause confusion.

In the case of a colour graphics display the white point of the monitor, i.e. the white with maximum luminance, could arbitrarily be given a Y value of 100, in which case $L_{max} = 100K$. Hence, $K = L_{max}/100$. For higher luminance factors Y for the white point is less than 100, as K is inversely proportional to Y.

When colours on the display are meant to represent surface colours, white points with Y greater than 100 would mean a colour with tristimulus values X,Y,Z would have a lower luminance than the same colour displayed with a luminance factor such that Y_{max} is less than 100. The problem with the latter case is that some light colours may be out of gamut. Turning up the brightness control on the monitor will also increase the luminance, but the chromaticity will also be affected. This problem is discussed further later.

7.8.4 LIGHTNESS

Humans' perception of the grey scale (lightness) is non-linear with respect to both reflectance and Y tristimulus value. The relationship between Y and lightness has been investigated by observations on the Munsell value (V) scale, which consists of steps from 0 (black) to 10 (white), the intervals being equally spaced visually. The crude data for V versus Y (Newhall *et al.*, 1943) has had a number of equations fitted to it, varying from Hunter's simple $V = Y^{0.5}$ to Judd's complex inverse 5th degree polynomial as used in ANLAB. In each case lightness is proportional to V.

The CIELAB equation is now the one generally used, lightness being L*.

$$L* = 116(Y/100)^{0.333} - 16 \qquad (4)$$

except at very low Y values.

Although the top limit for the original scale was 102.5, the maximum for L* is 100.

Another, little-known equation derived by Holdaway (1978) fits the data well, and has the advantage of easily being reversed for back-calculations.

$$L = 48.5\log_e(y + (y(y+2))^{0.5} + 1) \qquad (5)$$

where y = Y/33.4

$$Y = 0.334[((u + 1/u)/2) - 1]$$

where u = exp(L/48.5)   (6)

7.8.5   CHROMA

CIELAB uses the doubtful method of utilising the same power relationship developed for lightness for red versus green (a*) and yellow versus blue (b*) chromaticity, and also uses the Y conversion for both greenness and yellowness.

$$a* = 500[(X/X_n)^{0.333} - (Y/Y_n)^{0.333}]$$ (7)
$$b* = 200[(Y/Y_n)^{0.333} - (Z/Z_n)^{0.333}]$$ (8)

where X_n, Y_n, Z_n are the tristimulus values of the illuminant, Y_n being 100 in all cases.
   Chroma c* is then defined as follows:

$$c* = (a*^2 + b*^2)^{0.5}$$ (9)

7.8.6   BRIGHTNESS

Brightness is a perceptual scale for light sources similar to lightness for surface colours, but the limits of the scale have not been defined.

   Marsden has reviewed the relationship between perceived brightness and luminance for complex fields (Marsden, 1969), and reported his own work (Marsden, 1970). The experimental conditions under which the observers are asked to attempt to scale brightness as the luminance of the lighting changes is critical.

   In his review, Marsden (1969) compared the findings of several workers who used similar experimental conditions for the assessment of brightness. For instance, seven authors used direct estimation to obtain, among other things, a brightness scale for fairly small targets viewed in dim or dark surrounds. Plots of log luminance against log brightness were found to be approximately linear in each case, and in all but two, which were discounted for low observer numbers, the gradients all lay in the region 0.23–0.31 (Figure 7.8.3). Marsden summed up by saying 'there would appear to be ample evidence that brightness is proportional to some power of luminance, where that power is of the order of 0.3 for the dark-adapted eye'.

   It is interesting to reflect that in the calibration of monitors using gamma correction (Hawkyard and Wilkinson, 1990) a power relation is used to relate normalised luminance with normalised gun voltage (DAC values), the gradients of the linear log luminance against log gun voltage plots usually being 0.33–0.35.

   It is difficult to measure the response of the human optical system to light of different intensities, after various adaptation times, because connecting electrodes to human optic nerve fibres to measure discharges is very difficult. However, work on the Horse Shoe Crab (Gregory, 1990) has provided strong physiological evidence to support the claim that a power law relates sensation to stimulus. The rate of discharges was roughly in proportion to the log of the light intensity, and the rate of discharges increased with increasing dark adaptation times for a constant light intensity.

   The judgement of intensity is also affected by the background intensity, plots of DI against I being exponential (Weber's Law) (Gregory, 1990). DI is the difference in intensity between target light and background, and I is the intensity of the target. Similar exponential relationships also apply to intensity versus layer thickness (Lambert's Law) and colorant concentration (Beer's Law) for light absorption by transparent coloured materials. Here $\log_{10}(I_o/I_t)$, where I_o is the initial intensity, and I_t is the final intensity after absorption, is termed absorbance, and this is linearly related to thickness and concentration.

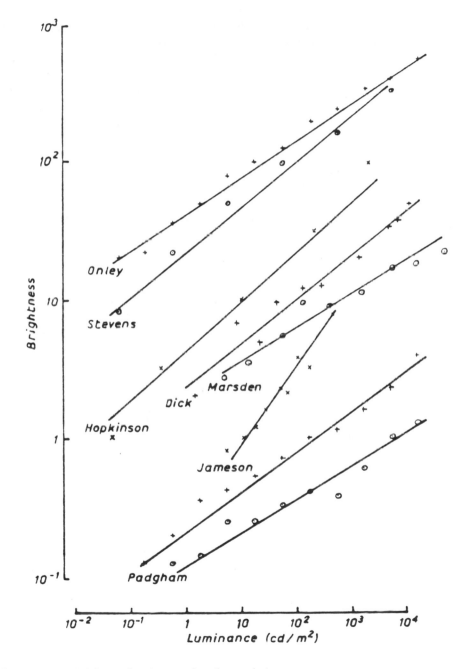

Figure 7.8.3. Brightness/luminance data (log scales).

Looking at a candle in a brightly lit room is equivalent to looking at one through a thick layer of Perspex!

7.8.7   COLOURFULNESS

It is a well-known fact that multi-coloured scenes appear to be more colourful under high levels of incident lighting than under dim lighting. When the sun comes out from behind the clouds the colours of the flowers look more vivid. This effect is also apparent when simulated scenes on computer-aided design (CAD) monitors are compared visually with surface colours under standard lighting conditions.

Thus, in the Shademaster System (Hawkyard and Oulton, 1991) the scene represented on screen is of the inside of a matching cabinet. When a visual match is attempted by placing a cabinet with surface colours in it immediately next to the screen in a dark room, good visual matches may be obtained for a fairly low light intensity in the cabinet. However, when the lights in the cabinet are brighter, as is often the case in the USA, the colours on screen appear muted by comparison. The answer is not just to increase the luminance of the foreground colours, but of the whole scene on the monitor, so that the luminance on the screen is equivalent to that in the cabinet.

Berns and Fairchild (1993) have calculated the relationship between colourfulness c, and the absolute luminance of the light source Y_n, derived from the trend of data presented by Takahama *et al.*, 1980. (Nayatani *et al*, 1980).

$$c = 0.219 - 0.0784\log_{10}(Y_n) \tag{10}$$

In their colour appearance model RLAB, Berns and Fairchild (1993) also suggest that the reference illuminant should be D65 with a luminance level of 318 cdm^{-2}, this being the luminance of a perfect reflecting diffuser viewed under an illuminance of 1000 lux.

7.8.8   ABSOLUTE Y

From the above summary it can be concluded that an absolute scale for Y would be very useful. Berns and Fairchild have hinted at this, without making a specific proposal. Following up their standard illuminant specifications, one suggestion is to set Y = 100 with a luminance of 318 cdm^{-2}. A simpler fixed point for the absolute scale would be Y = 100 for a luminance of 100 cdm^{-2}.

Marsden (1969) in his discussion of different methods of scaling brightness, wrote: 'For each of the criteria there is scope for variability in the size of brightness unit and/or the absolute value to be ascribed to the scale.'

Should the scale for luminance be linear, or would a logarithmic scale, or a power scale such as decibels for sound, be appropriate for the wide range of luminances encountered in practice? If a log scale were to be chosen it could be:

$$Y_{abs} = 50\log_{10}L \tag{11}$$

However, this would mean that luminances below 1 cdm^{-2} would produce negative Y_{abs} values. In order to avoid this, the equation is amended thus:

$$Y_{abs} = 20\log_{10}L + 60 \tag{12}$$

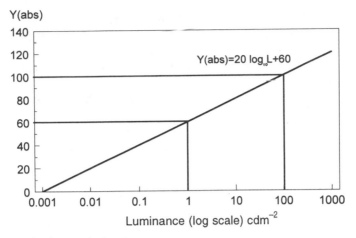

Figure 7.8.4. An absolute scale for Y.

The relationship between Y_{abs} and luminance would then be as shown in Figure 7.8.4.

7.8.9   CONSEQUENCES

The absolute Y tristimulus value would be useful in mapping lightness, brightness, chroma and colourfulness on a unified scale. Lightness and brightness would be functions of Y_{abs}, chroma would require X_{abs} and Z_{abs} in addition, whereas colourfulness would be a function of chroma and Y_{abs}. The choice of a log scale would probably simplify the relationships for lightness and brightness. The two are likely to be similar in any case, in that brightness tends to be judged by observations of objects viewed by reflectance. Such an absolute scale would also simplify colour appearance calculations.

Equation (10) for colourfulness, for instance would become:

$$c = 0.219 - 0.0784/20 \ (Y_{abs} - 60)$$
$$= 0.4542 - 0.00392 \ Y_{abs} \tag{13}$$

7.8.10   CIE STIMULI

The X,Y Z stimuli were designed such that:

1. The line XY touches the spectrum locus for a considerable length in the red–yellow region of the spectrum. In this region Z=0.
2. The line YZ touches the spectrum locus such that the area of the XYZ triangle is a minimum.
3. The X and Z stimuli lie on a line of zero luminance, the alichne, on a plane of zero luminance.

Thus the Y tristimulus value alone is a measure of luminance, the y colour matching function being identical in shape to the V_λ curve. The 1931 two degree data have been shown to be suspect (Kinney, 1983), but the effect of the new curve on Y has not been recalculated. X and Z are thus imaginary red and blue lights with zero luminance. A student of mine once commented that they must surely then be black. In fact, the power distributions of X, Y and Z have not been defined as far as I am aware, but will have negative as well as positive lobes. One suggestion, from an infinite number of possibles, is shown in Figure 7.8.5.

What is the value of defining the spectral power distribution of X, Y and Z? I will leave that for others to answer!

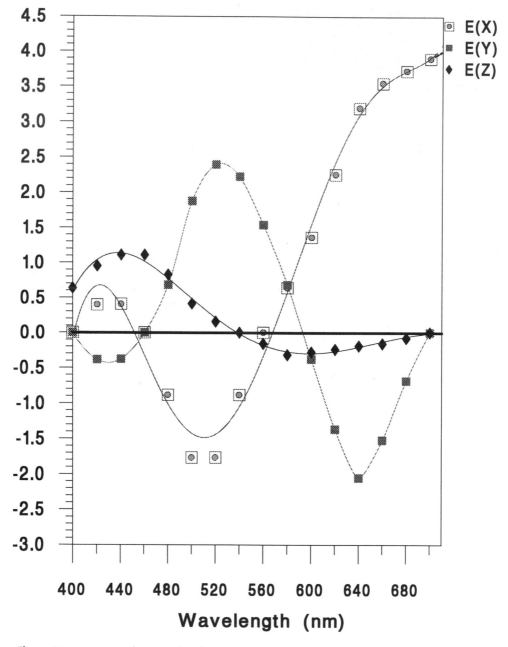

Figure 7.8.5.   Spectral power distribution for 'X', 'Y' and 'Z' primaries.

7.8.11 REFERENCES

BERNS, R. S. & FAIRCHILD, M. D. (1993) Color appearance specification for cross-media color reproduction, *Proceedings of the 7th Congress of the AIC, Budapest 1993*, Vol B, Chapter 11 1–5.

GREGORY, R. L. (1990) Seeing brightness, *Eye and Brain*, Chapter 6, London: Weidenfeld & Nicolson.

HAWKYARD, C. J. & WILKINSON, C. (1990) Accurate representation of the colour of physical samples on a cathode ray tube graphics monitor, *Journal of the Society of Dyers and Colourists*, **106**, 356–362; 1991, ibid., **107**, 83.

HAWKYARD, C. J. & OULTON, D. P. (1991) Colour in textile computer-aided design systems, *Journal of the Society of Dyers and Colourists*, **107**, 309–313.

HOLDAWAY, H. W. (1978) A suggested replacement of the Munsell function for colour-difference formulae, *Journal of the Society of Dyers and Colourists*, **94**, 260–261.

KINNEY, J. A. S. (1983) Brightness of colored self-luminous displays, *Colour Research and Applications*, **8**, 82–89.

MARSDEN, A. M. (1969) Brightness – a review of current knowledge, *Lighting Research and Technology*, **1**, 171–181.

MARSDEN, A. M. (1970) Brightness-luminance relationships in an interior, *Lighting Research and Technology*, **2**, 10–16.

NAYATANI, Y., TAKAHAMA K. & SOBAGAKI, H. (1980) *Acta Chromatica*, **3**, 172–175.

NEWHALL, S. M., NICKERSON, D. & JUDD, D. B. (1943) Final report of the OSA subcommittee on the spacing of the Munsell colors, *Journal of the Optical Society of America*, **33**, 385–418.

Section 8 – Colour Constancy

Colour Constancy from Colour Relations in the Normal and Colour-deficient Observer

David H. Foster, Sérgio M.C. Nascimento
and Karina J. Linnell

8.1.1   INTRODUCTION

The notion of colour constancy was known to Thomas Young (1807), who remarked that

> when a room is illuminated either by the yellow light of a candle, or by the red light of a fire, a sheet of writing paper still appears to retain its whiteness. (p. 456)

This notion is at the centre of the traditional interpretation of colour constancy; namely, the invariance of the perceived colour of a surface despite changes in the intensity and spectral composition of the light source. Von Helmholtz (1866) assumed that colour constancy was achieved by an unconscious elimination of the contribution of illumination, and a variety of mechanisms have been proposed for the production of illuminant-invariant colour percepts, mainly based on the adaptation or scaling of receptor responses (e.g. Helson and Jeffers, 1940; Judd, 1940; Land, 1959a, b; McCann *et al.*, 1976; von Kries, 1905). When colour constancy has been measured, typically by observers making matches between coloured surfaces in scenes illuminated by different light sources, the degree of colour constancy has been found to be limited or variable (Arend and Reeves, 1986; Cornelissen, 1994; Lucassen, 1993; Nascimento and Foster, this volume, pp. 491–499; Reeves, 1992; Tiplitz Blackwell and Buchsbaum, 1988; Troost and de Weert, 1991; Valberg and Lange-Malecki, 1990; for single-cell and animal behavioural data, see, for example, Zeki, 1983a,b; Carden *et al.*, 1992).

There is, however, an alternative approach to colour constancy based on a one-to-one correspondence between the ability to make matches that are invariant under illuminant changes and the ability to make discriminations between illuminant and non-illuminant changes in scenes (Foster and Nascimento, 1994, Appendix 1). Consideration of this discriminative capacity has been referred to as an operational approach to colour constancy (Craven and Foster, 1992; Foster *et al.*, 1992). The formal equivalence of the two approaches to colour constancy derives from a technically 'non-constructive' argument (Foster and Nascimento, 1994, Appendix 1): it does not provide algorithms or procedures for generating particular invariant colour quantities. This kind of equivalence is not special to colour constancy, it has analogies in other visual tasks: for example, two planar patterns related by a rigid motion in the plane may be recognised as being the same either because some spatially invariant quantity is visually associated with each or because it is possible to transform the visual representation of one pattern into the visual representation of the other by the equivalent of a rigid motion (Foster and Mason, 1979). The first process corresponds to the traditional approach to colour constancy; the second to the operational approach.

In practice, observers can make reliable discriminations between illuminant and non-illuminant changes in simultaneously presented coloured images (Foster *et al.*, 1992) and in sequentially presented coloured images (Craven and Foster, 1992). In this study, some experimental evidence for this ability is reviewed, along with a possible theoretical explanation based on a low-level coding of spatial colour relations. This explanation leads to a prediction about discriminating illuminant from non-illuminant changes by colour-deficient observers. An experimental test of this prediction is reported for two protanopes and two deuteranopes.

8.1.2   DISCRIMINATING ILLUMINANT FROM NON-ILLUMINANT CHANGES

The following experiment (Craven and Foster, 1992, experiment 3) was used to test the ability of observers to make discriminations between sequentially presented images of Mondrian patterns that had undergone either illuminant or illuminant and non-illuminant changes. Precisely the same method was used to test dichromatic observers, as described later. The illuminants used in the experiment were natural daylights, which, in the CIE (1931) (x, y)-chromaticity diagram, fall on a line slightly on the green side of the Planckian locus; they were labelled by a single co-ordinate, the x-co-ordinate. The spectral energy distributions of the daylights were taken from the principal components analysis by Judd *et al.* (1964). The surfaces used in the experiment were from the Munsell set, the spectral reflectances of which encompass those of a large set of natural coloured objects, such as flowers, flower clusters, leaves, and berries (Jaaskelainen *et al.*, 1990). The spectral reflectances of the Munsell surfaces were taken from the principal components analysis by Parkkinen *et al.* (1989).

Observers were presented with two sequential 1 s images: one was of a Mondrian pattern whose patches, drawn at random from the Munsell set, were illuminated spatially uniformly by a daylight with x-co-ordinate either 0.25 (30 000 K) or 0.37 (4400 K), chosen at random; the other image was of the same Mondrian pattern illuminated by a daylight of the same colour but shifted along the daylight locus. In conjunction with this spatially uniform change in illuminant, an additional spatially non-uniform change was imposed: for half of the patches in the pattern, selected at random, the daylight received a further shift Δx along the daylight locus in the positive direction, and, for the remaining half of the patches, an equal shift in the negative direction. In half of the trials the non-uniform shift Δx was set to zero. Observers had to report whether there was 'a change of material' (see below). The magnitude of the uniform shift in illuminant and the magnitude of the non-uniform shift Δx varied from trial to trial. In all, there were 18 experimental conditions: three uniform illuminant shifts by two directions of shift by three non-uniform illuminant shifts.

When the non-uniform shift was zero, the changes observed in the sequentially presented displays could be interpreted plausibly as being due to a shift in illuminant, an *illuminant* change; when the non-uniform shift was non-zero, the simplest interpretation was that there was an additional change in the spectral reflectance of the individual patches in the patterns, a *material* change.

Mean performance by three observers, all with normal colour vision, is shown by the solid lines in the graphs of Figure 8.1.1, where discrimination index d' from signal-detection theory is plotted against Δx (the open symbols refer to measurements by dichromats, described later). As is evident from the graphs, as Δx increased, d' increased. The effect of Δx was statistically significant ($F_{2,4} = 39.0, p = 0.002$), although it depended on the magnitude of the uniform shift ($F_{2,4} = 16.1, p = 0.01$) and on its starting point ($F_{1,2} = 39.8, p = 0.02$). Further discussion is given in Craven and Foster (1992).

8.1.3 SPATIAL COLOUR RELATIONS

The ability to distinguish between illuminant and material changes in a scene might be based on a visual coding of spatial colour relations within that scene; these relations might, in turn, be specified by the ratios of cone-photoreceptor excitations produced by light reflected from pairs of surfaces within the scene (Foster and Nascimento, 1994). Notice that these excitations refer to activity within rather than between cone classes. Cone-excitation ratios have been assumed to be computed in adaptational (von Kries, 1905) models of colour constancy, as part of a scaling mechanism, usually with respect to an explicit or inferred reference 'white' (Ives, 1912; West and Brill, 1982; Worthey and Brill, 1986); they have been incorporated into Retinex models, as sequential products relating each surface to one or more high-reflectance surfaces (Land and McCann, 1971; McCann et al., 1976); and they have been used in theoretical studies (see, e.g., Brill and West, 1981; West and Brill, 1982; Worthey and Brill, 1986) to set constraints on illuminant and surface reflectance spectra for colour constancy, although results from the last have yielded unrealistic data

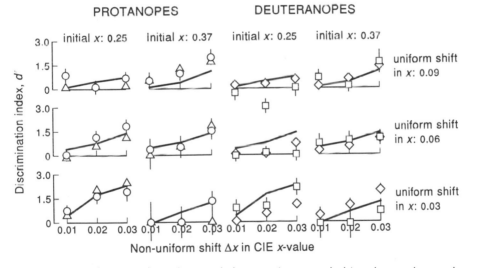

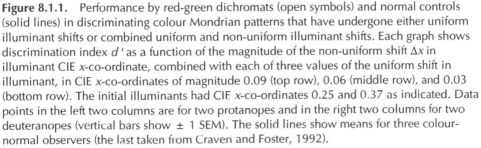

Figure 8.1.1. Performance by red-green dichromats (open symbols) and normal controls (solid lines) in discriminating colour Mondrian patterns that have undergone either uniform illuminant shifts or combined uniform and non-uniform illuminant shifts. Each graph shows discrimination index d' as a function of the magnitude of the non-uniform shift Δx in illuminant CIE x-co-ordinate, combined with each of three values of the uniform shift in illuminant, in CIE x-co-ordinates of magnitude 0.09 (top row), 0.06 (middle row), and 0.03 (bottom row). The initial illuminants had CIE x-co-ordinates 0.25 and 0.37 as indicated. Data points in the left two columns are for two protanopes and in the right two columns for two deuteranopes (vertical bars show ± 1 SEM). The solid lines show means for three colour-normal observers (the last taken from Craven and Foster, 1992).

(Brill and West, 1986, p. 198). The approach considered here is the converse of the last: given natural surfaces and illuminants, how constant are cone-excitation ratios under changes in illuminant?

Let r_i be the ratio of excitations in cone class i (i = 1, 2, 3 corresponding to short-, medium-, and long-wavelength-sensitive classes) produced by light from two surfaces drawn at random from the set of Munsell surfaces illuminated by a single illuminant e drawn at random from the daylight locus (correlated colour temperatures ranging over 4300–25 000 K); and let r'_i be the corresponding ratio for the same two surfaces illuminated by another illuminant e', also drawn at random from the daylight set. These two ratios r_i, r'_i were calculated 1000 times, the illuminants e, e' and surfaces being chosen afresh on each calculation. Figure 8.1.2 shows a scatterplot of the resulting points (r_i, r'_i) (open circles) for each cone class i (from Foster and Nascimento, 1994). If the ratios were invariant under changes in illuminant, that is, r_i = r'_i, then all the points would lie on the line of unit slope and zero intercept. The proportion of pairs of ratios r_i, r'_i within 10 per cent of each other did not fall below 0.96. When the illuminants were drawn instead from a Planckian radiator, at temperatures of 2000–100 000 K (small solid circles in Figure 8.1.2, plotted under open circles), the scatter was little changed, and the corresponding proportions of pairs of ratios within 10 per cent of each other again did not fall below 0.96. (The relevance of this limiting value of 10 per cent for proportions is discussed in Foster and Nascimento, 1994.) Also shown in Figure 8.1.2 are data for particular pairs of Munsell surfaces under two extreme Planckian illuminants, at temperatures of 2000 K and 100 000 K. These data give an indication of the colorimetric significance of departures from the line r'_i = r_i. The surfaces were either (1) of intermediate Chroma (in the Munsell system of notation, 5R 5/4, 5G 5/4, 5Y 5/4, 5B 5/4), separated by increments of perceptually similar magnitude of 2 units in Chroma, 1 in Value, and 2.5 in Hue (open squares); or (2) of extreme Chroma (5R 6/14, 5G 7/10, 5Y 7/12, 5B 7/8), in all six combinations (open triangles). The expanded scale of the insets to the figure shows more clearly that for only a few of the extreme-Chroma surfaces were there large departures from invariance.

These special cases excepted, the ratio of cone excitations produced by light from pairs of surfaces is therefore almost invariant under changes in natural illumination. Moreover, the proportion of pairs of ratios within 10 per cent of each other decreased only a little when spectral reflectances were random, and was still better than 0.93 for all cone classes (Foster and Nascimento, 1994).

8.1.4   LOSS OF A CONE CLASS

If the discriminability of illuminant from material changes were based on cone-excitation ratios, then, as these ratios involve signals within rather than between classes, the loss of one of the three cone classes should lead only to a modest impairment in this ability. The size of the supposed impairment depends on which cone class is lost. Because of the closeness of the long- and medium-wavelength-sensitive cone spectral sensitivities, if either one or other cone class were lost there would be little reduction in the coverage of the visible spectrum. But the reduction in coverage would be substantial if the short-wavelength-sensitive cone class were lost. Although a reduction in the coverage of the spectrum would not affect the stability of cone-excitation ratios under illuminant changes, the ability to discriminate between illuminant and material changes would be reduced, because more material changes could be accepted as illuminant changes.

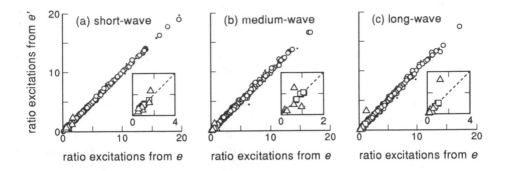

Figure 8.1.2. Scatterplot of ratios of cone excitations for each of the three cone classes: (a) short-, (b) medium-, and (c) long-wavelength sensitive. Each point represents a pair of ratios r_i, r'_i of excitations in cone class i produced by light from two surfaces drawn at random from the Munsell set, illuminated in turn by two illuminants e, e' drawn at random from the set of daylight spectra, with correlated colour temperatures of 4300–25 000 K (open circles) or from a Planckian radiator, with temperatures of 2000–100 000 K (small solid circles, plotted under open circles). Data for particular pairs of surfaces from the Munsell set are shown (on an expanded scale in the insets) for surfaces of intermediate Chroma (open squares) and extreme Chroma (open triangles; see text). Based on 1000 random samples of pairs of surfaces and pairs of illuminants in each condition. Reproduced, with permission, from Foster and Nascimento (1994, Figure 3).

To test the prediction concerning loss of the medium- and long-wavelength-sensitive cone classes, an experiment was undertaken that was identical to the one (Craven and Foster, 1992, Expt 3) summarised earlier, in which observers had to discriminate sequentially presented images of Mondrian patterns. The 18 experimental conditions were the same: three uniform illuminant shifts by two directions of shift by three non-uniform illuminant shifts. In this version of the experiment, which has not been previously reported, the observers were four red-green dichromats: two protanopes and two deuteranopes. They were aged 33–49 years and each wore spectacles. The colour deficiency of the observers was classified with anomaloscopy performed by J. D. Moreland. All were unpracticed in psychophysical procedures and were unaware of the purpose of the experiment. Results are shown by the open symbols in the graphs of Figure 8.1.1, where d' is plotted against Δx.

All four dichromats could perform the task. For sufficiently large non-uniform shifts Δx in illuminant, they were each able to make reliable discriminations of illuminant changes from material changes. An analysis of variance with repeated measures was applied to the data, and the main results were as follows. For the dichromats taken together, the effect of the non-uniform shift Δx in illuminant was highly significant ($F_{2,4} = 39.8$, $p = 0.002$), although the effect for deuteranopes was numerically slightly weaker than for protanopes. For the protanopes, deuteranopes, and controls taken as separate groups, there was little difference in the pattern of discrimination performance over the 18 experimental conditions ($F_{2,4} = 5.8$, $p = 0.07$), and no difference in the effects of Δx ($F_{4,8} = 1.6$, $p = 0.26$).

8.1.5 COMMENT

The tolerance of the visual system to changes in the colour of an illuminant is not unlimited: for sufficiently large departures from the spectral energy distribution of daylight, objects fail to maintain their perceived daylight colour (Judd, 1940). Despite sensitivity to these changes, the relations between the perceived colours of objects are, in general, preserved, and observers are able to reliably discriminate illuminant changes from material changes in a scene. Presumably, the stability of these relations enables one to maintain a stable percept of the spatial-chromatic structure of the environment under changes in illuminant, without loss of illuminant information (Jameson and Hurvich, 1989).

This ability could be based on the coding of spatial colour relations in terms of the ratios of cone excitations produced by light reflected from pairs of surfaces in a scene. When evaluated for a large class of pigmented surfaces or for surfaces with random spectral reflectances, these ratios are almost invariant under changes in illuminants drawn either from the daylight set or from Planckian radiators. A prediction of this explanation of discrimination of illuminant changes from material changes is that protanopic and deuter-anopic observers should be able to make such discriminations almost as well as normal controls. The protanopes and deuteranopes tested here were indeed able to achieve reliable discrimination performance at levels similar to those of normal controls.

In computing these ratios, the visual system need not make use of cone signals directly but some post-receptoral combination of them (Nascimento and Foster, 1994). One of the effects of post-receptoral opponent-colour processing is that it effectively sharpens (long- and medium-wavelength-sensitive) spectral sensitivity functions (Foster, 1981; Foster and Snelgar, 1983); such sharpening has been shown to lead to an improvement in the stability of the ratios of the processed signals (see Finlayson et al., 1994a,b; Nascimento and Foster, 1994), although given the already high stability of cone-excitation ratios in the absence of spectral sharpening, the effect should be small. For red-green dichromats, with no opponency of long- and medium-wavelength-sensitive cone signals, there can be no sharpening, and no improvement in the stability of cone ratios.

An approach to the measurement of colour constancy so far not considered here depends on the more cognitive task of colour naming of surfaces (e.g. Morland et al., this volume, pp. 463–468; Troost and de Weert, 1991). Colour naming of surfaces is indeed more robust under changes in illuminant (Troost and de Weert, 1991), but it is also less precise than matching, because one colour name may correspond to many discriminable colours. For colour-deficient observers, colour naming of surfaces under changes in illuminant may be difficult to interpret, for their use of colour names is different from that of colour-normal observers, even under constant illuminants. John Dalton found (1794) from his own experience that the apparent colours of some surfaces were not constant under illuminant changes:

> The flowers of most of the Cranesbills appear to me in the day, almost exactly sky blue, whilst others call them deep pink; but happening once to look at one in the night by candle light I found it of a colour as different as possible from day light; it seemed then very near yellow, but with tincture of red; whilst no body else said it differed from the daylight appearance. (p.115).

In a study of colour constancy using colour naming of surfaces in the presence of different illuminants (Morland et al., this volume, pp. 463–468) red-green dichromats were shown to perform markedly worse than normal controls: with performance quantified by the number of changes in colour names, the controls obtained a score of 3.0 ± 0.8 out of 36 (compare Troost and de Weert, 1991) and the dichromats a score of 11.3 ± 2.5 out of 36.

In principle, any shift of colours – spatially uniform or otherwise – along the dichromat's confusion lines due to changes in illuminant is likely to be unrecognised by the dichromat. The daylight and Planckian illuminant shifts used here, however, gave shifts in apparent surface colour that were generally not far from being orthogonal to the protanopic and deuteranopic confusion lines. It might be assumed that the apparent colour of any particular surface should therefore change no more on average than the apparent colours of the surrounding surfaces under changes in the illuminant. Even so, as was shown in the insets of Figure 8.1.2, failures in spatial colour relations can occur, and the flowers of the Cranesbill inspected by Dalton may fall into this category.

8.1.6 ACKNOWLEDGEMENTS

We thank M. G. A. Thomson and S. Westland for critical reading of the manuscript. We also thank J. P. S. Parkkinen, J. Hallikainen, and T. Jaaskelainen for supplying their data for the Munsell set. This work was supported by the Wellcome Trust (grant no. 034807), the Junta Nacional de Investigação Científica e Tecnológica (grant no. BD/1328/91-RM), and the Universidade do Minho, Braga, Portugal.

8.1.7 REFERENCES

AREND, L. & REEVES, A. (1986) Simultaneous color constancy, *Journal of the Optical Society of America*, A **3**, 1743–1751.

BRILL, M. & WEST, G. (1981) Contributions to the theory of invariance of color under the condition of varying illumination, *Journal of Mathematical Biology*, **11**, 337–350.

BRILL, M. H. & WEST, G. (1986) Chromatic adaptation and color constancy: a possible dichotomy, *Color Research and Application*, **11**, 196–204.

CARDEN, D., HILKEN, H., BUTLER, S. R. & KULIKOWSKI, J. J. (1992) Lesions of primate visual area V4 produce long-lasting deficits to colour constancy, *Irish Journal of Psychology*, **13**, 455–472.

CORNELISSEN, F. W. (1994) Light & Colour: Psychophysical studies on the use of lighting for visual rehabilitation and on spatial interactions in colour constancy, PhD thesis, Rijksuniversiteit Groningen.

CRAVEN, B. J. & FOSTER, D. H. (1992) An operational approach to colour constancy, *Vision Research*, **32**, 1359–1366.

DALTON, J. (1794) Letter by Dalton to his cousin dated 20th February 1794, *Memoirs and Proceedings of the Manchester Literary & Philosophical Society (Manchester Memoirs)*, **68**(9), 115, (1924).

FINLAYSON, G. D., DREW, M. S., & FUNT, B. V. (1994a) Spectral sharpening: sensor transformations for improved color constancy, *Journal of the Optical Society of America*, A **11**, 1553–1563.

FINLAYSON, G. D., DREW, M. S., & FUNT, B. V. (1994b) Color constancy: generalized diagonal transforms suffice, *Journal of the Optical Society of America*, A **11**, 3011–3019.

FOSTER, D. H. (1981) Changes in field spectral sensitivities of red-, green- and blue-sensitive colour mechanisms obtained on small background fields, *Vision Research*, **21**, 1433–1455.

FOSTER, D. H. & MASON, R. J. (1979) Transformation and relational-structure schemes for visual pattern recognition, *Biological Cybernetics*, **32**, 85–93.

FOSTER, D. H. & NASCIMENTO, S. M. C. (1994) Relational colour constancy from invariant cone-excitation ratios, *Proceedings of the Royal Society of London*, B **257**, 115–121.

FOSTER, D. H. & SNELGAR, R. S. (1983) Test and field spectral sensitivities of colour mechanisms obtained on small white backgrounds: action of unitary opponent-colour processes? *Vision Research*, **23**, 787–797.

FOSTER, D. H., CRAVEN, B. J. & SALE, E. R. H. (1992) Immediate colour constancy, *Ophthalmic and Physiological Optics*, **12**, 157–160.

VON HELMHOLTZ, H. (1866) *Handbuch der Physiologischen Optik*, 1st Edition, Vol. II. Translation 3rd Edition (*Helmholtz's Treatise on Physiological Optics*) J. P. C. Southall (Ed.) Republished (1962) New York: Dover Publications.

VON HELMHOLTZ, H. (1866) *Handbuch der Physiologischen Optik*, 1st Edition, Vol. II. Translation 3rd Edition (*Helmholtz's Treatise on Physiological Optics*) J. P. C. Southall (Ed.) Republished (1962) New York: Dover Publications.

HELSON, H. & JEFFERS, V. B. (1940) Fundamental problems in color vision. II. Hue, lightness, and saturation of selective samples in chromatic illumination, *Journal of Experimental Psychology*, **26**, 1–27.

IVES, H. E. (1912) The relation between the color of the illuminant and the color of the illuminated object, *Transactions of Illuminating Engineering Society*, **7**, 62–72.

JAASKELAINEN, T., PARKKINEN, J. & TOYOOKA, S. (1990) Vector-subspace model for color representation, *Journal of the Optical Society of America*, Optical Society of America, pp. 286–287, **A 7**, 725–730.

JAMESON, D. & HURVICH, L. M. (1989) Essay concerning color constancy, *Annual Review of Psychology*, **40**, 1–22.

JUDD, D. B. (1940) Hue saturation and lightness of surface colors with chromatic illumination, *Journal of the Optical Society of America*, **30**, 2–32.

JUDD, D. B., MACADAM, D. L. & WYSZECKI, G. (1964) Spectral distribution of typical daylight as a function of correlated color temperature, *Journal of the Optical Society of America*, **54**, 1031–1040.

VON KRIES, J. (1905) Die Gesichtsempfindungen. In: Nagel, W. (Ed.) *Handbuch der Physiologie des Menschen*, Vol. 3 of *Physiologie der Sinne*, Braunschweig: Vieweg und Sohn.

LAND, E. H. (1959a) Color vision and the natural image. Part I, *Proceedings of the National Academy of Sciences, USA*, **45**, 115–129.

LAND, E. H. (1959b) Color vision and the natural image. Part II, *Proceedings of the National Academy of Sciences, USA*, **45**, 636–644.

LAND, E. H. & MCCANN, J. J. (1971) Lightness and Retinex theory, *Journal of the Optical Society of America*, **61**, 1–11.

LUCASSEN, M. P. (1993) *Quantitative Studies of Color Constancy*, PhD thesis, Rijksuniversiteit Utrecht.

MCCANN, J. J., MCKEE, S. P. & TAYLOR, T. H. (1976) Quantitative studies in Retinex theory. A comparison between theoretical predictions and observer responses to the 'Color Mondrian' experiments, *Vision Research*, **16**, 445–458.

NASCIMENTO, S. M. C. & FOSTER, D. H. (1994) Illuminant invariants at receptoral and postreceptoral levels as a basis for relational colour constancy, *Perception*, **23**, 8–9.

PARKKINEN, J. P. S., HALLIKAINEN, J. & JAASKELAINEN, T. (1989) Characteristic spectra of Munsell colors, *Journal of the Optical Society of America*, **A 6**, 318–322.

REEVES, A. (1992) Areas of ignorance and confusion in color science, *Behavioral and Brain Sciences*, **15**, 49–50.

TIPLITZ BLACKWELL, K. & BUCHSBAUM, G. (1988) Quantitative studies of color constancy, *Journal of the Optical Society of America*, **A 5**, 1772–1780.

TROOST, J. M. & DE WEERT, C. M. M. (1991) Naming versus matching in color constancy, *Perception and Psychophysics*, **50**, 591–602.

VALBERG, A. & LANGE-MALECKI, B. (1990) 'Colour constancy' in Mondrian patterns: a partial cancellation of physical chromaticity shifts by simultaneous contrast, *Vision Research*, **30**, 371–380.

WEST, G. & BRILL, M. H. (1982) Necessary and sufficient conditions for Von Kries chromatic adaptation to give color constancy, *Journal of Mathematical Biology*, **15**, 249–258.

WORTHEY, J. A. & BRILL, M. H. (1986) Heuristic analysis of von Kries color constancy, *Journal of the Optical Society of America*, **A 3**, 1708–1712.

YOUNG, T. (1807) *A Course of Lectures on Natural Philosophy and the Mechanical Arts*, Vol. I, Lecture XXXVIII, London: Joseph Johnson.

ZEKI, S. (1983a) Colour coding in the cerebral cortex: the responses of wavelength-selective and colour-coded cells in monkey visual cortex to changes in wavelength composition, *Neuroscience*, **9**, 767–781.

ZEKI, S. (1983b) Colour coding in the cerebral cortex: the reaction of cells in monkey visual cortex to wavelengths and colours, *Neuroscience*, **9**, 741–765.

Colour Constancy in Acquired and Congenital Colour Vision Deficiencies

A.B.Morland, J.H. MacDonald and K.F. Middleton

8.2.1 INTRODUCTION

A feature of normal colour vision is the ability to perceive surfaces as invariant in colour appearance under spectrally different illuminations. The effect, known as colour constancy, is elicited most effectively for complex visual scenes in which there are a large number of different coloured surfaces. In contrast, an isolated surface with a black surround changes its apparent colour in line with the chromaticity shifts caused by a change in illuminant. Most studies of colour constancy have, therefore, employed arrangements of coloured surfaces in a two dimensional array, which due to their resemblance to the work of the artist Mondrian bear his name.

Three factors that contribute to colour constancy are: retinal adaptation to the overall spectral composition of the illuminant, the responses of neurones in prestriate cortical area V4 (which are selective for colour appearance rather than the spectral content of a stimulus), and finally cognitive factors that enable some objects to be used as references because of their known colour. Brief presentations of Mondrian stimuli have demonstrated that discrimination between changes in the Mondrian caused by illuminant changes and changes not caused by illuminant shifts is possible in the absence of retinal adaptation (Craven and Foster, 1992; Foster *et al.*, 1992). Lesion studies in primates have revealed that colour constancy is effectively lost in the absence of V4, whereas colour discrimination remains relatively intact (Walsh *et al.*, 1993; Wild *et al.*, 1985). In this study, we have examined colour constancy for observers with abnormal cone spectral sensitivities associated with congenital red-green colour vision deficiencies, and compared their responses with those of an observer who has normal retinal function, but who exhibits abnormal colour vision due to a lesion in pre-striate cortex.

8.2.2 SUBJECTS

The subjects who took part in the experiments are described below. One subject, BL, had an acquired colour vision deficiency, frequently described as achromatopsia, and the other subjects had normal or congenitally deficient red-green colour vision.

8.2.2.1 Case Report: subject BL

BL is a 56-year-old male, who had suffered an encephalitic illness attributed to a viral infection. Immediately following this illness, he suffered severely disrupted vision but most visual functions had returned to normal before the psychophysical experiments described here were conducted. There remained, however, a severe disturbance in his colour vision. The patient was acutely aware that colours no longer looked the same as they did before his illness, and he displayed abnormal colour naming. MRI scans revealed bilateral lesions of the fusiform and lingual gyri, areas known to be involved in the central processing of chromatic signals.

BL displayed near-normal responses to the Ishihara plates, with errors ranging from 0 to 3 on repeated testing, but he made abnormally large error scores (400–600) on the Farnsworth-Munsell 100 hue arrangement test, without a distinct axis in the error score distribution. The Wright colorimeter (Wright 1927–28) was used for colour matching and wavelength discrimination experiments. With a bipartite 1°20' square field, BL used a normal mixture of 530 nm and 650 nm spectral primaries in matching a 590 nm test stimulus, but with a larger than normal matching range. He accepted an age matched normal's mixture of 435 nm and 505 nm primaries to match a 490 nm test stimulus, a match that eliminates the effects of macular pigment absorption (Ruddock, 1963). He also made a normal Rayleigh match when the two halves of the colour matching field were presented sequentially for two seconds with a one second gap between them, although his matching range was enlarged relative to that for simultaneous presentation. With a 10° field, his matches were normal, with a smaller matching range than for the 1°20' field and, correspondingly, his wavelength discrimination improved for the large field. BL's wavelength discrimination for a 1°20' field was abnormal, with the values of his just discriminable wavelength step being between three and five times larger than normal values for all spectral stimuli examined. BL's discrimination of coloured stimuli from white was also sub-normal, his discrimination steps being significantly larger than those for a normal subject, although his discrimination ellipse had normal orientation in the chromaticity chart. A Maxwellian view optical system (Barbur and Ruddock, 1980) was employed in measuring both the blue sensitive π_3 spectral response function (Stiles, 1978), and the spectral sensitivity to monochromatic, 0.5 s duration targets presented on a 3 log troland white background (Sperling and Harwerth, 1971; King-Smith and Carden, 1976). BL's π_3 spectral sensitivity followed closely the corresponding normal function given by Stiles (1978). Furthermore, his spectral sensitivity for detection of a 0.5 s target flash presented on a 3.0 log troland white background was also normal, with the characteristic opponent notches in the function occurring at the same wavelengths as in the normal (approximately 500 nm and 600 nm). Other measurements revealed that BL responded normally to stimulus motion, and stereoscopic depth, and he was able to arrange a grey scale of 46 tiles (Robertson and Wright, 1965) with normal accuracy. BL continues to exhibit mild prosapagnosia, topographical agnosia and has a scotoma to small (0.25 mm² on Goldmann perimeter) targets in the upper left field, which phenomena are all commonly associated with colour vision deficiency of central origin (Meadows, 1974).

8.2.2.2 Control subjects

All the control subjects, nine normal adult observers, six anomalous trichromats (two protan and four deutan) and four dichromats (all deutan), made Rayleigh colour matches and wavelength discrimination measurements. In order to quantify the severity of the

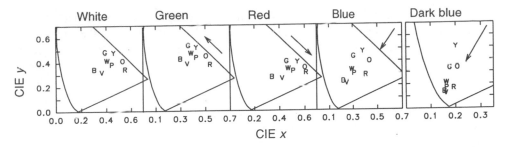

Figure 8.2.1. Chromaticity values of the patches comprising the Mondrian stimulus. Each patch colour is denoted by a letter, which corresponds to the colour name given to the patch under the white illuminant by normal observers, as follows: red, R; orange, O; yellow, Y; green, G; blue, B; purple, V; pink, P; and white, W. The notation is maintained in each of the panels, in which the data for the different illuminants (shown above each panel) are plotted.

congenitally deficient observers, we ranked them according to the size of their wavelength discrimination steps. The individual anomalous trichromats were ranked in terms of discrimination loss (ranks 2 and 7 corresponded to the least and most severe losses respectively). Normals were all ranked 1 and the dichromats were ranked 8.

8.2.3   METHODS

Colour constancy was measured using five Mondrian boards, each comprising 25–30 coloured patches with nine different colours repeated at least twice. Each board had a different spatial arrangement of the colour patches and was illuminated by one of five different illuminants. The illuminants were of approximately equal brightness and were coloured white, red, green, blue and dark blue. The nine patch colours were defined in terms of x and y chromaticity co-ordinates for each of the five illuminants, as shown in Figure 8.2.1. Each subject was required to name patches, indicated by the experimenter, on the five boards: first board 1 under the white illuminant, and subsequently boards 2, 3, 4 and 5 under the red, green, blue and dark blue illuminants respectively. Each patch colour was tested at least twice under any one illuminant to confirm the consistency of the subject response. The observers' responses were assessed in terms of an index that was defined as the number of name changes given to a colour patch under the four colour illuminants compared to that given under the white illuminant. There were four possible name changes for each patch, and therefore the total number of possible changes was 36, which represents the maximum index value and indicates complete absence of colour constancy. In light of BL's abnormal colour naming, two additional strategies were employed in his case. The first was to repeat the colour constancy measurements so that each patch was named no less than four times in any one session and also to repeat sessions on different days. The second was to obtain colour names for over 100 differently coloured test patches (presented twice), in order to define areas of the chromaticity chart that correspond to his colour names. Changes in colour naming were defined by reference to these areas of standard colours.

8.2.4   RESULTS

Indices for the normal subjects ranged from 2 to 4 with a mean of 3.0 ± 0.8 (1 s.d.). In contrast, values for the deuteranopes were higher, with a mean of 11.3 ± 2.5 (1 s.d.). The anomalous trichomats displayed the most varied response patterns, with one observer giving a normal index value of 4 and another giving 14. BL, however, gave the largest index value 20, which indicates very poor colour constancy. In Figure 8.2.2. we compare the index value achieved with the rank assigned to all observers. There is a strong dependence of the index on the discrimination rank for the control observers, the correlation coefficient of a linear regression between the two variables being 0.8.($p = 0.017$). One point on the plot (filled circle) represents the index of the subject BL plotted against the rank number, which was chosen on the basis of his wavelength discrimination steps compared to the anomalous trichomats. The position of this point clearly indicates that BL has a more severe loss of colour constancy than would be predicted on the basis of his loss of colour discrimination.

8.2.5 DISCUSSION

Previous assessments of colour constancy have involved normal observers, and variation of colour constancy with colour discrimination performance has not been examined. In this study, we have investigated the link between colour constancy and colour discrimination in order to give a true control data set for the study of a subject with a colour vision deficiency caused by cortical damage. The results of the control observers, however, also merit examination.

Subjects with sub-normal colour discrimination perceive fewer hues than normal and require a greater chromaticity change to detect a difference in hue. The perception of colour, therefore, involves fewer colour categories than normal and it could be argued that

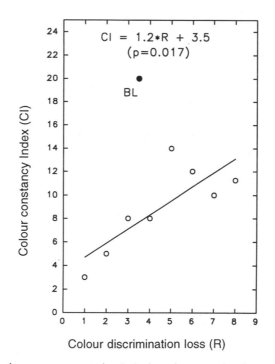

Figure 8.2.2. The colour constancy index (CI) plotted against the discrimination rank (R) assigned to each observer. Open circles represent data for the subjects with normal and congenitally deficient colour vision, and the filled circle denotes the data for subject BL.

such observers should exhibit greater colour constancy. This deduction is consistent with Jameson and Hurvich's (1989) argument, that colour constancy is a result of illuminant changes failing to produce chromaticity changes which cross categorical boundaries. The evidence of this study is, however, inconsistent with that postulate, as the colour constancy index increases systematically with loss in discrimination (Figure 8.2.2.).As discussed in the Introduction, there are three mechanisms (retinal, cortical and cognitive) that contribute to colour constancy. The cognitive element, which is almost entirely removed by employing a non-contextual stimulus such as a Mondrian display, is assumed to be available to all control observers. The remaining retinal and cortical mechanisms are clearly interrelated, with the former providing the input to the latter. The retinal contribution to colour constancy is probably due to adaptation to the illuminant. Adaptation of the retinal photoreceptors is not restricted to normal trichromatic colour vision, and is presumably a significant factor in colour constancy for observers with congenital colour vision deficiencies. Foster *et al.* (this volume, pp. 453–461) has shown that dichromatic observers have normal sensitivity in discriminating illuminant changes from non-illuminant changes to Mondrian stimuli, which was interpreted on the basis of cone excitation ratios. It seems probable, therefore, that the central processing of colour in subjects with congenital colour vision deficiencies is normal, and their impairment of colour constancy evident in our results reflects the effects of changes in the chromatic input from the abnormal peripheral mechanisms. The precise method by which the highly colour specific responses of V4 neurones are generated from the input signals is unknown, but requires considerable multiplexing (D'Zmura and Lennie, 1986). Surprisingly, congenital deficiencies of colour vision produce greater sensitivity to changes in illuminant, despite the fact that they reduce sensitivity to colour differences.

BL's visual function is documented in the case report, which establishes that although his colour vision is disturbed, the subject responds normally to other parameters of the light stimulus. Our data demonstrate that his photoreceptoral and post-receptoral opponent mechanisms are normal, but he exhibits abnormal colour discrimination and colour naming. BL's responses correspond to those of some patients with central achromatopsia, although there are significant differences between different patients who have been described as being achromatopsic. For example, some subjects with achromatopsia have residual colour discrimination (Heywood *et al.*, 1987), whereas others do not (see Meadows, 1974, for review). In addition, the blue sensitive response mechanism has been reported as being selectively impaired in some subjects (Pearlman *et al.*, 1979; Young and Fishman, 1980), but in our subject and others (Mollon *et al.*, 1980) it is normal. The absence of the colour opponent response in some subjects (Heywood *et al.*, 1994) has lead to the conclusion that residual discrimination is due to chromatic border detection by the achromatic M pathway. In this respect our subject is clearly different, because he is able to discriminate sequentially presented stimuli with no abutting borders.

BL has a higher value of the colour constancy index than would be predicted on the basis of his discrimination loss. We required our subjects to assign colour names to stimuli, a method that yields more robust colour constancy than matching paradigms (Troost and de Weert, 1991). Because, in our experiments, subjects were required to name colours, and as BL's colour naming is abnormal, we calibrated his colour naming against the CIE x-y chromaticity space as explained in the methods section and used this to determine changes in named colours. The abnormally high colour constancy index for BL confirms the involvement of his cortical lesion in colour constancy. The properties of the lesioned area appear to be very similar to that described by Zeki (1980) because BL's response pattern is in many respects similar to that of the macaques studied by Wild *et al.* (1985) and Walsh *et al.* (1993), which suffered V4 lesions.

8.2.6 REFERENCES

BARBUR, J.L. & RUDDOCK, K.H. (1980) Spatial characteristics of movement detection mechanisms in human vision I Achromatic vision, *Biological Cybernetics*, **37**, 77–92.

CRAVEN, B.J. & FOSTER, D.H. (1992) An operational approach to colour constancy, *Vision Research*, **32**, 1359–1366.

D'ZMURA, M. & LENNIE, P. (1986), Mechanisms of color constancy, *Journal of the Optical Society of America*, A **3**, 1662–1672.

FOSTER, D.H. CRAVEN, B.J. & SALE, E.R.H. (1992) Immediate colour constancy, *Ophthalmology and Physiological Optics*, **12**, 157–160.

HEYWOOD, C.A., WILSON, B & COWEY, A. (1987), A case study of cortical colour 'blindness' with relatively intact achromatic discrimination, *Journal of Neurology and Neurosurgical Psychology*, **50**, 22–29.

HEYWOOD, C.A., COWEY, A. & NEWCOMBE, F. (1994) On the role of parvocellular (P) and magnocellular (M) pathways in cerebral achromatopsia, *Brain*, **117**, 245–254.

JAMESON, D. & HURVICH, L. (1989) Essay concerning color constancy, *Annual Review of Psychology*, **40**, 1-22.

KING-SMITH P.E & CARDEN D. (1976) Luminance and opponent-color contributions to visual detection and adaptation and to temporal and spatial integration, *Journal of the Optical Society of America*, **66**, 709–717.

MEADOWS, J.C. (1974) Disturbed perception of colours associated with localised cerebral lesions, *Brain*, **97**, 615–632.

MOLLON, J.D., NEWCOMBE, F., POLDEN, P.G. & RATCLIFF, G. (1980) On the presence of three cone mechanisms in a case of total achromatopsia. In: Verriest, G. (Ed.) *Colour Vision Deficiencies V*, Bristol: Higler, pp. 130–135.

PEARLMAN, A.L., BIRCH, J. & MEADOWS, J.C. (1979) Cerebral color blindness; an acquired defect in hue discrimination, *Annals of Neurology*, **5**, 253–261.

ROBERTSON, A.R. & WRIGHT, W.D. (1965) International comparison of working standards for colorimetry, *Journal of the Optical Society of America*, **55**, 694–706.

RUDDOCK, K.H. (1963) Evidence for macular pigmentation from colour matching data, *Vision Research*, **3**, 417–429.

SPERLING, H.G. & HARWERTH, R.S. (1971) Red-green cone interactions in the increment-threshold spectral sensitivity of primates, *Science*, **172**, 180–184.

STILES, W.S. (1978) *Mechanisms of Colour Vision*, London: Academic.

TROOST, J.M. & DE WEERT, C.M.M. (1991) Naming versus matching in color constancy, *Perception and Psychophysics*, **50**, 591–602.

WALSH, V., CARDEN, D., BUTLER, S.R. & KULIKOWSKI, J.J. (1993) The effects of V4 lesions on the visual abilities of macaques: hue discrimination and colour constancy, *Behavioural Brain Research*, **53**, 51–62.

WILD, H.M., BUTLER, S.R., CARDEN, D. & KULIKOWSKI, J.J. (1985) Primate cortical area V4 important for colour constancy but not wavelength discrimination, *Nature*, **313**, 133–135.

WRIGHT, W.D. (1927–28) A trichromatic colorimeter with spectral primaries, *Transactions of the Optical Society*, **29**, 225.

YOUNG, R.S. & FISHMAN, G.A. (1980) Loss of colour vision and Stiles π_1 mechanism in a patient with cerebral infarction, *Journal of the Optical Society of America*, **70**, 1301–1305.

ZEKI, S. (1980) The representation of colours in the cerebral cortex, *Nature*, **284**, 412–418.

Adaptation or Contrast: The Controlling Mechanism for Colour Constancy

John J. McCann

8.3.1 INTRODUCTION

Light and dark adaptation is one of the most studied mechanisms in the human visual system. Alpern and Campbell (1963) showed that the light adaptation mechanism is located in the retina. Using the pupillary response, they showed that rods and cones continue to send a signal related to light absorption to the cortex until the receptors are dark adapted. Nevertheless, numerous experiments, such as those summarised by Yarbus (1967), document a neural suppression mechanism to render invisible images that are stabilised on the retina. Daw (1962) studied whether afterimages can affect the colour appearance of objects in real-life images. His experiment used red and white projections. He used a still-life image with a large red pillow and a teapot spout placed in front of the pillow. Daw used the tip of the spout as the fixation point. Observers stared at the tip to form the afterimage. Daw occluded the red projection, leaving the black and white colour separation in white light on the screen. He asked the observers to continue to look at the tip. They reported the expected cyan afterimage. What was not expected was that when Daw asked the observers to look at other objects in the projection, the afterimage vanished, but reappeared when the observer refixated on the tip of the teapot, and vanished again when the observer looked elsewhere. When one repeats the experiment with the conventional uniform white screen, the cyan pillow is visible for several minutes. Daw suggested that the presence of conflicting contours between the afterimage – fixed on the retina – and the 'live' image caused the visual system to suppress the afterimage.

Experiments show that rods and cones continuously send signals about their state of adaptation to the brain. Nevertheless, Daw's experiment raises questions about whether the visual system uses light/dark adaptation, or grey-world information in calculating colour appearances in complex images. The experiments in the next section are tests of the influence of averages in images exhibiting colour constancy.

8.3.2 GREY-WORLD EXPERIMENTS

McCann *et al.* (1976) made quantitative colour matching measurements of a colour constancy experiment. The 18-area Mondrian, a 30° display, was illuminated with 630, 546 and 450 nm narrow-band lights. The experimenters measured the triplet of radiance coming from a Munsell N/6.25 grey paper at a point. They asked observers to match all 18 areas in the display. The average of all observers for the grey paper was 5YR 6/1. This paper is a grey with a very slight warm cast. To make a red paper send the same triplet of radiances to the eye as the above grey paper, they changed the intensity of the three illuminants. They adjusted the 630, 546 and 450 intensities so that now the same radiance triplet came from a 10RP 6/10 red paper in the new illumination, as came from the grey paper in the old illumination. Despite the fact that the quanta catch by the retinal receptors was the same as from the grey paper, the observer match was 5R 6/6, a red paper.

8.3.2.1 Effect of total average radiance

Adaptation (Helson, 1964) and grey-world theories attempt to account for these results by normalising the receptor responses using an average of all the quanta caught over the entire field of view. Potentially such a mechanism could be used to explain that the red paper looked red despite the fact that it had the same quanta catch as the grey paper. Such theories could say the intensities of the three illuminants changed the grey-world average, which in turn caused a compensation equal to the shift in quanta catch.

In order to test whether the average of the entire field of view is used by the human visual system to compensate for changes in illumination, McCann, (1989) repeated the McCann, McKee and Taylor experiments, but this time holding the total average radiance constant. The total average radiance is the triplet of average quanta catch of each cone receptor, integrated over the entire field of view. McCann selected background paper that, when placed around the Mondrian, compensated for the change in illumination. In these experiments the Mondrian was surrounded by N/6 when the total average radiance triplets were measured. To get the same triplet of radiances from 10RP 6/10, he decreased the 630 nm and increased the 546 and 450 nm lights. Quantitative measurements showed that a very saturated red background paper increased the 630 nm and decreased the 546 and 450 nm average by an amount equal to the illumination change. The match under these conditions was 5R 7/4 for the same quanta catch and same average quanta catch as N/6.

There were five iterations in each of these experiments. Grey, red, yellow, green and blue papers were used. The observers' matches were 5YR 6/1, 5R 7/4, 5Y 8.5/8, 10 G 7/4, 2.5PB 4/6 for identical quanta catches, but *different* total average radiances (McCann *et al.*, 1976). They were N/6, 2.5R 7/4, 5Y 8.5/8, 7.5GY 7/4 and 10B 6/2 for identical quanta catches and *identical* total average radiances (McCann, 1989). If total average radiance was the parameter used by the human visual system to account for colour constancy, we would have expected all five matches to be identical. Instead, the matches show that the visual system is highly insensitive to total average radiance. The results cover nearly the entire gamut of the Munsell Book and are within experimental error of McCann *et al.*'s (1976) data with variable averages. So far, we find no evidence that change in average radiance effects appearance.

8.3.2.2 Effect of new average

What are the biggest changes we can induce by changing averages in real world images? The experiment introduced new background colours to the Mondrian; it used one grey and four of the most saturated papers available with constant illumination. The new Mondrian areas were made of the same papers but had half the dimensions. They were placed so that their centres had the same location as in the original Mondrian. The result was that each paper was surrounded by the new brightly coloured background. This experiment was an extreme test in several ways: it used the most saturated coloured papers available; it replaced 75 per cent of the area of each paper with the new 'average-changing' paper; and the new paper surrounded the old paper on all sides. The intent was to change the average significantly and to measure the magnitude of the influence of averages.

The changes in appearance were very small. They were the order of one or two chips in the Munsell book (McCann, 1987, 1994a). These changes were too small to account for the changes observed in colour constancy experiments.

8.3.3   CONTRAST WITH MAXIMA EXPERIMENTS

At first glance it should not matter whether an image is normalised using the average, the maxima or the minima. Each value can be used to scale radiances and in a linear model will render the same results. Land and McCann (1971) described a model for colour constancy that not only normalised the radiance array with the maximum, but also proposed that humans normalised each cone type independent of the others. Extensions of that model (Frankle and McCann, 1983; McCann, 1989, 1994b; McCann et al., 1976) have shown that a non-linear normalisation to the maxima mimics human processing as measured by matching. Recent experiments test the independent normalisation for each waveband hypothesis directly (McCann, 1992a,b). Experiments using the 'destroy the match' technique support the hypothesis that the normalisation process for colour constancy in human vision consists of three independent normalisations to the maxima in each of the long-, middle-, and short-wave cone quanta catch. These models are referred to as contrast with maxima mechanisms.

The previous 'destroy the match' experiments constructed arrays of papers that had the same relative reflectances, but different absolute values for each waveband. The experimenter chose two illuminants such that two different sets of reflectances with two different illuminants sent identical stimuli to the eye.

As both displays were identical, they looked the same. The experimenter then introduced a wide variety of new identical patches to both displays. The introduction of any paper that sent to the eye a higher quanta catch for any type of cone destroyed the match between corresponding areas. Papers that sent to the eye less light than those already in the display had no effect on the match. These results support the theory that the process controlling colour constancy normalises to the maxima in the field of view. Furthermore, they confirm that humans normalise not just to the white, but independently normalise to each waveband. A new, higher radiance white introduces three new maxima; a new *yellow*, *magenta* or *cyan* introduce two, and a new *red*, *green* or *blue* introduce one new maxima. Regardless, any new maxima change colour appearances of other areas.

The present experiment tests a different normalising strategy, namely using maxima. Here, we test to see if maxima show an influence on colour appearances, while the experimental design restricts the average of the entire field of view to be constant. Two different illuminants are chosen. Two different sets of reflectances are chosen such that the product of the reflectances and illumination produce two images that have equal radiances at all corresponding pixels. This is possible by making the ratio of reflectances in the first and second reflectance arrays be equal to the ratios of illuminants.

The control experiment creates two sets of reflectance and illuminations whose products are equal, at corresponding pixels. They must look alike – and they do. The experiment consists of adding identical reflectances to the control displays. This experiment has a new constraint. It introduced a new maximum, while not disturbing the average quanta catch of the whole field of view. The new area added to both reflectances is half maximum and half minimum. The average of this new area is middle grey. The question is whether a new maximum can still 'reset' the appearance when an equal area of minimum is used to hold the average of the scene constant. An average, or grey-world, hypothesis predicts that half-max/half-min area cannot cause a change: the average has not changed. The contrast with maxima mechanism predicts that the new maximum will destroy the match between the corresponding reflectances, regardless of the state of the average. The experimental results show that new maxima destroy the matches.

8.3.4   DISCUSSION

The first two experiments measured the changes in appearance due to changes in averages. The changes were very small. We found no evidence that the human eye's colour constancy mechanism uses an average or grey-world process. In all three experiments, the results support the contrast with maxima hypothesis.

The lack of evidence of adaptation is a very interesting paradox. The adaptation state of the rods and cones is controlled by the integration of quanta caught over time. That state of adaptation in the retina sends a signal to the brain. By monitoring the size of our pupils, we can monitor the level of this adaptation signal. Why does human vision not use it?

Daw's experiment on the visibility of afterimages provides an important insight into understanding colour appearances. The signals sent from the retina to higher levels are suppressed as stabilised images are suppressed. Colour appearance is calculated from the 'live image' incident at the moment while the average adaptation of the rods and cone signal shows no significant effect on colour appearance. Perhaps it is suppressed, just as Daw's afterimages were.

Adjusting adaptation levels does not produce changes large enough to explain colour constancy, but is there any detectable change in colour appearance that is driven by average quanta caught? McCann, McKee and Taylor measured changes in the appearance of the white area in the Mondrian, with many different levels of illumination. They reported very small changes in lightnesses of the white area with changes in absolute intensity. A change of intensity of four times (0.6 log units) caused a change of lightness of 0.8. At this rate, if we extended the changes in lightness to a range from white to black – nine lightness units would require [(9/.8)*0.6 log units]. This amounts to seven log units to change from white to black. This is in sharp contrast with the experimental fact that 2.0 log unit at the retina generates the change from white to black (Stiehl et al., 1983).

Rather than accounting for colour constancy, these tiny shifts around white might correlate with the state of adaptation of the cones. The normalisation to maxima hypothesis predicts the 'destroy the match', but does not predict the tiny shift in the colour of the white. A compromise mechanism could be that the state of adaptation controls the tiny changes about white and other maxima, while contrast mechanisms, insensitive to averages, control the appearance of the rest of the image. Further experiments are needed to test these hypotheses.

8.3.5 REFERENCES

ALPERN, M. & CAMPBELL, F.W., (1963) The behavior of the pupil during dark adaptation, *Journal of Physiology*, **165**, 5P.

DAW, N. (1962) Why afterimages are not seen in normal circumstances, *Nature*, **196**, 1143–1145.

FRANKLE, J. & McCANN, J.J. (1983) Method and apparatus of lightness imaging, US Patent, 4,384,336.

HELSON, H. (1964) *Adaptation Level Theory*, New York; Harper & Row.

LAND, E.H. & McCANN, J.J., (1971) Lightness and Retinex Theory, *Journal of the Optical Society of America*, **61**, 1–11.

McCANN, J.J., McKEE, S.P. & TAYLOR, T.H. (1976) Quantitative studies in Retinex theory, *Vision Research*, **16**, 445–458.

McCANN, J.J. (1987) Local/Global Mechanisms for Color Constancy, *Die Farbe*, **34**, 275–283.

McCANN, J.J. (1989) The role of nonlinear operations in modeling human color sensations, *SPIE Proceedings*, **1077**, 355–363.

McCANN, J.J. (1992a) Rules for color constancy, *Ophthalmic and Physiological Optics*, **12**, 175–177.

McCANN, J.J. (1992b) Color constancy: small overall and large local changes, *SPIE Proceedings*, **1666**, 310–321.

McCANN, J.J. (1994a) Psychophysical Experiments in Search of Adaptation and the Gray World, Proceedings of the IS & T 47th Annual Meeting.

McCANN, J.J. (1994b) Scene normalization mechanisms in humans, Proceedings of the IS &T/SID Color Imaging Conference, **2**.

STIEHL, W.A., McCANN, J.J. & SAVOY, R.L. (1983) Influence of intraocular scattered light on lightness-scaling experiments, *Journal of the Optical Society of America*, **73**, 1143–1148.

YARBUS, A.L. (1967) *Eye Movements and Vision*, New York: Plenum Press.

A Neurocomputational Model for Colour Constancy

Shiro Usui and Shigeki Nakauchi

8.4.1 INTRODUCTION

Colour appearances stay roughly constant under different illumination conditions. This ability to assign roughly constant colours to objects despite the variation in the illumination is called colour constancy. To attain colour constancy, the visual system must transform a triplet of cone responses varying with the illumination into the information about surface reflectances that remain fixed for a given object (Hurlbert, 1989). However, as this transformation is not unique, the visual system cannot recover the surface reflectances from only the cone responses in the absence of additional constraints.

This article describes an energy function under the computational assumptions for such an ill-posed problem of colour constancy and proposes a neurocomputational model that recovers the surface reflectances by minimising the energy. We show some simulation results for evaluating the proposed model using the images under the illuminants with colour and spatial variations.

8.4.2 FORMULATION OF THE PROBLEM OF COLOUR CONSTANCY

Consider a two-dimensional discretised scene illuminated by a source of light. The cone response at location (x,y) of a two-dimensional cone array is described as

$$\rho_k(x, y) = \int E(x, y, \lambda)S(x, y, \lambda)R_k(\lambda)d\lambda \tag{1}$$

where $E(x,y,\lambda)$ is an illuminant spectral power distribution, $S(x,y,\lambda)$ is surface reflectance, $R_k(\lambda)$ is k-th cone spectral sensitivity, and k is the number of cone types ($k = 1,2,3$).

Here, we assume that the $E(x,y,\lambda)$ and $S(x,y,\lambda)$ can be represented by a linear, three-dimensional model as follows:

$$E(x, y, \lambda_n) = \sum_{i=1}^{3} \varepsilon_i(x, y)E_i(\lambda_n). \tag{2}$$

$$S(x, y, \lambda_n) = \sum_{j=1}^{3} \sigma_j(x, y)S_j(\lambda_n). \tag{3}$$

where $E_i(\lambda)$ and $S_j(\lambda)$ are the basis functions for illuminant and surface reflectance, $\varepsilon_i(x,y)$ and $\sigma_j(x,y)$ are the coefficients for these basis functions. We used the basis functions $E_i(\lambda)$ for daylight derived by Judd *et al.* (1964). Surface reflectance curves can be represented by a similar technique (Maloney, 1986); we calculated principal component vectors as $S_j(\lambda)$ for a set of surface reflectances of 1569 Munsell colour chips.

Using equations (2) and (3), equation (1) is rewritten as

$$\rho_k(x,\ y) = \sum_{j=1}^{3} \sigma_j(x,\ y)\Lambda_{Ej,k}(x,\ y), \tag{4}$$

where,

$$\Lambda_{Ej,k}(x,\ y) = \sum_{i=1}^{3} \varepsilon_i(x,\ y)\Lambda_{i,j,k},$$

$$\Lambda_{i,j,k} = \sum_{n=1}^{N} E_i(\lambda_n)S_j(\lambda_n)R_k(\lambda_n).$$

The problem of colour constancy is then clearly formulated as recovering $\sigma_j(x,y)$ from a set of $\rho_k(x,y)$. However, additional constraints are needed to solve the problem, because $\Lambda_{Ej,k}(x,y)$ is also unknown in general.

8.4.3   ENERGY FUNCTION FOR COLOUR CONSTANCY

We adopt the following assumptions for solving the problem of colour constancy.

A: *Perceived colour is specified by recovered surface reflectance coefficients.*
B: *Surface reflectance coefficients are recovered by using contrast and spatially local averaged values only at edges of the input images and spreading across regions within the edges (Horn, 1974).*
C: *Grey-world assumption; average surface reflectance is close to grey (Land, 1959).*
D: *Spectrum of ambient light is close to white.*

Under these assumptions the energy function for colour constancy is represented by contrast and data-fitting terms, and a grey-world term as follows:

$$J = J_C + \lambda_1 J_D + \lambda_2 J_G \tag{5}$$

where,

$$J_C = \frac{1}{2}\sum_{j}^{3} \sum_{x,y}^{n,m} [L^{-1}\{T[\nabla^2\sigma_j(x,y)^{white}] - \nabla^2\hat{\sigma}_j(x,y)\}]^2, \tag{6}$$

$$J_D = \frac{1}{2}\sum_{j}^{3} \sum_{x,y}^{n,m} G[T[\nabla^2\sigma_j(x,y)^{white}]] \times \{\sigma_j(x,y)^{LDC} - \hat{\sigma}(x,y)\}^2, \tag{7}$$

$$J_G = \frac{1}{2}\sum_{j}^{3} [\sigma^{grey} - \frac{1}{n\times m}\sum_{x,y}^{n,m} \hat{\sigma}^j(x,y)]^2, \tag{8}$$

$$\text{Threshold operator}: T[x] = \begin{cases} x & \text{if } x > \text{ threshold} \\ 0 & \text{otherwise} \end{cases}$$

$$\text{Gating operator}: G[x] = \begin{cases} 1 & \text{if } x > \text{ threshold} \\ 0 & \text{otherwise} \end{cases}$$

$\sigma_j(x,y)^{white}$: pseudo-surface-coefficients given under the assumption that the illuminant is white

$\sigma_j(x,y)^{LDC}$: local DC value derived by Gaussian filtering to $\hat{\sigma}_j(x,y)^{white}$

$\hat{\sigma}_j(x,y)$: recovered surface reflectance coefficients

σ_j^{grey} : surface coefficient of standard grey surface

$L^{-1} = (\nabla^2)^{-1}$: inverse Laplacian operator

J_C and J_D require that the contrast (differentiation) and local DC values (LDC) of recovered surface reflectance coefficients are close to those of the input image. J_G enforces the constraint that the averages of the reflectance coefficients take a grey value, σ^{grey}.

Figure 8.4.1. shows the schematic diagram of the proposed model. σ^{white}, represented at A-plane, is computed from the input image, $\rho_i(x,y)$ under the assumption that the illuminant is white. $T[\nabla^2 \sigma_j(x,y)^{white}]$ at B-plane and σ^{LDC} at C-plane are derived by Laplacian-threshold operator and Gaussian filtering, respectively. Recovered surface reflectance coefficients $\hat{\sigma}_j(x,y)$ are represented at D-plane, which is the output plane of the model.

The proposed model recovers $\hat{\sigma}_j(x,y)$ dynamically by gradient descent method, that is,

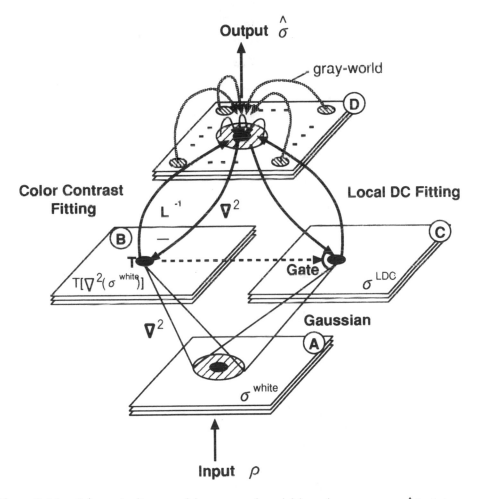

Figure 8.4.1. Schematic diagram of the proposed model for colour constancy $\hat{\sigma}_j(x,y)$ that minimises the energy recovered dynamically.

$$\frac{d\hat{\sigma}_j(x,y)}{dt} \alpha - \frac{\partial J}{\partial \hat{\sigma}_j(x,y)} \tag{9}$$

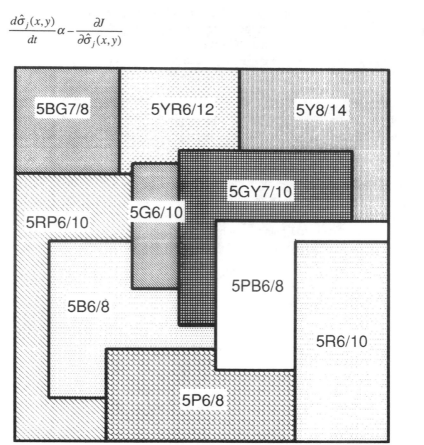

Figure 8.4.2.   A Mondrian as a testing image.

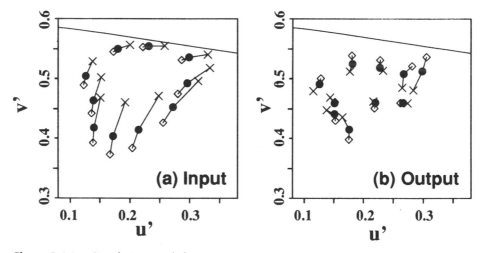

Figure 8.4.3.   Simulation result for removing illuminant colour. CIE $u'v'$ co-ordinates of 10 colour patches are indicated by: ×, incandescent light (4000K); ●, daylight (6774K); ◇, fluorescent light (10 000K). Upper solid line without symbol shows the spectrum locus.

At the beginning of calculation ($t = 0$), initial values of $\hat{o}_j(x,y)$ is set to D-plane by inverse Laplacian operation on $T[\nabla^2\hat{o}_j(x,y)^{white}]$. $-\partial J/\partial\hat{o}_j$ is then computed to update $\hat{o}_j(x,y)$ as follows; $-\partial J_C/\partial\hat{o}_j$ is derived by computing the differences between $\nabla^2\hat{o}_j(x,y)$ and $T[\nabla^2\hat{o}_j(x,y)^{white}]$ through the backward connections from D-plane to B-plane, and added to the initial value of $\hat{o}_j(x,y)$ at D-plane through the forward connections from B-plane to D-plane. $-\partial J_D/\partial\hat{o}_j$ is also computed by the similar way through the backward and the forward connections between D- and C-plane although this computation is carried only at edges of the input image. $-\partial J_G/\partial\hat{o}_j$ is computed through the inhibitory horizontal connections at D-plane.

8.4.4   SIMULATION RESULTS

The proposed model was evaluated using two-dimensional Mondrian images, that is, a flat surface covered with 10 different colour patches of uniform surface reflectance as shown in Figure 8.4.2.

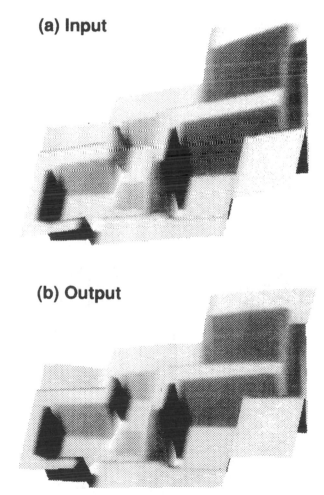

Figure 8.4.4.   Simulation result for removing the spatial non-uniformity of illumination. The Mondrian is illuminated from right side. Intensity then decreases gradually from right to left.

8.4.4.1 Removing the colour variations of the illuminant

First, we tried to recover the surface reflectance coefficients of the Mondrian under the illuminant with colour variations. Figure 8.4.3. shows the CIE $u'v'$ co-ordinates of 10 colour patches derived from (a) cone responses as the input and (b) recovered surface reflectance as the output. Co-ordinates of patches under the 4000K incandescent light, 6774K daylight and 10 000K fluorescent light are indicated by ×, • and ◊, respectively.

Cone responses shown in Figure 8.4.3(a) strongly depend on the illuminant colour, that is, co-ordinates of the patches under the incandescent light become yellowish and those of the fluorescent light become bluish. By contrast, co-ordinates derived from the recovered surface reflectance coefficients shown in Figure 8.4.3(b) remain roughly constant despite the variation of the illuminant colour. That is, the proposed model can explain the approximate colour constancy in the environment with colour variations of the illuminants.

8.4.4.2 Spatially non-uniform Illuminants

Next, the performance of the proposed model under the spatially varying illuminations was evaluated. The Mondrian shown in Figure 8.4.2. is illuminated from the right side in such a way that the intensity decreases gradually from right to left.

Figure 8.4.4. (a) and (b) display $\hat{\sigma}_1^{white}(x,y)$ and $\hat{\sigma}_1(x,y)$. Although spatial non-uniformity of illumination has influences on $\hat{\sigma}_1^{white}(x,y)$, these effects are removed in $\hat{\sigma}_1(x,y)$. Therefore,

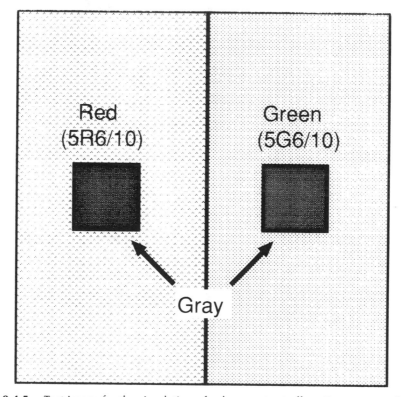

Figure 8.4.5. Test image for the simulation of colour contrast effect. Two grey patches which have the same reflectance seen to be different colours to human observer.

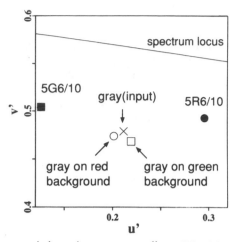

Figure 8.4.6. Simulation result for colour contrast effect. CIE $u'v'$ co-ordinates of each colour patch are indicated by: ●, red background; ■, green background; ×, inputted-grey; ○, recovered-grey on red background; □, recovered-grey on green background.

surface reflectance coefficients, which are constant within the patches, were recovered successfully despite the spatial non-uniformity of illumination.

8.4.4.3 Simultaneous colour contrast effect

Finally, simultaneous colour contrast effect was simulated using the image that consisted of two grey patches (flat spectral reflectance with value 0.5) on a red (5R6/10) and green (5G6/10) background as shown in Figure 8.4.5. These grey patches cause different colour sensations to the human observer although they are the same colour.

Figure 8.4.6 shows CIE $u'v'$ co-ordinates plotted in the same fashion as for Figure 8.4.3. Co-ordinates of recovered greys on a red background and a green background shift barely to greenish (○) and reddish (□) from the inputted grey (×); colour appearance shifts to the complementary colour of the background colour (● and ■).

Obtained results showed that our model could explain both phenomena, which produce opposing effects, by the same mechanism of colour information processing. This suggests that the colour contrast effect reflects the neural mechanism of colour constancy, that is, computing the colour contrast may play a key role to attain colour constancy.

8.4.5 CONCLUSIONS

We propose a neurocomputational model for colour constancy. The model minimises the energy based on the computational formulation of the problem of colour constancy. Computer simulation of the proposed model showed that surface reflectance coefficients were recovered successfully under the illuminants with colour variations, and that the spatial non-uniformity of the illumination was removed in the output image. Colour contrast effect was also simulated successfully by the proposed model. This result suggests that there exists strong connections between colour constancy and colour contrast effects.

8.4.6 REFERENCES

HORN, B.K.P. (1974) Determining lightness from an image. In: *Computer Graphics and Image Processing*, **3**, Academic Press, pp. 277–299.

HURLBERT, A.C. (1989) The computation of colour MIT AI Laboratory Technical Report, No. 1151.

JUDD, D.B., MACADAM, D.L. & WYSZECKI, G. (1964) Spectral distribution of typical daylight as a function of correlated colour temperature, *Journal of the Optical Society of America*, **A 54**(8), 1031–1040.

LAND, E.H. (1959) Experiments in color vision, *Scientific American*, **201**, 286–298.

MALONEY, L.T. (1986) Evaluation of linear models of surface spectral reflectance with small numbers of parameters, *Journal of the Optical Society of America*, **A 3**, 1673–1683.

A Functional View of Cone Pigments and Colour Vision

D. Osorio

The assertion that colour vision did not evolve to allow complete reconstruction of reflectance spectra, or even to distinguish the maximum possible number of objects, but rather to tackle the day to day challenges faced by our ancestors, is a piety of the kind that in most branches of psychology can give few insights. In general, we cannot adequately reconstruct past lifestyles or define natural constraints and optima (e.g. Barkow *et al.*, 1992), but colour vision may be the exception. Starting from the visual pigments, this chapter considers red-green vision as an adaptation for finding food. This functional hypothesis is extended to colour constancy, and I ask how the simplest mechanism will perform for a monkey foraging in a forest.

8.5.1 NATURAL SELECTION AND TUNING OF L AND M PIGMENTS

A recent article on great-ape pigment genes (Deeb *et al.*, 1994) concludes unreservedly that 'since duplication of the ancestral gene, natural selection operated to maintain the degree of separation in peak absorption between red and green genes that allowed for optimal chromatic discrimination in a particular environment'. In the absence of selection, gene conversion due to illegitimate recombination (the main cause of colour deficiencies) would otherwise wash out the spectral sensitivity difference between the M and L cones. Such bold claims for optimality are unusual, and this one is open to doubt; illegitimate recombination could not increase the spectral separation of the cones, and the L cone may in any case be close to the long wave limit for retinal based photopigments (Lythgoe and Partridge, 1989). It is still less clear whether there is any molecular constraint preventing the M-pigment from evolving to shorter wavelengths. Nonetheless the conservatism of M and L photopigment peaks at 535 nm and 563 nm in catarrhine (Old World) primates is indicative of a local optimum. This optimum seems to be general; it is shared by primates of diverse habits and habitats from guenon monkeys to macaques, baboons and man (Bowmaker, 1991), and it may be that selection against variants is quite strong (see Conclusion).

A plausible reason for the large spectral overlap of the M and L cones is that as both contribute to luminance vision, luminance and chromatic signals are inevitably confounded, at least at high spatial frequencies (Lennie and D'Zmura, 1988; Morgan, 1991; Williams *et al.*, 1991). Thus, chromatic information comes at the expense of luminance information (although the cost may be negligible relative to other sources of noise). Can the resulting trade-off between chromatic and luminance vision explain the specific tuning of the pigments?

Explanations of visual coding often make very general assumptions about how signals are used, implying either that the brain needs to reconstruct the spectra perfectly or alternatively that the number of discriminable images is maximised. Instances of such explanations in colour vision include estimates of the proportion of the chromatic signal encoded by three receptor classes (Maloney, 1986), or of the number of discriminable surfaces in a scene (Lythgoe and Partridge, 1989, 1991), and prediction of the optimal coding strategy for opponency channels (Buchsbaum and Gottschalk, 1983). It is possible that the compromise between luminance and chromatic vision given by our cone pigments optimises retinal information capacity, but it is difficult to see how maximisation of information could give a single optimal pair of cones rather than a set of optimal pairs. A less parsimonious, more biologically constrained approach may be appropriate.

8.5.2　RED-GREEN VISION AS A SPECIALISATION FOR FINDING FOOD

Measurements of natural spectra, and simulations of the effects of 'evolutionary' shifts in pigment sensitivities bear out the conjecture that red-green vision did not evolve as a general-purpose supplement to luminance vision. The L-M chromatic signal seems to be pessimal for general purpose colour vision in that for a given spectral separation the natural cone pair minimises the chromatic signal for the 'average' scene of living and dead vegetation, soil etc. (Figure 8.5.2a; Nagle and Osorio, 1993). One inference from this observation is that the cone peaks have been selected so as to minimise chromatic interference in the luminance signal, while at the same time maintaining a good L-M signal from the special colours of fruit (Mollon, 1989).

Catarrhines' diets are based on fruit, often orange or red, and young leaves (Gautier-Hion, 1988; Napier and Napier, 1967) for which colour is a good indicator of edibility. Even if we accept, a priori, that red-green vision is useful to a frugivore, to understand the advantages a catarrhine trichromat may enjoy over a dichromatic mammal it is important to specify rather precisely the task involved. Three plausible tasks that put significantly different demands on colour vision are: (1) detection of fruit, (2) judgement of its ripeness, and (3) identification of the species (Osorio and Vorobyev, 1995). Thus, discrimination for identification of fruit colours is barely improved by the acquisition of a third (i.e. M-type) visual pigment, whereas detection against leaves is helped by red-green vision because fruits often give a large L-M signal on a background of mature leaves when the L-S signal is small (Figure 8.5.1b; Osorio and Vorobyev, 1995.).

I focus here on judgement of ripeness, as a simple measure of the utility of a chromatic signal. Accurate judgement is important to help avoid under-ripe or rotten food, and as ripening is a continuous process the number of discriminable grades of ripeness is a measure of the 'functional bandwidth' of a chromatic channel. For ideal conditions the maximum number of discriminable grades is given by (or at least proportional to) the number of just noticeable differences (jnds) separating the least from the most ripe stage under a single illuminant (Figure 8.5.1b). Here, estimates of jnds are based on wavelength discrimination thresholds at 570 nm for the L–M (approximately red–green) signal, and 480 nm for the $\frac{1}{2}$(L + M)-S (approximately yellow-blue) signal. Thresholds will vary according to conditions but $\delta\lambda$ thresholds of 1 nm at each of the two loci are close to the upper limit of performance (Wyszecki and Stiles, 1982), giving chromatic contrast thresholds of around 0.01 for the L–M signal, and of 0.03 for the $\frac{1}{2}$(L + M)–S signal. It is quite clear that the L-M signal is significantly more useful than the $\frac{1}{2}$(L + M)–S at least for the fruit examined (banana, mango and pawpaw).

8.5.3   IS VON KRIES CONSTANCY ADEQUATE IN NATURAL CONDITIONS?

Selection does not act on the opsins alone, and functional specialisation of red-green vision should be manifested in other aspects of colour vision. Colour constancy has been treated formally as a general problem to be solved for all natural spectra and illuminants, and often requiring reconstruction of the illuminant (D'Zmura and Iverson, 1993; Maloney and Wandell, 1986), or tackled experimentally for a wide range of spectra, such as those of Munsell papers. But what kind of constancy mechanism is needed in nature?

Recently it has been argued that for Kirnov's (natural) spectra, a von Kries mechanism may give adequate constancy (Dannemiller, 1993). Von Kries pointed out that autonomous adaptation of receptors can contribute substantially to colour constancy (Wyszecki and Stiles, 1982), and lateral inhibition in the retina may give a functionally equivalent transformation in the spatial domain. This mechanism is imperfect, but if acceptable colour constancy is achieved as a by-product of retinal processes one might ask why higher level mechanisms are needed (Craven and Foster, 1992; D'Zmura and Iverson, 1993; Lennie and D'Zmura, 1988).

I take up this question for a frugivore in a model jungle. A uniform background of leaves gives a predictable mean reflectance (results are similar for an achromatic background), the illuminant is unknown, and target fruits of indeterminate ripeness are equiluminant with the background. Forest illuminants are from a recently published set (Figure 8.5.1a; Endler, 1993) and include direct sunlight, illumination by blue sky (north light), and green light beneath the forest canopy. A shift of more than one jnd in the chromatic signal for the fruit against its natural leafy background is indicative of imperfect colour constancy; this measure is intentionally rather stringent, the variations in illumination are large and the chromatic jnds are small.

It turns out that after complete receptor adaptation, residual shifts in chromatic signals due to variable illumination do have the potential to degrade colour vision; L-M signals for ripe fruit against a background of leaves can vary by up to 3 jnds (Figure 8.5.1b; Osorio and Vorobyev (1995) support these conclusions using different methods and a much larger dataset of fruit spectra). In other words, the number of discriminable stages of ripeness, and hence the 'functional bandwidth' of the chromatic channel, may be significantly reduced as a consequence of variations in illumination (Figure 8.5.1c).

Interestingly, the detrimental effects of variations in illumination could be a factor promoting the phylogenetic stability of the M and L pigment tunings. This is because variable illumination limits the improvement in the chromatic signal given by increases in pigment separation. In general (disregarding the L-S signal), such increases will give a larger L-M signal for fruit, but this improvement may be offset by the increased failures of colour constancy. For our simple model the number of reliably distinguishable grades of ripeness under variable illumination plateaus for pigment separations of around 30 nm (Figure 8.5.1c, 8.5.2b). By comparison, the amplitude of the chromatic signal for the

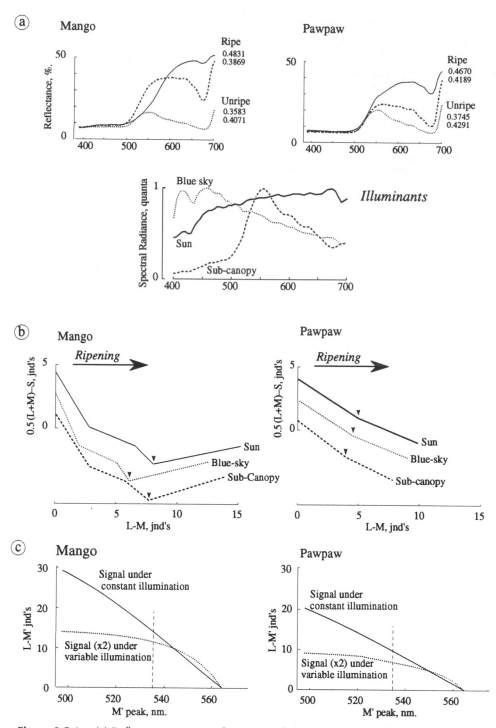

Figure 8.5.1. (a) Reflectance spectra of mango and pawpaw at three different stages of ripeness, and the illumination spectra used (from Endler, 1993). Fruit contain a small number of pigments so the form of the spectral changes illustrated are common to many that ripen from green to yellow-red. CIE (1931) loci are given for the least and most ripe samples.

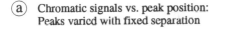

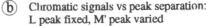

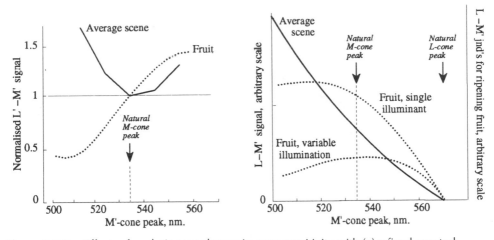

Figure 8.5.2. Effects of evolutionary change in cone sensitivity with (a) a fixed spectral overlap, or (b) with a fixed L-pigment and varied M' pigment. L'-M' signals, are estimated for general scenes (Nagle and Osorio, 1993) and for fruit (62 spectra).

(a) Effects of moving L' and M' pigment sensitivities along the spectrum with fixed overlap, signals normalised to those for the natural cones (Nagle and Osorio, 1993). For 'background' spectra the natural cones are at a pair of spectral points that minimise the L'-M' signal, and hence chromatic distortion of luminance vision. The fruit signal, (dotted line) gives the root mean square L-M signal separating ripe fruit from a leaf background (or unripe fruit), the largest signals are for long-wavelength pigment pairs.

(b) Summary of the effects of changing spectral separation for L-M' signals (i.e. L-cone tuning fixed M varied). The signal for the 'background' spectra increases exponentially with pigment separation, but the fruit signal tends to plateau. The utility of the L-M signal for judging ripeness under unpredictable illumination is an estimate based on results given in Figure 8.5.1c (assuming von Kries constancy, see text and Figure 8.5.1b) peaks close to the natural pigment separation. A more extensive treatment is given in forthcoming papers Osorio and Vorobyev (1995) and Vorobyev and Osorio, *in prep.*

(b) Plots of the L–M (red-green) and $\frac{1}{2}(L + M)$–S (yellow-blue) signals for ripening mango and pawpaw under varying illumination. For clarity, plots are arbitrarily displaced on the vertical (yellow-blue) axis. The eye is assumed to be adapted to a background of unripe fruit, which are very similar to leaves. The small vertical arrow shows the position of an intermediate sample. The distances, in jnds, separating a given sample under varying illumination indicates the corruption of the signal due to 'failure' of von Kries constancy. Cone sensitivities are based on standard fundamentals (Smith and Pokorny, 1975).

(c) The number of jnds (see text) separating the most from the least ripe samples give an indication of the degradation of the chromatic signal caused by variable illumination, with L pigment fixed and M' pigment varied. The dashed vertical line gives the natural M cone peak. For cones containing hypothetical pigments, sensitivities are obtained using a simple model of rhodopsin sensitivities (Stavenga *et al.*, 1993), filtered by the ocular media (Wyszecki and Stiles, 1982), with a cone optical density of 0.4.

'average scene', and hence the potential for chromatic signals to corrupt luminance vision increases exponentially with pigment separation (Figure 8.5.2b; Nagle and Osorio, 1993).

8.5.4 CONCLUSION

Whereas explanations of the roots of human psychology tend to be speculative (Barkow *et al.*, 1992), hypotheses concerning the function of colour vision can be raised on firm foundations of the visual pigments. The L and M pigments are a pair that is common to all catarrhines studied, and are selectively favoured (Bowmaker, 1991; Deeb *et al.*, 1994). Interestingly, it may be possible to obtain a measure of the relative strength of selection against natural variants, as frequencies of occurrence of anomalous trichromacies and dichromacies between species should give an accurate measure of the strength of selection for normal pigments (absolute estimates would require knowledge of mutation rates). One might predict, for example, that the gelada baboon, a species which lives on grasses, has higher rates of colour deficiency than other catarrhines.

I have suggested that neither information criteria nor the need to reconstruct reflectance (or illumination) spectra suffice to explain the tuning of the cone pigments. The stability of pigment tuning indicates that the red-green signal rather than being a general source of visual information, is an adaptation for finding food which compromises luminance based vision (Nagle and Osorio, 1993; Osorio and Bossomaier, 1992; Osorio and Vorobyev, 1995).

The way in which this functional perspective might inform work on colour vision is illustrated with a simple discussion of colour constancy. Constancy may be important for a monkey foraging in variegated light, where variation in illumination may limit the number of discriminable stages of fruit ripeness. Using a fairly stringent theoretical limit on discrimination thresholds, photoreceptor adaptation fails to give satisfactory colour constancy, with unpredictable illumination leading to failures of colour constancy, which could cause stomach ache.

8.5.5 ACKNOWLEDGEMENTS

I thank R.H. Douglas of City University for the loan of his spectroradiometer, and L. Chittka for spectral data.

8.5.6 REFERENCES

BARKOW, J.H., COSMIDES, L. & TOOBY, J. (1992) *The Adapted Mind: Evolutionary Psychology and the Generation of Culture*, New York: Oxford University Press.

BOWMAKER, J.K. (1991) Visual pigments and colour vision in primates. In: Lee, B.B. & Valberg, A. (Eds) *From Pigments to Perception*, New York: Plenum Press, pp. 1–9.

BUCHSBAUM, G. & GOTTSCHALK, A. (1983) Trichromacy, opponent colours coding and optimum colour information transmission in the retina, *Proceedings of the Royal Society of London*, **B 220**, 89–113.

CRAVEN, B.J. & FOSTER D.H. (1992) An operational approach to colour constancy, *Vision Research*, **32**, 1359–1366.

DANNEMILLER, J.L. (1993) Rank orderings of photoreceptor photon catches from natural objects are nearly illuminant-invariant, *Vision Research*, **33**, 131–40.

DEEB, S.S., JORGENSEN, A.L., BATTISTI, L., IWASKI, L. & MOTULSKY, A.G. (1994) Sequence divergence of the red and green visual pigments in great apes and humans, *Proceedings of the National Academy of Science USA*, **91**, 7262–7266.

D'ZMURA, M. & IVERSON, G. (1993) Color constancy. I. Basic theory of two-stage linear recovery of spectral descriptions for lights and surfaces, *Journal of the Optical Society of America*, **A 10**, 2148–2165.

ENDLER, J.A. (1993) The color of light in forests and its implications, *Ecological Monographs*, **63**, 1–27.

GAUTIER-HION, A. (1988) The diet and dietary habits of forest guenons. In: Gautier-Hion, A., Bourlière, F. & Gautier, J-P. (Eds) *A Primate Radiation: Evolutionary Biology of the African Guenons*, Cambridge: Cambridge University Press, pp. 257–283.

LENNIE, P. & D'ZMURA, M. (1988) Mechanisms of color vision, *CRC Critical Reviews in Neurobiology*, **3**, 333–399.

LYTHGOE, J. N. & PARTRIDGE, J.C. (1989) Visual pigments and the acquisition of visual information, *Journal of Experimental Biology*, **146**, 1–20.

LYTHGOE, J. N. & PARTRIDGE, J.C. (1991) Modelling the optimal visual pigments of dichromatic teleosts in green coastal waters, *Vision Research*, **31**, 361–371.

MALONEY, L.T. (1986) Evaluation of linear models of surface spectral reflectance with small numbers of parameters, *Journal of the Optical Society of America*, **A 3**, 1673–1683.

MALONEY, L.T. & WANDELL, B.A. (1986) Color constancy: a method for recovering surface spectral reflectance, *Journal of the Optical Society of America*, **A 3**, 29–33.

MOLLON, J.D. (1989) 'tho' she kneel'd in that place where they grew ...'. The uses and origins of primate colour vision, *Journal of Experimental Biology*, **146**, 21–38.

MORGAN, M. (1991) Decoding the retinal colour signal, *Current Biology*, **1**, 215–217.

NAPIER, J.R. & NAPIER, P.H. (1967) *A Natural History of Primates*, London: Academic Press.

NAGLE, M.G., OSORIO, D. (1993) The tuning of human photopigments may minimize red-green chromatic signals in natural conditions, *Proceedings of the Royal Society of London*, **B 252**, 209–213.

OSORIO, D. & BOSSOMAIER, T.R.J. (1992) Human cone-pigment spectral sensitivities and the reflectances of natural surfaces, *Biological Cybernetics*, **67**, 217–222.

OSORIO, D. & VOROBYEV, M. (1995) Red-green vision as an adaptation to frugivory, *Animal Behaviour*, submitted.

SMITH, V.C. & POKORNY, J. (1975) Spectral sensitivities of human foveal cone photopigments between 400 and 500 nm, *Vision Research*, **15**, 161–171.

STAVENGA, D.G., SMITS, R.P. & HOENDERS, B. J. (1993) Simple exponential functions describing the absorbance bands on visual pigments spectra, *Vision Research*, **33**, 1011–1017.

VOROBYEV, M. & OSORIO, D. (1995) In preparation.

WILLIAMS, D.R., SEKIGUCHI, N., HAAKE, W., BRAINARD, D. & PACKER, O. (1991) The cost of trichromacy for spatial vision. In: Lee, B.B. & Valberg, A. (Eds) *From Pigments to Perception*, New York: Plenum Press, pp. 11–22.

WYSZECKI, G. & STILES, W.S. (1982) *Color Science: Concepts and Methods, Quantitative Data and Formulae*, 2nd edn., New York: Wiley.

Dependence of Colour Constancy on the Time-course of Illuminant Changes

Sérgio M. C. Nascimento and David H. Foster

8.6.1 INTRODUCTION

The spectral properties of the light reflected from a collection of object surfaces depend on the interaction of the spectral reflectances of the surfaces with the spectral power distribution of the light source. Changes in illuminant give rise to changes in the light reaching the eye; yet, in everyday experience, the colours of objects are usually perceived as being unchanged. This phenomenon is referred to as colour constancy; it was commented on and variously analysed by Young (1807), von Helmholtz (1866), Hering (1878), and von Kries (1905), and, more recently, by Helson and Jeffers (1940), Judd (1940), Land (1959a, 1959b), Land and McCann (1971), and many others.

In the laboratory, measurements of the human perception of coloured surfaces under different illuminants have shown that colour constancy is less than perfect (Arend and Reeves, 1986; Cornelissen, 1994; Lucassen and Walraven, 1993; McCann et al, 1976; Tiplitz Blackwell and Buchsbaum, 1988; Valberg and Lange-Malecki, 1990; Walraven et al., 1987); but it does not fail completely, and the extent or degree of constancy can be quantified, for example, by comparison of the changes in perception of surfaces in a coloured surround with the changes in perception of those surfaces in a void, as the illuminant is altered. A variety of experimental approaches have been used, which have demonstrated various degrees of constancy, but they have usually considered pairs of illuminants that were stable in time. In natural viewing conditions, however, illuminants vary in time; for example, when a cloud covers the sun or when an artificial light is suddenly switched on. Little attention has been directed to the issue of the stability of surface colour percepts when illuminants are not steady. The present work addresses this question in three experiments.

The first experiment, essentially a control, established the degree of constancy with steady illuminants. A family of steady illuminants, the colours of which defined a circular pattern in (u', v') chromaticity space around the colour of a white illuminant, were applied individually to a coloured sample patch embedded in three different surround fields: a void; a multicoloured surround field under the same illuminant as the sample patch; and a multicoloured surround field under an illuminant different from the sample patch (the second and third conditions are referred to as *consistent* and *inconsistent* illuminants, respectively). Changes in the perceived colour of a set of such sample patches were measured with a haploscopic matching technique; the degree of constancy was quantified by comparing these perceptual changes under the three surround conditions. As in previous studies, partial colour constancy was obtained.

The second experiment determined the effect of varying the time-course of changes in illuminant. Sensitivity to changes in the perceived colour of just one coloured sample patch in each of the three surround fields was measured under an illuminant whose colour varied according to each of three time-courses. Sensitivity was little affected by either background condition or time-course of illuminant changes. The third experiment extended the second one to cover the full range of illuminant colours used in the first experiment, but the slowest time-course was always used and the inconsistently illuminated surround was omitted. Although sensitivity to changes in the sample patch varied with the direction of illuminant change, the two surround fields had indistinguishable effects. Some implications of these findings for the assessment and interpretation of colour constancy are briefly considered.

8.6.2   GENERAL METHODS

Colour images were generated by an RGB colour-graphics system, with 8-bit resolution selected on each gun (Ramtek UK Ltd, Basingstoke, Hampshire, 4660 series), under the control of a computer (Sun Microsystems Inc, Mountain View, CA, USA; type 3/160) and displayed on a 19-inch colour monitor (Sony, Japan; Trinitron) with a resolution of 1280×1024 pixels and a frame rate of 60 Hz. The colour-graphics system allowed images to be displayed with a time-course controlled locally and independent of further intervention by the host computer. The system was calibrated with a telespectroradiometer, the calibrations of which were in turn traceable to the UK National Physical Laboratory.

The stimuli were coloured square patches subtending $1.5°$ visual angle (viewed at a distance of 0.7 m from the monitor screen) presented either on their own or in the centre of a square Mondrian pattern of side $10.5°$ and consisting of 48 coloured patches. The coloured patches were simulations of Munsell surfaces from the *Munsell Book of Color* (1976) illuminated by light with spectral power distribution drawn from the collection generated with a set of basis functions obtained from a principal components analysis by Judd *et al.* (1964) for daylight illuminants. The spectral reflectances of the simulated Munsell surfaces were drawn from the collection generated with a set of basis functions obtained from principal components analysis by Parkkinen *et al.* (1989). The set of surfaces that formed the surround Mondrian, which was the same in all conditions of all experiments, was chosen so that its space average-colour when illuminated by the CIE Standard Illuminant D_{65} was the same as the colour of the illuminant. There were two observers, GP and ME; each had normal colour vision, as assessed with the Farnsworth-Munsell 100-Hue test and Ishihara plates, and normal Snellen acuity. Each was unaware of the purpose of the experiments.

8.6.3   EXPERIMENT 1

This experiment determined the degree of colour constancy of a set of sample patches presented in a void and in a consistently illuminated Mondrian surround field and in an inconsistently illuminated Mondrian surround field. The illuminants were all steady.

8.6.3.1 Methods

The observer viewed the sample coloured patch in the given surround field with the left eye; a comparison patch, always in a void, was viewed with the right eye. The observer's task was to adjust the comparison patch so that it appeared to have the same colour as the sample patch. The sample patch was variously a simulation of a Munsell red (5R 7/4), green (5G 7/4), blue (5B 7/4), or white surface (with a constant spectral reflectance function) illuminated by one of nine illuminants: a white illuminant, namely, the CIE Standard Illuminant D_{65}, and a family of eight coloured illuminants, distributed in the (u', v') chromaticity diagram around a circle with radius $d = 0.0283$ centred on the colour of the white illuminant. These illuminants were generated by weighting appropriately the three basis functions derived by Judd *et al.* (1964) for daylight illuminants. In each trial the sample patch could be illuminated by any of the nine illuminants, and surrounded by any one of three fields, namely, a void, a Mondrian pattern under the same illuminant (the consistent condition), and a Mondrian under the white illuminant (the inconsistent condition).

8.6.3.2 Results and comment

Figure 8.6.1 shows in (u', v') space the matches made by observer GP for the red sample patch under each of the nine illuminants tested. Similar performance was obtained with the other sample patches and by the second observer ME. Each symbol represents the mean of five matches and the vertical and horizontal bars show ± 1 SEM where sufficiently large. Data for the void condition are shown by the open circles in both (a) and (b); for the consistent-surround condition, by solid squares in (a) and, for the inconsistent-surround condition, by solid triangles in (b). Data in a similar format were reported by Walraven *et al.* (1987) and by Lucassen and Walraven (1993), although the distribution of points in those studies corresponded to a set of surfaces illuminated by one illuminant rather than as here to the same surface illuminated by different illuminants.

The distributions of the matches in (u', v') space for each condition were almost circular, but the diameter of the circle for the consistent-surround condition was smaller than that for the void condition and the diameter of the circle for the inconsistent-surround condition was larger than that for the void condition. A systematic colour-biasing effect of the Mondrian surround field was evident in the translations of the corresponding distributions for the non-void conditions relative to the distribution for the void condition.

A measure of the contraction or expansion of each distribution of matches obtained with non-void surround fields is given by the mean distance of the data points to the central D_{65} point relative to the corresponding distance for the void condition. Table 8.6.1 shows these values for the two observers and all conditions of the experiment. For the consistently illuminated surround field, there was a contraction of about 0.7–0.8 in the distribution obtained with each coloured sample patch, and an expansion of about 1.1 in the distribution obtained with the white sample patch. For the inconsistently illuminated surround field, there was an expansion of about 1.2–1.5 in the distribution obtained with each coloured sample patch, and an expansion of about 1.7 in the distribution obtained with the white sample patch.

The contractions in the distributions of the matches with the coloured sample patches and consistently illuminated surround fields are compatible with a limited colour constancy: perfect colour constancy would correspond to a contraction to a single point. The

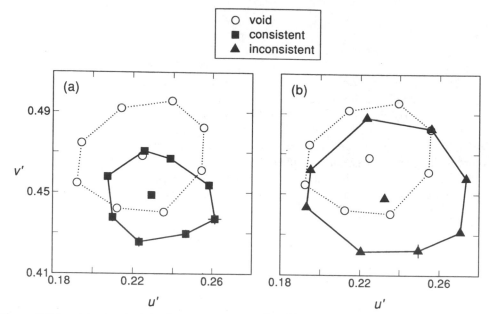

Figure 8.6.1. Matches in (*u'*, *v'*) space to a Munsell red (5R 7/4) sample patch in three kinds of surround field under each of nine illuminants. Each symbol is the mean of five matches; the bars show ± 1 SEM where sufficiently large.

expansions in the distributions with inconsistently illuminated surrounds are considered later.

8.6.4   EXPERIMENT 2

Given that some colour constancy occurs with steadily and consistently illuminated Mondrian surrounds, this second experiment determined the effect of varying the time-course of the illuminant; specifically, whether sensitivity to a change in illuminant was less

Table 8.6.1. Mean distance between matches to a sample Munsell surface under eight coloured illuminants to a match to the surface under a white illuminant (D_{65}). The matches were obtained in the presence of consistently illuminated and inconsistently illuminated fields surrounding the sample surface, and corresponding distances are expressed in relation to those obtained in a void surround

Observer	Surface	Illuminant	
		consistent	inconsistent
ME	red	0.841	1.265
	green	0.802	1.342
	blue	0.853	1.211
	white	1.127	1.666
GP	red	0.820	1.243
	green	0.819	1.494
	blue	0.721	1.240
	white	1.104	1.700

when the surround was illuminated consistently than when it was not. One plausible expectation is that a consistently illuminated surround should make illuminant changes less obvious by virtue of its stabilising effect on colour matches.

8.6.4.1 Methods

The observer binocularly viewed the sample patch, and, as in Experiment 1, the surround field was either a void or the Mondrian. The sample patch was always the simulation of the Munsell red (5R 7/4) surface, which was one of the surfaces eliciting some degree of constancy in Experiment 1. During an initial adaptation period of 5 s, the illuminant was D_{65} after which it changed continuously in the direction defined by a vector from it to one of the family of eight illuminants used in Experiment 1. As in Experiment 1, the illumination on the surround field was either consistent with the sample patch or not (D_{65} in the latter condition). Discriminability of changes in appearance of the sample patch under changes in illuminant as a function of the size of the illuminant change was measured by the method of constant stimuli for three time courses: an instantaneous (step) change in illuminant, a fast ramp change with speed 0.0036 s^{-1}, and a slow ramp change with speed 0.0018 s^{-1}, where speeds were expressed in units of distance in (u', v') space per second. In half of the trials the illuminant varied in time and in half it did not. The task was then interpreted as a discrimination of 'signal' (change of appearance of the sample surface under illuminant change) from 'noise' (no change of appearance of the sample surface); discrimination was quantified by the discrimination index d' from signal detection theory, and SDs were calculated by the method of Gourevitch and Galanter (1967).

8.6.4.2 Results and comment

Figure 8.6.2 shows for each observer the discriminability d' of changes in appearance of the red sample patch as a function of the size of the illuminant change for the three time-courses, as indicated. No clear effect of the background was found. An analysis of variance (ANOVA) of the data showed no significant difference between the Mondrian surround fields at the two higher speeds tested and a weakly significant effect at the lower speed ($F_{2,18} = 4.0, p = 0.04$). Sensitivity to changes in illuminant on a sample patch seems to be little impaired by a consistently illuminated surround field, despite the effects of that field in modifying colour matches.

8.6.5   EXPERIMENT 3

The results of the preceding experiment may have been affected by the choice of the particular direction of illuminant colour change. In this experiment, the direction in (u', v') space of the illuminant change could be any of the eight directions defined by the positions of the family of coloured illuminants of Experiment 1 relative to the white illuminant.

8.6.5.1 Methods

Sensitivity to changes in perceived colour were measured as in Experiment 2, also for the red patch, but only for the lowest speed (0.0018 s^{-1}) and for the void and consistent-

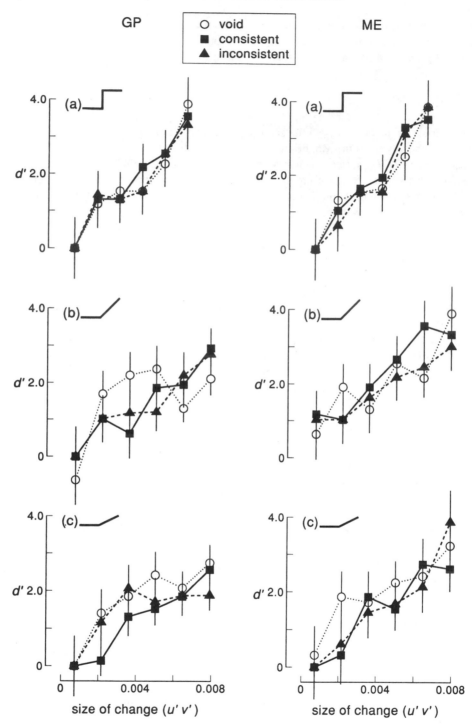

Figure 8.6.2. Discriminability d' of changes in appearance of a Munsell red (5R 7/4) sample patch as a function of the size of illuminant change according to three time courses: (a) an instantaneous (step) change in illuminant; (b) a fast ramp change with speed 0.0036 s^{-1}; and (c) a slow ramp change with speed 0.0018 s^{-1}, where speeds were expressed in units of distance in (u', v') space per second.

surround conditions. Discriminability was again expressed in terms of d'. Threshold values of illuminant change were derived by fitting to the d' data a quadratic function of distance in (u', v') space and setting a criterion performance level of $d' = 2.0$. Standard errors were computed by a bootstrap procedure (Foster and Bischof, 1991).

8.6.5.2 Results and comment

Figure 8.6.3 shows, for each observer, threshold values for detecting a change in the appearance of the red sample patch for each of the eight directions of illuminant change. The distributions of values were slightly elliptical in both the void and consistent-surround conditions: thresholds were least along an approximately red-green axis. An ANOVA applied to the d' data showed no significant difference ($F_{1,96} = 42$, $p = 0.1$) between the void and the consistently illuminated surround fields.

8.6.6   DISCUSSION

The effect of a family of nine steady illuminants on the apparent colour of a sample patch, as specified by its match to a comparison patch, depends on the surround field: when the surround field was illuminated consistently with the sample patch, the apparent colour of the sample patch was more stable than when the surround was illuminated inconsistently or when it was void. This stability was quantified by the contraction of the circular distribution in (u', v') space of the haploscopic matches to the sample patch under the eight non-white illuminants. If perfect colour constancy did hold, the distribution of matches should have collapsed to a single point. The contractions, of about 0.7–0.8, obtained with each of the three coloured sample patches (red, green, and blue) are quantitatively compatible with the findings of other studies (Tiplitz Blackwell and Buchsbaum, 1988; Lucassen and Walraven, 1993; Valberg and Lange-Malecki, 1990; Walraven et al., 1987), in which limited colour

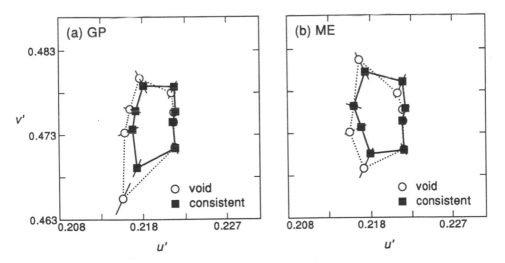

Figure 8.6.3.   Threshold values for detecting a change in the appearance of a Munsell red (5R 7/4) sample patch in two kinds of surround field under illuminant changes in eight directions in (u', v') space.

constancy was obtained by matching measures. There was no contraction of the distribution of matches with the white sample patch, a result that may be explained by the assumed role of whites in defining a reference in multicolour displays (see e.g. Land and McCann, 1971; McCann, 1992; McCann et al., 1976). For the inconsistently illuminated steady surround, there was an expansion of the distribution of matches, of about 1.2–1.5. The fact that this effect is the opposite of that obtained with the consistently illuminated surround may be a consequence of chromatic contrast between the sample patch and its surround, but it is not clear why the expansion should have been uniform, as the background was identical for all surfaces and had average co-ordinates in (u', v') space, the co-ordinates of the white illuminant (D_{65}).

The results of the second two experiments showed that a surround field had little effect on sensitivity to changes in apparent colour of a sample patch due to changes in illuminant, for any of the temporal profiles tested. In particular, sensitivity to illuminant changes was little impaired by a consistently illuminated surround, despite its stabilising effects on colour matches. In this sense, colour constancy in the time-domain seems to be absent.

A possible reason for the disparity between the results for steady and time-varying illuminants may be a difference in the temporal characteristics of the mechanisms responsible for stabilising colour percepts in multicoloured fields under steady illuminants and the mechanisms responsible for detecting changes in those illuminants. As has been argued elsewhere (Craven and Foster, 1992; Foster and Nascimento, 1994; Foster et al., 1992; Jameson and Hurvich, 1989) in a different context, we can detect a change in illuminant on a scene, or on part of it, and at the same time recognise – albeit to a limited degree – the stability of the colours in that scene, despite the illuminant change.

8.6.7 ACKNOWLEDGEMENTS

We thank K. J. Linnell, M. G. A. Thomson and S. Westland for critical reading of the manuscript. We also thank J. P. S. Parkkinen, J. Hallikainen, and T. Jaaskelainen for supplying their data for the Munsell set. This work was supported by the Wellcome Trust (grant no. 034807), the Junta Nacional de Investigação Científica e Tecnológica (grant no. BD/1328/91-RM), and the Universidade do Minho, Braga, Portugal.

8.6.8 REFERENCES

AREND, L. & REEVES, A. (1986) Simultaneous color constancy, *Journal of the Optical Society of America*, **A 3**, 1743–1751.

CRAVEN, B. J. & FOSTER, D. H. (1992) An operational approach to colour constancy, *Vision Research*, **32**, 1359–1366.

CORNELISSEN, F. W. (1994) *Light & Colour: Psychophysical studies on the use of lighting for visual rehabilitation and on spatial interactions in colour constancy*, PhD thesis, Rijksuniversiteit Groningen.

FOSTER, D. H. & BISCHOF, W. F. (1991) Thresholds from psychometric functions: superiority of bootstrap to incremental and probit variance estimators, *Psychological Bulletin*, **109**, 152–159.

FOSTER, D. H. & NASCIMENTO, S. M. C. (1994) Relational colour constancy from invariant cone-excitation ratios, *Proceedings of Royal Society, London*, **B257**, 115–121.

FOSTER, D. H., CRAVEN, B. J. & SALE, E. R. H. (1992) Immediate colour constancy, *Ophthalmic and Physiological Optics*, **12**, 157–160.

GOUREVITCH, V. & GALANTER, E. (1967) A significance test for one parameter isosensitivity functions, *Psychometrika*, **32**, 25–33.

VON HELMHOLTZ, H. (1866) *Handbuch der Physiologischen Optik, 1st Edition, Vol. II.* Translation 3rd Edition (*Helmholtz's Treatise on Physiological Optics*) J. P. C. Southall (Ed.), Optical Society of America, pp. 286–287. (Re-published (1962) New York: Dover Publications.)

HELSON, H. & JEFFERS, V. B. (1940) Fundamental problems in color vision. II. Hue, lightness, and saturation of selective samples in chromatic illumination, *Journal of Experimental Psychology*, **26**, 1–27.

HERING, E. (1878) Collected works in: *Outlines of a Theory of the Light Sense*, Cambridge, MA: Harvard University Press. (Translated (1964) by L. M. Hurvich and D. Jameson, pp. 7–8.)

JAMESON, D. & HURVICH, L. M. (1989) Essay concerning color constancy, *Annual Review of Psychology*, **40**, 1–22.

JUDD, D. B. (1940) Hue saturation and lightness of surface colors with chromatic illumination, *Journal of the Optical Society of America*, **30**, 2–32.

JUDD, D. B., MACADAM, D. L. & WYSZECKI, G. (1964) Spectral distribution of typical daylight as a function of correlated color temperature, *Journal of the Optical Society of America*, **54**, 1031–1040.

VON KRIES, J. (1905) Die Gesichtsempfindungen, in *Handbuch der Physiologie des Menschen*, Vol. 3, *Physiologie der Sinne*, W. Nagel (Ed.), Braunchschweig: Vieweg und Sohn.

LAND, E. H. (1959a) Color vision and the natural image. Part I, *Proceedings of the National Academy of Sciences, USA*, **45**, 115–129.

LAND, E. H. (1959b) Color vision and the natural image. Part II, *Proceedings of the National Academy of Sciences, USA*, **45**, 636–644.

LAND, E. H. & McCANN, J. J. (1971) Lightness and Retinex theory, *Journal of the Optical Society of America*, **61**, 1–11.

LUCASSEN, M. P. & WALRAVEN, J. (1993) Quantifying color constancy: evidence for nonlinear processing of cone-specific contrast, *Vision Research*, **33**, 739–757.

McCANN, J. J. (1992) Rules for colour constancy, *Ophthalmic and Physiological Optics*, **12**, 175–177.

McCANN, J. J., McKEE, S. P. & TAYLOR, T. H. (1976) Quantitative studies in Retinex theory. A comparison between theoretical predictions and observer responses to the 'Color Mondrian' experiments, *Vision Research*, **16**, 445–458.

Munsell Book of Color–Matte Finish Collection (1976) Baltimore, MD: Munsell Color Corporation.

PARKKINEN, J. P. S., HALLIKAINEN, J. & JAASKELAINEN, T. (1989) Characteristic spectra of Munsell colors, *Journal of the Optical Society of America*, A **6**, 318–322.

TIPLITZ BLACKWELL, K. & BUCHSBAUM, G. (1988) Quantitative studies of color constancy, *Journal of the Optical Society of America*, A **5**, 1772–1780.

VALBERG, A. & LANGE-MALECKI, B. (1990) 'Colour constancy' in Mondrian patterns: a partial cancellation of physical chromaticity shifts by simultaneous contrast, *Vision Research*, **30**, 371–380.

WALRAVEN, J., BENZSCHAWEL, T. & ROGOWITZ, B. E. (1987) Color-constancy interpretation of chromatic induction, *Die Farbe*, **34**, 269–273.

YOUNG, T. (1807) *A Course of Lectures on Natural Philosophy and the Mechanical Arts*, Vol I, Lecture XXXVIII, London: Joseph Johnson.

Space-average Scene Colour Used to Extract Illuminant Information

Karina J. Linnell and David H. Foster

8.7.1 INTRODUCTION

Human observers are able to determine whether changes in the colour appearance of a complex scene are consistent with a change in the spectral composition of the illuminating light or of the reflecting properties of its constituent materials (Craven and Foster, 1992; Foster et al., 1992). When an illuminant change is sufficiently large, it is perceived as a change in the space-average colour of the scene; in other words, it appears as though a wash of a different colour had been applied uniformly across the scene. The two experiments reported here were designed to investigate the capacity of human observers both to extract information about space-average colour and to use it to provide information about illuminant colour.

8.7.2 EXPERIMENT 1

If information about space-average colour is extracted from a scene, it should be possible to detect a change in illuminant over *different* as well as *identical* scenes, providing that the surfaces in each scene are sampled sufficiently uniformly to ensure that, on average, they reflect approximately the same amounts of energy in all regions of the visible spectrum. This experiment tested observers' capacity to detect a change in illuminant over two different random samples of reflecting surfaces, and how that capacity depended on the chromatic uniformity of the samples as determined by the number of surfaces in each sample. A practical analogy is provided by our everyday experience of walking from one room into another: can we detect a difference in illuminant between the two rooms, and, if we can, how does detection performance depend on the number of different reflecting surfaces in the two rooms? Clearly, in the limit where each room has only one reflecting surface, it is impossible to disambiguate a difference in illuminant from a difference in the spectral reflectance of the surfaces.

8.7.2.1 Method

Apparatus

Stimuli were generated by an RGB colour-graphics system with 8-bit resolution selected on each gun (Ramtek UK Ltd, Hampshire; 4660 series) under the control of a computer (Sun Microsystems Inc, CA, USA; type 3/160) and displayed on a 19-inch RGB monitor (Sony, Japan; Trinitron). Screen resolution was 1280×1024 pixels. Calibration procedures were as detailed in Craven and Foster (1992).

Stimuli

Stimuli were computer simulations of illuminated, square Mondrian patterns presented in a black surround. The individual colour patches physically comprising the Mondrian patterns were square and subtended on each side 0.86° visual angle. There were 49, 25 or 9 patches in each pattern; the pattern therefore subtended on each side 6.0°, 4.3°, or 2.6° respectively. Colour patches had the reflectance characteristics of Munsell surfaces. Surfaces were randomly selected from the 1976 *Munsell Book of Color*, and their spectral reflectances were taken from the basis-function decomposition by Parkkinen *et al.* (1989).

The illuminants were all formed from different combinations of the basis functions derived from the family of daylight illuminants (Judd *et al.*, 1964). Illuminant shifts were from a whitish origin, at $u' = 0.20$ on the daylight locus in the CIE (u', v') chromaticity diagram, to a range of points radiating out from this origin along four different colour directions: 'blue', 'orange', 'green', and 'pink' (in Figure 8.7.1, these directions are indicated by ' + ' signs). Specifically, blue and orange shifts were from the whitish origin at $u' = 0.20$ to various points along the tangent to the daylight locus at $u' = 0.20$, ranging to $u' = 0.18$ and to $u' = 0.22$ respectively; green and pink shifts were from the origin to equivalently spaced points along the normal to the daylight locus at $u' = 0.20$.

Procedure

On each trial one Mondrian was presented for 1 s and it was immediately replaced by a second Mondrian which was also presented for 1 s. Observers were asked to decide which change accounted for the change in the two Mondrians: either a change in the random sample of reflecting surfaces and their geometry, or a change in the illuminant *in addition to* a change in the random sample of reflecting surfaces and their geometry. The two alternatives were equally likely. When a change in illuminant occurred, it could have a magnitude represented by one of five different Euclidian distances in (u', v') space: 0.0066, 0.0131, 0.0197, 0.0263, 0.0438, in any one of the four different colour directions. An experimental session consisted of eight blocks of 80 trials. Within sessions, the number of colour surfaces from which each pattern was built remained the same, but across sessions it varied. In all, observers completed three sessions with each number of surfaces.

Observers

There were two naive observers, GP and TH; each had normal colour vision, as assessed with the Farnsworth-Munsell 100-hue test, and normal Snellen acuity.

Table 8.7.1. Values of the discrimination index d' as a function of increasing size of illuminant shift in the green direction. (SEMs of d' values ranged from 0.2, for d' values less than 1.0, to 1.0 or greater for the largest d' values between 2.0 and 3.0.)

Observer	Number of surfaces	Illuminant shift				
		0.0066	0.0131	0.0197	0.0263	0.0438
TH	49	0.3	1.4	1.9	2.9	2.9
	25	−0.1	0.6	0.9	1.6	2.7
	9	0.3	0.2	0.4	0.8	2.6
GP	49	−0.2	1.0	1.4	2.9	2.9
	25	0.0	0.5	1.3	1.4	2.7
	9	0.1	0.2	0.5	1.1	2.7

8.7.2.2 Results

Detection performance was quantified in terms of the discrimination index d' from signal-detection theory. Table 8.7.1 shows for each of the two observers d' values with the 49-surface, 25-surface and 9-surface patterns and illuminant shifts in the green direction. The d' values for illuminant shifts in the three other colour directions were similar.

For both observers, d' values were generally greater than zero, and increased with increasing size of illuminant shifts and number of colour surfaces.

8.7.2.3 Discussion

To determine whether these results are consistent with the assumption that observers relied upon estimates of space-average colour, a calculation was made of the performance of an ideal observer who was capable of perfectly extracting space-average colour. The ideal observer was presented with exactly the same stimuli as one of the real observers (TH). The first step to the calculation was to derive the space-average colour of each Mondrian pattern. If the Euclidian distance between the space-average colours of any two sequentially presented Mondrian patterns was greater than some criterion value, the ideal observer responded that an illuminant change had occurred, and if it was less than this criterion value the ideal observer responded that no illuminant change had occurred. Criterion values were chosen so that the false-alarm rates of the ideal observer were the same as those of the real observer; modest alterations to the criterion values did not substantially affect the outcome.

The d' values calculated from these hypothetical responses for 49-surface Mondrian patterns and illuminant shifts in the green direction through the five Euclidian distances in order of increasing magnitude were 0.6, 1.6, 2.9, 2.9 and 2.9 (2.9 was the maximum numerical value of d', given the false-alarm rate determined by the chosen criterion value). The d' values that observer TH (see Table 8.7.1) actually produced were of the same order of magnitude as these hypothetical ones, based on the assumption that space-average colour information and information about shifts in space-average colour were perfectly extracted. There was similar agreement between hypothetical and actual d' values for illuminant-shifts in the other directions and for the smaller patterns.

Even so, these results do not constitute evidence that space-average colour is the source of the observer's knowledge about the colour of the illuminant. There is another cue to illuminant colour that generally covaries with the space-average cue, namely, the colour of the highest-luminance patch in the pattern (McCann, 1992). Monte-Carlo simulations of Experiment 1 showed that the two observers' hit and false-alarm rates were predicted not only by shifts in space-average colour but also by shifts in the colours of the patches with the highest luminances.

To determine whether illuminant information can actually be derived from estimates of space-average colour alone, it was necessary to ensure that the information provided by the space-average cue was different from that provided by the highest-luminance patch. To this end, a second experiment (employing a different paradigm) was performed in which space-average colour was deliberately made a poor cue to illuminant colour while the cue provided by the colour of the highest-luminance patch remained good.

8.7.3   EXPERIMENT 2

The space-average colour cue was biased by building ('dual-cue') Mondrian patterns from a sample of 49 Munsell surfaces that, on average, reflected more light in one (orange) region of the visible spectrum than in any other region. One of the 49 surfaces was, however, a whitish surface that reflected light at all wavelengths approximately equally, and had the highest luminance under all the illuminants used to illuminate the dual-cue pattern. In the hypothetical case, in which observers used space-average colour to extract information about the colour of the illuminant, their information would differ substantially from that extracted in a second hypothetical case in which they used the colour of the highest-luminance patch.

To determine what colour observers actually assumed the illuminant to have, they were required to adjust the colour of the illuminant on a second ('comparison') Mondrian pattern until the illuminant was judged the same as that illuminating the dual-cue Mondrian pattern (see Beck, 1959, 1961, for description of a similar paradigm in which observers adjusted the luminance of a light illuminating various grey-level or essentially monochrome patterns). The two patterns were presented haploscopically; thus they could be compared simultaneously, but without interaction, in that the comparison pattern did not influence adaptation to the dual-cue pattern, and vice versa. An unbiased sample of 49 Munsell surfaces was used to build the comparison Mondrian pattern, for which both space-average colour and the colour of the highest-luminance patch were good predictors of illuminant colour. If observers adjusted the colour of the illuminant on the comparison pattern so that its space-average colour (which was effectively equivalent to the colour of the illuminant on the comparison pattern) approximated the space-average colour of the dual-cue pattern, then it could be concluded that they used space-average colour to extract illuminant information, even though space-average colour was not a good cue to illuminant colour. If, conversely, they set the colour of the illuminant on the comparison pattern so the colour of its highest-luminance patch (which was also effectively the colour of the illuminant on the comparison pattern) approximated the colour of the highest-luminance patch in the dual-cue pattern, then it could be concluded that they used the cue offered by the highest luminance patch to extract illuminant information.

At the limit, when individual colour patches are so small as to be unresolvable, only the space-average colour cue is available. In this experiment, although the dimensions of the square patches were always the same in the comparison and dual-cue patterns, they varied across experimental conditions from side 1 pixel (0.03°) to side 32 pixels (1.0°). (In Experiment 1, each patch had side slightly less than 1.0°.) To keep pattern size from varying with patch size, the number of individual patches generated from each of the 49 Munsell surfaces associated with each pattern was increased as patch size decreased. Mondrian patterns with 1-pixel patches appeared textured and it was impossible to identify individual colours; therefore, the only colour information available was from the space-average. In this case, observers were expected to set the colour of the comparison illuminant so that the space-average colour of the comparison pattern approximated the space-average colour of the dual-cue pattern. As patch size increased, however, individual colours, including the colour of the highest-luminance patch, were more and more easily identified. It then became an empirical issue whether space-average colour was still available and was still used to provide information about illuminant colour. The corresponding question for grey-level (or monochrome patterns) with only sparsely sampled grey-levels was addressed by Beck (1959, 1961), who considered patterns with and without clearly identifiable patches. Beck (1961) concluded that for patterns in which there are no clearly identifiable patches with high luminance, judgments about the illuminant are strongly influenced by space-average luminance, whereas for patterns in which there are clearly identifiable patches with high luminance, judgments about the illuminant are strongly influenced by the luminance of those patches.

8.7.3.1 Method

Apparatus

As in Experiment 1.

Stimuli

Stimuli were computer simulations of Mondrian patterns of illuminated Munsell surfaces. The simulations relied on the same basis-function descriptions of spectral reflectances and illuminants as used in Experiment 1.

Two square Mondrian patterns, each of side 7.0°, were presented side-by-side on a black background with their inside vertical edges separated by 3.0°. The comparison Mondrian pattern, presented on the left side of the display, and the dual-cue Mondrian pattern, presented on the right side, had equal numbers of colour patches. Across different conditions of the experiment, patch size varied from side 1 pixel (0.03°), through 2, 4, 8 and 16 pixels, to side 32 pixels (1.0°), but patch colour was always equally likely to be the colour of one of the 49 Munsell surfaces associated with each pattern. In Mondrian patterns with patches of side 32 pixels, each of the 49 Munsell surfaces associated with the pattern occurred only once, whereas in Mondrian patterns with 1-pixel patches, each of the 49 surfaces occurred 1024 times.

The 49 Munsell surfaces associated with the comparison pattern reflected on average the same amount of light in all regions of the visible spectrum, whereas those associated with the dual-cue pattern reflected on average more light in the orange region of the visible spectrum than in any other single region. One of the 49 surfaces associated with both comparison and dual-cue patterns was, however, a whitish sample which reflected light at all wavelengths approximately equally, and which was the highest-luminance surface under all the coloured illuminants used to illuminate the dual-cue pattern.

In total there were eight different illuminants used to illuminate the dual-cue Mondrian pattern across different trials: two blue, two orange, two green, and two pink. Like the illuminants in Experiment 1, they all fell along either the tangent or the normal to the daylight locus at the whitish point $u' = 0.20$ in (u', v') space. The two blue illuminants fell on the tangent to the daylight locus and had u' values of 0.18 (more saturated) and 0.19 (less saturated). The two orange illuminants also fell on the tangent to the daylight locus but had u' values of 0.22 (more saturated) and 0.21 (less saturated). The two green and the two pink illuminants fell at equivalently spaced points on the normal to the daylight locus, each side of the whitish point. The (u', v') co-ordinates of all of these illuminants except the more saturated orange one are plotted as the colours of the highest-luminance patch in the dual-cue pattern in each of the graphs in Figure 8.7.1.

Procedure

On each trial, comparison and dual-cue Mondrian patterns were presented simultaneously to the left and right eyes respectively. The dual-cue pattern was illuminated by one of the eight 'dual-cue' illuminants. Observers were required to adjust the colour of the illuminant on the comparison Mondrian pattern (the illuminant being set initially to be whitish) until it was judged the same as the illuminant on the dual-cue Mondrian pattern. While making these adjustments, they were encouraged to switch attention from one pattern to the other. In each experimental session the six patch-size conditions were undertaken in random order. For each condition, observers made eight matches, one for each of the eight dual-cue illuminants. There were six experimental sessions in all, and therefore observers repeated matches for each combination of illuminant and patch size six times. Different random arrangements of patches were used in different patch-size conditions and in different sessions.

Observers

There were two naive observers, GP and ME (one of whom participated in Experiment 1); each had normal colour vision, as assessed with the Farnsworth-Munsell 100-hue test, and normal Snellen acuity.

8.7.3.2 Results

Figure 8.7.1 shows the average matching performance (over six matches) of each of the two observers for each of seven of the eight dual-cue illuminants and three of the six patch sizes. Matching performance is represented by the space-average colour of the comparison pattern after matching. Each of the graphs in Figure 8.7.1 shows both the illuminant colour predicted by the space-average colour of the dual-cue pattern and the illuminant colour predicted by the colour of the highest-luminance patch in the dual-cue pattern for each illuminant. (Data are not presented for the more saturated of the two orange illuminants on the dual-cue patterns because when the illuminant on the comparison patterns was judged the same colour to observers, it was so saturated that the colour of the reflected light from some surfaces could not be reproduced by the monitor.)

8.7.3.3 Discussion

The colour of the illuminant on the comparison Mondrian pattern was set in such a way that the space-average colour of the comparison pattern was close to the space-average colour of the dual-cue pattern over most of the range of sizes of the patches making up the patterns. But with the largest patch size (1° side), the space-average colour of the comparison pattern was displaced part-way along a straight line joining the space-average colour of the dual-cue pattern and the colour of its highest-luminance patch (see Figure 8.7.1). It appears that

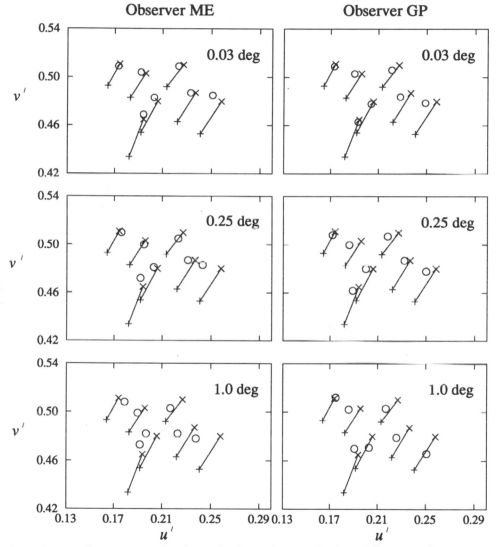

Figure 8.7.1. Illuminant matches for each of two observers for three different patch sizes. Each graph shows, for each of seven of the eight dual-cue illuminants, the average illuminant match made by the observer, defined as the average space-average colour of the comparison pattern after matching (O), and the illuminant matches predicted by both the space-average colour of the dual-cue pattern (×) and the colour of the highest-luminance patch in the dual-cue pattern (+). For each dual-cue illuminant, a straight line joins the matches predicted by the two cues. Patch size is indicated at the top right of each graph.

observers had access to information about space-average colour in patterns with the largest patches, even if they weighted this information less strongly than when the patches were smaller (compare Beck, 1959, 1961). Not only does space-average information appear to be extracted by the observer, it also appears to be extracted remarkably efficiently: performance altered little as patches increased in size from side 0.03° to side 0.25°.

8.7.4 SUMMARY AND CONCLUSIONS

The presence of different illuminants on different scenes can be reliably detected. Experiment 1 showed that observers' performance in this task increased with increasing size of illuminant change on the scenes and number of surfaces within them, and in a way that was similar to that shown by an ideal observer using space-average scene colour as the cue to the illuminant colour. But, in this experiment, as in naturally occurring scenes, space-average colour and the colour of the highest-luminance region covaried, and, in principle, human observers could have used either as the cue. In Experiment 2, these two cues were made to conflict with each other. In these circumstances, space-average colour was the preferred cue with patterns in which the constituent patches ranged in size from 0.03° to 0.5° across, and was a strong cue, if not the preferred one, with patterns in which the patches were 1.0° across (larger than the patches in Experiment 1).

If patch size had been increased further, and the gamut of colour surfaces decreased, the cue offered by the colour of the highest-luminance patch could have become more important in judging illuminant colour. In sparsely sampled grey-level patterns with clearly identifiable patches, the luminance of the highest-luminance patch has been shown to strongly influence illuminant matches (Beck, 1959, 1961). In a rather different task, the appearance of 'colour tautomi' arrays of just five colour patches has been shown to depend strongly on the presence of a white in the array (McCann, 1992). It is also possible that if the denser and more richly sampled Mondrian patterns used here had contained shape-from-shading information and the whitish patches were interpreted as highlights, observers might have attached greater significance to these local cues, and correspondingly less to space-average ones. For the two-dimensional Mondrian images used here, however, space-average colour seems to be the preferred cue to illuminant colour.

8.7.5 ACKNOWLEDGEMENTS

This work was supported by the Wellcome Trust (grant no. 034807). We thank J. J. McCann and S. M. C. Nascimento for helpful discussion; M. G. A. Thomson and S. Westland for critical review of the manuscript; and J. P. S. Parkkinen, J. Hallikainen and T. Jaaskelainen for providing their data for the spectral reflectances of the Munsell surfaces.

8.7.6 REFERENCES

BECK, J. (1959) Stimulus correlates for the judged illumination of a surface, *Journal of Experimental Psychology*, **58**, 267–274.

BECK, J. (1961) Judgments of surface illumination and lightness, *Journal of Experimental Psychology*, **61**, 368–375.

CRAVEN, B. J. & FOSTER, D. H. (1992) An operational approach to colour constancy, *Vision Research*, **32**, 1359–1366.

FOSTER, D. H., CRAVEN, B. J. & SALE, E. R. H. (1992) Immediate colour constancy, *Ophthalmic and Physiological Optics*, **12**, 157–160.

JUDD, D. B., MACADAM, D. L. & WYSZECKI, G. (1964) Spectral distribution of typical daylight as a function of correlated color temperature, *Journal of the Optical Society of America*, **54**, 1031–1040.

McCANN, J. J. (1992) Rules for colour constancy, *Ophthalmic and Physiological Optics*, **12**, 175–177.

PARKKINEN, J. P. S., HALLIKAINEN, J. & JAASKELAINEN, T. (1989) Characteristic spectra of Munsell colors, *Journal of the Optical Society of America*, **A6**, 318–322.

Colour Constancy, Excitation Purity and a Test of the Coefficient Theory

Mark F. Tritsch

Colour constancy mechanisms function to preserve the colour appearance of surfaces of given spectral reflectance when the spectrum of their illuminant changes. In systems restricted to colour representation in few dimensions, however, such as biological organisms, no mechanism can achieve perfect constancy. Many popular colour constancy models employ a lightness algorithm in which the final step involves normalisation of signals in three independent lightness channels (Hurlbert, 1986). This may be accomplished by dividing the response in each channel by the response produced in the same channel when the illuminant is reflected by a reference white surface (McCann *et al.*, 1976; Worthey and Brill, 1986), or by the average response in that channel for the entire scene (Buchsbaum, 1980). In the organism this might be realised through a combination of von Kries receptor adaptation and eye movements (D'Zmura and Lennie, 1986). However, the exact process or even the level of the visual system at which normalisation occurs has no significant bearing on the deviations from constancy that will be described below. The von Kries coefficient rule (also extensively reviewed in Wyszecki and Styles, 1982) does produce by definition perfect 'white' constancy for the shade of white or grey to which it has been normalised. Significantly enough, commercially available video cameras employ a similar adjustment to compensate for spectral variation in the illuminant and call it the 'white balance'.

Is the 'colour constancy' produced by the von Kries coefficient rule as good as the 'white constancy'? A thought experiment shows that it is not, and that excitation purity (a measure of the distance from the white point in the chromaticity diagram) has an important effect on the degree of constancy. A (purely theoretical) surface of almost monochromatic spectral reflectance is lit by two illuminants with differing broad-band spectral power distributions (SPDs). As the surface can only 'sample' the illuminant in one very narrow wavelength region, the absolute maximum of the SPD of the resulting stimulus may change considerably when the illuminant is exchanged, but its shape and position on the wavelength abscissa will remain almost unaltered. As a result, the chromaticity co-ordinates of the stimuli produced by the two illuminants will also remain unchanged, giving automatic colour constancy. However, if the visual system then also follows the von Kries coefficient rule for the two illuminants and adjusts the receptor responses accordingly, the visual sensations will be altered when the illuminants are exchanged and cease to be colour constant.

As monochromatic reflectance spectra do not exist, the principles of the thought experiment were applied to a computer simulation, in which the effect on human colour constancy of varying the bandwidth of reflectance spectra was investigated with and without application of von Kries coefficients to the receptor responses. Additionally, psychophysical experiments were carried out to measure the degree of colour constancy present for human observers estimating unique hues in saturated and unsaturated colour chips. Both these experiments examined the effect of excitation purity on colour constancy.

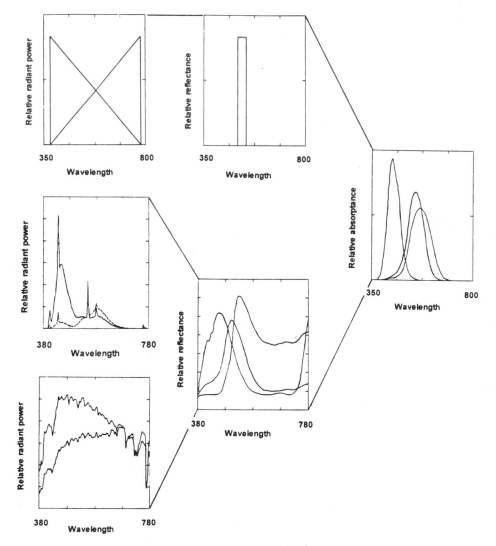

Figure 8.8.1. Spectral data for illuminants (left column), artificial or DIN chip colours (middle column) and human cone photoreceptors (right column). The combination of all three used for the simulation is connected by a line in the upper track, that used for the unique hue experiment is in the middle track, and that used for daylight simulation is in the lower track.

Finally, a computer simulation of the problem as it may occur under natural viewing conditions was carried out.

8.8.1   SIMULATING VARIATIONS IN REFLECTANCE SPECTRUM BANDWIDTH

Bandwidth was varied systematically using artificial surface colours whose reflectance was either 0 or 1 with maximally two transitions. Bandwidths of 40 nm, 100 nm, 240 nm and 400 nm (equal energy white) were used, the colours being distributed along the spectrum at appropriate intervals between 380 nm and 780 nm. Two illuminants were simulated by triangular SPDs (as shown in the upper track of Figure 8.8.1) with a base of 380–780 nm and an apex at either 380 nm (mainly short-wavelength, SWL) or 780 nm (mainly long-wavelength, LWL). Receptor responses were computed using Smith-Pokorney fundamentals (normalised to produce equal responses for an equal-energy white stimulus) and projected into the s + m + l = 1 plane of human receptor space (Smith and Pokorny, 1975); in the figures shown here, m is plotted against l. The effect of adjustment of the receptor responses by von Kries coefficients for the chosen illuminants was examined by performing the appropriate multiplication and plotting the resulting receptor responses once again (in the figures the spectrum locus is not adjusted). The von Kries coefficient k_j for the jth receptor is given by

$$k_j = \frac{1}{\sum_\lambda S(\lambda) q_j(\lambda)}$$

where $S(\lambda)$ is the SPD of the illuminant and $q_j(\lambda)$ is the spectral sensitivity of the jth photoreceptor.

The results are plotted in Figure 8.8.2, where the arrows show the shift in receptor responses when the SWL light is replaced by the LWL light. The von Kries adjusted responses are on the right. The 40 nm bandwidth unadjusted response shows almost no shift in receptor response when the illuminant is exchanged. The adjusted response, however, shows a very large shift with an increase in the s cones when the illuminant contains more long-wavelength light. This confirms the loss of colour constancy when von Kries adjustment is used with narrow-band reflectance spectra. As this shift would make the stimulus appear more blue under long-wavelength illumination, this is an overcompensation for the effects of the illuminant. Of special interest is the 100 nm bandwidth simulation, which shows a shift in the von Kries adjusted responses (in the direction of overcompensation) of approximately the same size as the shift in the opposite direction in the unadjusted responses. If natural spectra of this kind were to exist, the advantages and disadvantages of a colour constancy mechanism using the von Kries rule would cancel each other out. The receptor responses for the 400 nm bandwidth simulation (not shown) showed simply the shift between the two illuminants when unadjusted and exhibited perfect constancy when adjusted by the von Kries coefficients.

8.8.2   COLOUR CONSTANCY IN UNIQUE HUES

Shifts in the colour appearance of chips from the 24-hue DIN colour atlas were measured at two different levels of saturation by identifying unique hues (blue, green and yellow) under two different illuminants. The chips were mounted next to each other in order of hue number on a strip of white card for each saturation level. One strip contained chips from saturation level 2 and darkness level 1, the other (more highly saturated) strip contained chips from saturation level 5 or 6 (level 5 was the highest for some hues) and darkness levels 1–4 (using the lowest available). Eight subjects identified the chip that most closely approached the definition of the given unique hue (e.g. for yellow, neither reddish nor greenish), or else interpolated an imagined choice between two chips. Illumination was

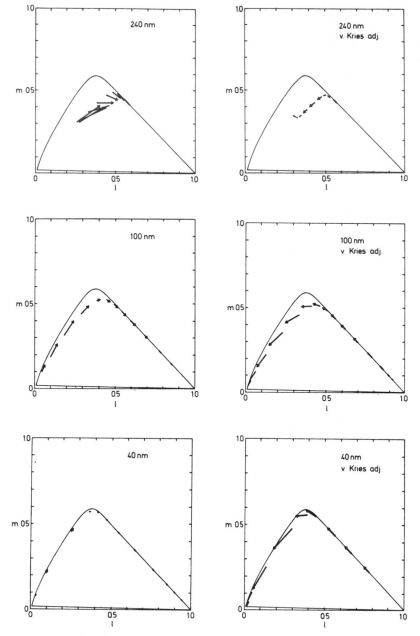

Figure 8.8.2. Results of the simulation of varying reflectance spectrum bandwidth (as described in the text).

provided by blue, green and yellow fluorescent lights mixed in one of two different ratios but at constant brightness, to give approximately SWL and LWL illuminants. Figure 8.8.1 (middle track) shows the spectra of the two illuminants and of some of the chips used. The subjects were encouraged to make their judgements briskly and the illuminant was switched between judgements, so that adaptation times were between 5 and 20 seconds.

The theory above leads one to expect overcompensation for all colours, but it should be greater for saturated colours (which have greater excitation purity). The results in Figure 8.8.3 show that overcompensation did indeed occur. When the illumination was switched from SWL to LWL, the subjects all chose unique yellows that were shifted towards the red and unique blues that were shifted towards the green. This was the case for both unsaturated and saturated colours, but the hue shift was in fact less for saturated than for unsaturated colours. In the case of unique green, there was no significant shift for the unsaturated colour (almost perfect constancy) and undercompensation for the saturated colour. The shifts were significant at the $p < 0.01$ level (t-test).

Figure 8.8.4 shows the results in terms of von Kries adjusted receptor responses (m plotted against l as above). The filled circles represent the chip chosen as unique hue under SWL illumination, the arrowheads represent the same chip under LWL illumination and the crosses represent the chip actually chosen as unique hue under LWL illumination. If the results were exactly as predicted by the von Kries rule, the crosses would lie on the circles. If the results showed perfect constancy (i.e. no overcompensation), the crosses would lie on

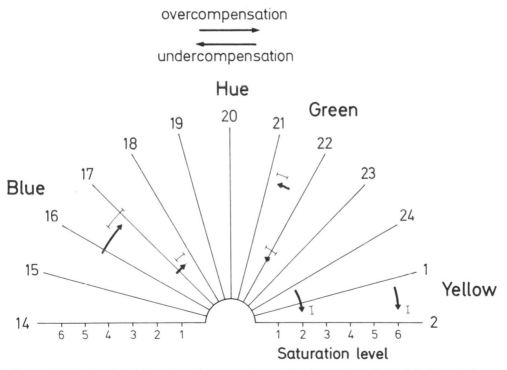

Figure 8.8.3. Results of the unique hue experiment. The figure shows half of the hue circle, containing the DIN colour chips 14–24 and 1–2. Saturation level is shown radially, and approximate positions of unique hues are as labelled. The arrows show the mean shift in judgement of unique hue when the illuminant was changed from SWL to LWL. The error bars are SEMs.

the arrowheads. In fact the results did deviate from perfect constancy in the direction of overcompensation predicted by the von Kries rule (except for green), but not by very much. The unsaturated colours conform more closely to the von Kries rule than the saturated ones, as indicated by the greater degree of overcompensation for them in Figure 8.8.3.

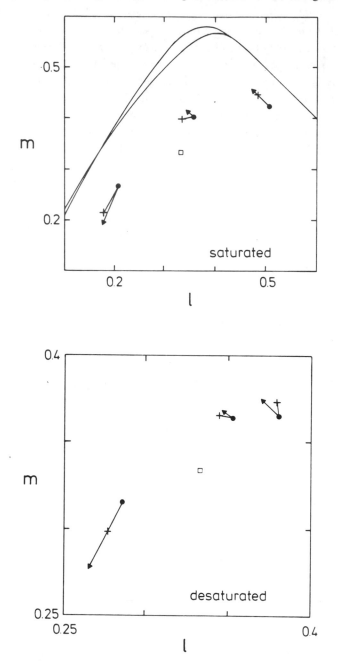

Figure 8.8.4.   Results of the unique hue experiment in terms of von Kries adjusted receptor responses for saturated (above) and unsaturated chips (below). The symbols are as described in the text. The lower plot is scaled to show a smaller section of the receptor diagram. The upper plot also shows the shift in the spectrum locus caused by the von Kries adjustment.

8.8.3   DAYLIGHT SPECTRA AND VON KRIES COEFFICIENTS

What relevance does this have for natural viewing conditions under daylight? Figure 8.8.5 (top) shows receptor response shifts calculated for saturated blue, green and yellow chips

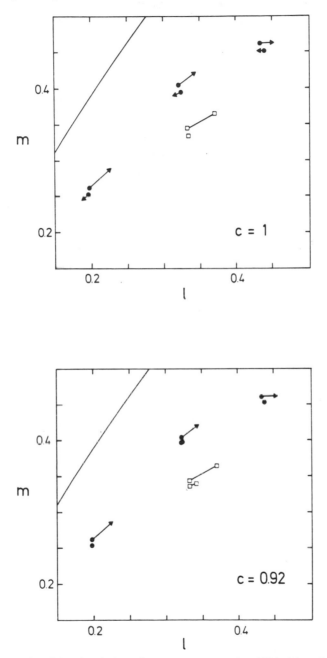

Figure 8.8.5.   Results of the simulation of receptor responses to DIN chips viewed in different phases of daylight. The symbols are as described in the text. In the upper plot the von Kries rule is applied with c − 1. In the lower plot the effect of the von Kries coefficients is moderated using the factor c = 0.92.

under two phases of daylight (the filled circles are for morning light from the western sky, the arrowheads for afternoon light from the same). The reflectance spectra and SPDs are shown in the bottom track of Figure 8.8.1. The big shifts (to greater m and l) are produced by the unadjusted responses and the smaller shifts in the opposite direction by the von Kries adjusted responses. The open squares show the responses for white. Here also, therefore, the theory predicts overcompensation for coloured surfaces but perfect constancy for white.

8.8.4   DISCUSSION

The simulation showed that, with a von Kries coefficient rule for colour constancy, surface colours that have high excitation purity depart from constancy because of overcompensation. The results of the unique hue experiment, however, showed that human colour constancy is better than this model would predict and exhibits only some of the overcompensation expected. The amount of overcompensation in the receptor responses is, unexpectedly, more for unsaturated than for saturated colours, and there are differences between unique green and unique yellow or blue. In his analysis of the McCann *et al.* (1976) experiment, Worthey (1985) also noted that overcompensation predicted by the von Kries rule did not occur in the experimental subjects. A possible explanation for the reduced overcompensation in human subjects is that the operation of the von Kries coefficients is somehow moderated in its effect. Figure 8.8.5 (bottom) shows the shift in receptor responses for different phases of daylight when the von Kries coefficients are moderated by a further factor *c*. The new coefficients a_j are then given by

$$a_j = \frac{3ck_j}{\sum_\lambda k_j} + (1 - c)$$

where $c = 1$ for full adjustment, and $c = 0$ for no adjustment. With $c = 0.92$ the model yielded almost perfect constancy for the colour chips, but a significant undercompensation for white.

The von Kries adjusted receptor responses of trichromats do in fact contain information about the excitation purity of the stimulus. Therefore, a later stage of the visual system could reverse the overcompensating effect of the von Kries coefficients for stimuli of high excitation purity, but leave the response for stimuli close to the white point unaltered. This could explain the unexpectedly small amount of over-compensation found for saturated colour chips. A candidate is the second-stage of the constancy mechanism suggested by Jameson and Hurvich (1989). Of course, this is an option that would not even theoretically have been available to a dichromat like John Dalton. The potential for better colour constancy might therefore be an additional difference between dichromats and trichromats.

8.8.5   REFERENCES

BUCHSBAUM, G. (1980) A spatial processor model for object colour perception, *Journal of the Franklin Institute*, **310**, 1–26.

D'ZMURA, M. & LENNIE, P. (1986) Mechanisms of colour constancy, *Journal of the Optical Society of America*, **A 3**, 1662–1672.

HURLBERT, A. (1986) Formal connections between lightness algorithms, *Journal of the Optical Society of America*, **A 3**, 1684–1693.

JAMESON, D. & HURVICH, L.M. (1989) Essay concerning colour constancy, *Annual Review of Psychology*, **40**, 1–22.

McCANN, J.J., McKEE, S.P. & TAYLOR, T.H. (1976) Quantitative studies in retinex theory, *Vision Research*, **16**, 445–458.

SMITH, V.C. & POKORNY, J. (1975) Spectral sensitivity of the foveal cone photopigments between 400 and 500 nm, *Vision Research*, **15**, 161–171.

WORTHEY, J.A. (1985) Limitations of colour constancy, *Journal of the Optical Society of America*, **A 2**, 1014–1026.

WORTHEY, J.A. & BRILL, M.H. (1986) Heuristic analysis of von Kries colour constancy, *Journal of the Optical Society of America*, **A 3**, 1708–1712.

WYSZECKI, G. & STYLES, W.S. (1982) *Color Science*, New York: Wiley.

Average Colour Constancy and Categorical Hues

J.J. Kulikowski, L. Routledge, H. Jordan and P. Laycock

8.9.1 INTRODUCTION

Colour constancy is the perceived stability of the colour of objects under different illuminants (see review by Pokorny, 1991). In terms of survival, it is advantageous to readily identify objects (e.g. fruits and their ripeness, flowers, and other animals, which either signal their presence, or warn predators, or use camouflage), despite changes in illumination. This ability is possessed by a wide range of species, ranging from insects to vertebrates (Ingle, 1985; Neumeyer et al., this volume, pp. 55–62). Most mammals have only dichromatic colour vision, but primates, including humans, have trichromatic colour vision with colour constancy. There are several mechanisms that make it possible to minimise the effects of illuminant changes, one of the more important being adaptation of the photoreceptors. Several recent models have shown that this receptoral component is dominant under 'natural' viewing conditions. Under such conditions daylight illumination does not change rapidly nor to any great extent, particularly in many places in the Northern hemisphere (e.g. Dannemiller, 1992; Jepson et al., 1989; Krinov, 1953).

Colour constancy in primates has probably evolved under more challenging conditions of illumination, which resulted in the development of other specialised mechanisms, including those in the visual cortex (Zeki, 1980, 1983). The top performance in colour constancy cannot be achieved if visual cortical area V4 is damaged (Carden et al., 1993; Walsh et al., 1993; Wild et al., 1985). V4 probably contains a 'constancy-expertise' centre, but a loss of constancy with a V4 lesion does not imply a total loss of colour vision. Walsh et al. (1992) have shown that monkeys with V4 lesions (like normal monkeys – Sandell et al., 1979) are capable of learning to discriminate between hues of different categories faster than between hues of the same basic category, provided that white illumination is used. Thus, colour categorisation appears to precede constancy and probably contributes to its operation.

Basic colour categories – red, yellow, green and blue can be defined by several methods, e.g. verbally (Boynton and Gordon, 1965), or as unique hues (Jameson and Hurvich, 1968); for review see Pokorny (1991). These hues can be determined for each subject by using a simple method of choosing five 'typical' colours (see Methods). Adoption of five basic colours follows recent studies (Mullen and Kulikowski, 1990; see also Jordan and

Kulikowski, this volume, pp. 421–430), which showed that there are five discriminable spectral regions, whose borders can be established by using strict psychophysical discrimination, at detection threshold.

These findings prompted our preliminary investigation of how 'constant' are categorical colours under different illuminants as compared with intermediate or border colours (Kulikowski and Walsh, 1993a,b). The same question is pursued here with several refinements of the method. In particular, the opportunity for the receptors to adapt to a change in illuminant is minimised. Colour constancy in this situation is poorer than after a period of prolonged adaptation (Kulikowski and Walsh, 1993b). The present preliminary report deals with a specific task of colour constancy, with a quantitative evaluation of our ability to match or identify a coloured surface under a variable illuminant with a surface under standard illuminant (C).

8.9.2   METHOD

There are obvious advantages associated with the 'reflecting surface' approach adopted here, in that it refers to physical objects, in this case Munsell chips. As physical objects, Munsell chips make the task of 'object colour constancy' very direct and avoid many problems associated with colour simulation and they do not require frequent calibration. The system is common enough to be easily replicated in other studies.

8.9.2.1 Apparatus

A display box consisted of two separate parts: the left illuminated by either one of two illuminants (either A or g, see below), and the right by a reference 'daylight white' close to illuminant C. Subjects adapted to illuminant C and only briefly glanced at a test Munsell chip under the variable illuminant A or g. All chips were displayed on neutral backgrounds of values: 9 ('light'), then 5 ('dark'). Each test chip under the variable illuminant is to be matched with one of the several chips (several Munsell hues and Munsell chromas) displayed under reference illuminant C. (The uniform backgrounds, rather than 'mondrians' in the preceding studies, were used in order to simplify the analysis, see Valberg and Lange-Malecki, 1990.) This study tested constancy of 40 Munsell chips of value 7 and chroma 8. Luminance of Munsell chips of the same value (7) is not completely constant under illuminants either A or g, but these differences did not exceed 15 per cent (in most cases were within 10 per cent), and could be minimised by adjusting the angle of incident light (care was taken to avoid specular reflections). Two complete sets of Munsell chips were used in matching tasks.

Illuminant A was a tungsten bulb. Its chromaticity co-ordinates (measured originally by Bentham Spectral analyser) were $x,y = 0.46,0.41$ and $u',v' = 0.26,0.53$, colour temperature of approximately 2800 K. Illuminant g (illuminant C covered by a green filter), was introduced to represent greenish illumination. Its chromaticity co-ordinates on the $u'v'$ plane were chosen to form a vector Cg approximately orthogonal to CA (the angle is close to 90°): $u',v' = 0.161,0.492$ ($x,y = 0.285,0.387$). These parameters were checked periodically using SpectraScan/PR650 analyser and their variations were found to be minimal. Broadly speaking, illuminant changes between C and A simulate partly daylight variations, whereas changes from C to g are not connected with any natural illuminant (although they may mimic reflectance from green foliage). Note (Figure 8.9.1) that the illuminants A and g are close to the loci of the Munsell chips: 7.5YR and 2.5G, respectively.

8.9.2.2 Procedure

The experiments consisted of two parts. In the first part, the subjects were asked to specify 'typical' hues: red, yellow, green, blue and violet among the Munsell chips used in further studies (value 7, chroma 8). This modified version of estimation of unique hues, parallelled the method that studied 'typical' colours among spectral hues and their categorical borders (Jordan and Kulikowski, this volume, pp. 421–430; see also a clinical version, Schefrin *et al.*, 1991). The subjects viewed a range of 7/8 test chips; their task was to specify a chip whose hue would not contain components of the adjacent basic hues. Thus, yellow should not contain components of red-orange, or green, green would not have yellow or blue, and blue would not contain green or violet. The results were then averaged for all subjects.

In the second part, the method of successive matching in free viewing was used, after the subject adapted to a reference illuminant C. After spending some time (at least 10 min) in a dim room, a subject was instructed to adapt to C for at least 60 s, then glance at a test chip under the variable illuminant and point to the 'matching' chip under C. The matching chips (providing a best match) were of various hues, chromas (saturations) and values. Subjects were also encouraged to interpolate between chips if none ideally matched the test chip. By restricting adaptation time to the variable illuminant, it is possible to simplify the interpretation of the matched hues with reference to the standard (C). In the preceding experiments Kulikowski and Walsh (1993b) found substantial differences in colour constancy performance when each eye was allowed to adapt to a different illuminant for at least 30 s. (Adaptation to a second illuminant alters the position of the hue on any colour

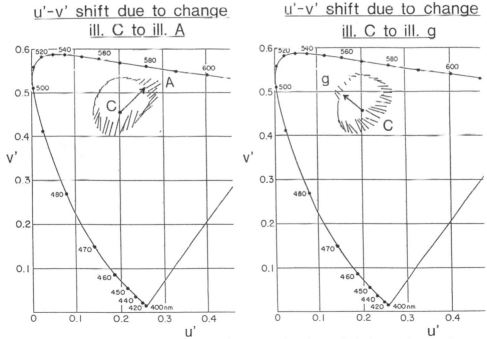

Figure 8.9.1. Representation of 40 Munsell hues used in the study (value 7; chroma 8) on the *u'v'* chromaticity plane (dark background). The subject (LR, 20) matched each chip under the illuminant A or g with one of many chips shown under the standard illuminant C; the chromaticity co-ordinates of this matched chip is then specified for the illuminant C. Note the chromaticity coordinates of illuminants (C, A and g) and the near orthogonality of vectors CA and Cg.

plane used to compute the perceived hue change; these control experiments are mentioned in Discussion.)

The effect of changes in luminance, brightness, or value of Munsell chips are not included in this study. Fine adjustment in these parameters were achieved by changing the angle of the chips in relation to the observer by means of an adjustable 'chip-holder'. The subject had to re-adapt to C before making the final match.

Our procedure is substantially different from those adopted in other studies (Arend *et al.*, 1991; Lukassen and Walraven, 1993; Troost and de Weert, 1991; Valberg and Lange-Malecki, 1990) and it resembles more the 'immediate constancy' experiments (Barbur *et al.*, 1992; Foster *et al.*, 1992).

8.9.2.3 Subjects

A total of six subjects participated in the experiment, all with normal colour vision. One was an experienced observer, the remainder were inexperienced young observers. In addition to the matching tasks, each subject had to point to Munsell hues representing typical colours, red, yellow, green, blue and violet, under illuminant C on both light and dark backgrounds. The performance of all subjects was averaged (see the letters in Figures 8.9.2, 8.9.3 and 8.9.4).

8.9.2.4 Analysis

The chromaticity plane utilised in this study is the CIE (1932) $u'v'$ plane, as it represents an equal discriminability scale. As colour appearance of Munsell chips under different illuminants is assessed by matching of hues and saturations, it is possible to measure colour constancy in terms of a hue and saturation change of a matched chip. A high degree of constancy means that the same chip is selected as a match under a different illuminant; poor constancy means that a matching chip (under C) is several Munsell steps apart from the test chip. This 'perceptual shift' could be described in terms of Munsell steps, but it is more convenient to use the chromaticity co-ordinates. The co-ordinates of the matched Munsell chip (matched with the test chip) under the standard illuminant, can be plotted on the $u'v'$ chromaticity plane. The variability of appearance of particular hues under different illuminants can simply be calculated by measuring the apparent chromaticity shift in the chip location on the chromaticity plane. The computations of shifts as a function of illuminant with reference to illuminant C and to $u'v'$ chromaticity co-ordinates are obviously arbitrary (xy co-ordinates could also be used). Hence, as an alternative measure, we used a relative shift, namely the ratio of $u'v'$ perceptual shift (as above) to the physical $u'v'$ shift. The physical shift was a change of $u'v'$ co-ordinates from those under illuminant C and A or g, measured by SpectraScan PR650. Note that our shift ratio, R, is related to a 'one-dimensional Brunswick ratio' (Troost and de Weert, 1991), Br, by $R = 1 - Br$.

8.9.3   RESULTS

8.9.3.1 Matching of Munsell chips

Figure 8.9.1 shows an example of the performance of one subject under two illuminants: A, g. These graphs illustrate how changes in chip appearance are measured, analysed and represented.

The 40 Munsell hues are arranged along a pseudo-ellipsoid. When a chip is presented under illuminants A (or g) it is matched with a reference chip under illuminant C (see Methods). The newly chosen match with a chip under illuminant C is then described in terms of its $u'v'$ coordinates. Constancy (or inconstancy) is characterised here by the length of a vector whose other parameters are the origin (the initial co-ordinate of each Munsell chip under illuminant C) and angle (measured in radians with respect to the u' axis). The vector length is specified by a difference between initial and final perceptual (matched) position of a chip. Figure 8.9.1 shows these shift vectors as well as illuminant shifts (measured for the neutral backgrounds, CA and Cg).

It might be thought that the vector shifts tend to have an orientation similar to that of the illuminant. However, it is approximately so only for hues whose positions on the $u'v'$ plane is close to those of variable illuminants. In other words, angles of hue shifts are nearly the same as angles of illuminants only for hues close to A or g respectively. It will be seen that other vectors have variable orientation, which may change in clusters (see Figure 8.9.2).

Second, the length of a shift is not even for all hues. It is generally smaller for greens and yellows and greatest for the violets and purples. This length is one measure of constancy – ideal constancy is when length is zero (but see below).

Third, it was found by averaging the results of all six subjects that the background (either light or dark) makes relatively little difference to the results. Consequently the results for both backgrounds were averaged.

These averaged results are quantitatively illustrated in Figures 8.9.2 and 8.9.3. Hues are enumerated starting from purple, through blue, green, yellow, red and ending on red-purple: No.1 = 10P, No.2 = 7.5P, No.3 = 5P, No.4 = 2.5P, No.5 = 10PB, ... No.40 = 2.5RP (only hues 5P, 5B, 6G, 5Y and 5R are marked on the abscissa in Figures 8.9.2–8.9.4). Note that the numbers between 4 (2.5P) and 36 (2.5R) denote hues with dominant wavelengths in the spectral region (400–625 nm); the remainder are non-spectral purples.

Mean of 6 subjects & 2 backgrounds

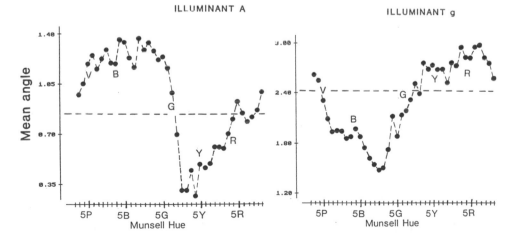

Figure 8.9.2. Mean angle of chromaticity shifts (in radians, $u'v'$ plane). The data for two illuminants (A and g) are shown. The results are averages for six subjects, each performed matching using two neutral background (N9 and N5). Note the typical colour (indicated by the initials): Violet, Blue, Green, Yellow and Red. The horizontal dashed lines indicate shift-angles for neutral backgrounds.

8.9.3.2 Angle of the shift

Figure 8.9.2 illustrates the mean angles of shifts (in radians, with reference to u'-axis) for various hues when seen under illuminants A and g, respectively. The angles of the illuminant shift for the neutral backgrounds were angle (CA) = 0.843 radian and angle (Cg) = 2.435 radian (marked by the dashed lines). It is obvious that very few hues (e.g. around green) have similar angles of shifts as the angle of illuminant shifts. The angle is a fairly regular function of the Munsell hue with possible 'ripples' around 'typical' hues (marked V, B, G, Y and R). These irregularities are, however, within noise level and cannot be regarded only as a residual effect of categorisation.

8.9.3.3 Absolute and relative length of a shift

Figure 8.9.3 shows the lengths of apparent (matched) shifts ($u'v'$) for various hues. As was seen for an individual subject, the shift-lengths are shortest for greens and yellows, longest (worst constancy) for violets and red-purples, so that the length functions form u-shaped curves.

However, these shifts must be compared with physical ($u'v'$) shifts that vary for different hues. For example, the 'physical hue shift' measured colorimetrically in the case of illuminant change CA is up to 0.12 for purples, about 0.09 for blue, but only around 0.055 for the green-orange range. Hence, after normalisation, the relative shifts are different than absolute. For illuminant A the ratio of apparent/physical shifts is smallest for blue (about 0.32), slightly greater for the yellow-green range and the largest (about 0.58) for orange around the position of illuminant A. Thus, the shift-ratio, or 'relative inconstancy index' varies at best around 0.3–0.4; 0 defines ideal constancy.

The ($u'v'$) shifts for illuminant g are smaller, both perceptual (0.017–0.036) and physical (0.039–0.069). Consequently, the variations of both absolute and relative shifts for various hues are less pronounced. The minimum 'relative inconstancy index' for blue is about 0.42, maximum 0.62 (for purples) and rather large (0.5) around the position of illuminant g.

Figure 8.9.3 illustrates a certain pattern of the $u'v'$ shifts. Both the averaged lengths and shift-ratios show that local 'dips' (i.e. better constancy) occur near typical hues (B, G, Y and R). However, the significance of these irregularities is obscured by substantial inter-subject differences (also in specifying typical hues); the standard deviations of the mean lengths of shifts are large: for illuminant A about 0.005 and for illuminant g about 0.004, i.e. of the same order as the above mentioned irregularities or 'dips'.

8.9.3.4 Grand average of all shifts

Figure 8.9.4 shows the length shifts and shift ratios (i.e. relative shifts) averaged for both illuminants A and g. These graphs, especially shift-ratio, give some measure of how hue appearance is distorted when the illuminant changes. It seems that the mean of all of the subjects under two illuminants and against two backgrounds shows similar irregularities in the form of smaller shifts for colours regarded as typical. There is only one additional hue that shows relatively good constancy, although it belongs to intermediate hues, namely blue-green (2.5BG), or cyan. Conversely, the largest shifts are observed for violet/purples and for hues near the illuminants of A and g.

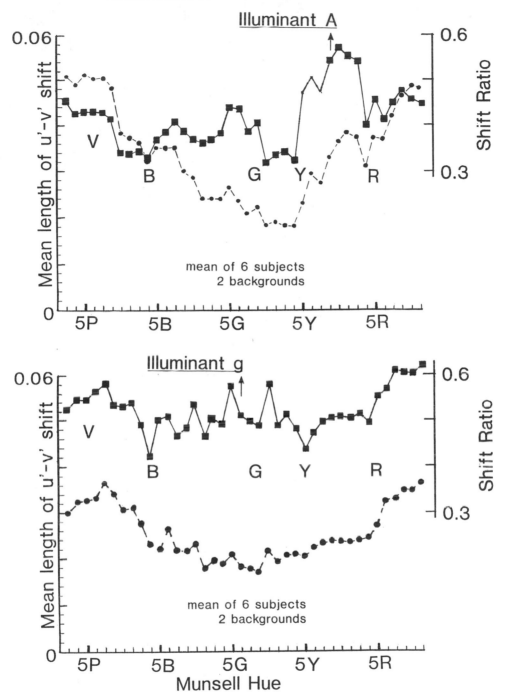

Figure 8.9.3. The filled circles mark the mean lengths of chromaticity shifts (*u'v'* plane; average of six subjects and two backgrounds) for illuminants A and g (the arrowheads indicate the positions of these illuminants with respect to the nearest chips). Note a generally encountered U-shape of the *u'y'* shift characteristics and slight 'dips' near 'typical' colours (B, G, Y and R, averaged for six subjects).

The filled squares mark the relative shifts, i.e. *ratios* of perceptual-to-physical shifts of Munsell hues under illuminants A (top) and g (bottom); the 'dips' are now more conspicuous because the 'shift ratio' characteristics are relatively flat. Note that the Brunswick ratio Br = 1 - 'shift-ratio'.

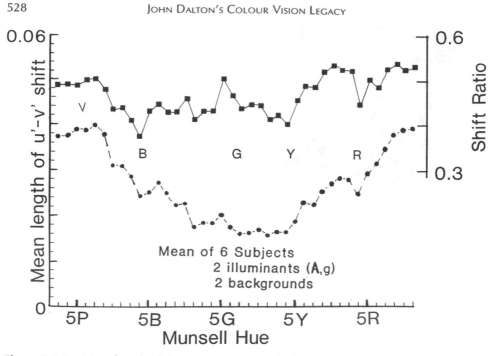

Figure 8.9.4. Mean length of chromaticity shifts for both illuminants (A, g), two backgrounds (N9 and N5) and 6 subjects (40 test Munsell chips 7/8). The filled squares mark the relative shifts (ratios: perceptual/physical) averaged for all conditions.

8.9.4 DISCUSSION

8.9.4.1 Rules of colour constancy

The most conspicuous outcome of the present experiments is that colour constancy shows a certain regularity for both illuminants (A, g), both backgrounds (Light, Dark) and both methods of assessment. Whether constancy is evaluated by a shift (absolute length on the $u'v'$ plane), or by a shift-ratio, namely the ratio of perceptual-to-physical shifts (relative index), it is relatively good for typical hues, marked as B, G, Y and R (but not for violet, V) and poorest in the range of purples and for hues resembling the illuminants.

   These typical colours, marked in Figures 8.9.2, 8.9.3 and 8.9.4, are averaged for six subjects (each chosen from a range of Munsell hues of the same value and chroma, 7/8); they are broadly related to the typical spectral colours obtained under different conditions (Jordan and Kulikowski, this volume, pp. 421–430).

   It will be seen that under the present conditions the ratio of perceptual-to-physical shift, i.e. 'inconstancy index' is moderate: 0.3–0.4 (which corresponds to the Brunswick ratios of 0.7 and 0.6), even though minimisation of the effects of adaptation should make constancy poorer (some matches of these hues were often a fraction of a Munsell step and the match was interpolated). Other observers simply accepted the same Munsell chip as a match that could be interpreted as complete colour constancy (Brunswick ratio of 1). This suggests the extraordinary ability of colour constancy to operate even under minimum adaptation (i.e. without long-term adaptation, see below). For other hues, the relative shift increases less than shifts shown in Figure 8.9.3, being around 0.4 and exceeding this value only for the purples.

In the present study, the 'dips' are not statistically significant, due to the inter-subject variability of the data (see below); moreover, there are more 'dips' than typical colours. Thus the possible greater robustness of categorical (rather than non-categorical) colours may only be of a residual nature. Among other studies, only Troost and de Weert (1991) have addressed the relationship between categories and colour constancy, but they used different conditions of adaptation.

8.9.4.2 Limitations of the test with Munsell chips

The use of colour systems of the physical type has a common disadvantage, namely a limited number of available chips, so that it is impossible to avoid discontinuities in hue saturation and value space, which are perceptible by the human visual system. Hence it is necessary to allow the subjects to interpolate between the chips available for matching. Moreover, the better constancy, the more Munsell steps would be required to match the test chip.

In the present study the quantisation errors (due to restricted number of Munsell chips) do not seriously limit the matching performance, because inter-subject variations are relatively large and constancy is moderate, partly due to a restricted adaptation time. However, if the number of test hues were reduced, the salient points might have been missed. Thus if only the odd numbers of samples were used, the minima in Figure 8.9.4 for B, Y and R would pass unnoticed.

Inter-subject variations in the length of the shift on the $u'v'$ colour plane as a result of the change in illuminant are statistically significant ($p > 0.05$). Thus, bearing in mind the small number of subjects in this study, it is surprising that any consistent pattern emerges (the results with similar 'dips' have been obtained in follow-up studies).

8.9.4.3 Effect of adaptation time

This effect of prolonged (monocular) adaptation in the haploscopic paradigm was reported by Kulikowski and Walsh (1993b) and will be dealt with separately. However, it is worth stressing that the present results with immediate constancy are substantially altered when the subject's eyes are allowed to adapt, each to a different illuminant, e.g C and A. The change is best noticeable for the $u'v'$ shifts in the region of blue-green hues, for which adaptation brings about almost perfect constancy. Thus, even only 30 s adaptation (followed by successive matching that does not disrupt adaptation) results in an almost flat reduction of the $u'v'$ shifts by about 0.02. Moreover, the hues between 5G-5Y show a zero shift, or ideal constancy, partly due to a floor effect. Still longer adaptation results in these zero shifts becoming negative, which means over-constancy (see also Troost and De Weert, 1991).

8.9.5   CONCLUSION

Immediate colour constancy holds best for hues corresponding to 'typical' colours, as compared with the adjacent hues; however, this effect must be considered as residual, probably resulting from greater proportions of cells being tuned to typical spectral hues. On average, the shift-ratio ('inconstancy index') varies around 0.53 (Brunswick ratio of 0.47) in the worst cases of purples and hues near illuminants A, g. The smallest shift ratios

0.38–0.45 (Brunswick ratio of 0.62–0.55) are for typical colours (B, G, Y and R) and, unexpectedly, for a blue-green.

8.9.6   ACKNOWLEDGEMENTS

We wish to thank Professor H. Vaitkevicius of the Vilnius University, Lithuania, for helpful criticism of this study and the Royal Society for sponsoring this collaboration.

8.9.7   REFERENCES

AREND, L.E., REEVES, A., SCHIRILO, J. & GOLDSTEIN, R. (1991) Simultaneous color constancy: papers with diverse Munsell values, *Journal of the Optical Society of America*, A **8**, 661–672.

BARBUR, J.L., FORSYTH, P.M. & WILLIAMS, C.B. (1992) Measurements of colour constancy under realistic and unnatural changes of illuminant, *Perception*, **21**, 11.

BOYNTON, R.M. & GORDON, J. (1965) Berzold-Brücke hue shift measured by color naming technique, *Journal of the Optical Society of America*, **55**, 78–86.

CARDEN, D., HILKEN, H., BUTLER, S.R. & KULIKOWSKI, J.J. (1992) Lesions of primate visual area V4 produce long-lasting deficits to colour constancy, *Irish Journal of Psychology*, **13**, 455–472.

DANNEMILLER, J.L. (1992) Spectral reflectance of natural objects: how many basis functions are necessary? *Journal of the Optical Society of America*, A **9**, 507–515.

FOSTER, D.H., CRAVEN, B.J. & SALE, E.R.H. (1992) Immediate colour constancy, *Ophthalmic and Physiological Optics*, **12**, 157–160.

INGLE, D. (1985) The goldfish as a retinex animal, *Science*, **227**, 651–654.

JAMESON, D. & HURVICH, L. (1968) Opponent response functions related to measured cone pigments, *Journal of the Optical Society of America*, **58**, 429–430.

JEPSON, A.D., GERSHON, R. & HALLETT, P.E. (1989) Cones, colour constancy and photons. In: Kulikowski, J.J., Dickinson, C. & Murray, I.J. (Eds) *Seeing Contour and Colour*, Oxford: Pergamon Press, pp. 768–776.

KRINOV, E.L. (1953) Spectral reflectance properties of natural formations, Technical Translation TT-439, National Research Council of Canada, Ottawa.

KULIKOWSKI, J.J. & WALSH, V. (1993a) Colour vision: isolating mechanisms in overlapping streams, *Progress in Brain Research*, **95**, 417–426.

KULIKOWSKI, J.J. & WALSH, V. (1993b) Colour constancy for categorical centroid and border colours, *Perception*, **22** (suppl), 13.

LUKASSEN, M.P. & WALRAVEN, J. (1993) Qualifying color constancy: Evidence for nonlinear processing of cone-specific contrast, *Vision Research*, **33**, 739–757.

MULLEN, K.T. & KULIKOWSKI, J.J. (1990) Wavelength discrimination at detection threshold, *Journal of the Optical Society of America*, A **7**, 733–742.

POKORNY, J. (1991) Color appearance and color constancy. In: Gouras, P. (Ed.) *The Perception of Color*, Basingstoke: Macmillan, pp. 43–61.

SANDELL, J.H., GROSS, C.G. & BORNSTEIN, M.H. (1979) Color categories in macaques, *Journal of Comparative Physiology and Psychology*, **93**, 626–635.

SCHEFRIN, B.E., ADAMS, A.J. & WERNER, J.S. (1991) Anomalies beyond sites of chromatic opponency contribute to sensitivity losses of an S-cone pathway in diabetes, *Clinical Vision Sciences*, **6**, 219–228.

TROOST, J. & DE WEERT, C.M.M. (1991) Naming versus matching in color constancy, *Perception & Psychophysics*, **50**, 591–602.

VALBERG, A. & LANGE-MALECKI, B. (1990) Colour constancy in Mondrian patterns: a partial cancellation of physical chromaticity shifts by simultaneous contrast, *Vision Research*, **30**, 371–380.

Walsh, V., Kulikowski, J.J,, Butler, S.R. Carden, D. (1992) The effects of lesions of area V4 on the visual abilities of macaque: colour categorization, *Behavioral Brain Research*, **52**, 81–89.

Walsh, V., Carden, D., Butler, S.R. & Kulikowski, J.J. (1993) The effects of lesions of area V4 on the visual abilities of macaque: hue discrimination and colour constancy, *Behavioral Brain Research*, **53**, 51–62.

Wild, H.M., Butler, S.R., Carden, D. & Kulikowski, J.J. (1985) Primate cortical area V4 important for colour constancy, but not wavelength discrimination, *Nature*, **313**, 133–135.

Zeki, S.M. (1980) The representation of colours in the visual cortex of rhesus monkey, *Nature*, **284**, 412–418.

Zeki, S.M. (1983) Colour coding in the cerebral cortex: the reaction of cells in monkey cortex to wavelengths and colours, *Neuroscience*, **9**, 741–765.

Surface Colour and Colour Constancy

A.P. Petrov

8.10.1 INTRODUCTION

In spite of the significant progress in colour science made over some 200 years, we still have no clear definition of colour agreed upon by all the researchers. Misunderstandings begin when any specific behaviour controlled by spectral characteristics of light is claimed as a proof of colour vision (Thomson *et al.*, 1990) and with attributing colour to light fluxes. Meanwhile, no employment of spectral 'devices' can be recognised as producing specific colour perception and there is a problem of exact bounding of the colour phenomena.

Here we consider colour as a phenomenon of the human visual field and attribute colour to surfaces of objects. It does not mean that colour is assumed to be perceptually equivalent to reflectance. The human visual system does not estimate reflectances and explicitly perceived colour is not a function of the reflectance alone (Gilchrist, 1977; Nikolaev, 1975).

The classical statement of the colour constancy problem refers to a certain range of illumination changes, the choice of which is often questionable (Maximov, 1984). Meanwhile there is a natural set of illuminant variations. They occur when a surface rotates or undergoes deformations in a scene with fixed illumination conditions (sources, etc). It is clear that such colour constancy under shape changes is absolutely necessary for adequate shape perception and this colour constancy is as perfect as the perceived shape is accurate.

To define surface colour a colourimetrical procedure is used as the basis of the construction and the colour space H in the following sections is a factor-space F/R of the real linear space F of light fluxes by an equivalence relation R established in colourimetry by definition. Note that H does not bear any natural metrics and so the colour space has an arbitrary structure.

8.10.2 ILLUMINATION SPACE

Usually the illumination is complex and depends not only on the geometry of light sources but also on the layout of all reflecting surfaces. To describe the illumination conditions we use a new approach to the task.

Let us place a small white Lambertian sphere at some point P of the scene and measure the intensity, $I(n; P,\lambda)$, of the light scattered from different parts of this probe sphere. Here λ and n, as usual, denote the wavelength of light and the normal vector on the sphere.

It is important that for a scene illuminated by a combination of a diffuse source and a set of arbitrarily located and spectrally different point sources, $I(n; P,\lambda)$ is a spherical function of a special kind

$$I(n; P, \lambda) = s(P, \lambda) \cdot n + I^d(P, \lambda) \tag{1}$$

for each region G of the probe sphere illuminated by the same set of the sources visible from all points of the region, the last term is a diffused light component. Note that illuminations of equation (1) form a three-dimensional family of spectral functions independently of the number and spectral quality of the light sources. This fact allows us to expect a relation between the dimensions of the regular physical and colour spaces.

Instead of using spectral energy distributions, we can write the illumination formulae as a vector-function mapping our probe sphere into the colour space

$$h(n; P) = H_0 \cdot n + h_0^d \tag{2}$$

where h, h_0^d are vectors in the colour linear space H and H_0 is a 3×3 matrix. The matrix H_0 depends on P and n but is constant as a function of n in each region G.

8.10.3   IMAGE IRRADIANCE EQUATION AND SURFACE COLOUR

In the above section describing the illumination, we used a standard probe body, the white Lambertian sphere. It is obvious that if instead we take another uniformly coloured spherical surface, we get the same formula with different matrix H_0 and vector h_0^d

$$h(n; P) = H \cdot n + h^d \tag{3}$$

The function $h(n; P)$ on the left-hand side of equation (3) can be thought of as a colour image after substitution of co-ordinates in the retina for the variable P and, hence, equation (3) is the image irradiance equation for the case of colour image and complex illumination

$$h(x,y) = H \cdot n(x,y) + h^d \tag{4}$$

Here, x,y are co-ordinates in the image h; the normal vector n of the surface is the function of x and y.

By definition, let us call *surface colour* the matrix C in the following equation

$$C \cdot H_0 = H \tag{5}$$

C is the colour matrix defined in Petrov (1984, 1993) as a mapping $H \to H$, which describes changes in colour images when the white surface is substituted with the coloured one. The black surface will obviously have the null colour matrix and the white one will get the unit matrix independently of the basis in the colour space.

Equation (4) is analogous to the image irradiance equation of Horn (1985) but written for complex colour illumination, colour objects and with psychophysical variables. Let us make a note about the left-hand side of equation (4), i.e. the image h(x,y). In biological visual systems the cell responses are non-linear for photopic stimuli and moderate contrasts. Hence, it makes no sense to consider the retinal response as an element of a linear space, and we prefer to define the input image as the results of a colourimetric procedure carried out upon the scene.

Using reflectances of samples as functions of wavelength and characteristics of the standard viewer, one can calculate colour matrices of these samples. Figure 8.10.1 shows the reflectances of differently coloured papers and the corresponding colour matrices for the samples. The data for calculations were taken from Judd and Wyszecki (1975).

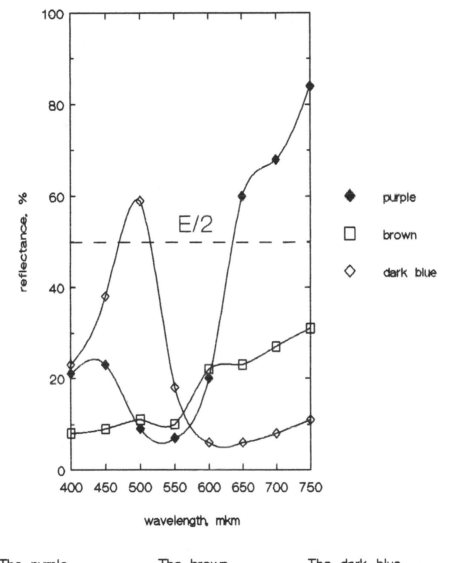

The purple	The brown	The dark blue
0.65,−0.44, 0.02	0.30,−0.14, 0.00	−0.30, 0.24, 0.01
0.16, 0.01, 0.01	0.10, 0.06, 0.00	−0.19, 0.43, 0.02
0.05,−0.06, 0.21	0.00, 0.00, 0.10	−0.11, 0.14, 0.46

Figure 8.10.1. Reflectances and colour matrices.

8.10.4   THE COLOUR SET AND COLOUR CONSTANCY

From equation (5) it follows that we define the surface colour as a linear operator acting in the colour space. To each surface patch there corresponds its colour, i.e. a numeric colour matrix C. The set of surface colours is a region in the corresponding space of matrices. It can be easily shown that:

- the elements $c_{i,j}$ of the colour matrix are bounded;
- the colour set is convex;
- the colour set is symmetrical with the centre E/2;
- the dimension of the colour set is nine;
- there is a partial order relation in the colour set;
- there is no natural metric in the colour set.

In the study by Petrov (1993), it is shown that the colour set represents all the perceived colours adequately. This means that any two surfaces with equal colour matrices look alike for a viewer with normal colour vision and vice versa two samples looking the same colour have equal colour matrices. The proof (omitted here) is based on the assumption of perfect constancy of colour perception for the scenes of the following types:

1. the scene consists of uniformly coloured matt spherical bodies against no background (the black background); all the spheres are the same size;
2. there is a white sphere in the scene located in a known position;
3. illumination is produced by three far pointwise light sources, controlling intensities that cover all variants of coloured illumination;
4. contribution of inter-reflections into illumination is not significant.

Scenes of this type preclude any 'recognition' of colour based on shape differences of objects but on the other hand in such scenes there are still enough clues for computation of the correct (constant) colours. We admit, of course, that we do not have an experimental proof that would show the colour constancy in these scenes and in reality our assumption may not be accurate or valid. The idea of the proof consists in analysis of visible changes in such scenes caused by replacements of spherical surfaces observed with other ones of different or the same colour. This analysis can be easily performed for the set of scenes formalised above.

Also, it is concluded from the consideration that the surface colour sets obtained in the scenes illuminated by linear combinations of different 3D spaces of illumination are the same, i.e. by means of transition to a new illumination space we cannot evoke perception of a colour that could never be perceived under the former 3D illumination.

8.10.5   ON METRICS IN THE COLOUR SET

The concept of surface colour outlined in the above sections allows us to reconsider metrics in the colour space. Literature on the perception of lightness (Arend and Goldstein, 1987; Hurlbert, 1989; Land and McCann, 1971) makes the topic important and interesting.

If it were possible to introduce metrics into the conventional colour space H, we could easily define the norm in the surface colour set

$$\|C\| = \overset{max}{_h} \|C \cdot h\| / \|h\| \qquad (6)$$

Such a norm of surface colour can be called *lightness*. It estimates the fraction of energy reflected by the surface under optimal illumination. The 'white' chromatic class ($det C \neq 0$)

contains surface colours with different norms or lightnesses. It is convenient to select as the basic white sample a surface with the largest norm. Then other samples will have norms $\|C\| < 1$. Note that the norm of the basic white always equals one and the norm of the black is zero.

It is well-known that there is no natural global metric in the colour space H. Nevertheless, we consider two ways of introducing a norm into the colour space.

The first way to define norm in H is to return to the linear space of the light fluxes and for each vector $h \in H$ select the colourimetrically equivalent light with minimal energy. The value of this energy can be used as a norm. Then the difference between two vectors h_1 and h_2 is measured by the minimal total energy of two light fluxes, the additions of which make h_1 and h_2 colourimetrically equivalent. Consistency of this definition can be easily proved but, unfortunately, we cannot find any arguments supporting it in colour perception.

The other way of metricising the colour space seems more promising. We shall not try to define a universal metric in H. Instead, we shall construct an induction of the metrics in the ordinary physical space of the scene on H and hence, the obtained metrics in H relate to the corresponding scene only and it will change if the scene or illumination conditions change.

Let us define

$$\|h\| = \min_{n} \{k : k \geq 0, h = k \cdot H_0 \cdot n\} \tag{7}$$

as the *norm* in H. It can be easily shown that this norm is invariant under transformations of the basis in H and the norm is defined over all the image of the scene. Obviously, if $det H_0 \neq 0$ then it follows from the definition that $\|H_0 \cdot n\| = 1$ and, using equation (6) for the norm (lightness) of surface colour we can write

$$\|C\| = \max_{n} \|C \cdot H_0 \cdot n\| \tag{8}$$

The above metrics (the ratio k) in H correspond to measuring differences of some colour vectors by the value of the minimal angle between two equally coloured surface patches producing these colour vectors in the scene. To consider the case of different chromaticities let h_1 and h_2 be two colour vectors corresponding to points n_1 and n_2 on the probe sphere

$$h_1 = H_0 \cdot n_1 + h_0^d$$

and

$$h_2 = H_0 \cdot n_2 + h_0^d$$

Now we can measure the distance between h_1 and h_2 by the value of the angle between n_1 and n_2. If the mapping of the sphere into H is of a one-to-one type, the defined function is a metric on the image of this mapping. More general cases can be analysed and no major problems are anticipated.

It means that if we adjust several sequent rectangular chips from, for instance, the Munsell Neutral Value Scale whose steps keep the above difference constant then an observer will see a homogeneously coloured surface of a prism with equal angles between its faces. And vice versa, if asked to set the brightness of a face of the prism simulated on a screen to make the prism look right and uniformly coloured the observer does it in accurate correspondence with the Scale.

We can conclude a deep relation of the structure of the colour space and the structure of the encompassing physical space and that not only the dimension of the colour space should be explained by the dimension of the physical space but also its metrical structure arises from the metrics of the physical space.

8.10.6 ACKNOWLEDGEMENTS

The author is indebted to N.D. Nuberg and A.L. Yarbus for stimulating his interest in colour; heartfelt thanks to J.J. McCann and A.C. Hurlbert for inspiring discussions and help; for friendly and careful criticism, thanks to M.H. Brill (1991); thanks to A. Gilchrist and L. Arend for helpful discussions on lightness and colour perceptions. He thanks his colleagues A. Prussakov, A. Akhriev, G. Antonova for help in the experimentations and A. Bonch-Osmolovski for improving the manuscript.

8.10.7 REFERENCES

AREND, L.E. & GOLDSTEIN, R. (1987) Lightness models, gradient illusions, and curl, *Perception and Psychophysics*, **42**, 65–80.

BRILL, M.H. (1991) Photometric models in multispectral machine vision. In: Rogowitz, B.E., Brill, M.H. & Allebach, J.P. (Eds) *Human Vision, Visual Processing and Digital Display II*, SPIE-91, **1453**, 369–80.

GILCHRIST, A.L. (1977) Perceived lightness depends on perceived spatial arrangement, *Science*, **195**, 185–87.

HORN, B.K.P. (1985) *Robot Vision*, MIT Press and McGraw-Hill.

HURLBERT, A. C. (1989) The computation of color, MIT Artificial Intelligence Laboratory, Technical Report 1154.

JUDD, D.B. & WYSZECKI G. (1975) *Color in Business, Science and Industry*, New York: J. Wiley & Son.

LAND, E.H. & MCCANN, J.J. (1971) Lightness and retinex theory, *Journal of the Optical Society of America*, **61**, 1–11.

MAXIMOV, V.V. (1984) *Color Transformations Under Changing Illumination*, Moscow: Nauka (in Russian).

NIKOLAEV, P.P. (1975) Algorithms for recognition of surface colors. In: *Models of Learning and Behavior*, Moscow: Nauka, pp. 121–151 (in Russian).

PETROV, A.P. (1984) Structure of the set of perceived colors, Preprint IAE N 4050/15, Moscow, Kurchatov Institute of Atomic Energy (in Russian).

PETROV, A.P. (1993) Surface color and color constancy, *Color, Research and Application*, **14**(4), 236–240.

THOMSON, E., PALACIOS, A. & VARELA, F. (1990) Ways of Coloring, Rapport N9008 B, Groupe de Recherche sur la Cognition, Ecole Politechnique, Paris.

Age-related Changes in Saturation of Non-spectral Lights

James M. Kraft and John S. Werner

8.11.1 INTRODUCTION

In one sense, the data presented here on age-related changes in the saturation of non-spectral lights are quite unremarkable, but in another sense they are quite surprising. The data are unremarkable in that lights of higher colourimetric purity appeared to be more saturated. Colourimetric purity is a physical correlate of saturation, so this result merely represents veridical perception. The result is quite surprising, however, in that short-wavelength lights equated in colourimetric purity at the retina were perceived as more saturated by older observers, or more precisely, by individuals with denser ocular media. This finding suggests that the visual system has information concerning its own sensitivity to short-wavelength light, and further, that it uses this information to partially compensate for any discrepancy from the norm. This behaviour is strikingly similar to colour constancy, a process by which the visual system codes the colour of an object consistently despite illumination changes that dramatically alter the spectral power distribution it reflects. Previous research from our laboratory has demonstrated compensation for age-related increases in the density of the ocular media in other contexts as well.

Colour constancy across the life span requires compensation for age-related increases in ocular media density known from many studies (Mellerio, 1971; Pokorny *et al.*, 1987; Weale, 1988; Werner, 1982). Figure 8.11.1 shows estimated ocular media density spectra for an average 20-year-old (solid curve) and 80-year-old (dashed curve) based on model fits to heterochromatic flicker photometry (HFP) data (Kraft and Werner, 1994). Between these ages, the density of the ocular media increases by an average of 1.3 log units at 420 nm, and by 0.3 log units at 500 nm. To achieve the same retinal illuminance, a 420-nm light must be 20 times more intense for an average 80-year-old than for an average 20-year-old, while a 500 nm light must be two times more intense. These data agree well with Weale's (1988) measurements from excised lenses. Analysis of heterochromatic brightness matching data from the same observers showed a smaller reduction in brightness sensitivity than would have been predicted by the reduction in retinal illuminance. The retinal brightness sensitivity of lights from 420-560 nm increases by 0.05 log unit per decade. Over a 60-year period, this sensitivity increase is equivalent to 0.3 log units, a factor of two. As a result of this enhancement, brightness sensitivity to 420 nm at the cornea falls by a factor of seven

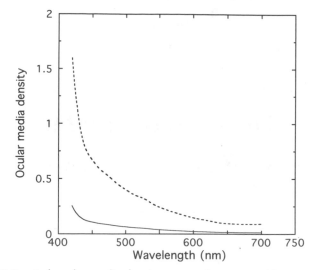

Figure 8.11.1. Estimated ocular media density spectra for average 20-year-olds (solid curve) and 80-year-olds (dashed curve) as determined by Kraft and Werner (1994).

instead of 20, while brightness sensitivity at 500 nm is roughly constant instead of falling by a factor of two. The sensitivity enhancement partially compensates for the reduction in available short-wavelength light, and therefore provides some degree of colour constancy over the life span.

Werner and Schefrin (1993) provide further evidence for colour constancy across the life span. Observers adjusted the proportion of unique blue light in a mixture with unique yellow light so that the mixture appeared achromatic. The proportion of unique blue light in the achromatic mixture did not change significantly with age, although a sizable change would have been expected given the aforementioned increases in ocular media density. This result suggests that a compensatory process preserves the blue-yellow hue balance of chromaticities around the achromatic point. If there were no compensation, a broadband light that appears achromatic to a younger observer would appear progressively more yellow with age, but this does not occur. Given that the brightness of short wavelength lights and that the hue of certain broadband lights tend to be maintained across the life span, one might also expect the saturation of pale violet and blue lights to be enhanced relative to increasing ocular media density. A method expected to be sensitive to a compensatory process was devised to test this hypothesis.

Observers scaled the saturation of mixtures of broadband and monochromatic light. Monochromatic light intensities were determined by each observer's HFP function. The mixture lights were composed of 200 td of broadband light and 50 td of monochromatic light. Because the retinal illuminance of the spectral lights was equated by HFP, each set of mixture lights was physically different, but provided an approximately equivalent physical stimulus at the observer's retina. These lights could be said to have a *retinal* colourimetric purity of 20 per cent for the observer who scaled them. If the saturation of violet and blue lights were not enhanced over the life span by a compensatory process, then under these conditions, scaled saturation functions from older observers should be similar to those of younger observers because the test lights were equated at the retina. If older observers compensate for their higher ocular media densities and perceive the lights as they are at the cornea rather than at the retina, however, then they should perceive the violet and blue lights as more saturated. A positive result is evidence for compensation, therefore, even though it merely indicates that lights of higher colourimetric purity were perceived as more saturated. This method is sensitive to the existence of a compensatory mechanism, but it does not specify the magnitude of the compensation in physical terms.

8.11.12   METHODS

8.11.2.1 Observers

In this paper, we present preliminary data from 11 younger observers (six female and five male, average age 28 years, range 20–42 years) and 10 older observers (five female and five male, average age 74 years, range 64–87 years). Observers reported no history of ocular disease. The American Optical HRR pseudoisochromatic plates, the Farnsworth Panel D-15 test, the F-2 plate, and the Neitz anomaloscope indicated the observers to be normal trichromats. Older observers were also screened by funduscopic examination.

8.11.2.2 Stimuli

Stimuli were presented foveally in Maxwellian view to one eye as 1.5 s flashes with 3 s interstimulus intervals. The stimuli were circular, with a diameter of 1.2° of visual angle. A wavelength range of 420–700 nm was covered, and the stimuli were composed of broadband and monochromatic light as specified earlier.

8.11.2.3 Apparatus

Stimuli were created by two channels of a conventional Maxwellian-view optical system. A holographic grating monochromator (Instruments SA, Model H-20, 8-nm bandpass at half power) produced monochromatic light. The final Maxwellian-view image was 2.0 mm in diameter. Observers were aligned using a bite-bar assembly and an adjustable chair so that the pupil, viewed through an auxiliary optical system, was centred with respect to a reticle aligned to the optical axis of the Maxwellian-view system. Optical corrections, if needed, were provided by appropriately selected spherical lenses or the observer's own spectacles (if transparent). HFP measurements from Kraft and Werner (1994) were used when possible. For observers who had not participated in the previous experiment, the same apparatus and methods were used to measure HFP sensitivity.

Spectral lights, neutral density filters and wedges were calibrated radiometrically with a silicon photodiode and linear readout system (United Detector Technology, 81 Optometer) calibrated relative to standards traceable to the National Institute of Standards and Technology. A Minolta photometer (LS-100) was used for photometric calibration, and retinal illuminance was computed by the method of Westheimer (1966). Other details of apparatus calibration are given elsewhere (Kraft and Werner, 1994).

8.11.2.4 Procedures

While dark adapting for 10 minutes, observers were told that they would see coloured lights, and were asked to rate the saturation of the lights as a percentage of chromatic colour in relation to the total chromatic plus achromatic sensation. Twelve practice trials were performed to ensure that observers understood the task and were performing it consistently.

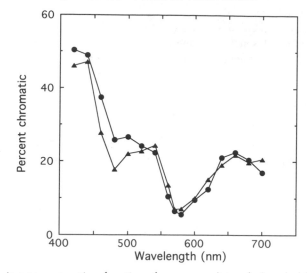

Figure 8.11.2. Average saturation functions for younger (triangles) and older (circles) groups.

Each mixture was scaled twice. The 16 test lights were presented in a random order, and then again in the opposite order after a short break. The logit transformation, which equalises variances by weighting percentages near 100 and zero more heavily than percentages near 50, was used to average the ratings for each wavelength, and for all subsequent averages and statistical tests (Judd and McClelland, 1989).

8.11.3 RESULTS

Figure 8.11.2 shows average saturation for the younger (triangles) and older (circles) observers plotted as a function of wavelength. Both functions have the typical shape of a

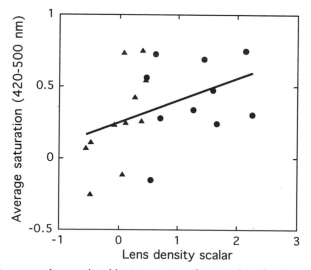

Figure 8.11.3. Average of normalised logit saturation for wavelengths from 420–500 nm plotted as a function of wavelength for younger (triangles) and older (circles) observers. The solid line displays the linear regression equation.

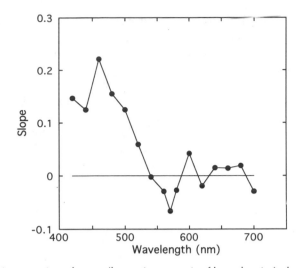

Figure 8.11.4. Logit saturation change (log units per unit of lens density) plotted as a function of wavelength. The horizontal line at zero indicates no age-related change.

saturation function (see Kaiser *et al.*, 1976) with a maximum at short wavelengths, a shoulder around 500 nm, a minimum at about 580 nm, and a somewhat higher plateau at longer wavelengths. The functions cover a range of 10–1, from roughly 5–50 per cent. Saturations for wavelengths from 420–500 nm are somewhat higher for the older group, suggesting the predicted enhancement of short-wavelength saturation for older observers. As presented in this figure, however, the difference does not appear terribly robust.

To analyse the short-wavelength difference, each observer's data were normalised to an average value over the range 620–700 nm. This normalisation corrects for overall differences in the functions without obscuring differences at short wavelengths. Figure 8.11.3 shows normalised saturation averaged over 420–500 nm for each observer plotted as a function of the ocular media density estimated from the observer's HFP function (see

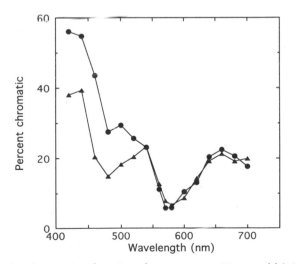

Figure 8.11.5. Extrapolated saturation functions for an average 20-year-old (triangles) and 80-year-old (circles). See text for a description of how these functions were derived.

Kraft and Werner, 1994 for a discussion of this method). Circles represent older observers, and triangles represent younger observers. The solid line shows the best-fitting linear regression. The observed change in short-wavelength saturation as a function of ocular media density is marginally significant ($r = 0.42$, $p < 0.06$). Figure 8.11.3 also suggests that the rather small difference between the younger and older groups may be due to the fact that four of the older observers (plotted as circles) have ocular media densities that are more similar to those of the younger observers than to others in their own age group. This unlucky coincidence, while not surprising given known individual variation in ocular media density, dilutes the difference between the age groups.

Figure 8.11.4 shows the estimated change in saturation corresponding to a unit change in ocular media density at each wavelength. Only the third point (460 nm) is statistically different from zero ($r = 0.50$, $p < 0.02$), but the uniformity of six contiguous positive slopes at wavelengths of 420–520 nm suggests that they are not spurious. The best estimates of the slope are roughly zero at longer wavelengths. These slopes provide further evidence for an increase in short-wavelength saturation to compensate for increasing ocular media density.

Figure 8.11.5 shows extrapolated saturation functions for observers with ocular media densities of an average 20-year-old (triangles) and 80-year-old (circles), as determined by Kraft and Werner (1994). These ocular media densities fall at the extremes of the distribution of densities found in the present experiment, so differences between the saturation functions of the younger and older groups are magnified. The functions shown in Figure 8.11.5 were derived from the data gathered in this experiment by substituting ocular media densities for average 20- and 80-year-olds into regression equations specifying saturation as a function of ocular media density. The slopes of these regression equations were presented in Figure 8.11.4. Figure 8.11.5 more clearly shows that short-wavelength lights that are equated at the retina appear more saturated for observers with higher ocular media densities. These observers must be compensating for their higher ocular media densities in order to perceive the lights as do others with lower ocular media densities.

This result demonstrates a third aspect of a compensation mechanism maintaining colour constancy over the life span relative to increasing ocular media density. These three aspects all concern different visual dimensions and different parts of chromaticity space. The brightness of short-wavelength lights is enhanced at the spectrum locus; the hue balance of chromaticities around the achromatic point is maintained; and the saturation of pale violet and blue lights is enhanced at intermediate points between the spectrum locus and the achromatic point. The relation of compensatory mechanisms to the aging process becomes clearer when all of these aspects are considered as a whole.

8.11.4 ACKNOWLEDGEMENTS

Supported by grant AG04058 from the National Institute on Aging.

8.11.5 REFERENCES

JUDD, C. & McCLELLAND, G. (1989) *Data Analysis: A Model Comparison Approach*, San Diego: Harcourt Brace Jovanovich.

KAISER, P.K., COMERFORD, J.P., & BODINGER, D.M. (1976) Saturation of spectral lights, *Journal of the Optical Society of America*, **66**, 818–826.

KRAFT, J.M. & WERNER, J.S. (1994) Spectral efficiency across the life span: flicker photometry and brightness matching, *Journal of the Optical Society of America*, **A11**, 1213–1221.

MELLERIO, J. (1971) Light absorption and scatter in the human lens, *Vision Research*, **11**, 129–141.

POKORNY, J., SMITH, V.C., & LUTZE, M. (1987) Aging of the human lens, *Applied Optics*, **26**, 1437–1440.

WEALE, R.A. (1988) Age and the transmittance of the human crystalline lens, *Journal of Physiology*, **395**, 577–587.

WERNER, J.S. (1982) Development of scotopic sensitivity and the absorption spectrum of the human ocular media, *Journal of the Optical Society of America*, **72**, 247–258.

WERNER, J.S. & SCHEFRIN, B.E. (1993) Loci of achromatic points throughout the life span, *Journal of the Optical Society of America*, **A 10**, 1509–1516.

WESTHEIMER, G. (1966) The Maxwellian view, *Vision Research*, **6**, 669–682.

Section 9 – Models of Colour Vision

Predicting Colour Appearance of Simple and Complex Stimuli

Mark D. Fairchild

9.1.1   INTRODUCTION

The accurate reproduction of colour images in different media has a number of requirements (Fairchild, 1994). One of the most notable is the need to specify and reproduce colour
appearance across a range of media and viewing conditions. This cannot be accomplished
using traditional colourimetry, which is only capable of predicting colour matches under
identical viewing conditions for the original and reproduction. When viewing conditions
such as the luminance level, white-point chromaticity, surround relative luminance, and
cognitive interpretation of the medium vary, a colour-appearance model is necessary to
predict the appropriate image transformation required to produce an image that closely
resembles the colour appearances of the original.

The RLAB colour-appearance space was developed by Fairchild and Berns (1993) for
cross-media colour reproduction applications in which images are reproduced with differing white points, luminance levels, or surrounds. Since its development, the RLAB space
has been subjected to an extensive series of psychophysical comparisons with other colour-
appearance models. This chapter reviews the RLAB space, briefly describes the results of
some visual evaluations of its performance, and outlines the derivation of a revised version
of RLAB. The revisions result in a simpler formulation of RLAB with performance equal
to or better than the original in all applications evaluated to date.

9.1.2   OVERVIEW OF RLAB

For a detailed derivation of the original RLAB equations, the reader is referred to Fairchild
and Berns (1993). A descriptive summary of the philosophy and implementation of the
RLAB colour-appearance space is given below.

RLAB was derived to have colour-appearance predictors similar to those of the CIELAB
colour space including lightness, L^R, redness-greenness, a^R, yellowness-blueness, b^R,
chroma, C^R, and hue angle, h^R. These appearance predictors are calculated using equations
virtually identical to the CIELAB equations after the stimulus tristimulus values are
transformed to the corresponding tristimulus values for a reference viewing condition

549

(D65, 318 cdm^{-2}, hard copy). The transformation is accomplished using a modified von Kries-type chromatic adaptation transformation previously formulated by Fairchild (1991). The end result is that the RLAB colour space is identical to (and takes advantage of the excellent performance of) the CIELAB colour space for the reference viewing conditions. However, for other viewing conditions, the more accurate chromatic-adaptation transform replaces the normalisation of tristimulus values inherent in the CIELAB equations.

The chromatic-adaptation transform utilised in RLAB has several unique features. The first is the capability to predict incomplete levels of chromatic adaptation that result in highly chromatic 'white-points' retaining some of their chromatic appearance. In addition, the incomplete-chromatic-adaptation feature can be turned on and off depending on whether or not cognitive 'discounting-the-illuminant' mechanisms are active. These mechanisms are active when viewing hard-copy images in an illuminated environment and inactive when viewing soft-copy images. A final unique feature is a matrix in the transformation that modelled interaction between the cone-types allowing the prediction of luminance-dependent appearance effects such as the Hunt effect.

Another feature of the RLAB model is that the power-function non-linearities in the CIELAB equations (cube root) are allowed to vary depending on the image-surround conditions. This is to model the change in image contrast caused by changes in the relative luminance of the image surround. For example, the dark surround in which projected slides are typically viewed causes the perceived contrast to be lower than if the same image luminances were presented in an average surround as is typical of a printed image.

9.1.3   VISUAL EVALUATION OF RLAB

A series of experiments have been undertaken to visually evaluate the performance of various colour-appearance models under a variety of viewing conditions using both complex stimuli (images) and simple colour patches. This section reviews and summarises the results of five such studies. The performance of the RLAB colour-appearance model relative to the other models in these experiments has provided a greater understanding of its relative strengths and weaknesses.

9.1.3.1 Print-to-print image reproduction

Experiment 1 examined the reproduction of printed images viewed under different light sources at different luminance levels. Details of this experiment were described by Kim *et al.* (1993). Four pictorial images were used in this experiment. The originals were viewed under a CIE illuminant A simulator at a luminance level (white) of 214 cdm^{-2}. Reproductions were viewed under fluorescent CIE illuminant D65 simulators at one of three different luminance levels (71, 214, and 642 cdm^{-2}). The reproductions were produced by applying colour-appearance transformations as described by each of eight models. The reproductions were viewed pairwise in every possible combination and 30 observers were asked to choose which image in each pair was a better reproduction of the original. The data were then analysed using Thurstone's Law of Comparative Judgements to derive interval scales of model performance. Confidence limits were also calculated about each of the scale values. The images were viewed using a successive-*Ganzfeld* haploscopic viewing technique (Fairchild *et al.*, 1994). The rank order of each model's performance (averaged over all images and conditions) is given in Table 9.1.1. Models that did not perform significantly differently than one another are given identical ranks. Only the data for the 5 appearance models common to all of the experiments is given in Table 9.1.1. In experiment 1, the RLAB, CIELAB, Hunt, and von Kries models all performed similarly, while the Nayatani model performed significantly worse. The other three models performed worse than each of these 5, which is why they were not included in further experiments.

9.1.3.2 Simple object-colour reproduction

Experiment 2 was virtually identical to experiment 1 with the exception that simple colour patches on grey backgrounds were used as stimuli rather than pictorial images. Details of this experiment were described by Pirrotta (1994). Ten different original colours, chosen to maximise differences between the appearance-model predictions, were used. The originals were viewed under a CIE illuminant A simulator at a luminance level (white) of 73 cdm^{-2}. Reproductions were viewed under fluorescent CIE illuminant D65 simulators at a luminance of 763 cdm^{-2}. Nine different colour-appearance transformations were evaluated using the same experimental procedure and analysis as experiment 1 and viewed via the successive-*Ganzfeld* haploscopic technique by 26 observers. The rank order of each model's performance (averaged over all colours) is given in Table 9.1.1. In experiment 2, the Hunt model performed significantly better than the others followed by the Nayatani, von Kries, and CIELAB models with similar performance. The RLAB model performed significantly worse than all of the other models in this experiment. It is of interest that the RLAB model performed best for pictorial images and worst for simple colour patches under similar experimental conditions.

Further analysis of the RLAB model showed that it introduced an unwanted shift in the lightness of the colour samples upon changes in luminance level. This resulted in the poor performance of RLAB for the simple colour patches. This problem was not apparent in the experiments using pictorial images because the lightness shift occurred for all of the image colours and the image contrast was properly reproduced. This deficiency in the RLAB model was traced to the C matrix, which models interactions between the cone types. The problem is corrected by removal of the C matrix in the revised formulation of RLAB given below.

9.1.3.3 Print-to-CRT image reproduction

Experiment 3 examined the performance of five colour-appearance transformations for reproductions of printed original images as CRT-displayed images. The experiment was carried out using five different viewing techniques to determine which was most appropriate for such comparisons (Braun and Fairchild, 1994). A memory-matching technique was determined to be the best. Thus, the memory-matching results are summarised below. Five different pictorial images were used as originals. In one session, the originals were

Table 9.1.1. Rank order of model performance in each of the four visual experiments

Model	Exp. 1	Exp. 2	Exp. 3	Exp. 4
RLAB (Fairchild and Berns, 1993)	1	5	1	1
CIELAB (CIE, 1986)	1	2	2	2
von Kries (1902)	1	2	3	2
Hunt (1994)	1	1	4	4
Nayatani *et al.* (1990)	5	2	5	(5)

viewed under a fluorescent CIE illuminant D50 simulator. In the second session, the originals were viewed under a CIE illuminant A simulator. The reproductions were viewed on a CRT monitor with CIE illuminant D65 white-point chromaticities. The luminance of white for all conditions was 75 cdm^{-2}. Both the originals and reproductions were viewed with white borders, grey backgrounds, and dark surrounds. Fifteen observers took part in this experiment. A paired-comparison experiment with data analysis similar to the first two experiments was used. The model-performance rank order (averaged over images and print white points) is given in Table 9.1.1. This experiment proved to be the most sensitive test of model performance with each model performing significantly differently than the others. The order of performance from best to worst was RLAB, CIELAB, von Kries, Hunt and Nayatani. The problems exhibited by RLAB in experiment 2 were not apparent in this experiment due to the use of equal luminance levels and complex images.

9.1.3.4 CRT-to-projected slide image reproduction

Experiment 4 was carried out in a manner similar to experiment 3. However, the original images were presented on a CRT display with white-point chromaticities of either CIE illuminant D65 at 53 cdm^{-2} or CIE illuminant D93 at 60 cdm^{-2}, and the reproductions were projected 35mm transparencies with a white-point correlated colour temperature of 3863K at a luminance of 109 cdm^{-2}. The CRT images were viewed in a dim surround of office lighting and the projected transparencies were viewed in a dark surround to test the models' abilities to predict surround effects. Fifteen observers completed the experiment. The data were collected using a memory matching technique and analysed in a way similar to the first three experiments. The Nayatani model was excluded from the psychophysical experiments as the images produced by it were clearly inferior to those produced by other models. The rank order results (averaged over three pictorial images) are given in Table 9.1.1. The RLAB model performed best followed by CIELAB and von Kries in a tie, and Hunt performed the worst of the models actually evaluated.

9.1.3.5 Image and colour dependence

It should be noted that the results described in this chapter are the overall average results for each experiment. There are many details worthy of further investigation in the complete results of each experiment. For example, the performance of the models is typically somewhat image dependent. Usually the rank order of the models remains approximately the same, but occasionally more drastic dependencies can be noted. For example, CIELAB performs poorly for blue hues. Thus, if an experiment were designed using images that all had a preponderance of blue, the performance of CIELAB would likely be much worse than indicated by the results summarised above. The same is also true for experiment 2 in which simple colour patches were used. The models' performance differed for the various colours investigated. This colour dependency is likely to be a major cause of the observed image dependency.

9.1.4　EVOLUTION OF RLAB

The RLAB model performs as well as, or better than, all of the other colour-appearance transformations in the experiments dealing with images. As the original objective in the derivation of RLAB was to develop a simple model that would perform at least as well as more complicated models in colour reproduction applications it seems that it has been successful. However, the poor performance of RLAB in experiment 2 highlighted a flaw in the model that could easily be corrected without affecting the good performance in the other experiments. In addition, further simplifications of the equations have been derived to allow easier implementation and inversion of the model (both necessary for imaging applications). This was accomplished by replacing the 'if-then' linear/power functions of the CIELAB equations with approximately equivalent simple power functions that do not require the 'if-then' implementation and its complex inversion. Further flexibility was added to RLAB by allowing the cognitive 'discounting-the-illuminant' mechanisms to be partially active. This is likely to be the case in situations such as large projected transparencies in a darkened room. Finally, the capability to express hue as percentage combinations of the unique hues was added to provide a more precise definition of perceived hue. These changes are detailed below in the new RLAB equations.

9.1.5   SUMMARY OF RLAB EQUATIONS

The following equations describe the forward implementation of the new RLAB equations. Changes are described as they are presented. One begins with a conversion from CIE tristimulus values ($Y = 100$ for white) to fundamental tristimulus values as illustrated in equations 1 and 2.

$$\begin{vmatrix} L \\ M \\ S \end{vmatrix} = \mathbf{M} \begin{vmatrix} X \\ Y \\ Z \end{vmatrix} \tag{1}$$

$$\mathbf{M} = \begin{vmatrix} 0.4002 & 0.7076 & -0.0808 \\ -0.2263 & 1.1653 & 0.0457 \\ 0.0 & 0.0 & 0.9182 \end{vmatrix} \tag{2}$$

The next step is calculation of the $\mathbf{A}$ matrix that is used to model the chromatic adaptation transformation.

$$\mathbf{A} = \begin{vmatrix} a_L & 0.0 & 0.0 \\ 0.0 & a_M & 0.0 \\ 0.0 & 0.0 & a_S \end{vmatrix} \tag{3}$$

$$a_M = \frac{p_M + D(1.0 - p_M)}{M_n} \tag{4}$$

$$p_M = \frac{(1.0 + Y_n^{1/3} + m_E)}{(1.0 + Y_n^{1/3} + 1.0/m_E)} \tag{5}$$

$$m_E = \frac{3.0(M_n/98.47)}{L_n/102.70 + M_n/98.47 + S_n/91.82} \tag{6}$$

The a terms for the short- (S) and long-wavelength (L) sensitive systems are derived in a similar fashion using analogous functions. Y_n is the absolute adapting luminance in cdm^{-2}. Terms with n subscripts refer to values for the adapting stimulus. The D factor was added in equation 4 to allow various proportions of cognitive 'discounting-the-illuminant'. D should be set equal to 1.0 for hard-copy images, 0.0 for soft-copy displays, and an intermediate value such as 0.5 for situations such as projected transparencies in completely darkened rooms.

After the **A** matrix is calculated, the tristimulus values for a stimulus colour are converted to corresponding tristimulus values under the reference viewing conditions using equations 7 and 8.

$$\begin{vmatrix} X_{ref} \\ Y_{ref} \\ Z_{ref} \end{vmatrix} = \textbf{RAM} \begin{vmatrix} X \\ Y \\ Z \end{vmatrix} \tag{7}$$

$$\textbf{R} = \begin{vmatrix} 186.01 & -112.95 & 21.98 \\ 36.12 & 63.88 & 0.0 \\ 0.0 & 0.0 & 108.89 \end{vmatrix} \tag{8}$$

The RLAB co-ordinates are then calculated using equations 9–13.

$$L^R = 100(Y_{ref}/100.00)^\sigma \tag{9}$$

$$a^R = 430[(X_{ref}/95.05)^\sigma - (Y_{ref}/100.00)^\sigma] \tag{10}$$

$$b^R = 170[(Y_{ref}/100.00)^\sigma - (Z_{ref}/108.88)^\sigma] \tag{11}$$

$$C^R = \sqrt{(a^R)^2 + (b^R)^2} \tag{12}$$

$$h^R = \tan^{-1}(b^R/a^R) \tag{13}$$

Equations 9–11 have been simplified as described above to avoid complexities in the implementation and inversion of the CIELAB-style equations. The exponents have changed slightly, but their ratios have remained the same. For an average surround $\sigma = 1/2.3$, for a dim surround $\sigma = 1/2.9$, and for a dark surround $\sigma = 1/3.5$. The hue composition, H^R, can be calculated via linear interpolation of the values in Table 9.1.2. These were derived based on the notation of the Swedish Natural Colour System (NCS). Example values are listed in Table 9.1.2 in italics. The inversion of the revised RLAB equations is straightforward.

9.1.6   COMPARISON OF NEW AND OLD RLAB EQUATIONS

To compare the new and old RLAB equations, a sample of 125 colours was generated (five levels each of X, Y and Z). The RLAB co-ordinates of each of these colours were calculated

Table 9.1.2.   Data for conversion from hue angle to hue composition

h^R	R	B	G	Y	H^R
24	100	0	0	0	R
0	*82.6*	*17.4*	*0*	*0*	*R17B*
270	*17.4*	*82.6*	*0*	*0*	*R83B*
246	0	100	0	0	B
180	*0*	*21.4*	*78.6*	*0*	*B79G*
162	0	0	100	0	G
90	0	0	0	100	Y
24	100	0	0	0	R

with both the old and new equations and then the RLAB (i.e. CIELAB) colour differences between the old and new predictions were calculated. For an average surround the mean colour difference was 6.18 units with a maximum of 12.17. The mean colour differences were 5.49 and 4.94 with maximums of 11.40 and 10.56 for dim and dark surrounds respectively. While these changes might seem large, they are not significant when compared to the inter-observer variability in colour-appearance judgements, which can often exceed 20 CIELAB units (Hunt and Luo, 1994), and the differences between similarly-performing colour-appearance models, which are even larger. It should also be noted that the gamut of the $5 \times 5 \times 5$ XYZ sampling (a simulation) far exceeds the gamut of physically realisable colours, thus producing a more rigorous comparison of the equations.

9.1.7 CONCLUSION

The RLAB colour-appearance space performs as well as, or better than, more complex appearance models in imaging applications. This is most likely to be due to the complex nature of image-colour appearance judgements in comparison with judgements of simple colour patches. The added complexity in other appearance models might be useful for predicting subtle colour-appearance effects. However, these effects are apparently masked in image judgements. The RLAB equations have been further simplified while at the same time improving their performance for all types of applications.

The Hunt model performed very well in experiment 2 on simple patches. Thus, it is surprising that it did not perform equally well in other situations. One reason for this is some ambiguity in deciding the values of the various parameters in the Hunt model for a particular application. The model was implemented exactly as published in the above experiments. However, it is clear that the Hunt model can perform as well as the RLAB model if its various parameters are optimised to the particular viewing conditions (Hunt and Luo, 1994). An advantage of the RLAB model is that its simplicity leaves little room for ambiguity in its implementation.

9.1.8 ACKNOWLEDGEMENTS

This research was supported by the NSF-NYS/IUCRC and NYSSTF-CAT Center for Electronic Imaging Systems.

9.1.9 REFERENCES

Braun, K. & Fairchild, M.D. (1994) Viewing environments for cross-media image comparisons, *IS&T's 47th Annual Conference/ICPS*, pp. 391–396.

CIE (1986) *Colorimetry*, CIE Publication 15.2, Vienna: CIE.

Fairchild, M.D. (1991) Formulation and testing of an incomplete chromatic adaptation model, *Color Research Applications*, **16**, 243–250.

Fairchild, M.D. (1994) Some hidden requirements for device-independent color imaging, *SID International Symposium*, pp. 865–868.

Fairchild, M.D. & Berns, R.S. (1993) Image colour-appearance specification through extension of CIELAB, *Color Research Applications*, **18**, 178–190.

Fairchild, M.D., Pirrotta, E. & Kim, T.G. (1994) Successive-Ganzfeld Haploscopic Viewing Technique for Color-Appearance Research, *Colour Research Applications*, **19**, 214–221.

Hunt, R.W.G. (1994) An improved predictor of colourfulness in a model of color vision, *Colour Research Applications*, **19**, 23–26.

Hunt, R.W.G. & Luo, M.R. (1994) Evaluation of a model of color vision by magnitude scalings: Discussion of collected results, *Color Research Applications*, **19**, 27–33.

Kim, T.G., Berns, R.S. & Fairchild, M.D. (1993) Comparing appearance models using pictorial images, *IS&T/SID Color Imaging Conference*, pp. 72–77.

Kries, J. von (1902) Chromatic adaptation, Festschrift der Albrecht-Ludwig Universität, Fribourg, (Translated by D.L. MacAdam (1970) *Sources of Color Science*, Cambridge, MA, MIT Press.

Nayatani, Y., Takahama, K., Sobagaki, H. & Hashimoto, K. (1990) Color-appearance model and chromatic adaptation transform, *Color Research Applications*, **15**, 210–221.

Pirrotta, E. (1994) Testing chromatic adaptation models using object colors, unpublished MS Thesis, Rochester Institute of Technology.

Coefficient Channels for Colour Constancy

Graham D. Finlayson and Brian V. Funt

9.2.1 INTRODUCTION

The mechanisms for achieving colour constancy are the source of much research and debate (D'Zmura and Lennie, 1986; Finlayson et al., 1993, 1994; Forsyth, 1990; Land, 1977; Land and McCann, 1971; Maloney and Wandell, 1986; West and Brill, 1982). Here we concentrate on the *coefficient* approach to colour constancy. Advocates of coefficient solutions believe that sufficient colour constancy can be achieved by applying simple scaling coefficients to the sensor responses. At the outset, we ally ourselves with this view and then proceed to consider the consequences. The coefficient approach in mathematical notation is as follows:

$$\begin{bmatrix} d_1 \\ d_2 \\ d_3 \end{bmatrix} = \begin{bmatrix} c_1 & 0 & 0 \\ 0 & c_2 & 0 \\ 0 & 0 & c_3 \end{bmatrix} \begin{bmatrix} p_1 \\ p_2 \\ p_3 \end{bmatrix} \tag{1}$$

here p_i denotes the response of the ith cone class for some surface viewed under an unknown illuminant. Each p_i is scaled by a coefficient c_i to discount the effect of the illuminant. The vector of components d_i, which we call a descriptor, describes illuminant-independent properties of the surface.

It has already been shown (D'Zmura and Lennie, 1986; West and Brill, 1982) that scaling coefficients applied to cone responses cannot account for illuminant change very accurately: equation (1) is a poor model for colour constancy. In this chapter we ask if this failure can be mitigated by first transforming the cone responses to a new basis before applying the scaling coefficients. We call the coupling of a change of sensor basis with equation (1) the *generalized coefficient model of colour constancy*:

$$\begin{bmatrix} t_{11} & t_{12} & t_{13} \\ t_{21} & t_{22} & t_{23} \\ t_{31} & t_{32} & t_{33} \end{bmatrix} \begin{bmatrix} d_1 \\ d_2 \\ d_3 \end{bmatrix} = \begin{bmatrix} c_1 & 0 & 0 \\ 0 & c_2 & 0 \\ 0 & 0 & c_3 \end{bmatrix} \begin{bmatrix} t_{11} & t_{12} & t_{13} \\ t_{21} & t_{22} & t_{23} \\ t_{31} & t_{32} & t_{33} \end{bmatrix} \begin{bmatrix} p_1 \\ p_2 \\ p_3 \end{bmatrix} \tag{2}$$

Computational methods are developed to find the *best* linear combination of the cones, the *coefficient channels*, for use in equation (2). We present experimental simulations that demonstrate that simple scalings applied to the coefficient channels provide excellent colour constancy. The experimental adequacy of the generalised coefficient model leads us to predict that the human visual system employs these coefficient channels. Indeed if the coefficient channels exist then they provide a plausible explanation for the results of many experimental, stimulus-response, studies (Foster, 1981; Foster and Snelgar, 1983a,b; Jaeger *et al.*, 1983; Kalloniatis and Harwerth, 1990; Sperling and Harwerth, 1971; Wyszecki and Stiles, 1982).

In section 9.2.2, we formalise the derivation of coefficient channels as a combinatorial optimisation problem. The experimental performance of the derived channels is examined in section 9.2.3. We relate our derived coefficient channels to experimental studies in section 9.2.4. The chapter finishes with some conclusions in section 9.2.5.

9.2.2   DERIVING COEFFICIENT CHANNELS

Our goal is to find linear combinations of the cone responses, the coefficient channels, which are *optimal* in the sense that equation (2) is a good model of illuminant change. It is well known (Forsyth, 1990) that, without restricting the spectral characteristics of either reflectance or illuminant spectra, equation (2) is a perfect model if and only if the transformed cone basis consists of three narrow-band sensors. Of course there does not exist a linear combination of the cones that are narrow-band. Therefore, to derive coefficient channels we simply set out to find the linear combination of cones that behaves most like a set of narrow-band sensors.

9.2.2.1 Colour response

The response of the cone with spectral sensitivity function $R_k(\lambda)$ to a reflectance $S(\lambda)$ illuminated by a spectral power distribution $E(\lambda)$ is equal to:

$$p_k = \int_\omega E(\lambda)S(\lambda)R_k(\lambda)d\lambda \ (k = 1,2,3) \qquad \text{(3 } Colour\ observation\text{)}$$

where the integral is taken over the visible spectrum ω. We call the 3-vector of cone responses, denoted $\underline{p}$, a *colour observation*. The product of reflectance multiplied by the illuminant, $E(\lambda)S(\lambda)$, is called a *colour signal*. The response of a narrow-band sensor set,

$\alpha_k\delta(\lambda - \lambda_k) \ (k = 1, 2, 3)$, will be called a *narrow observation*:

$$q_k = \int_\omega E(\lambda)S(\lambda)\alpha_k \ \delta(\lambda - \lambda_k)d\lambda = \alpha_k E(\lambda_k)S(\lambda_k) \ (k = 1,2,3)$$

$$\text{(4 } Narrow\ observation\text{)}$$

The scalars α_k mediate the sensitivity of the narrow-band sensors.

Let us assume that the visible spectrum can be represented adequately by samples taken 10nm apart over the range 400–700nm[1]. By adopting this convention, the integrals in equations (3) and (4) can be replaced by summations. Representing the response functions of the eye and narrow-band sensor sets as 31×3 matrices R and N and a colour signal by a 31-vector $\underline{c}$ we can rewrite equations (3) and (4) as:

$$\underline{p} = R^t\underline{c} \qquad\qquad\qquad\qquad (5)$$

$$\underline{q} = N^t\underline{c} \qquad\qquad\qquad\qquad (6)$$

where t is the transpose operation. Let the columns of the $31 \times n$ matrix C denote a calibration set of n colour signal spectra. The eye and narrow-band response to the entire calibration set are captured by the $3 \times n$ observation matrices P and Q:

$$P = R^t C \tag{7}$$

$$Q = N^t C \tag{8}$$

9.2.2.2 Optimal coefficient channels

Our goal is to find the linear transform of the cones, the coefficient channels, which behaves most like a narrow-band sensor set. However, we must take care in constructing our measure of similarity. For example, suppose we derived the coefficient channels that minimised the difference (maximised the similarity) defined in equation (9).

$$\|T_{i,j,k}P - Q_{i,j,k}\|_F \ (i,j,k \in , ..., 31) \ i \neq j, 1 \neq k, j \neq k \qquad (9 \ Naive \ formulation)$$

Here (and henceforth) the subscripts i, j, k denote wavelengths i, j and k; $Q_{i,j,k}$ is the observation matrix for the narrow-band sensor set with delta functions placed at i, j and k. $\|\cdot\|_F$ in (9) denotes the Frobenius norm – the square root of the sum of squares difference between $T_{i,j,k}P$ and $Q_{i,j,k}$; $T_{i,j,k}$ is a 3×3 matrix mapping the cone responses to the coefficient channels. Let $Q_{a,b,c}$ and $Q_{u,v,w}$ denote the observation matrices for two different sets of narrow-band sensors. Let us assume that:

$$\|T_{a,b,c}P - Q_{a,b,c}\|_F > \|T_{u,v,w}P - Q_{u,v,w}\|_F \tag{10}$$

Trivially there exists a scalar $\gamma, 0 < \gamma < 1$ such that:

$$\|T_{a,b,c}P - Q_{a,b,c}\|_F < \|\gamma T_{u,v,w}P - \gamma Q_{u,v,w}\|_F \tag{11}$$

A more serious problem with the measure defined in equation (9) lies in maintaining the full dimensionality of the data set under the transform $T_{i,j,k}$. Let us suppose that the rows in an observation matrix differ only by a scaling so that $Q_{i,j,k}$ has a rank of only 1. In this case the matrix $T_{i,j,k}$ minimising equation (9) will also have rank 1 and the 3-dimensional cone responses are mapped onto a 1-dimensional subspace.

Both the problem of trivial scaling and rank deficiency result from treating the row vectors of P and $Q_{i,j,k}$ as if they were fixed quantities. Rather they are simply the sensor responses for *a particular pair of sensor bases*. A more informed measure of similarity treats all possible vectors in the row spaces of P and $Q_{i,j,k}$ as equal. A useful tool in developing this notion of similarity is the projection operation π. The projection of a matrix X is defined as:

$$\pi(X) = X^t[XX^t]^{-1}X \tag{12}$$

For an arbitrary $n \times 1$ vector $\underline{v}$, the $n \times 1$ vector $\pi(P)\underline{v}$ is the vector in the row space of P, which is closest in the least-squares sense to $\underline{v}$. The projection of a matrix is independent of basis: $\pi(X) = \pi(MX)$ for arbitrary matrix M of full rank. This is a useful property given the definition of similarity. We say that the row spaces of matrices P and $Q_{i,j,k}$ are similar if $\pi(P)\underline{v}$ and $\pi(Q_{i,j,k})\underline{v}$ are *expected* to be similar.

Let Z denote an n-row matrix where each n-vector occurs with equal probability. Under the equi-probability assumption, the autocorrelation matrix of ZZ^t is equal to the $n \times n$ identity matrix I. The difference $d(P, Q_{i,j,k})$ between the row spaces of P and $Q_{i,j,k}$ is defined as:

$$d(P, Q) = \|[\pi(P) - \pi(Q)]Z\|_F \tag{13}$$

(the expected distance between $\pi(P)\underline{v}$ and $\pi(Q_{i,j,k})\underline{v}$). Our goal is to find the three narrow-band sensors that minimise this difference. In fact equation (13) can be rewritten independently of Z, using the well-known identity:

$$\|M\|_F^2 = trace(MM')$$

(14)

which yields

$$d(P,Q)^2 = trace([\pi(P) - \pi(Q)]ZZ'[\pi(P) - \pi(Q)]')$$

(15)

As, by assumption $ZZ' = I$, (15) can be rewritten as:

$$d(P,Q)^2 = trace([\pi(P) - \pi(Q)][\pi(P) - \pi(Q)]')$$

(16)

Using the identity in equation (14) in the reverse direction:

$$d(P,Q) = \|[\pi(P - \pi(Q)]\|_F$$

(17)

For a given calibration set C and a given set of narrow-band sensors it is easy to calculate P and $Q_{i,j,k}$ (equations (7) and (8)). Consequently the difference (or gap (Chatelin, 1993)) between the row spaces of P and Q defined in equation (17) can be computed. To find the optimal triplet of narrow-band sensors we must find the i, j and k, which minimise

$$d(P,Q_{i,j,k}) \ (i, j, k \in 1, ..., 31) \ i \neq j, 1 \neq k, j \neq k$$

(18 *The optimisation*)

Both matrices P and $Q_{i,j,k}$ are $n \times n$ making equation (17) and the whole optimisation appear computationally expensive. We show elsewhere (Finlayson and Funt, 1994), however, that equation (17) can be evaluated by simple operations on a pair of 3×3 matrices. Thus, even though there are $\binom{31}{3} = 4495$ distinct narrow band-sensor sets, the optimisation is readily solved.

While the minimisation based on equation (13) does not suffer from the trivial scaling or rank deficiency problem, it does not define a cone basis that will meet our goal of behaving like a set of narrow-band sensors. Such a basis is easily determined, however. If $N_{x,y,z}$ is the optimal set of narrow-band sensors then the least-squares fit mapping the cone observations to narrow observations defines the desired basis: equations (19) and (20).

$$TR'C \approx N'_{x,y,z}C$$

(19)

$$T_{x,y,z} = N'_{x,y,z}C\pi(R'C)C'R$$

(20)

The cones transformed by $T_{x,y,z}$ are the *coefficient channels*.

9.2.3 PERFORMANCE OF COEFFICIENT CHANNELS

For our calibration set we use the 426 Munsell spectra (Newhall *et al.*, 1943), multiplied by eight typical illuminants: five Judd (Judd *et al.*, 1964) daylight phases (D48, D55, D65, D75 and D100) and CIE standard illuminants A, B and C. Solving the general optimisation it was found that the optimal narrow-band sensors are positioned at 460nm, 540nm and 610nm. The derived coefficient channels are contrasted with the cones in Figure 9.2.1. In line with our intuition, the coefficient channels appear narrower.

Let us presuppose that the goal of colour constancy is to map colour responses under an arbitrary illuminant to those observed under a fixed canonical illuminant. We will consider three candidate mappings: the simple coefficient model (equation (1)), the generalised coefficient model (equation (2)) and the general linear model (equation (21)) defined below:

$$\underline{d} = M\underline{p}$$

(21 *General linear model*)

where M is *any* 3×3 bijective map. The general linear model must perform better than either the simple or generalised coefficient models and serves as a control for our simulations.

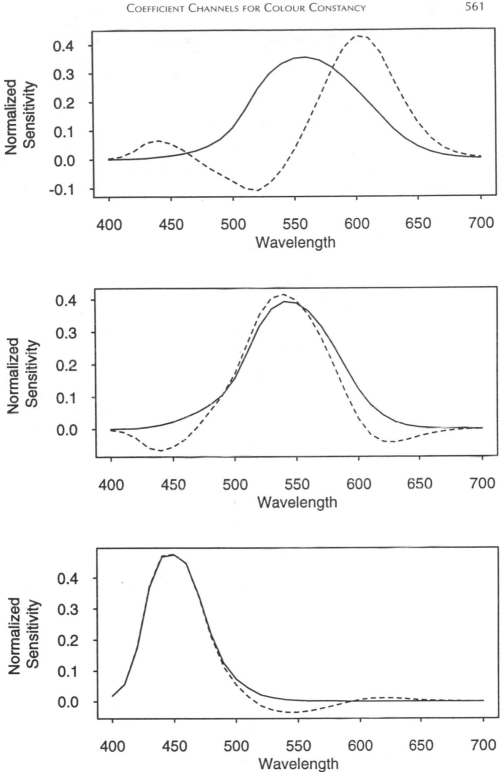

Figure 9.2.1. The cone sensitivities (solid lines) are contrasted with the coefficient channels (dashed lines).

Table 9.2.1. Theoretical performance limits on linear models of colour constancy.

Model	< 1	< 2	99% less than
Linear	82.2%	93.5%	$6\Delta_{Lab}$
Simple coefficient	41.3%	68.3%	$13\Delta_{Lab}$
Generalised coefficient	72.1%	90.0%	$8\Delta_{Lab}$

Under each of the eight illuminants the XYZ observations of the 462 Munsell reflectances (Newhall *et al.*, 1943) are calculated. Arbitrarily we choose D65 as the canonical illuminant. For each test illuminant we find the mappings minimizing the error norms:

$$\|H^{D65} - X^{-1}D^{test}XP^{test}\|_F \qquad (22 \text{ Simple coefficient})$$

$$\|H^{D65} - T^{-1}D^{test}TH^{test}\|_F \qquad (23 \text{ Generalised coefficient})$$

$$\|H^{D65} - M^{test}H^{test}\|_F \qquad (24 \text{ General linear})$$

where H denotes a matrix (here 3×462) of XYZ responses and the superscript denotes the illuminant. The superscript *test* is one of D48, D55, D75, D100, CIE A, CIE B, CIE C. The 3×3 matrix X takes the XYZ basis onto the cone basis so equation (22) provides a bound for the best performance possible using the simple coefficient rule. The 3×3 matrix T maps the XYZ sensors onto the coefficient channels so equation (23) bounds the performance of the generalised coefficient model.

Although we minimise equation (22) through equation (24) using a least-squares criterion, it is more informative to consider performance relative to a perceptual measure. We calculate the distance between each XYZ canonical descriptor and mapped counterpart using the CIELAB metric (Wyszecki and Stiles, 1982). For practical purposes (outside the laboratory) a CIELAB difference of 2 or less is not noticeable (Stokes *et al.*, 1992). We histogrammed the CIELAB errors for the complete set of test illuminants and summarise the results in Table 9.2.1 and Figure 9.2.2.

The general linear model performs very well; 93.5% of XYZ observations are mapped to within two CIELAB units of their D65 counterparts. Increase the error to six CIELAB units and 99 per cent of the data has been accounted for. The simple coefficient model performs much more poorly than the general model. Only 68.3 per cent of mapped cone observations are within two CIELAB units. Moreover for a 99 per cent fit the CIELAB error must be increased to 13 units. On the other hand, the performance of the coefficient channels is not much worse than that of the general linear model; 90 per cent are mapped to less than two CIELAB units and the 99 per cent threshold is reached at the eight CIELAB unit mark.

9.2.4   EXPERIMENTAL EVIDENCE FOR COEFFICIENT CHANNELS

The experiments of section 9.2.3 validated our initial hypothesis; a coefficient model provides a very good vehicle for colour constancy. This result would be of more interest if there were evidence of coefficient channels in the human visual system. Indeed this is the case and in this section we provide a brief review of the related stimulus-response experimental studies.

Stiles (Wyszecki and Stiles, 1982) endeavoured to determine the sensitivity of the human cones in his test- and field-spectral sensitivity experiments. The sensor (or π) mechanisms he isolated in his experiments correspond well with cone sensitivities derived by other means (e.g. colour matching experiments with dichromats (Wyszecki and Stiles, 1982)) and are in broad agreement with absorption functions of the cone photopigments (Bow-maker and Dartnall, 1980). However, his experiments also isolated mechanisms other than the cones. In Stiles' π_1 mechanism there is a peak around 600 nm that does not coincide with any of the cone peaks: 440, 540 or 570 nm. If, in fact, what the test-spectral sensitivity experiments isolated were coefficient channel mechanisms, then we would expect a peak around 600 nm.

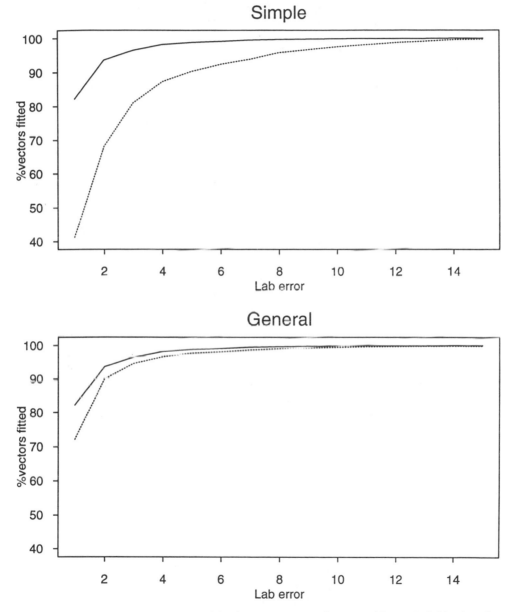

Figure 9.2.2. The graph at the top of the figure compares the general linear (solid line) and simple coefficient (dashed line) colour constancy models. CIE Lab error is plotted against the percentage of colour observations accounted for. The graph at the bottom of the figure compares the general linear and generalized coefficient (real calibration set).

The test-spectral sensitivity experiments of Sperling and Harwerth (1971) also appear to isolate mechanisms other than the cones. Their test-spectral sensitivity curves show a sharp peak around 610 nm and a notch (the trough between successive peaks) around 580 nm. Sperling and Harwerth suggest that this peak can be explained by a new mechanism formed by taking a linear combination of the cones. Our red coefficient sensor peaks at 610 nm and is dominant (most sensitive) at wavelengths greater than 580 nm with the green coefficient channel dominating at shorter wavelengths. This would be sufficient to explain both the peak at 610 nm and the notch at 580 nm. Sperling and Harwerth also observed a sharp peak (sharper than the green cone sensitivity) at 530 nm that can also be explained by the coefficient channels. More recently Foster (Foster, 1981; Foster and Snelgar, 1983a,b) has reported similar test- and field-spectral sensitivities.

If coefficient channels exist, and we could design an experiment to isolate them, we would expect their shape to be invariant to a change in the spectral power distribution of the illuminant (because colour constancy requires only a scaling of the coefficient channels). Jaeger et al. (1983) have measured spectral field sensitivities under changing illumination. In those experiments, illumination was changed by placing coloured filters in front of the eye. A similar test spectral sensitivity curve is measured under both a reddish and bluish illuminant. This curve, as before, matches well with our results; sharp peaks are recorded at 530 nm and 610 nm. We would also expect that the shape of the coefficient channels be invariant to the intensity of light entering the eye. Kalloniatis and Harwerth (1990) have measured test spectral sensitivities under white adapting fields of different intensity and found that the shape of the spectral sensitivity curve is maintained. Again this is in agreement with our coefficient channels.

9.2.5   CONCLUSION

We began with the hypothesis that there exists a linear combination of the cones – the coefficient channels – with respect to which a coefficient model is sufficient for colour constancy. Methods were developed to determine the cone combinations most consistent with this hypothesis. Simulation experiments indicated that derived coefficient channels provide an excellent vehicle for colour constancy based on a coefficient rule. Test- and field-spectral sensitivities obtained under many different experimental conditions are consistent with the derived coefficient channels.

9.2.6   NOTE

1 This assumption is routine and forms the basis for the linear systems approach to colour vision.

9.2.7   REFERENCES

BOWMAKER, J.K. & DARTNALL, H.J.A. (1980) Visual pigments of rods and cones in the human retina, *Journal of Physiology*, **298**, 501–511.

CHATELIN, F. (1993) *Eigenvalues of Matrices*, New York: Wiley.

D'ZMURA, M. & LENNIE, P. (1986) Mechanisms of color constancy, *Journal of the Optical Society of America*, **A 3**, 1662–1672.

FINLAYSON, G.D. & FUNT, B.V. (1994) Coefficient channels: Derivation and relationship to other theoretical studies, Simon Fraser University: School of Computing Science Technical Report.

FINLAYSON, G.D., DREW, M.S. & FUNT, B.V. (1993) Diagonal transforms suffice for color constancy. In *Proceedings of Fourth International Conference on Computer Vision*, IEEE Computer Society & European Vision Society, May.

FINLAYSON, G.D., DREW, M.S. & FUNT, B.V. (1994) Spectral sharpening: Sensor transformations for improved color constancy, *Journal of the Optical Society of America*, A 11(5), 1553–1563.

FORSYTH, D. (1990) A novel algorithm for color constancy, *International Journal of Computational Vision*, **5**, 5–36.

FOSTER, D.H. (1981) Changes in field spectral sensitivities of red-, green- and blue-sensitive colour mechanisms obtained on small background fields, *Vision Research*, **21**, 1433–1455.

FOSTER, D.H. & SNELGAR, R.S. (1983a) Initial analysis of opponent-colour interactions revealed in sharpened field sensitivities. In Mollon, J.D. & Sharpe, L.T. (Eds) *Colour Vision: Physiology and Psychophysics*, London, New York: Academic Press, pp. 303–312.

FOSTER, D.H. & SNELGAR, R.S. (1983b) Test and field spectral sensitivities of colour mechanisms obtained on small white backgrounds: action of unitary opponent-colour processes? *Vision Research*, **23**, 787–797.

JAEGER, W., KRASTEL, H. & BRAUN, S. (1983) An increment-threshold evaluation of mechanisms underlying colour constancy. In Mollon, J.D. & Sharpe, L.T. (Eds) *Colour Vision: Physiology and Psychophysics*, London, New York: Academic Press, pp. 545–552.

JUDD, D.B., MACADAM, D.L. & WYSZECKI, G. (1964) Spectral distribution of typical daylight as a function of correlated color temperature, *Journal of the Optical Society of America*, **54**, 1031–1040.

KALLONIATIS, M. & HARWERTH, R.S. (1990) Spectral sensitivity and adaptation characteristics of cone mechanisms under white-light adaptation, *Journal of Optical Society of America*, A 7, 1912–1928.

LAND, E.H. (1977) The retinex theory of color vision, *Scientific American*, **237** 108–129.

LAND, E.H. & McCANN, J.J. (1971) Lightness and retinex theory, *Journal of the Optical Society of America*, **61**, 1–11.

MALONEY, L.T. & WANDELL B.A. (1986) Color constancy: a method for recovering surface spectral reflectance, *Journal of Optical Society of America*, A, 29–33.

NEWHALL, S.M., NICKERSON, D. & JUDD, D.B. (1943) Final report of the OSA subcommittee on the spacing of the Munsell colors, *Journal of the Optical Society of America*, A 33, 385–418.

SPERLING, H.G. & HARWERTH, R.S. (1971) Red-green cone interactions in the increment-threshold spectral sensitivity of primates, *Science*, **172**, 180–184.

STOKES, M., FAIRCHILD, M.D. & BERNS, R.S. (1992) Precision requirements for digital color reproduction, *ACM Transactions on Graphics*, **11**(4), 406–422.

WEST, G. & BRILL, M.H. (1982) Necessary and sufficient conditions for von Kries chromatic adaption to give colour constancy, *Journal of Mathematical Biology*, **15**, 249–258.

WYSZECKI, G. & STILES, W.S. (1982) *Color Science: Concepts and Methods, Quantitative Data and Formulas*, New York: Wiley 2nd ed.

Colour Sensations in Honeybees?

Werner Backhaus

9.3.1 INTRODUCTION

The subjective colour space of the honeybee possesses two chromatic dimensions, comparable to our colour space, but has no brightness dimension. Also the geometry of the colour space of the bee is slightly different from the Euclidean geometry of the human colour space. The colour space of the bee possesses a city-block metric (Backhaus, 1987; Backhaus et al., 1987), i.e. the subjective difference between two colours is simply derived as the sum of the absolute differences on the two psychophysical scales (dimensions A and B). The two abstract scales A and B were found to be interpretable as the excitation values of the two spectral types of tonic colour opponent coding interneurons (Backhaus, 1991), which were exclusively found in the honeybee brain by intracellular recordings (Kien and Menzel, 1977).

The colour theory allows very precise prediction of the choice proportions of the bee in colour training experiments, just from the measured spectral light intensity distributions of the colour stimuli used (Backhaus, 1993). Further investigations showed that the colour space of the honeybee is indeed best represented by the two-dimensional colour opponent coding (COC) diagram spanned by the two excitation scales A and B of the two types of colour opponent coding neurons. Even the colour shifts due to greater light intensity changes, known from human colour vision as the Bezold-Brücke effect, were quantitatively accurately predicted to exist also in the bee (Backhaus, 1992a). This supports the results of earlier investigations on photoreceptor models that colour shifts in honeybees as well as in humans would be exclusively due to the non-linear transduction process of the photoreceptors (see Backhaus, 1987; Backhaus and Menzel, 1987). Also colour constancy, which occurs when the spectral composition of white light illumination of coloured plates is varied within certain limits, is explained in honeybees by colour theory to be exclusively due to adaptation of the photoreceptors to the average light reflected by the arrangement.

The colour theory describes colour vision and colour choice behaviour of the bee as exclusively related to the electrical excitations of the neuronal colour coding system. But, is the behaviour of the honeybee exclusively based on the electrical excitations of the neuronal system that codes colour information, or do honeybees possess colour sensations in addition, comparable to ours? The predictions from a quantitative model of colour sensations show that this question is answerable by multiple colour training experiments, if the bee indeed learns a specific unique-colour instead of the entire colour as a food signal. First results of double colour training experiments (Backhaus and Kratzsch, 1993) support the hypothesis that unique-colours and thus colour sensations also exist in honeybees. Furthermore, bee colour names are derived from the COC diagram in terms of the predicted unique-colours. For easier communication about bee colours, human 'false colour' names are derived in addition.

9.3.2   COLOUR OPPONENT CODING IN THE HONEYBEE

The honeybee brain contains about 850 000 neurons, of which approximately 450 000 are located in the optic lobes. The honeybee compound eye possesses three different spectral classes of photoreceptor cells that are most sensitive in the UV, blue, and green range (λ_{max}: 340 nm, 440 nm, and 550 nm). The bee is able to see in the UV range, which appears dark to us, but cannot discriminate lights at the longer wavelength scale, which appear reddish to us, from dark. Thus, the spectral range of colour vision in the bee (300–550 nm) appears to be shifted by about 100 nm to the shorter wavelengths. Although the transduction processes in vertebrates and invertebrates are quite different, the light intensity/potential functions of the bee photoreceptor cells (Lipetz, 1971) have the same form as in humans (Rodieck, 1973; Rushton, 1972). Photoreceptor cells of the same spectral class feed into respective monopolar cells (first interneurons), which mainly amplify the excitations (graded potentials) of the photoreceptor cells (Menzel, 1974; Ribi, 1987; de Souza et al., 1992). The monopolar cells feed into colour opponent coding cells via excitatory and inhibitory synapses (Kien and Menzel, 1977).

Colour vision and colour choice behaviour of the honeybee (*Apis mellifera*) worker is very well described by the theory of colour vision in honeybees (Backhaus, 1991, 1992a, 1993; see Figure 9.3.1). This is because the theory is based on: (1) the results of psychophysical (colour training and multiple colour choice) experiments performed with bees (Backhaus et al., 1987); (2) electrophysiological properties of photoreceptors of honeybees, i.e. spectral sensitivity (best estimates of measured functions, Backhaus, 1991; Menzel and Backhaus, 1991), and other insects, i.e. adaptation properties (Backhaus, 1987; Backhaus and Menzel, 1987); and (3) colour opponent coding interneurons (light intensity/ potential functions (Kien and Menzel, 1977)). The upper part (above dashed line) of Figure 9.3.1 is related to the physiology of the colour vision system, while the lower part represents the psychophysical model of colour vision. The complete mathematical description (right side) as well as the neuronal interpretation (left side) of the theory is presented. Also the psychophysical part of the theory (lower part, right side) allows for a complete interpretation by neurons with simple (linear) properties. The term $_Kd_{ij}$ represents a judgment value neuron which realises the city block metric by adding the results from pairs of (>0)-neurons. In the example, exclusively the two alternatives S_2 and S_3 are shown, and the rewarded stimulus s_1 is not presented to the bee. The judgement value neuron calculates the difference between the two colour differences between the excitation values A_1 and B_1 of the learned colour stored in memory and the excitation values A_2, A_3 and B_2, B_3 corresponding to the alternatives. If $_Kd_{ij}$ is greater than zero at the instant of decision, stimulus S_3 is chosen. If $_Kd_{ij}$ is less than zero, stimulus S_2 is chosen (from Backhaus, 1993, Figure 3).

9.3.3 THE MODEL OF COLOUR SENSATIONS IN HONEYBEES

Human colour sensations consist of six unique-colours: blue-yellow and red-green, and black and white (Hering, 1878, 1905). The many colour nuances we experience, differ only in the amounts of these six unique-colours. As blue-yellow and red-green are never simultaneously visible in any colour sensation, i.e. appear to exclude or oppose each other, these unique-colours are called opponent colours (indicated above by a hyphen). Thus, in

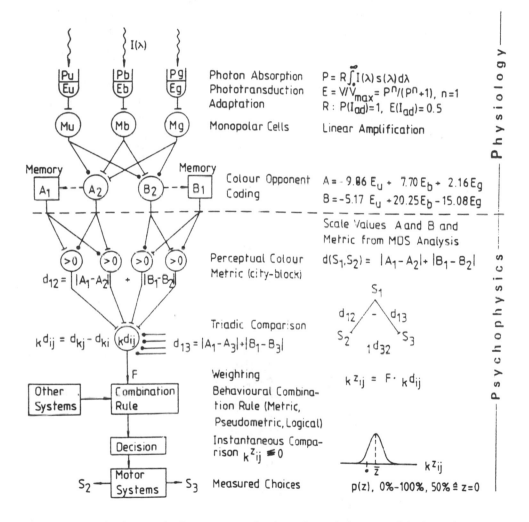

Figure 9.3.1. The theory of colour vision and colour choice behaviour of the honeybee. $I(\lambda)$, spectral light intensity distribution; u,b,g, photoreceptor cell types; R, range sensitivities; $s(\lambda)$, spectral sensitivity; P, absorbed photon flux; E, cell excitation; V, cell potential; M, monopolar cell; A,B, excitations of colour opponent coding neurons (circles: interneurons, boxes: memories); d_{ki}, colour difference of two stimuli S_k and S_{ij}; k_{ij}^d, judgment values of stimuli S_i and S_j with respect to the training stimulus S_k; F, experiment type dependent scaling factor; $_k d_{ij}$, weighted judgment values; p(z), inverse z-transformation to choice percentages p.

a first step, the colour theory for the bee was extended by the unique-colours hypothesis (Backhaus and Kratzsch, 1993; Backhaus, 1995). As colour vision in honeybees has no brightness dimension, only five unique-colours are postulated to exist, namely two pairs of chromatic opponent unique-colours, A^-/A^+, B^-/B^+, and one achromatic unique-colour 0. In human colour vision, the subjective colour space is equi-spaced in terms of the Munsell space as well as in terms of unique-colours (e.g. Hurvich and Jameson, 1956).

The concentric squares in Figure 9.3.2 represent loci of colours that are subjectively equi-distant from the centre point. The centre point is the locus of the adaptation light. As the COC diagram is equi-spaced, the difference between two arbitrary colours can be directly graphically derived just by counting the numbers of squares that are crossed by moving from one colour to the other on a straight line. The example shows that the graphical result is identical to the calculated sum of the absolute values of the differences ΔA and ΔB (from Backhaus, 1991, Figure 4).

As shown in Figure 9.3.2, in honeybees the two colour opponent coding neurons A and B span the equi-spaced two-dimensional colour opponent coding (COC) diagram. Thus, a linear relationship between the excitations of each of the two opponent coding neurons and the amounts of the unique-colours of each opponent pair of unique-colours is postulated (Backhaus and Kratzsch, 1993; Backhaus, 1995).

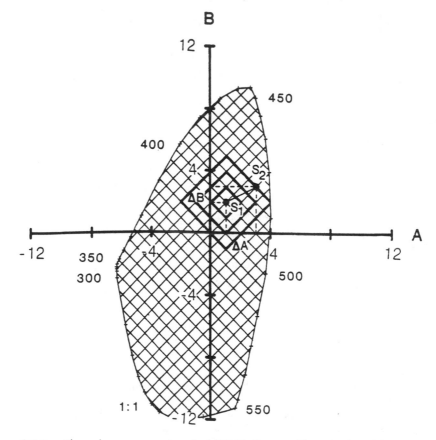

Figure 9.3.2.   The colour opponent coding (COC) diagram. The axes A and B represent the excitation values (relative spike frequencies) of the two types of colour opponent coding neurons.

The unique-colours hypothesis for the honeybee predicts colour sensations to consist of the pure unique-colours A^- or A^+ when neuron A shows minimum ($A = -12$) or maximum ($A = 12$) relative excitation and neuron B is at rest ($B = 0$). On the other hand, colour sensations consist exclusively of B^- and B^+ respectively when neuron B shows minimum ($B = -12$) or maximum ($B = 12$) relative excitation and neuron A is at rest ($A = 0$) (see Figure 9.3.3a). When both neurons are at rest ($A = 0$ and $B = 0$), which is only the case when the bee sees natural daylight or darkness, the corresponding colour sensation consists exclusively of the achromatic unique-colour 0. Intermediate excitations of the neurons A and B should lead to colour sensations that are mixed from three out of the five possible unique-colours.

It is assumed that pure chromatic colour sensations, i.e. 100 per cent A^- (B^-) and 100 per cent A^+(B^+), occur at the extreme excitation values -12 and 12. A pure achromatic sensation, i.e. 100 per cent 0, occurs only when both neurons show their resting potential, $A = B = 0$, which occurs when the bee is exposed to natural daylight or to darkness. For intermediate excitation values, the percentage of unique-colours can be directly read from the diagram. The piechart shows typical examples (A^-: dashed, A^+: black, and 0: white).

In Figure 9.3.3(b), the amounts of unique-colours are proportional to the relative excitation values A and B. The amount of achromatic grey in a colour sensation is assumed to be the complement to 100 per cent, as shown in the example. As far as the electrical excitation values A and B are considered, the colour loci of each of the concentric squares in the COC diagram are equally distant (city-block metric) from the achromatic centre point (see Figure 9.3.2). But, if the colour choice behaviour of the bee is related exclusively to one unique-colour, this is not at all the case. Moving along one side of a square shows that the amount of unique-colour changes drastically over the entire range of possible amounts from 0–100 per cent. This allows us to test the existence of unique-colours and thus colour sensations in bees, if the bee can be trained exclusively to one unique-colour.

9.3.4 COLOUR NAMES FOR COLOUR SENSATIONS IN HONEYBEES

It is suggested that the predicted colour sensations in bees are named, as in human colour vision, simply by composing the names of the respective unique-colours in increasing order of relative amount. $0\,A^-B^+$, for example, denotes a colour sensation in the bee that consists mainly of unique-colour B^+ and secondary of unique-colour A^-, which, in addition, is slightly achromatic 0, i.e. unsaturated. For quick and easy communication, it might be more convenient to denote bee colour sensations in terms of 'false colours' using human colour names for describing the lights that stimulate almost pure colour sensations, which consist mainly of one unique-colour. The 'false colour' names are obtained with the help of coloured cardboards (HKS, Hostmann-Steinberg) under daylight conditions, which possess colour loci closer to the ends of the axes of the COC-diagram (Figure 9.3.1). The following names might be used instead of the more accurate but abstract COC-nomenclature: A^-, UV; A^+, green; B^-, yellow; B^+, violet; and 0, grey (see Figure 9.3.3b). The colour sensation of the example above reads in this terminology: unsaturated UV-violet. The lines 45° to the axes of the COC diagram are the loci of 50:50 mixtures of two unique-colours and thus represent the predicted categorical boundaries for the dominant unique colour in a colour sensation. The 50 per cent grey square around the 0 point is the boundary for dominance of the achromatic unique-colour 0 (grey). It has to be pointed out that the predicted unique-

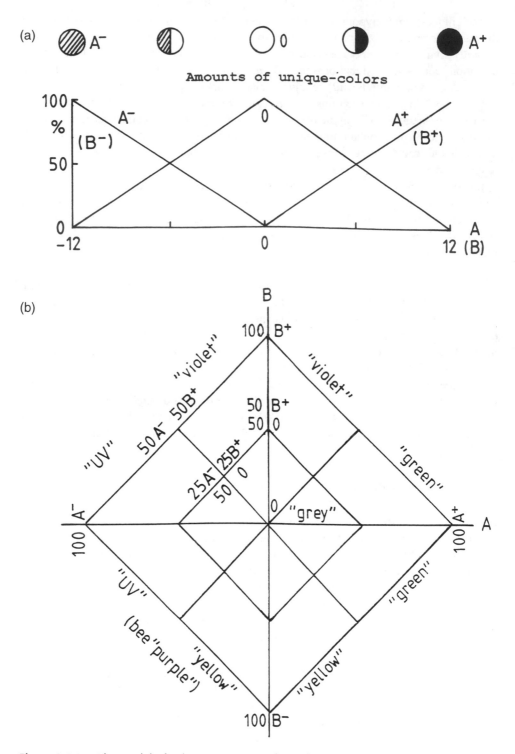

Figure 9.3.3. The model of colour sensations in honeybees. (a) The relationship between the amounts of unique-colours and the excitation values A and B. (b) The amounts of all five unique-colours are shown in the COC-diagram (see Figure 9.3.2).

colours in honeybees are most different from the colours caused by the monochromatic lights, for which the three photoreceptor cell types are most sensitive, because of the weighting of the colour opponent coding (COC) system. The crossing points of the spectral curve in Figure 9.3.2 and the axes A and B are the loci of (mixed) monochromatic lights (372 nm, 415 nm, 493 nm, and 7 per cent 300 nm and 93 per cent 550 nm; see Backhaus, 1992b) which affect only one of the two colour opponent coding neurons A and B and, thus, are predicted to cause colour sensations that consist only of one unique-colour and grey. Obviously, these four (mixed) monochromatic lights are quite different from the only three maxima of the spectral sensitivities of the three photoreceptor cell types (see above).

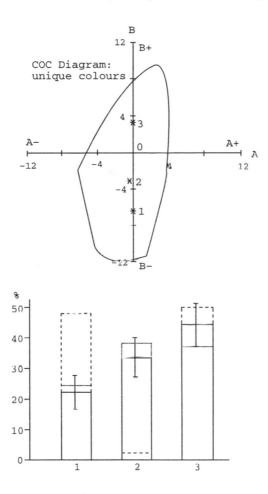

Figure 9.3.4. Results of a double colour training experiment. (a) Colour opponent coding (COC) diagram of the honeybee showing the excitation values A and B of the two types of colour opponent coding neurons due to monochromatic light (closed spectral curve) and to three colour stimuli (1–3). (b) Comparison of the choice percentages measured in the double colour training experiment (solid line) and the predictions of the common colour theory for the honeybee (see Figure 9.3.1) (dashed line), and of the colour theory extended by the unique-colours hypothesis for the bee with the assumption that the bee learns the unique-colour that both the rewarded colours have in common, i.e. the achromatic unique colour 0 (dotted line). (From Backhaus and Kratzsch, 1993, Figure 1–2.)

9.3.5 THE MODEL OF UNIQUE-COLOUR CHOICE BEHAVIOUR

If honeybees posses colour sensations comparable to ours, it should be possible to train an individual bee to a specific unique-colour by reward on several colour stimuli shortly after each other. The bee might learn under these conditions the specific unique-colour as a food signal and furthermore might choose the alternatives presented in the tests according to the amounts of these unique-colours. The choice percentages calculated from this model are indeed very different from the choice percentages predicted from the standard colour theory. Thus, multiple colour training experiments allow us to test in principle whether the choice behaviour of the honeybee is, under certain conditions, related to the electrical excitations of the neuronal colour coding system or to specific unique-colours.

9.3.6 TESTS

First tests of the unique-colours hypothesis are performed in the form of double colour training experiments (Backhaus and Kratzsch, 1993). A bee was rewarded on two different colour stimuli (grey violet and grey yellow) alternatingly, which were predicted from the colour theory extended by the model of colour sensations to have just the achromatic unique-colour 0 (grey) in common. The measured choice behaviour of the bee was in agreement with the predictions of the model of unique-colour choice behaviour (see Figure 9.3.4).

In Figure 9.3.4a, A⁻, A⁺ and B⁻, B⁺ represent the locations of the four hypothetical (pure) 'chromatic' unique-colours and of a hypothetical (pure) 'achromatic' unique-colour (0). Three colour stimuli (1–3) were selected, which are well discriminated (> 94 per cent) by the bee from each other and from the grey background. The stimuli differ only for neuron type B. According to the unique-colours hypothesis for the bee, colour 1 consists of 47 per cent 0 and 53 per cent B⁻, colour 2 consists of 74 per cent 0 and 26 per cent B⁻, and colour 3 consists of 72 per cent 0 and 28 per cent B⁺. An individual bee was alternately trained to the two stimuli, 1 and 3. In the unrewarded tests, all three stimuli were presented.

In Figure 9.3.4b, the measured choice percentages do not agree with the predictions of the common colour theory on the basis of the electrical properties of neurons alone. Instead, the results agree well (v^2, 5 per cent-level) with the predictions from the colour theory extended by the unique-colours hypothesis for the bee. These results thus support the hypothesis that unique-colours also exist in the colour vision of the honeybee.

9.3.7 REFERENCES

BACKHAUS, W. (1987) Color vision in bees: similarity measures and metric scales of the perceptual space. Dissertation, Freie Universität Berlin.

BACKHAUS, W. (1991) Color opponent coding in the visual system of the honeybee, *Vision Research*, **31**, 1381–1397.

BACKHAUS, W. (1992a) The Bezold-Brücke effect in the color vision system of the honeybee, *Vision Research*, **32**, 1425–1431.

BACKHAUS, W. (1992b) Color vision in honeybees, *Neuroscience and Biobehavioral Reviews*, **16**, 1–12.

BACKHAUS, W. (1993) Color vision and color choice behaviour of the honeybee. In: *Recent Progress in Neurobiology of the Honeybee*, **24**, 309–331.

BACKHAUS, W. (1995) Unique-colors in honeybees? In: Drum, B. (Ed.) *Color Deficiencies*, vol 12, Dordrecht: Kluwer.

BACKHAUS, W. & KRATZSCH, D. (1993) Unique-colors in color vision of the honeybee? In: Elsner, B. & Heisenberg, M. (Eds) *Gene-Brain-Behavioral Proceedings of the 21st Göttingen Neurobiology Conference*, **39**, New York: Thieme, Heidelberg.

BACKHAUS, W. & MENZEL, R. (1987) Color distance derived from a receptor model of color vision in the honeybee, *Biological Cybernetics*, **55**, 321–331.

BACKHAUS, W., MENZEL, R. & KREISSL, S. (1987) Multidimensional scaling of color similarity in bees, *Biological Cybernetics*, **56**, 293–304.

HERING, E. (1878) *Zur Lehre vom Lichtsinn*, Vienna: Carl Gerold's Sohn.

HERING, E. (1905) *Grundzüge einer Theorie vom Lichtsinn*, Leipzig: Engelmann. [*Outlines of a Theory of the Light Sense*, translated by L.M. Hurvich and D. Jameson, (1964) Cambridge, MA: Harvard University Press].

HURVICH, L.M. & JAMESON, D. (1956) Some quantitative aspects of an opponent-colors theory. IV. A psychological color specification system, *Journal of the Optical Society of America*, **45**, 416–421.

MENZEL, R. & BACHAUS, W. (1991) Colour vision in insects. In: Cronly-Dillon, J. (Ed.) *Vision and Visual Dysfunction*, vol 6, chapter 14, London: Macmillan, pp 262–293.

LIPETZ, L.E. (1971) The relation of physiological and psychological aspects of sensory intensity. In: Loewenstein, W.R. (Ed.) *Principles of Receptor Physiology. Handbook of Sensory Physiology*, vol. I, Berlin: Springer, pp. 191–225.

MENZEL, R. (1974) Spectral sensitivity of monopolar cells in the bee lamina, *Journal of Comparative Physiology*, **93**, 337–346.

RIBI, W.A. (1987) The structural basis of information processing in the visual system of the bee. In: Menzel, R. & Mercer, A. (Eds) *Neurobiology and Behavior of Honeybees*, Berlin: Springer.

RODIECK, R.W. (1973) *The Vertebrate Retina*, San Francisco: Freeman.

RUSHTON, W.A.H. (1972) Pigments and signals in colour vision, *Journal of Physiology*, **220**, 1–31.

SOUZA, J.M. DE, HERTEL, H., VENTURA, D.F. & MENZEL, R. (1992) Response properties of stained monopolar cells in the honeybee lamina, *Journal of Comparative Physiology*, **A 170**, 267–274.

A Model of Spatial and Chromatic Processing in Early Vision

Ian R. Moorhead

9.4.1 INTRODUCTION

The visual world varies in both colour and luminance and many visual systems have evolved to exploit these variations to obtain information about the location and nature of objects. Although colour and luminance co-vary in an image (Burton and Moorhead, 1987) the majority of research has tended to concentrate on either the processing of spatial (luminance) information, or the processing of colour. The reasons for this have been pragmatic, by separating out colour and luminance it was easier to understand the visual mechanisms involved. However, some attempts have been made to understand how colour and luminance information is jointly processed by the early stages of vision. Early work by van der Horst (1969) measured the contrast sensitivity of the different colour channels. More recently, Losada and Mullen (1994) have measured the characteristics of chromatic channels. Atick et al. (1992), using an information theoretic approach to visual processing, have shown that receptive fields, which are spatially and spectrally selective, are optimal for processing natural scenes. Ingling and Martenez-Uriegas (1985) showed theoretically that simple opponent receptive fields could be viewed as multiplexing together luminance and colour information, in such a way that colour information was effectively handled as a lowpass spatial signal, while luminance information was carried as a bandpass signal. Since psychophysical experiments (Gouras, 1984) have shown that human vision appears to have different characteristics when presented with purely colour information, compared with purely luminance information, it has become fashionable to consider that a demultiplexing process operates at cortical level to separate out the colour and luminance signals that have been combined at the retinal ganglion stage. Recently, De Valois and De Valois (1993) published a model that suggested an explicit three stage model of how the retina combines information from the different cone types and how cortical units then extract separate luminance and colour channels from this representation. The model is linear and brings together ideas from previous work (D'Zmura and Lennie, 1986). The model differs from previous ones in that the authors propose that linear combinations of the common 'red-green' single opponent operators are modulated by a single opponent operator receiving inputs from short wavelength cones. Depending upon which linear combinations are taken then determines the spatial and spectral characteristics of the derived channels.

The work reported here was a preliminary attempt to produce a computer simulation of the De Valois and De Valois model in a form that is able to directly process full 2D colour images. The purpose was first to examine whether the mechanism for demultiplexing colour and luminance information would work as suggested, and second to determine whether the signals from the colour channels might be useful for generating colour descriptors for natural scenes.

The implementation of the model highlighted the fact that a number of aspects of the model had not been made explicit in the original paper.

Section 9.4.2 describes the De Valois and De Valois model briefly and explains a number of aspects that needed to be quantified in a computational version. Section 9.4.3 illustrates how the different stages of the model respond qualitatively to a simple colour image. Section 9.4.4 shows the results of simulating two classical psychophysical experiments and illustrates that the model can be used to predict threshold performance.

9.4.2   DESCRIPTION OF THE MODEL

This section will summarise the main components of the De Valois and De Valois model and highlight certain modifications and additions that were necessary to create a working computational scheme. The principle components of the model are illustrated schematically in Figure 9.4.1. The input is a retinal image consisting of signals from the three types of cone. The relative proportions of the long (L), medium (M) and short (S) cones is specified to be 10:5:2. In the retina it is only physically possible to have a single cone at any one location, but for simplicity in the computational version each cone type was assumed to exist at every location. The inputs to the next stage were weighted according to the relative abundance of each cone type. (It can be argued that the point spread function of the eye effectively spreads the same signal over a number of cones (Haig, 1993).) Future work will examine the effect of only having a single cone type at each location in the input. Cone spectral sensitivities corresponded to the Smith and Pokorny fundamentals.

The second stage of the model corresponds to the retinal ganglion cells. Receptive fields are constructed that have a single cone type input to the centre and one or more cone types as inputs to the surround. De Valois and De Valois designated these units according to the type of cone that formed the input to the centre of the receptive field, thus a unit with L cone inputs to the centre is an L_0 unit. Similarly M_0 and S_0 units receive inputs to the centre of their receptive fields from M cones and S cones respectively. The centre and surround are antagonistic. Figure 9.4.2 illustrates schematically the kinds of unit that result. The spatial structure of the receptive field was arranged to be a difference-of-Gaussian, to conform with other models of ganglion cells (Rodieck, 1965). The units at this stage are of two polarities: ON units with receptive field centres, which are excited by a particular cone type, and OFF units whose centres are inhibited by a particular cone type.

When actually producing a computer implementation of spatiochromatic operators of this kind it is necessary to decide exactly how the centre and surround responses will be weighted relative to each other. In the case of models of spatial vision difference-of-Gaussian operators are generally arranged to be balanced, i.e. to produce no response to a uniform field (e.g. Watt, 1988). This concept can be generalised to spatiochromatic operators like those described here, and they can be set up to produce no response to a uniform field *of a particular colour*. If R_c represents the response from the centre of the receptive field and R_s the response from the surround, then we require that $R_c = R_s$. These can be computed by summing spatially and spectrally, for each cone contribution to that part of the receptive field, thus:

$$R_c = \sum_{x \in Centre} \sum_{i=1}^{3} \int_{380}^{750} c_i(x,\lambda) S(x,\lambda) d\lambda$$

$$R_s = \sum_{x \in Surround} \sum_{i=1}^{3} \int_{380}^{750} c_i(x,\lambda) S(x,\lambda) d\lambda$$

where $c_i(x,\lambda)$ is the spectral sensitivity of the ith cone at position $\mathbf{x}$ and wavelength λ and $S(\mathbf{x}, \lambda)$ is the spectral power at position $\mathbf{x}$ and wavelength λ of the stimulus that is being used to weight the centre and surround. Note that this general formulation makes no assumption about which types of cone contribute to the centre and surround.

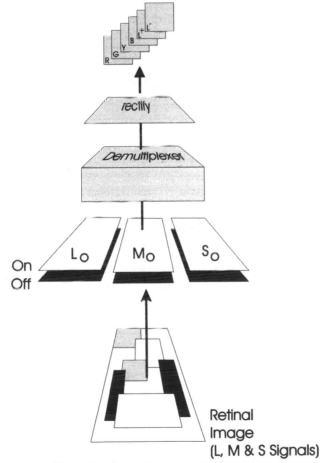

Figure 9.4.1. Diagram illustrating the various stages in the De Valois and De Valois model. The input image is specified in terms of L, M and S cone signals. These are then processed to produce six arrays that correspond to the responses of the single opponent (ganglion cell) operators designated by L_0, M_0 and S_0. Both ON- and OFF-centre types are computed. These signals are then demultiplexed and rectified to form a set of six arrays: four containing colour signals and two that contain lightness signals.

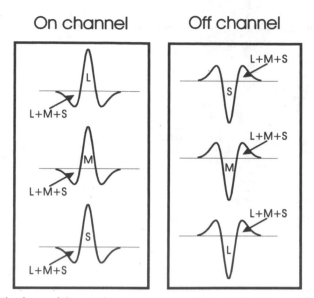

Figure 9.4.2. The form of the single opponent operators used in the model. Each has a single cone type as input to the centre, and a linear combination of three cone types to the surround. They have a difference-of-Gaussian spatial sensitivity. In the current implementation the standard deviation of the centre Gaussian was 0.68, and that of the surround was twice the centre value. The operators were implemented by direct convolution.

Whilst computationally this scheme is easy to achieve, it is not so clear that retinal ganglion cells operate in the same manner. The process, in fact, is a simple form of local colour constancy. This aspect of the model was not considered by De Valois and De Valois (1993).

The next stage of the model simulates the process of demultiplexing the colour and luminance information encoded by the retinal ganglion cell signals.

Figure 9.4.3, adapted from De Valois and De Valois (1993), summarises the process. What happens is that linear combinations of the various types of single opponent units are used to generate two lightness channels and four colour channels. The basic process combines L_0 and M_0 units. These are then further modulated by contributions from S_0 channels. The linear combination stage is followed by a non-linear half-wave rectification process. The linear combination process proposed by De Valois and De Valois requires that the single opponent L_0, M_0 and S_0 units be combined in a particular ratio (10:5:2). If this is not done, the model no longer provides an accurate prediction of the unique hue values. It is not made explicit in their model whether these units are combined from a single location in the visual field or whether, for example, ten L_0 units are summed over a region of the image. Again for simplicity, the units were combined at a single spatial location, but with the appropriate weighting factor.

9.4.2.1 Implementation details

The input to the model consisted of three arrays (which could be of any size) of cone signals. These were computed using image spectral information (CIE tristimulus values were computed and then transformed to the corresponding Smith and Pokorny cone

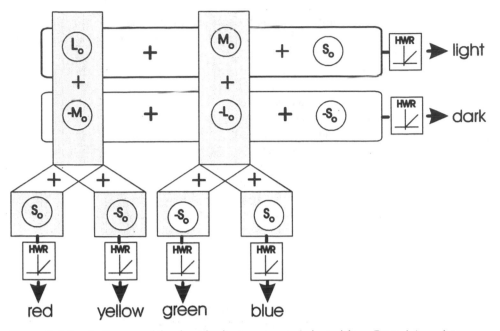

Figure 9.4.3.   A diagram of the demultiplexing process (adapted from De Valois and De Valois, 1993). Vertical combinations create the colour responses, while horizontal combinations produce the lightness responses. Negative symbols in front of the opponent channel labels indicate OFF-centre units.

signals). Generally images consisting of 64×64 or 128×128 values were used to reduce the time of computation. The single opponent filters were 15×15 pixels in size with a standard deviation for the centre of 0.68 pixels (this corresponds to a 1.5 octave (HWHH) filter with a centre frequency of 0.32 cycles/pixel). The standard deviation of the surround was twice this value. Responses were computed by direct convolution from the cone 'image' arrays.

9.4.3   QUALITATIVE BEHAVIOUR

In this section it will be demonstrated qualitatively how the different stages of the model respond to a simple coloured image. The image consisted of a set of coloured tiles, arranged as a grid consisting of six rows and four columns. For the 128×128 pixel image used as an example, each tile was 32×21 pixels (this leaves a small margin at the top and bottom of the image). The reflectance spectrum of each tile was chosen from the set of Munsell colours. The tiles were assumed to be uniformly illuminated by a D_{65} illuminant of a particular luminance. For the data that will be presented here, the image consisted of tiles that all had the same red hue (R2.5, in Munsell notation), but varied in value and chroma. The tiles making up the image were arranged so that the same set of 12 colours were present in the top half of the image as the bottom half. This arrangement was used in order to allow the top half of the image to be set to be isoluminant (for the CIE standard observer). This image structure allows one to examine the behaviour of the model under normal and isoluminant conditions simultaneously.

Figure 9.4.4 shows the response of the L cones to this test image.[1] The front axis corresponds to the top of the image. One can see that the cone signals directly reproduce the tiled structure of the input image. This is because the model does not incorporate any simulation of the optical point spread function. The three rows of tiles at the top of the image, which were set to be isoluminant, produce very similar responses and results from the fact that the cones are responding to colour differences only, whereas the bottom three rows are responding to colour and luminance differences.

Figure 9.4.5 illustrates the responses of a single opponent L_0 channel to the same test image. In the lower part of the image the responses are typical of a centre-surround single opponent filter. There is a mixture of band-pass, 'edge' responses, resembling those produced by a conventional luminance difference-of-Gaussian filter, and low-pass 'DC' responses. These operators produce particularly strong responses at corners when there are both luminance and colour differences. In the isoluminant portion of the image where there are now no luminance edges, only the 'DC' responses can be seen. This graph re-emphasises the fact that these kinds of operators multiplex together low-pass colour signals and band-pass luminance signals. The responses of the other types of single opponent

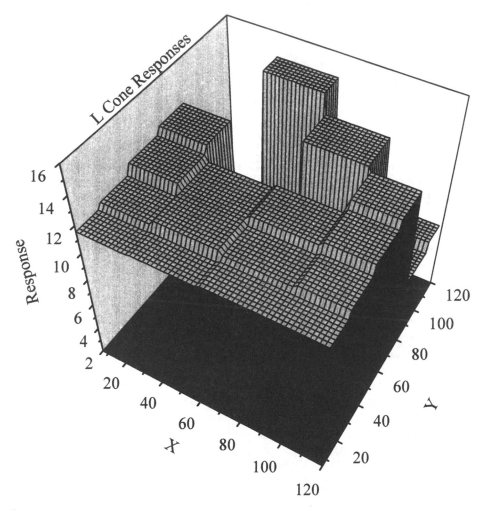

Figure 9.4.4. 3D plot of the responses of L cones to the test image. In this and subsequent plots the front (X) axis corresponds to the top of the image, while the right (Y) axis corresponds to the left side of the image.

operators are similar. It is the function of the next stage to separate out these two types of response.

If the subsequent demultiplexing stage operated to separate these two signals, the response of the colour channels should appear as a low-pass representation of the input image. Figure 9.4.6 shows the response from the 'red' channel of the model for this particular test image. It is clear that there are still significant 'edge transients' present in the bottom part of the image that contains both luminance and colour information. Not surprisingly, the isoluminant part of the image does show a low-pass representation of the input image.

These results demonstrate that the demultiplexing process is incomplete. By experimenting with the relative weighting of the single opponent channel inputs to the demultiplexing stage of the model, it was possible to achieve much better separation of the colour and luminance signals. To achieve this, equal contributions from the L_0 and M_0 units, without contributions from the S_0 units, were used. Unfortunately, this new scheme no longer provides an accurate prediction of unique hue wavelengths.

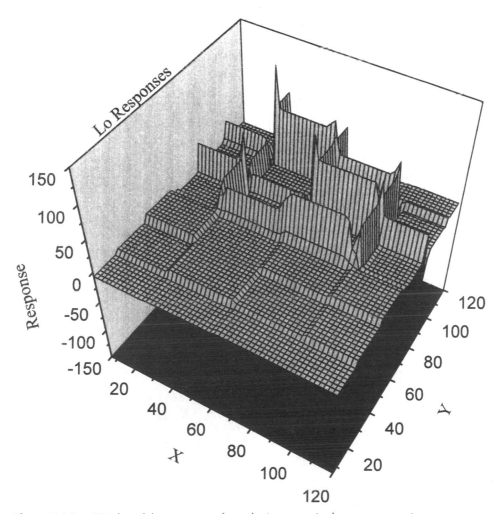

Figure 9.4.5.   3D plot of the responses from the L-centre single opponent unit.

9.4.4 QUANTITATIVE PREDICTIONS

In order to examine whether the model could reliably predict actual performance, two psychophysical experiments were simulated: an increment threshold experiment and a hue naming experiment. This section describes the methods and results.

9.4.4.1 Increment threshold

Increment threshold experiments generally involve an observer detecting a monochromatic increment on a white background. This was simulated as follows. A 64×64 pixel uniform white image was created, with a luminance of 50 cdm^{-2}. The colour temperature of the image could be set to any value required. A circular test spot measuring 10 pixels in diameter was added to this adapting field. The test spot could be of any wavelength and had a Gaussian spectral distribution with a standard deviation of 2 nm. The radiance of the test spot could be set also, and for the data presented here it was set arbitrarily to $1.0 \times e^6$ units.

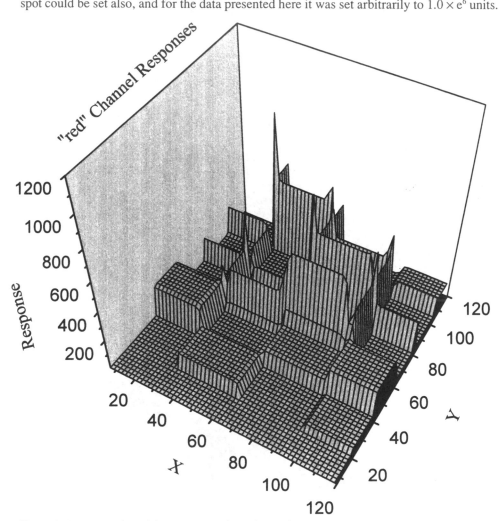

Figure 9.4.6. 3D plot of the responses from the 'red' colour channel (after the half-wave rectification).

Images were created for test spots with centre wavelengths ranging from 400 to 700 nm in steps of 10 nm. In order to obtain a single number that could be used to estimate the response of the model to the test stimulus, a number of different schemes were implemented. The simplest involved taking the maximum value from all of the channel responses at the centre of the test spot. A second method computed a root mean square value of all of the channel outputs at the centre of the test spot. Finally, a Gaussian weighted spatial average of the root mean square signal was also computed. This could either include just the colour channels or lightness and colour channels. The standard deviation of the Gaussian was set to be 2.0 pixels.

The results of one such experiment are plotted in Figure 9.4.7. The background colour temperature in the test images was set to 6500 K (D_{65}). The figure shows the responses computed using the different criteria described, as well as a typical set of human psychophysical data obtained by Kranda and King-Smith (1979). All of the data have been normalised before plotting. The data from the model reproduce the three-peaked increment threshold response typically found with human observers. In particular, the responses calculated as a Gaussian spatially weighted root mean square of the colour channels match the psychophysical data very closely, except towards the short wavelength end of the spectrum. In fact all of the model responses show a poor fit below wavelengths of 470 nm. In addition, the method of computing the maximum response does not reproduce the dip (Sloan's notch) in the psychophysical data at around 570 nm. These results are only achieved if the single opponent channel responses are normalised in the manner described

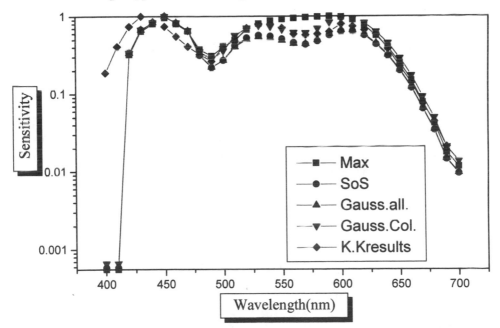

Figure 9.4.7.   Results of simulating an increment threshold experiment. The filled diamonds are the data taken from Kranda and King-Smith. Other plots correspond to the different methods used to compute a model response. Max (filled squares) is based on taking the maximum channel response at the centre of the image, SoS (filled circles) is a sum of squares calculation over all of the channels, Gauss all (filled triangles) is the sum of squares response taken over a small region of the centre of the image. Values were weighted according to a Gaussian window (sd 2 pixels). Gauss coll (inverted triangles) is the Gaussian weighted sum of squares for the colour channels only. Each curve was normalised separately.

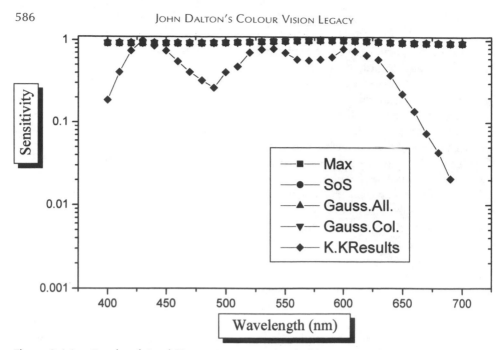

Figure 9.4.8.   Results of simulating an increment threshold experiment, but without the filter balancing at the single opponent stage (see Figure 9.4.7 for explanation of symbols).

in section 9.4.2. Figure 9.4.8 shows the predictions made by the model for the same increment threshold experiment when the normalisation process is not used. Here, the responses are virtually independent of wavelength.

A number of experiments were carried out in which the various parameters were manipulated. In general, the results appear to be quite robust as long as the single opponent channels are balanced in the manner described earlier. For example, if the colour temperature of the adapting field is set to that of illuminant A, the relative heights of the peaks at 550 nm and 620 nm are reduced compared with the blue peak. This is consistent with the fact that illuminant A has a lower colour temperature than D_{65} and therefore produces more adaptation at the red end of the spectrum.

9.4.4.2 Hue naming

Boynton and Gordon (1965) describe psychophysical data on the relative proportions of red, green, yellow and blue light used by observers to describe monochromatic lights. The outputs from the model should correspond in some fashion to these responses. In order to compare the model with the results of Boynton and Gordon, a monochromatic test spot on a low intensity background (10 cdm^{-2}) was used as an input to the model. In order to calculate the relative contributions from the different channels, a chromatic response was calculated by taking each colour channel response and dividing it by the sum of all of the colour channel responses. As in the previous experiment, this could also be done using a Gaussian spatial weighting function. The results are plotted in Figure 9.4.9.

The results are not unlike those of Boynton and Gordon (1965), in that the model predicts distinct responses from different parts of the spectrum, for each of the colour channels. In addition the red channel shows a distinct contribution at the shorter wavelength end of the

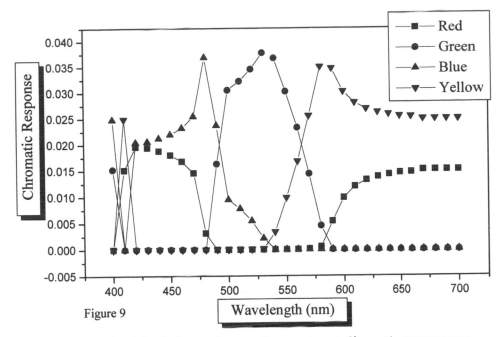

Figure 9

Figure 9.4.9. Results of simulating a colour naming experiment. Chromatic response was computed as the ratio of the signal from a particular channel to the sum of the responses from all of the other channels.

spectrum. However there are discrepancies between the model responses and the psychophysical results. In particular, the psychophysical data show the proportion of red increasing or perhaps levelling off for wavelengths above 600 nm, whereas the model response actually falls and then levels off in this region of the spectrum. This is similar for the yellow channel responses. Also, the widths and cross-over points for the data are different. Finally, as in the case of the increment threshold simulations, when the normalisation process is removed, the predictions become virtually independent of the wavelength.

9.4.5 DISCUSSION

The model described here is tantalising. In some respects it appears to represent well the processes of human colour vision, and yet, on the other hand, it makes erroneous predictions. As already shown by De Valois and De Valois (1993), the model predicts the unique hue locations correctly. Here, it has been shown that it can also provide a close approximation to the increment threshold function. On the other hand, the predictions made in the hue naming experiment are less convincing. In addition, the qualitative results of processing a simple tiled image suggest that the demultiplexing process is incomplete. Finally the quantitative data appear to rely upon the correct balancing of the centre and surround of the single opponent responses in order to provide good predictions of performance. This aspect was not made explicit in the original model. What has not been considered yet is whether the model can predict the effects of changing the spatial parameters of the stimulus, although some preliminary work examining increment threshold performance for small test spots suggests that the model does not predict the shift to a VV-shaped function as occurs psychophysically.

Another aspect not illustrated by the figures here is the fact that the type of response by a colour channel (the green output, for example) changes its characteristics according to the wavelength being used as a test stimulus in the increment threshold experiment. At shorter wavelengths, for example, the responses tend to be low-pass in form, but at longer wavelengths they appear much more like a band-pass response.

There are a number of parameters that can be manipulated in this model. The data presented here represent a first attempt at setting them. It seems likely that attempts to model other sets of psychophysical data will more strongly define the possible ranges of these parameters.

The incomplete demultiplexing of colour and luminance is problematic. It may be that there is a more appropriate linear combination of the single opponent responses that would not only separate the colour and luminance responses, but would leave the unique hue predictions intact. Alternatively, it may be that a non-linear mechanism is required to achieve correct demultiplexing. A third possibility, however, is that the model actually represents how human vision works. In this case, there may be stimuli and experiments that support the idea of incomplete demultiplexing of colour and luminance signals.

Although the prediction made for the increment threshold experiments is very good over the middle to long range of the spectrum, the prediction is poor at the short wavelength end. Not only is the blue peak in the wrong place, but the sensitivity is significantly poorer than that measured psychophysically. It is possible that these discrepancies arise from the fact that the S cone single opponent unit is an inappropriate model. There is some evidence that only certain types of S cone unit exist, and these may well have different sensitivities compared to the L cone and M cone units. Kranda and King-Smith (1979), for example, required a different slope for the blue-yellow channel when fitting an opponent channel model to their data. Future work will examine some of the uncertainties in the present version of the model and will extend the quantitative predictions to experiments in which space and colour effects interact.

9.4.6　NOTE

1. All 3D plots have been subsampled to 64×64 points to improve clarity.

9.4.7　REFERENCES

ATICK, J.J., LI, Z. & REDLICH, A.N. (1992) Understanding retinal color coding from first principles, *Neural Computation*, **4**, 559–572.

BOYNTON, R.M. & GORDON, J. (1965) Bezold-Brücke hue shift measured by color-naming technique, *Journal of the Optical Society of America*, **55**, 78–86.

BRAINARD, D.H. & WANDELL, B.A. (1986) Analysis of the retinex theory of color vision, *Journal of the Optical Society of America*, **A3**, 1651–1661.

BURTON, G.J. & MOORHEAD, I. R. (1987) Color and spatial structure in natural scenes, *Applied Optics*, **26**, 157–170.

DE VALOIS, R.L. & DE VALOIS, K.K. (1993) A multi-stage color model, *Vision Research*, **33**, 1053–1065.

D'ZMURA, M. & LENNIE, P. (1986) Mechanisms of color constancy, *Journal of the Optical Society of America*, **A3**, 1662–1672.

GOURAS, P. (1984) Color vision, *Progress in Retinal Research*, **3**, 227–261.

HAIG, N.D. (1993) Local gain control and focal accommodation in the self similar stack vision model, *Spatial Vision*, **7**, 15–34.

Horst van der, G.J.C. (1969) Transfer of spatial chromatic contrast at threshold in the human eye, *Journal of the Optical Society of America*, **59**, 1260–1266.

Ingling Jr., C.R. & Martenez-Uriegas, E. (1985) The spatiotemporal properties of the r-g X-cell channel, *Vision Research*, **25**, 33–38.

Kranda, K. & King-Smith, P.E. (1979) Detection of coloured stimuli by independent linear systems, *Vision Research*, **19**, 733–745.

Lennie, P. & D'Zmura, M. (1988) Mechanisms of Color Vision, *CRC Critical Reviews in Neurobiology*, **3**, 333–400.

Losada, M.A. & Mullen, K.T (1994) The spatial tuning of chromatic mechanisms identified by simultaneous masking, *Vision Research*, **34**, 331–341.

Rodieck, R. W. (1965) Quantitative analysis of cat retinal ganglion cell response to visual stimuli, *Vision Research*, **5**, 583–601.

Smith, V.C. & Pokorny, J. (1975) Spectral sensitivity of the foveal cone photopigments between 400 and 500 nm, *Vision Research*, **15**, 161–171.

Watt, R.J. (1988) *Visual Processing: Computational, Psychophysical and Cognitive Research*, Hove: Lawrence Erlbaum Associates.

Invariant Relationships Between Achromatic Colour, Apparent Illumination and Shape of Surface: Implications for the Colour Constancy Theories

A Logvinenko

The perceived colour of an object is believed to be closely associated with object reflectance rather than with the spectral distribution of light reflected to the eye by the object. When the incident illumination changes the perceived colour remains approximately the same despite the changing retinal illumination. This phenomenon, referred to as colour constancy, gives rise to a problem because the spectral distribution of reflected light is determined by both the surface reflection and incident illumination:

$$(reflected\ illumination) = (surface\ reflection) \times (surface\ illumination) \qquad (1)$$

It is still not clear how the visual system resolves this equation (1), involving only one known (the reflected illumination) and two unknowns (the surface reflection and illumination), although a few elegant computational algorithms have been recently proposed (D'Zmura and Iverson, 1993; Hurlbert, 1986).

However, there are other problems with colour constancy. One of the most important, and often overlooked, problem is that colour constancy from its earliest measurements (see, for review, Woodworth, 1938) has never been found to be perfect. As a matter of fact, colour matching as observed and measured in colour constancy experiments is always a compromise between complete constancy and a match based on the proximal stimulus (Arend and Reeves, 1986; Tiplitz Blackwell and Buchsbaum, 1988; Valberg and Lange-Malecki, 1990). Furthermore, considerable inter-individual differences have always been registered (Arend and Reeves, 1986; Woodworth, 1938). So, if the visual system really does solve equation (1) why does it do this so inaccurately?

The problem is more tractable within the context of a more general phenomenon, namely, veridicality of percept, which implies the invariance of relationships between various perceptual dimensions (Logvinenko, 1993). Particularly, it has long been realised that the apparent relief of a surface, its achromatic colour, and apparent illumination are mutually interdependent. For instance, an apparent transformation of the spatial relief of a surface affects its achromatic colour (Buckley *et al.*, 1994; Gilchrist, 1977; Katona, 1935; Knill and Kersten, 1991; Mach, 1959). A misperception of the surface illumination causes a change in the colour of the surface (Gelb, 1929; Logvinenko and Menshikova, 1994; Wallach, 1963). In other words, there is a kind of perceptual interaction between these perceptual dimensions which Hochberg called a 'percept-percept coupling' (Epstein, 1982; Hochberg, 1974).

These phenomenological observations have been formalised in terms of the albedo hypothesis (Beck, 1972; Koffka, 1935) that suggests the invariant relationship between perceived achromatic colour and perceived illumination is as follows:

$$(apparent\ illumination) \times (surface\ achromatic\ colour) \propto (retinal\ illumination)$$

(2)

However, experimental testing of the albedo hypothesis revealed contradictory results. Whereas some investigators claimed they found evidence in favour of the albedo hypothesis (Kozaki and Noguchi, 1976; Noguchi and Kozaki, 1985), others failed to verify it (Beck, 1961; Kozaki, 1973; MacLeod, 1940; Oyama, 1968).

It has been suggested recently that the failure to confirm the quantitative relationship between an observer's judgements of achromatic colour and perceived illumination may be due to errors in measuring the latter (Logvinenko, 1993; Logvinenko and Menshikova, 1994). As a matter of fact, all previous investigators took either brightness, defined as the subjective intensity of reflected light from a surface, or, a subjective magnitude of direct illumination from the light source, as an appropriate index of illumination. However, neither is an adequate indicator of the perceived illumination of a surface because both are really subjective characteristics of a light (or a light source) rather than the characteristics of a reflective surface. The following problem thus arises. How is illumination represented in a percept?

It should be pointed out that the answer depends on whether an absolute or relative illumination is meant. As for the absolute illumination, it is still not clear which perceptual dimensions represent it, if any. All the previous investigations have shown that human observers are not good at evaluating the absolute illumination of a scene (e.g. Beck, 1972).

On the contrary, there are no doubts of the ability of humans to perceive differences in the illumination of various parts of a scene. In other words, there is a relative illumination specific dimension of a perceived surface. However, there is no suitable term for it in the visual science vocabulary. The closest seems to be 'shading', but the polarity of shading is just the reverse to one of apparent relative illumination. Indeed, when illumination falling on a surface is screened, we say the surface grows shadowy, or its shading becomes stronger. So the term 'shading' is opposite to apparent relative illumination of surface. Nevertheless, we will use it equally with apparent relative illumination.

Notice that shading depends on both the physical illumination and spatial relief of a surface (and of spatial layout of surfaces). For instance, the shading of a surface changes as the slant (relative to the direction of prevailing illumination) changes. Hence, shading characterises both illumination of a surface and its spatial arrangement at the same time. It is a subjective correlate of a differentially illuminated surface or a relative-illumination-at-surface.

An attempt has been recently made to find out whether achromatic colour and perceived relative, rather than absolute, illumination are related, as the albedo hypothesis suggests (Logvinenko and Menshikova, 1994). It has been found that looking at a white paper cone attached to a vertical white screen through a pseudoscope induces an inversion of apparent depth, namely, it makes the cone look like a conical hole in the screen. This in turn causes the shadow that the now 'invisible' cone casts on the screen to change its appearance and to look like a pigmented area. In other words, under pseudoscopic vision a border between the shadowed area and the other part of screen is no longer perceived as an 'illumination edge'. On the contrary, it is perceived as an 'achromatic colour (or reflectance) edge', i.e. the shadowed area is perceived as an insertion with different achromatic colour. Therefore, the same gradient in retinal illumination might be interpreted by the visual system either as an illumination edge or as an achromatic colour edge depending on the sign of the apparent spatial relief. It has been hypothesised that these are two extreme cases and that normally a brightness contrast determines a combination of both illumination and colour edges so that a total amount of contrast holds constant. In other words, a sort of a conservation contrast law exists; if a certain amount of illumination (shading) contrast disappears at one area of a surface for some reason (e.g. due to pseudoscopical inversion of the apparent depth) then the same amount of achromatic colour contrast appears at the same area of the surface.

Although it was shown in this experiment that achromatic colour and perceived relative illumination are inversely proportional to each other so long as the retinal illumination is constant, equation (2) was not confirmed. It should be noted, however, that the albedo hypothesis in its classical form (2) can by no means be true because it implies that when the apparent illumination of a surface is constant, its greyness varies in direct proportion with the retinal illumination. Consequently, under constant physical illumination greyness of a chip should be proportional to its reflectance. In other words, equation (2) predicts the linearity of grey scale for achromatic colours so long as the illumination is veridically perceived. However, it is well established that the grey scale is non-linear (e.g. Wyszecki and Stiles, 1982).

To account for the data obtained in this experiment (Logvinenko and Menshikova, 1994) the albedo hypothesis is to be modified as follows:

$$(apparent\ relative\ illumination) \times (surface\ achromatic\ colour) \propto (brightness) \qquad (3)$$

Equation (3) differs from equation (2) in two points. Relative, rather than absolute, apparent illumination, and brightness, rather than retinal illumination, are involved. In other words, it is suggested that the perceived illumination and neutral colour co-vary in direct proportion to brightness rather than to retinal illumination, given that one of the two terms is kept constant. The latter modification is similar to that made by McCready (1986) to reconcile the size-distance invariance hypothesis (Kilpatrick and Ittelson, 1953).

More evidence that brightness rather than luminance is a real determinant of an achromatic colour–relative illumination product in equation (3) comes from the 3D Cornsweet-O'Brien effect (Pessoa et al., 1995). A classical, 2D Cornsweet-O'Brien effect is produced with a luminance cusp displayed on a flat area of constant luminance, which is experienced as two regions of different brightness (Cornsweet, 1970). When created on a 3D curved surface (e.g. cylinder or ellipsoid), it is perceived as two regions either of different colour under the same illumination, or of the same colour but differently illuminated. Thus, this brightness illusion brings about the alteration of colour and/or shading in the manner that equation (3) predicts.

Furthermore, sometimes the same luminance cusp is perceived as a distortion of spatial relief; that is, as a sort of dent on the surface, with both colour and shading being unaltered. This fact, as well as the one mentioned earlier, namely, that the apparent spatial relief of a surface may affect its achromatic colour, allows the hypothesis that there may be an analogous invariant relationship connecting apparent shape and colour on the one hand and brightness on the other hand.

Hence, the same perceptual dimension may be involved in different invariant relationships like equation (3). As a matter of fact, many other invariant perceptual relationships have been found, namely, the ones relating to apparent size and distance (Kilpatrick and Ittelson, 1953), apparent slant and shape (Epstein and Park, 1963), apparent depth and distance (Foley, 1967) and some others (see for review Epstein, 1973, 1982).

Such invariant relationships are to be distinguished from the psychophysical functions that link a subjective variable, such as brightness, and some physical attributes of the proximal stimulus, such as retinal illumination. First, these relationships link the perceptual dimensions of an object to the sensory dimensions of light rather than to the characteristics of the proximal stimulus. Second, the very nature of this connection is different. Whereas a sensory dimension is entirely determined by the proximal stimulus, there is no strict functional relationship between sensory dimensions (and consequently a proximal stimulus) and perceptual dimensions. Ambiguous figures such as Necker's cube prove that various percepts resulting from different perceptual contexts may have the same sensory basis. It was hypothesised that the connection between the sensory basis of percept and its perceptual context is rather similar to the connection between the sounds of language and the meanings of words (Logvinenko, 1985, 1993). The role that an invariant relationship such as equation (3) plays in perception is to function as a special normative rule (like grammatical ones), governing the link between the sensory basis and perceptual context (Logvinenko, 1981). Equation (3) exemplifies one such rule. It says that, although the same brightness may induce many combinations of achromatic colour and shading, all these must be in inverse proportion to each other.

All this has a strong implication for a theory of surface colour perception in general and colour constancy in particular. First of all, note that a relation between the perceptual dimensions of an object such as a surface colour and the physical dimensions of a proximal stimulus does not have to be psychophysical in nature. Hence, there may not be such a thing as psychophysics of surface colour. In particular, there is no point in trying to establish a psychophysical scale for surface colours, because it follows from equation (3) that, even if all other perceptual dimensions (e.g. apparent shape, apparent illumination etc.) are kept constant, achromatic colour would co-vary with the retinal illumination in the same way as brightness. In other words, as the link between achromatic colour and retinal illumination is mediated by brightness in the way equation (3) predicts, a grey scale cannot but have the same form as a brightness scale provided apparent illumination is fixed. This conclusion, no doubt, may be considered by some visual scientists as surprising; however, overlooking this fact has brought about a lot of conceptual confusion in the history of colour science.

The very existence of invariant relationship (3) contradicts the idea that colour can be processed separately irrespective of processing other perceptual dimensions as shading, shape, etc. In other words, it is unlikely that there may exist an independent module responsible for computation of only surface colour in the visual system (Marr, 1982).

In particular, equation (3) shows that perception of colour is determined by an apparent relative illumination to the same extent as by the retinal illumination. It undermines those psychophysical theories that account for colour solely in terms of retinal stimulation without any reference to perceived illumination, such as those of Jameson and Hurvich (1964) and Cornsweet (1970).

A 'taking-into-account' approach (Woodworth, 1938) is supposed to be an alternative to the psychophysical one (Epstein, 1973). It was claimed that the visual system takes into account the apparent illumination during computation of colour (Beck, 1972; Epstein,

1973; Helmholtz, 1867). To put it in another way, a 'taking-into-account' approach suggests that the visual system derives a surface colour from equation (2) in two steps. First, an apparent illumination is evaluated by using somehow, hypothetical 'cues' of illumination, and then a surface colour is derived from equation (2). However, adherents of this approach did not actually manage to find the appropriate cues for apparent illumination. Moreover, they treated apparent illumination as an auxiliary dimension compared to colour. However, there are fewer reasons to believe that colour could be in turn taken into account in order to compute an apparent illumination. As a matter of fact, equation (2) includes two unknowns – colour and apparent illumination – and they are symmetrically involved in it. Curiously enough, many efforts have been made in order to disentangle how the visual system solves the equation in respect to only one of the two unknowns, namely colour, the other variable (apparent illumination) being ignored. However, as every-day-life experience shows, the human visual system does somehow solve the equation in both unknowns; our capacity to perceive illumination is hardly poorer than colour.

So, the grave drawbacks of the 'taking-into-account' approach are as follows. First, the wrong equation was addressed. It is equation (3) that the visual system deals with rather than equation (2). Second, it attempts to reduce an equation involving two unknowns (colour and apparent illumination) to an equation with one unknown (colour).

On the other hand, the obvious fact is that equation (3) cannot be solved uniquely either because the number of unknowns is greater than the number of knowns. However, it should be kept in mind that the perceptual dimensions entered in it are also involved in other perceptual equations. Therefore, the visual system seems to face a whole system of perceptual equations where the number of unknowns (perceptual dimensions) may exceed the number of knowns (sensory dimensions). Such a system may allow a unique solution.

Moreover, there is evidence, coming from the experiments on perceptual conflicts, to suggest that perceptual equation solving is not a metaphor (Logvinenko, 1993). In the case of contradictory sensory information (such as pseudoscopical vision brings about) it has been revealed that the visual system attempted to resolve a contradictory set of perceptual equations by a trial-and-error method similar to the way a computer does (Logvinenko, 1981).

As a matter of fact reversing the sign of binocular disparity for a complex 3D visual scene produces an insurmountable perceptual conflict in the sense that there is not any non-contradictory 3D visual image consistent with these retinal patterns. So seeing a natural scene through a pseudoscope gives rise to a kaleidoscopic sequence of different perceptual images that gradually supersede each other. All these images may be thought of as variants of solution of the perceptual equations system. Under normal viewing conditions it takes very little time for the visual system to find an appropriate perceptual image that is in line with the sensory basis. Under pseudoscopical viewing, when such a solution does not exist, the process of putting forward and testing perceptual hypotheses (i.e. various versions of the perceptual image) may last long enough to be monitored by an observer.

In conclusion, getting back to the problem of colour constancy, note that one possible source of the deviation from perfect constancy may be concerned with the fact that colour is not only determined by information from retinal stimuli but is conditional on other perceptual dimensions, in particular, on apparent relative illumination. It follows that the achromatic colour of a surface is constant as long as the incident illumination is correctly perceived, any under-estimation of the surface illumination being accompanied by an over-estimation of surface colour and vice versa.

Therefore, perceptual constancy is a particular case of a more general phenomenon: veridicality of perception. In other words, a capital characteristic of visual perception is not that various perceptual dimensions, such as colour and apparent illumination, are constant, but that they are in constant veridical relationships, such as a revised albedo hypothesis (3). Veridicality means here that these relationships are similar to those of their physical counterparts.

9.5.1   REFERENCES

AREND, L. & REEVES, A. (1986) Simultaneous color constancy, *Journal of the Optical Society of America*, **A3**, 1743–1751.

BECK, J. (1961) Judgments of surface illumination and lightness, *Journal of Experimental Psychology*, **61**, 368–375.

BECK, J. (1972) *Surface Color Perception*, Ithaca and London: Cornell University Press.

BUCKLEY, D., FRISBY, J.P. & FREEMAN, J. (1994) Lightness perception can be affected by surface curvature from stereopsis. *Perception*, **23**, 869–881.

CORNSWEET, T. (1970) *Visual Perception*, New York: Academic Press.

D'ZMURA, M. & IVERSON, G. (1993) Color constancy, *Journal of the Optical Society of America*, **A10**, 2148–2180.

EPSTEIN, W. (1973) The process of 'taking-into-account' in visual perception, *Perception*, **2**, 267–285.

EPSTEIN, W. (1982) Percept-percept couplings, *Perception*, **11**, 75-83.

EPSTEIN, W. & PARK, J. (1963) Shape constancy: functional relationships and theoretical formulations. *Psychological Bulletin*, **60**, 265–288.

FOLEY, J. M. (1967) Binocular disparity and perceived relative distance: an examination of two hypotheses, *Vision Research*, **7**, 655–670.

GELB, A. (1929) Die 'Farbenkonstanz' der Sehdinge, *Handbuch der Normalen und Patologischen Physiologie*, **12**, 594–678.

GILCHRIST, A. L. (1977) Perceived lightness depends on perceived spatial arrangement, *Science*, **195**, 185–187.

HELMHOLTZ, H. VON (1867) *Handbuch der Physiologischen Optik*, Leipzig: Voss.

HOCHBERG, J. E. (1974) High-order stimuli and inter-response coupling in the perception of the visual world. In: MacLeod, R.B. & Pick, Jr., H.L. (Eds) *Perception. Essays in Honor of James J. Gibson*, Ithaca and London: Cornell University Press, pp. 17–39.

HURLBERT, A. (1986) Formal connections between lightness algorithms, *Journal of the Optical Society of America*, **A3**, 1684–1693.

JAMESON, D. & HURVICH, L. M. (1964) Theory of brightness and colour contrast in human vision, *Vision Research*, **4**, 135–154.

KATONA, G. (1935) Color contrast and colour constancy, *Journal of Experimental Psychology*, **18**, 49–63

KILPATRICK, F. P. & ITTELSON, W. H. (1953) The size-distance invariance hypothesis, *Psychology Review*, **60**, 223–231.

KNILL, D. C. & KERSTEN, D. (1991) Apparent surface curvature affects lightness perception, *Nature*, **351**, 228–230.

KOFFKA, K. (1935) *Principles of Gestalt Psychology*, New York: Harcourt, Brace.

KOZAKI, A. (1973) Perception of lightness and brightness of achromatic surface color and impression of illumination, *Japanese Psychological Research*, **15**, 194–203.

KOZAKI, A. & NOGUCHI, K. (1976) The relationship between perceived surface-lightness and perceived illumination, *Psychological Research*, **39**, 1–16.

LOGVINENKO, A. D. (1981) *Visual Space Perception*, Moscow: Moscow University Press (in Russian).

LOGVINENKO, A. D. (1985) *Sensory Basis of Space Perception*, Moscow: Moscow University Press (in Russian).

LOGVINENKO, A. D. (1993) Perceptual equations: implications for computer vision, *The Irish Journal of Psychology,* **14**, 330–342.

LOGVINENKO, A. D. & MENSHIKOVA, G. YA. (1994) Trade-off between achromatic colour and perceived illumination as revealed by using pseudoscopic inversion of apparent depth, *Perception*, **23**, 1007–1023.

MACH, E. (1959) *The Analysis of Sensations*, (translated from the 5th German edition by S. Waterlow), New York: Dover Publications.

MACLEOD, R. B. (1940) Brightness constancy in unrecognised shadows, *Journal of Experimental Psychology*, **27**, 1–22.

MARR, D. (1982) *Vision*, San Francisco: W. H. Freeman.

MCCREADY, D. (1986) Moon illusion redescribed, *Perception and Psychophysics*, **39**, 64–72.

NOGUCHI, K. & KOZAKI, A. (1985) Perceptual scission of surface-lightness and illumination: an examination of the Gelb effect, *Psychological Research*, **47**, 19–25.

OYAMA, T. (1968) Stimulus determination of brightness constancy and the perception of illumination, *Japanese Psychological Research*, **10**, 146–155.

PESSOA, L., GRUNEWALD A. & ROSS, W. (1995) The Craik-O'Brien lightness effect on 3D surfaces: curvature and highlights, *Investigative Ophthalmology and Visual Science*, **36**(4), S476.

TIPLITZ BLACKWELL, K. & BUCHSBAUM, G. (1988) Quantitative studies of color constancy, *Journal of the Optical Society of America*, **A5**, 1772–1780.

VALBERG, A. & LANGE-MALECKI, B. (1990) Color constancy in Mondrian patterns: a partial cancellation of physical chromaticity shifts by simultaneous contrast, *Vision Research*, **30**, 371–380.

WALLACH, H. (1963) The perception of neutral colours, *Scientific American*, **208**, 107–116.

WOODWORTH, R. S. (1938) *Experimental Psychology*, New York: Holt.

WYSZECKI, G. & STILES, W. S. (1982) *Color Science. Concepts and Methods, Quantitative Data and Formulae*, 2nd edn, New York: John Wiley & Sons.

A Model of Cone Interaction for Coding Chromatic Information

M. C. Morrone and L. Bedarida

9.6.1 INTRODUCTION

Ample experimental evidence points to the existence of three cardinal axes in colour space, corresponding to three independent visual channels: one luminance channel and two chromatic channels (Krauskopf *et al.*, 1982). Although it is clear that the chromatic channels must be created by combinations of the cone outputs in an opponent fashion (such as L-M and S-(L + M)), the exact form of the opponency required to explain the psychophysical and physiological data is still unclear. Classical models of linear opponency of the cone signals (Hurvich and Jameson, 1957) face difficulties in predicting the independence of the chromatic and luminance modulation signals over a range of average chromaticities. Non-linear models that combine Weber fractions of the cone signals (Stromeyer *et al.*, 1985) overcome some of these difficulties, but fail to simulate quantitatively the constancy of chromatic thresholds over an extended range of average chromaticities. To explain these and other phenomena, a second stage of chromatic adaptation has been proposed (Stromeyer *et al.*, 1985)

In this chapter we propose a new model for the creation of the L/M chromatic channel by a non-linear combination of cone signals, and show how this model predicts quantitatively a range of psychophysical data that has posed difficulties for other models. We will also describe a biologically plausible implementation of the model, which closely simulates the characteristics of double-opponent cells of the primate visual cortex.

9.6.2 THE RATIONALE

We commence by considering some simple and well-known contrast sensitivity data. Figure 9.6.1 reports contrast sensitivity measurements for detecting a red-green modulated grating of low spatial frequency as a function of *colour-ratio*, the ratio of red to total luminance. In close agreement with the original results of Mullen (1985), detection thresholds vary symmetrically about the V_λ equiluminance point, both for stationary gratings (filled squares) and for the 15 Hz contrast-reversed gratings (open triangles). The modulation of the red and green phosphors is given by:

$$R(x,y) = rI_0(1 + k/2 \cos(2\pi\omega y) \cos(2\pi\overline{\omega}t))$$
$$G(x,y) = (1 - r)I_0(1 - k/2 \cos(2\pi\omega y)\cos(2\pi\overline{\omega}t)) \qquad (1)$$

where r is the ratio of the average luminance of the red phosphors to the overall average luminance given by I_0. The modulation is green-black for $r = 0$, red-black when $r = 1$, and red-green when $r = 0.5$. The equiluminance point, assessed by standard flicker photometry, was at $r = 0.5$ for both subjects. The stimulus extended over $60 \times 60^\circ$ of visual field and comprised two periods of the grating. The CIE co-ordinates for the red and green phosphors were $x = 0.651$, $y = 0.348$ and $x = 0.403$, $y = 0.59$ respectively (when viewed through a Kodak Wratten filter 16).

Measurements were made with a two alternative forced-choice technique, using the QUEST procedure (Watson and Pelli, 1983) to home in near threshold. The final threshold estimate was obtained by fitting cumulative Gaussian functions to the probability of seeing data. Standard errors, calculated by repeated estimates of the partial data, were on average 0.03 log units.

The symmetry of the sensitivities for stationary gratings (that advantage the chromatic system) implies that the optimal response of the L-M chromatic channel occurs at the equiluminance point, where the stimulus luminance contrast is, by definition, zero. This is a general finding that has been verified over a large range of stimulus conditions (Mullen, 1985) and also observed in the response of visual evoked potential (Fiorentini et al., 1991). It is also a very intuitive result: the L-M chromatic channel, insensitive to luminance modulation, is maximally sensitive to modulation of pure chromaticity ($r = 0.5$), and decreases its response when the chromatic modulation of the stimulus is reduced, reaching

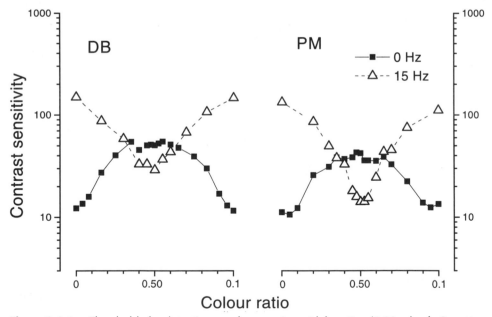

Figure 9.6.1. Thresholds for detecting a red-green sinusoidal grating (0.03 cdeg^{-1}, Gaussian vignetted exposure of time constant 1 s) when presented stationary (filled squares) or alternating in counter-phase at 15 Hz (open triangles) on a Barco Calibrator monitor.

minima at $r = 0$ and $r = 1$. However, this simple and intuitive result is not readily predictable from the textbook-type linear model of chromatic opponency.

Figure 9.6.2 (top) depicts schematically how the amplitude of the response of a classical linear (L–αM) mechanism should vary with colour-ratio. Given the CIE co-ordinates of the two phosphors, with $\alpha = 1$ a local minimum of the response is predicted for $r = 0.31$. The best approximation to a symmetrical curve is obtained with $\alpha = 2.85$, which produces a flat response at all colour ratios. However, no value of α can create a peak near $r = 0.5$. Non-linear models, such as the difference of L and M cone Weber fractions ($\Delta L/L - \Delta M/M$) (Stromeyer et al., 1985), also face difficulties, predicting maximum response not at $r = 0.5$ (as observed), but at $r = 0.58$.

9.6.3   THE MODEL

What interaction between cones could produce a response curve with maximum activity at equiluminance and zero at the two extremes? Figure 9.6.2 (bottom) shows the L and M cone activity for the stimuli of Figure 9.6.1. In this domain, the maxima and minima of luminance-modulated stimuli ($r = 0.0$ and $r = 1.0$) are represented by collinear vectors (falling on the same line passing through the origin, as shown by the points labelled with A and B). Equiluminant stimuli ($r = 0.5$) fall, by definition, on lines with slope of -1 ($L + M = $ constant). Stimuli with different ratios describe segments of various orientations and lengths. Note that the area enclosed by the stimulus segments and the vectors from the origin is zero for pure luminance-modulated stimuli, and increases with colour ratio (of constant modulation depth (k)) to a maximum at equiluminance (ratio 0.5). In principle, this area could be a useful measure of chromatic modulation.

The modulus of the vectorial product of the vectors corresponding to the extremes of the stimulus in the $<L,M>$ space is a simple measure of the parallelogram area. To normalise the chromatic modulation to a dimensionless value, we divide the vectorial product by the square of the mean luminance and term this output as *Chromatic Contrast* (C_c), by analogy to the luminance response characterised by the Michelson contrast:

$$C_c = 2 \frac{|\bar{v}_1 {}^\wedge \bar{v}_2|}{I_0^2}$$

(2)

where v_1 and v_2 represent the vectors associated with the extremes of visual stimuli in L and M cone space and I_0 is the average luminance given by the sum of the average activity of the L and M cones. The factor 2 is introduced to obtain a maximum C_c of 1 for stimuli that correspond to vectors separated by 45° (the maximum physical realisable chromatic modulation, given the superposition of the L and M spectral sensitivity curves (Smith and Pokorny, 1975)).

The function C_c is graphically represented by the continuous curve in Figure 9.6.2 (top). It is apparent that it satisfies the requirements of symmetry around the equiluminance point, and provides at least a qualitative fit to the data. The rest of the paper will be devoted to testing quantitatively the predictions of this model of colour contrast for a variety of psychophysical results, and showing how this definition is consistent with the notion of independent mechanisms for luminance and chromatic modulation.

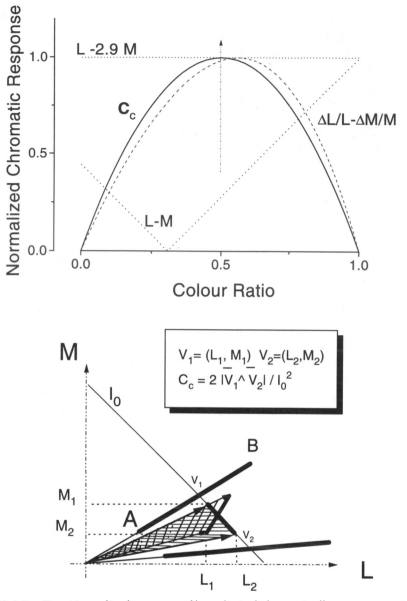

Figure 9.6.2. Top: Normalised response of hypothetical chromatically opponent units to the stimuli of Figure 9.6.1, as a function of the colour ratio *r*. The dotted lines are the prediction from linear models that combines the L and M cone outputs with a weight equal to 1 or 2.85. The dashed curve is a model that subtracts the L and M cone Weber fractions ($\Delta L/L - \Delta M/M$), and the thick continuous curve is the prediction from the chromatic contrast of equation 1. Bottom: Stimulus representation in the <L,M> cone activity space (calculated from the fundamentals of Smith and Pokorny, 1975). The thick segments represent the locus of cone activity elicited by gratings of *r* = 0, 1, 0.5 and 0.125 (modulation *k* = 0.5). The modulus of the vectorial product (equation (2)) is proportional to the shaded areas for each stimulus. For further details see text.

9.6.4   INDEPENDENT RESPONSE TO LUMINANCE AND CHROMATIC MODULATION

Equation (2) can be expressed in various ways, perhaps the most intuitive being:

$$C_c = 2\frac{|L_1M_2 - L_2M_1|}{I_0^2} = 2\frac{|\Delta L \cdot M - \Delta M \cdot L|}{I_0^2}$$

(3)

where (L_1,M_1) and (L_2,M_2) are the cone activity for the most chromatically different points of the stimulus and ΔL, ΔM, L and M are the variation and the average of the cone activity respectively.

Using one of the expressions in (3) it is easy to show that the response to stimuli of various colour ratio (r) and modulation (k) is simply given by:

$$C_c = 2kr(1 - r)|m_g l_r - l_g m_r|$$

(4)

where m_g, l_g, m_r, l_r are the McLeod-Boynton (1979) normalised cone activity to the pure red and green stimuli. The term within the absolute value brackets is a constant that depends on the spectral composition of the primitive lights. The Michaelson contrast associated with these stimuli can be expressed as:

$$M_c = 2k(r - 0.5)$$

(5)

Equations (4) and (5) can be used to calculate the amount of chromatic and Michaelson contrast in the stimuli of Figure 9.6.1 at threshold. Figure 9.6.3 shows the results for the two observers at the two temporal frequencies. The maximum C_c is obtained for stimuli with ratios near to equiluminance, and the maximum M_c for the stimuli with ratios near 0 and 1. All the other data are distributed over rectangular-like shapes. The thick continuous curves are the predictions derived from considering two independent detectors (for each stimulus condition), one sensitive to luminance contrast and the other to chromatic contrast, with probability summation between the two. The predictions fall quite close to the experimental observations.

9.6.5   SIMULATION OF 'SECOND-SITE' CHROMATIC ADAPTATION RESULTS

Stromeyer *et al.* (1985) have shown that the classical two-colour incremental thresholds can be modified by adding lights of different wavelength to the uniform chromatic adapting fields, and have used this result as evidence for a second-site chromatic adaptation. Figure 9.6.4A (adapted from Stromeyer *et al.*, 1985) shows thresholds for different adapting fields plotted in the L and M cone Weber-fraction space. The threshold data form different ellipses for different wavelengths of the adapting field, with the 636 nm field producing a much broader ellipse along the -45° direction. Any mechanism that combines linearly cone Weber fractions will fail to predict simultaneously all the pooled data, forcing the hypothesis of later-stage adaptation mechanisms.

However, while changing the adapting field does induce a change in the single cone Weber fractions, it leaves invariant C_c as defined in equations 2 and 3. Figure 9.6.4B shows the data of Figure 9.6.4A plotted as luminance contrast (M_c) against colour contrast (C_c). The different symbols refer to different wavelengths of the adapting field. For both subjects, the different stimulus conditions produce very similar values of C_c at threshold, about 0.002. Interestingly, this value of C_c is very similar to that for Figure 9.6.1, despite the differences in experimental conditions (monochromatic against broad-band, spots versus sine-wave gratings). As before, the data in Figure 9.6.4B all fall near the continuous curve given by the probability summation model of two independent detectors for luminance and colour.

Stromeyer *et al.* (1985) also measured detection thresholds for stimuli along the $\Delta M/M = 0$ direction, for a wide range of chromaticity and luminance. Figure 9.6.5 replots their data as $\Delta L/L$ versus M_c (open symbols) and C_c versus M_c (filled symbols), for the range 520–640 nm of the adapting fields (in the Rayleigh region). The triangles and the circles refer to different levels of luminance. While the Weber fraction varied by more than a factor of seven with adapting field, the C_c measure was practically constant. The data are again predictable by assuming probability summation between independent detectors.

9.6.6 COLOUR DETECTION ALONG THE EQUILUMINANT L-M AXES

The experiments described previously measured detection threshold for various stimulus conditions that contain both luminance and chromatic contrast. In a recent paper, Krauskopf and Gegenfurtner (1992) have measured colour detection along the $(S-(L+M)) = 0$ axis and shown that this varies little with adaptation. Figure 9.6.6 reproduces their results, showing that over the range of 0.6–0.85 l units of MacLeod-Boynton space, thresholds are constant. The thick continuous and the dotted lines are the prediction of a Helmholtz type

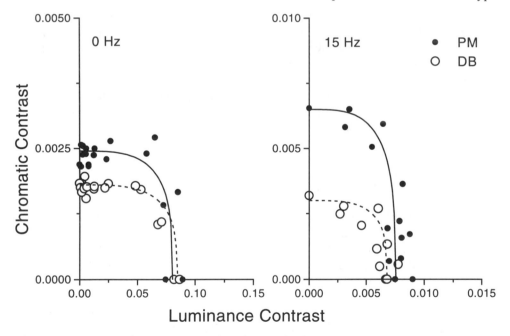

Figure 9.6.3. Data of Figure 9.6.1 replotted as Michaelson (luminance) contrast threshold against Chromatic contrast threshold (as defined in equation 2). The filled symbols refer to the data for subject DB and squares for PM (0 Hz at left, 15 Hz at right). The thick and dotted curves are predictions from probability summation between independent detectors whose response is proportional to M_c and C_c:

$$[(M_c/M_{ct})^\beta + (C_c/C_{ct})^\beta]^{1/\beta} = 1 \qquad (6)$$

where M_c and C_c are the two independent contrast variables and M_{ct} and C_{ct} are the contrast thresholds for the stimuli modulated in luminance and colour respectively. β is the slope of the psychometric function taken to be 3.5 (e.g. Pelli, 1987).

of model and of the difference cone Weber fraction respectively. None of these models predicts the invariance of the thresholds.

However, if colour detection is proportional to the C_c of the stimulus, and a fixed amount of contrast is needed to reach threshold, it is easy to predict the invariance. Given that the stimuli of Figure 9.6.6 are equiluminant and fall on the axes $\Delta L + \Delta M = 0$, equation (4) can be written as:

$$C_c = 2|m \cdot \Delta l - l \cdot \Delta m|2\Delta l \qquad (7)$$

where l and m are the MacLeod-Boynton normalised variables. From equation (7) it follows that the chromatic contrast of the threshold of Figure 9.6.6 is constant and equal to 0.0022, a value similar to that evaluated in the previous sections.

9.6.7   BIOLOGICALLY PLAUSIBLE IMPLEMENTATION

The previous section shows that when chromatic contrast is defined by equation (2), many thresholds for colour detection are readily predictable, and in fact become quite similar, despite the different conditions under which the data were collected. With this definition of colour contrast, all the thresholds examined can be explained by the action of independent luminance and colour channels that mediate detection. It is reasonable at this point to ask

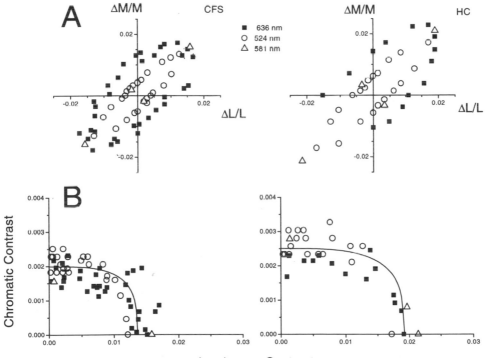

Figure 9.6.4.   A: Detection thresholds for 1.2° light spots superimposed on various adapting backgrounds of 636 (square), 524 (circles) and 581 nm (triangles) plotted in the L and M cone Weber fraction space. The data are replotted from Stromeyer *et al.* (1985, Figure 4). B: The data of Figure 9.6.4A plotted as threshold luminance contrast (M_c: $\Delta l/l_0$) against chromatic contrast (C_c). The thick lines show the prediction of probability summation between luminance and chromatic detectors (described by equation (6)).

how the visual system could compute this form of Chromatic Contrast and what particular properties it needs to do so. Equation (2) essentially requires a second-order or multiplicative non-linearity together with an automatic gain control mechanism for the overall mean luminance. Both these operations are biologically plausible and are common in many neurones at various levels of the visual system.

Of the many possible biologically plausible implementations, we would like to put forward one that closely resembles a multiplexing operation, needed to separate the chromatic from the luminance information transmitted by single opponent neurones (for review see Mullen and Kingdom, 1991). Let us consider that a neuronal operator responds to the local value of C_c as defined by:

$$R_c(x,y) = 2\frac{\bar{M} \cdot L(x,y) - \bar{L} \cdot M(x,y)}{(\bar{M} + \bar{L})^2}$$

(8)

where $L(x,y)$, $M(x,y)$ are the local values of the L and M cone activity and $\bar{M}$ and $\bar{L}$ are the average over a wider region of space.

Each of the two multiplicative terms can be well approximated by a multiplicative interaction between the centre and periphery response of a neuronal receptive field with a L-M or M-L single opponency. The inset of Figure 9.6.7 shows a diagrammatic illustration

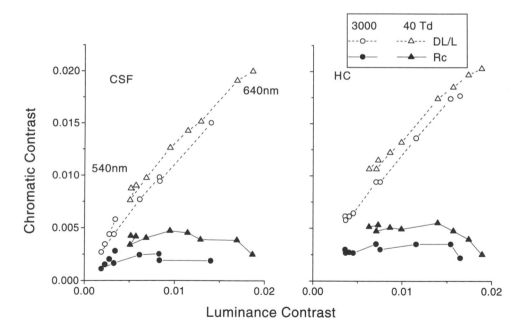

Figure 9.6.5. Thresholds from Stromeyer *et al.* (1985, Figure 7) for test stimuli that do not modulate M cones, presented on adapting backgrounds varying from 520 nm to 640 nm. The open symbols plot the L cone Weber fraction as a function of the luminance contrast (defined as luminance Weber fraction $\Delta I/I_0$) of the threshold stimulus, the filled symbols show the chromatic contrast calculated from equation 2. The 640 nm adapting field had a luminance of 3000 td (circles). The triangles refer to data collected with field components reduced by a factor of 75.

of the possible neuronal connection. If we consider that each simple opponent neurone has a luminance gain control (see for review Shapley and Enroth-Cugell, 1984), the simple difference of the two elements is generating a new operator that selectively responds to the chromatic contrast of the stimulus, ignoring the luminance contrast content. This new mechanism will effectively operate as a multiplexer, mimicking closely the properties of the double-opponent neurones. Note that the existence of the multiplicative interaction between the centre and the surround does not preclude the possibility of the classical subtractive linear opponency. After the combination of the two elements, the linear signals related to the single receptive field opponency will become small and their contribution in the overall response could be ignored.

To illustrate how the new operator will respond to a visual input, we implemented the algorithm and calculated its output to a scene that creates a classic colour illusion. Regions that are of the same yellow hue will appear more reddish or greenish if seen adjacent to a green or red region. This is schematically illustrated in Figure 9.6.7A where the lower yellow circles and the lower part of the ellipse will be perceived as reddish given that the surrounding region has a green average chromaticity. The stimulus is equiluminant except for a luminance border on the left (grey area), as shown by the sliced luminance profile in

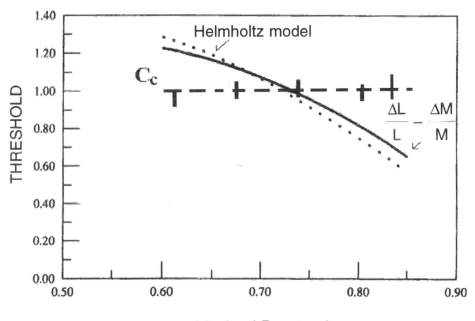

Figure 9.6.6. Thresholds for detecting red or green pulses on an equiluminant background varying along the L-M axis. The heavy vertical lines plot ± 1 SE, and thresholds are expressed in arbitrary units (1 unit corresponding to 0.0011 Δl). The three curves indicate predictions from three different models: the dotted line is the prediction from a Helmholtz-type model; the thick solid curve the prediction from the difference of L and M Weber fractions; and the thick dashed line the prediction from the chromatic contrast of equation (7). This figure has been reproduced with permission from Krauskopf and Gegenfurtner (1992).

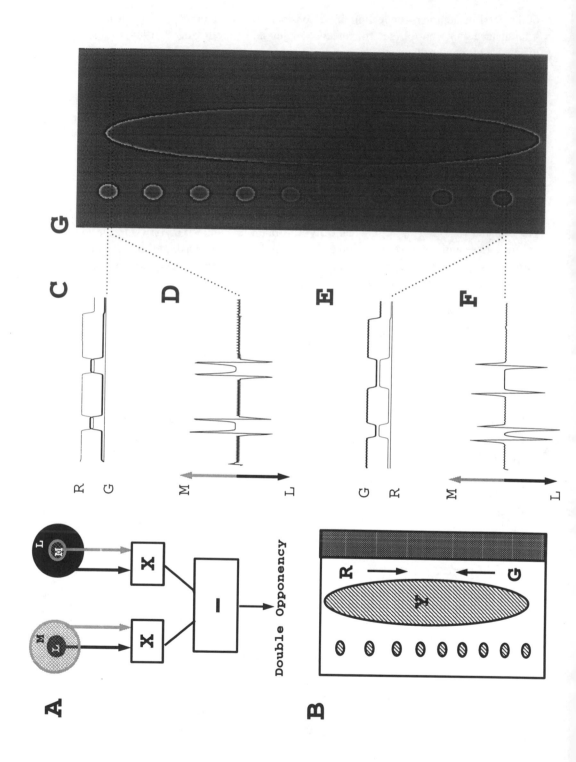

Figure 9.6.7.   A: Schematic diagram of how to generate the hypothetical units described by equation 8 from L-M and M-L single opponent receptive fields. The centre and the periphery of the two input receptive fields should first interact multiplicatively, and their outputs subtract to obtain a response proportional to the local chromatic contrast of equation 8. It is assumed that each single opponent unit has luminance control mechanisms that produce the luminance normalisation over a region equivalent to the receptive field size. B: Schematic representation of a stimulus given by several yellow disks and an ellipse surrounded by a background varying in colour from red to green from top to bottom. The stimulus is equiluminant except for a luminance border on the left illustrated by the grey region. The slice of the luminance profile of the red and green lights are illustrated in C and E by the thin and thick lines respectively. G: The output of the model described in equation 8, implemented by single opponent receptive fields as illustrated in diagram 7A. The centre and the periphery of the fields have been modelled with a 2D-Gaussian function of s = 0.5 and 1 pixels respectively (input image is 500 × 260 pixels), with the integral of the centre and surround being equal. The plots of D and F show the response of the model for the same rows whose luminance profile is illustrated in C and F. Note the inversion of the chromatic edge polarity between the outputs in D and F and the absence of the response to the luminance contrast.

Figures 9.6.7C and E for the red and green phosphors. Figure 9.6.7G shows the output of the model. All the chromatic borders are detected, with decreasing strength as the adjacent region becomes of similar wavelength, but the luminance border has been ignored. Note how the chromatic edges for the upper and lower disks (or for the upper and lower halves of the ellipse) have different polarity, as illustrated by the sliced profile in Figure 9.6.7D and F. The model therefore predicts that a red disc should be perceived in the lower half, while a green disc should be perceived in the top, qualitatively simulating the perceived pattern.

9.6.8   ACKNOWLEDGEMENTS

We thank David Burr and Adriana Fiorentini for help during the research and for fruitful discussion. This work was supported by CNR Target Grant Robotica (N. 92.00926PF67) and by the National Research Programme for Bioelectronics (contract MURST and SGS Thompson Microelectronics).

9.6.9   REFERENCES

FIORENTINI, A., BURR, D.C. & MORRONE, M.C. (1991) Spatial and temporal characteristics of colour vision: VEP and psychophysical measurements. In: Valberg, A. & Lee, B.B. (Eds) *From Pigment to Perception: Advances in Understanding Visual Processing*, New York: Plenum Press, pp. 139–150.

HURVICH, L.M. & JAMESON, D. (1957) An opponent-process theory of color vision, *Psychological Reviews*, **64**, 384–404.

KRAUSKOPF, J. & GEGENFURTNER, K. (1992) Color discrimination and adaptation, *Vision Research*, **32**, 2165–2175.

KRAUSKOPF,J., WILLIAMS, D.R. & HEELEY, D.W. (1982) Cardinal directions of color space, *Vision Research*, **22**, 1123–1131.

MACLEOD, D.I.A. & BOYNTON, R.M. (1979) Chromatic diagram showing cone excitation by stimuli of equal luminance, *Journal of the Optical Society of America*, **69**, 1183–1186.

MULLEN, K.T. (1985) The contrast sensitivity of human colour vision to red-green and blue-yellow gratings, *Journal of Physiology*, **359**, 381–400.

Mullen, M.T. & Kingdom, F.A.A. (1991) Colour contrast in form perception. In: Gouras, P. (Ed.) *Vision and Visual Dysfunction: The Perception of Colour*, London: MacMillan, pp. 198–217.

Pelli, D.G. (1987) On the relation between summation and facilitation, *Vision Research*, **27**, 119–123.

Shapley, R. & Enroth-Cugell, C. (1984) Visual adaptation and retinal gain controls. In: Osborn, N.N. & Chadler, J.G. (Eds) *Progress in Retinal Research*, Vol 3, Oxford: Pergamon Press.

Smith, V.C. & Pokorny, J. (1975) Spectral sensitivity of the foveal cone photopigments between 400 and 500 nm, *Vision Research*, **15**, 161–171.

Stromeyer, C.F. III, Cole, G.R. & Kronauer, R.E. (1985) Second-Site adaptation in the red-green chromatic pathways, *Vision Research*, **25**, 219–237.

Watson, A.B. & Pelli, D.G. (1983) QUEST: A bayesian adaptive psychometric method, *Perceptions and Psychophysics*, **33**, 113–120.

Linear Models of Dichromacy

Horst Scheibner and Arnd Orazem

9.7.1   DICHROMACY REDUCED FROM TRICHROMACY

It is well known that reducing trichromacy to a dichromacy may be accomplished by means of the missing colour (German: *Fehlfarbe* (see, for example, Nuberg and Yustova, 1958; Scheibner, 1968)). For the purpose of illustration, we consider the colour triangle (assumed to be rectangular) of Wright (1946) (Figure 9.7.1). In this colour system, a colour is represented by a vectorial equation of the form

$$C = B \cdot \mathbf{B} + G \cdot \mathbf{G} + R \cdot \mathbf{R} \tag{1}$$

where B, G, R are instrumental tristimulus values and $\mathbf{B}$, $\mathbf{G}$, $\mathbf{R}$ are the so-called primaries and stand for real reference stimuli. In a visual tristimulus colourimeter (ours was according to Guild and Bechstein (Beck and Richter, 1958)), these primaries are realised by monochromatic radiations of wavelengths $\lambda = 460$ nm (blue, B), $\lambda = 530$ nm (green, G) and $\lambda = 630$ nm (red, R). The chromaticity co-ordinates b, g, r are derived from the tristimulus values B, G, R according to the well-known rules

$$b = \frac{B}{B + G + R}, \quad g = \frac{G}{B + G + R}, \quad r = \frac{R}{B + G + R} \tag{1a,b,c}$$

The reduction turns the three-dimensional colour space into a two-dimensional one. Hence, the reducing mapping must be of the form:

$$\begin{bmatrix} B' \\ R' \end{bmatrix} = A \cdot \begin{bmatrix} B \\ G \\ R \end{bmatrix} \tag{2}$$

where the triple of the right hand side is a trichromatic colour vector, the pair on the left hand side is a dichromatic one; A is a matrix consisting of two rows and three columns. The notation of equation (2) fits the case of deutcranopia, which we preferredly treat as an example. The mapping (i.e. matrix A) is determined if we know a special colour vector

$$\begin{bmatrix} B_D \\ G_D \\ R_D \end{bmatrix} \tag{3}$$

for which

$$\begin{bmatrix} 0 \\ 0 \end{bmatrix} = A \cdot \begin{bmatrix} B_D \\ G_D \\ R_D \end{bmatrix} \tag{4}$$

holds. This special colour vector is the missing colour and can be measured (e.g. Kröger and Scheibner, 1977; Kröger-Paulus, 1980; Scheibner, 1976). In linear algebra, it (more exactly, the one-dimensional subspace spanned by it) is called the kernel of the (homomorphic) mapping in equation (2).

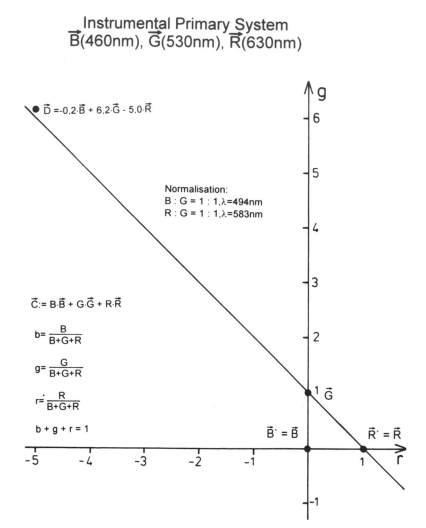

Figure 9.7.1. Instrumental primary system according to W. D. Wright (1946). In the left top corner, the chromaticity locus of a typical deuteranopic missing colour **D** is shown under the condition of the normalisation indicated. (**B'**, **R'**) is a possible set of remaining deuteranopic primaries.

The difference between the deuteranope and the normal trichromat is explained by the finding (Rushton, 1965) that the middle or 'green'-absorbing visual cone pigment is absent in the deuteranope. Therefore, one could in a simplified way conclude that, in Figure 9.7.1, the two-dimensionality is just achieved by discarding the 'green' primary **G**. The experiment shows, however, that the *real* colour **G** is *not* the missing colour but an *imaginary* colour vector **D** whose typical locus is indicated in Figure 9.7.1. A more convenient representation of **D** results by changing the normalisation of **R** in relation to **G** so that the locus of **D** is in a shorter distance from **G**. This will be done in the consecutive figures.

The missing colour is measured by the dichromat's applying the perceptual criterion 'indistinguishably equal', i.e. *his* colour match. In Figure 9.7.2 (Kröger-Paulus, 1980; Scheibner and Paulus, 1978), this method is demonstrated: two colours, distinctly different for a normal trichromat, may be (or are made) indistinguishably equal for the dichromat. Their vectorial difference, therefore, has the meaning of a null vector for the dichromat. This null vector is the vectorial missing colour (**D** in Figure 9.7.1). It owns a certain direction within the colour space and, therefore, a certain chromaticity locus. It lies coplanarly within the dichromat's null-luminance plane, the so-called alychne plane according to Schrödinger (1925), and its chromaticity locus is, therefore, incident on the dichromat's alychne trace. In general, the colour triangle side opposite to the locus of the missing colour lends itself to the dichromat's remaining chromaticity diagram, in Figure

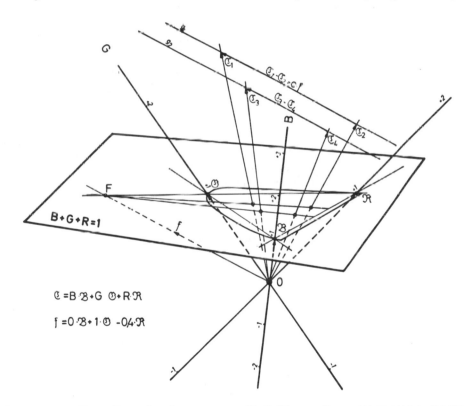

Figure 9.7.2. Three-dimensional vector space (**B, G, R**) according to W. D. Wright (1946) and pertaining chromaticity diagram within the plane B + R + G = 1. The two difference vectors C_1–C_2 and C_3–C_4 being null vectors are parallel to **f**, the deuteranopic missing vector, which pierces the chromaticity plane in point F, the co-punctal point (from Kröger-Paulus, 1980).

9.7.1, the join between **B** and **R**, which can be interpreted as a binary colour mixture line.

9.7.2   DICHROMACY REDUCED FROM TRICHROMACY DUALLY

The adjective 'dual' is understood here as in geometry, in particular as in projective geometry (see, for example, Coxeter, 1974). There is a way to approach trichromacy as well as dichromacy by means of perceptual criteria different from the colour match. The perceptual criteria applied are 'neither blue nor yellow', 'neither green nor red', and 'heterochromatically equally bright'. These criteria define loci within the chromaticity chart in the form of straight lines. The trichromatic reference is, then, not a triangle but a trilateral, and a reduction to dichromacy amounts to discarding a side of the trilateral. The constellation remaining to the dichromat is, then, not a binary mixture line but a pencil of straight lines, the vertex of which is the trilateral vertex opposite to the trilateral side discarded. It is obvious that such a procedure is a direct way to a system of opponent-colour vision.

In the chromaticity chart, which may be conceived of as a projective plane, straight lines are elements dual to points. Thus, we operate in a space dual to the colour vector space. In Figure 9.7.3, the procedure is demonstrated for deuteranopia.

Let us assume that we determine, by means of a visual tristimulus colourimeter, two chromaticity loci of which one obeys the perceptual criterion 'neither blue nor yellow', the other obeys the criterion 'heterochromatically equally bright'. Lochner and Scheibner (1991) and Knottenberg and Scheibner (1993) have reported on such experiments. In a good approximation, the chromaticity loci are straight lines. They can be expressed in the form

$$g = m \cdot r + h \tag{5}$$

where the variables r and g are chromaticity co-ordinates. But, as dual vectors are nothing other than linear forms (Kostrikin and Manin, 1989), it will prove to be advantageous to express the straight lines as homogeneous linear forms, say

$$\beta_1 \cdot B + \gamma_1 \cdot G + \rho_1 \cdot R = 0 \tag{5a}$$

for the first perceptual criterion,

$$\beta_2 \cdot B + \gamma_2 \cdot G + \rho_2 \cdot R = 0 \tag{5b}$$

for the second perceptual criterion.

Here, B, G, R are, again, the instrumental tristimulus values considered, however, as homogeneous projective co-ordinates. β_i, γ_i, ρ_i, $i = 1,2$, are the components of the dual vectors characterising the straight lines. The transition from equations (5) to (5a,b) is done through the relations (1a,b,c). The two straight lines intersect in a point that obeys the two equations (5a) and (5b). This leads again to the condition (4) we already had, namely

$$\begin{bmatrix} 0 \\ 0 \end{bmatrix} = A \cdot \begin{bmatrix} B_D \\ G_D \\ R_D \end{bmatrix}$$

Thus, the intersection point is given by the missing colour vector. It is the copunctal point of the two straight lines (5a) and (5b). For more mathematics, one may consult, for example, Rees (1983).

As the missing colour lies co-planarly in the null luminance plane (= alychne plane), the various different colour qualities captured by the different perceptual criteria converge into indistinguishability when approaching the (imaginary!) missing colour.

If the missing colour is known, the reducing mapping may be gained in an especially simple way, Figure 9.7.3. Beside the two lines determining the missing colour **D**, the co-punctal point, we plot a line joining **D** and **R** and a line joining **D** and **B**. They are described by the simpler homogeneous linear forms:

$$0 = \beta_B \cdot B + \gamma_B \cdot G$$
$$0 = \qquad \gamma_R \cdot G + \rho_R \cdot R \qquad\qquad (6)$$

Reduction to Deuteranopia in dual terms

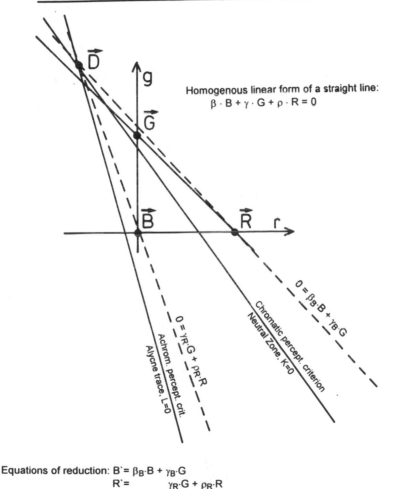

Homogenous linear form of a straight line:
$$\beta \cdot B + \gamma \cdot G + \rho \cdot R = 0$$

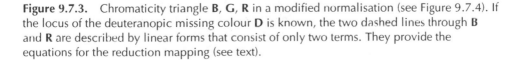

Equations of reduction: $B' = \beta_B \cdot B + \gamma_B \cdot G$
$$R' = \qquad \gamma_R \cdot G + \rho_R \cdot R$$

Figure 9.7.3. Chromaticity triangle **B**, **G**, **R** in a modified normalisation (see Figure 9.7.4). If the locus of the deuteranopic missing colour **D** is known, the two dashed lines through **B** and **R** are described by linear forms that consist of only two terms. They provide the equations for the reduction mapping (see text).

The reducing mapping equations then read

$$B' = \beta_B \cdot B + \gamma_B \cdot G$$
$$R' = \qquad\qquad \gamma_R \cdot G + \rho_R \cdot R \tag{7}$$

because all trichromatic colour vectors, in particular also those outside the kernel, are admitted to the mapping of equation (2).

In summary, the reduction from trichromacy to dichromacy in dual terms leads to a ray pencil, the carrier point of which is given by the locus of the missing colour. The rays, which are straight lines, describe dichromatic chromaticities directly. In contrast to the points of a dichromatic binary mixture line, they show how trichromatic chromaticities collapse into one dichromatic chromaticity. Thus, the dual representation of a dichromacy is more comprehensive than that in the colour space proper.

Figure 9.7.4 gives a numerical illustration for the male deuteranope A.O. Let us neglect, for our purpose, the line joining **R** and **G**. The remaining two straight lines were determined by means of the perceptual criteria mentioned. They are characterised through linear forms, i.e. through dual vectors. The triples of numerical coefficients are the dual vectors. The coefficients of the neutral zone, where a hue change from blue to yellow takes place, are the chrominance coefficients (K meaning chrominance); the coefficients of the alychne trace, where a sign change of luminance takes place, are the luminance coefficients (L meaning luminance). The intersection points of these rays with the abscissa (r-axis) fix the mapping from the deuteranopic instrumental system (**B'**, **R'**) into the deuteranopic opponent-colour system (**K**, **L**).

9.7.3 THE FUNDAMENTAL COLOUR SPACE AND ITS REDUCTIONS

According to the idea of Arthur König (1897), the missing colour of the protanope, deuteranope and tritanope can be made the three primaries of a colour space, the so-called fundamental colour space or cone excitation space (Figure 9.7.5). Transformation equations that achieve the transition into the fundamental colour space are well known (see, for example, Pokorny and Smith, 1986).

Within the fundamental system, the reduction to a dichromacy is simplified both for the colour space and its dual space. In the first, one vertex point of the fundamental colour triangle is discarded; the side opposite to it remains as the dichromatic binary mixture line. This remaining element is situated in the region of imaginary colours. In the second, one side of the fundamental trilateral is discarded. There remains the opposite pencil of straight lines. These remaining elements are the well-known confusion lines and cover the region of real colours.

9.7.4 CONNECTIONS BETWEEN FUNDAMENTAL COLOUR SPACE AND OPPONENT-COLOUR SPACE

Figure 9.7.6 (Scheibner and Bruckwilder, 1989) shows the three classical dichromacies in comparison. The fundamental colour triangle is assumed to be equilateral. The vertices P, D, T are the protanope's, deuteranope's and tritanope's locus of the missing colour. These loci are also the carrier points of the pertinent dichromatic ray pencils. A locus of a missing colour is always incident on the pertaining alychne trace. In protanopia and deuteranopia, the pertaining alychne traces form sides (p, d) of the fundamental colour triangle, but not so for tritanopia (t). Therefore, tritanopia must be of a different nature. Within the framework of the colour space, the missing colours P, D, T are determined by colour matches. Within the framework of the dual space, the alychne traces p, d, t are determined by hetero-chromatic brightness matches, the neutral zones n_P and n_D by the criteria *neither blue nor*

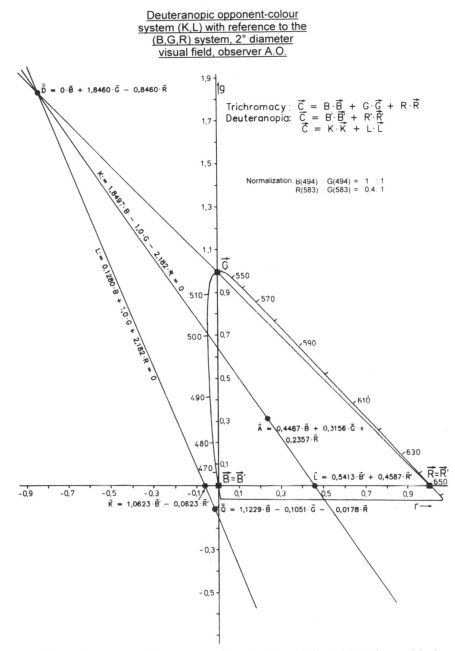

Deuteranopic opponent-colour system (K,L) with reference to the (B,G,R) system, 2° diameter visual field, observer A.O.

$\vec{D} = 0 \cdot \vec{B} + 1,8460 \cdot \vec{G} - 0,8460 \cdot \vec{R}$

Trichromacy: $\vec{C} = B \cdot \vec{B} + G \cdot \vec{G} + R \cdot \vec{R}$
Deuteranopia: $\vec{C} = B' \cdot \vec{B'} + R' \cdot \vec{R'}$
$\vec{C} = K \cdot \vec{K} + L \cdot \vec{L}$

Normalization: B(494) : G(494) = 1 : 1
R(583) : G(583) = 0.4 : 1

$\vec{K} = 1,8497 \cdot \vec{B} - 1,0 \cdot \vec{G} - 2,182 \cdot \vec{R} = 0$

$\vec{L} = 0,1280 \cdot \vec{B} + 1,0 \cdot \vec{G} + 2,182 \cdot \vec{R} = 0$

$\vec{A} = 0,4487 \cdot \vec{B} + 0,3156 \cdot \vec{G} + 0,2357 \cdot \vec{R}$

$\vec{K} = 1,0623 \cdot \vec{B'} - 0,0623 \cdot \vec{R'}$

$\vec{L} = 0,5413 \cdot \vec{B'} + 0,4587 \cdot \vec{R'}$

$\vec{R} = \vec{R'}$

$\vec{Q} = 1,1229 \cdot \vec{B} - 0,1051 \cdot \vec{G} - 0,0178 \cdot \vec{R}$

Figure 9.7.4. Chromaticity diagram according to W. D. Wright (1946). The modified normalisation is indicated. The neutral zone K = 0 and the alychne trace L = 0 are characterised by homogeneous linear forms, i.e. numerically by line co-ordinates. $\bar{A}$ and $\bar{Q}$ are averaged vectors. The loci of **K** and **L** are characterised by vectors, i.e. numerically by point co-ordinates (from Orazem and Scheibner, 1992).

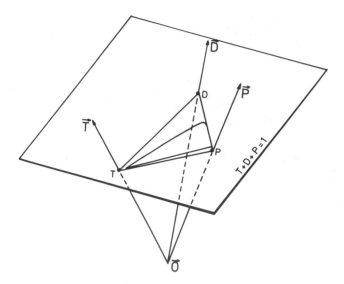

Figure 9.7.5. Three-dimensional fundamental colour space with primaries **P, D, T** and the pertaining chromaticity triangle within the plane P + D + T = 1.

yellow, the neutral zone n_T by the criterion *neither green nor red*. The copunctal point of a neutral zone and an alychne trace also determine the locus of the missing colour. Whereas the fundamental primary T is incident on t, by definition, T is incident on p and d only if the blue mechanisms in protanopia and deuteranopia do *not* carry brightness. The change of reference from dichromatic fundamental colour vision to dichromatic opponent-colour vision is given by the neutral zones n_P, n_D, n_T and the alychne traces p, d, t. They work as new referential chromaticities.

9.7.5   TRANSFORMATIONAL PROPERTIES

The physiologically interesting excitation transfer is represented by the mapping from the fundamental colour space onto the opponent-colour space. In Figure 9.7.7, the deuteranopic transfer is demonstrated in distimulus values (P, T) and (K, L) as well as in chrominance and luminance coefficients (π, τ) = (pi, tau) and (κ, λ) = (kappa, lambda). The reference system is the fundamental colour triangle P, D, T, assumed to be rectangular. The additive mixture of deuteranopic colours takes place on the mixture line joining **P** and **T**. As an example, two colours are added:

$$\mathbf{C}_1 = 0.2 \cdot \mathbf{P} + 0.8 \cdot \mathbf{T}$$

$$\mathbf{C}_2 = 0.6 \cdot \mathbf{P} + 0.4 \cdot \mathbf{T}$$

$$\mathbf{C}_1 + \mathbf{C}_2 = 0.8 \cdot \mathbf{P} + 1.2 \cdot \mathbf{T}$$

or renormalized

$$\mathbf{C}_1 + \mathbf{C}_2 = 0.4 \cdot \mathbf{P} + 0.6 \cdot \mathbf{T}$$

Dichromatic vision

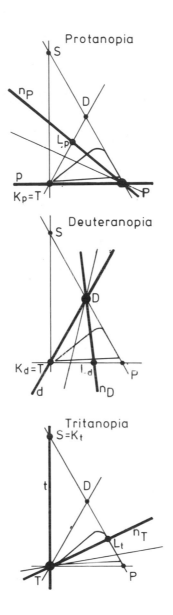

Figure 9.7.6. A triangle assumed to be equilateral is drawn three times. P, D, T are the copunctal points of the protanope, deuteranope, tritanope; n_P, n_D, n_T are their 'neutral' confusion lines, p, d, t are their alychne traces. Trace t is assumed to obey (in distimulus values) $D + 2 \cdot P = 0$, or (in chromaticity co-ordinates) $d = -2p$. (K_i, L_i), $i = p,d,t$ are the dichromatic opponent-colour systems, where K = chrominance, L = luminance. The point S may be interpreted as co-punctal point of a hypothetical fusion deuteranope exhibiting brightness vision of the normal trichromat (and the tritanope) (from Scheibner and Bruckwilder, 1989, modified).

The same event when taking place in the dual space reads:

$$\Gamma_1 : 0.8P - 0.2 \cdot T = 0$$

$$\Gamma_2 : 0.4 \cdot P - 0.6 \cdot T = 0$$

$$\Gamma_1 + \Gamma_2 : 1.2 \cdot P - 0.8 \cdot T = 0$$

or renormalized

$$\Gamma_1 + \Gamma_2 : 0.6 \cdot P - 0.4 \cdot T = 0$$

Transformation of Deuteranopic Spaces

Deuteranopic homogeneous linear forms: $\pi \cdot P + \tau \cdot T = 0$

$$\kappa \cdot K + \lambda \cdot L = 0$$

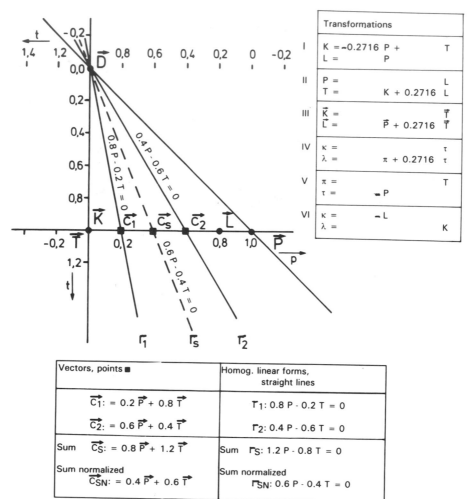

Transformations			
I	$K =$ -0.2716 P +		T
	$L =$	P	
II	$P =$		L
	$T =$	K + 0.2716	L
III	$\vec{K} =$		$\vec{T}$
	$\vec{L} =$	$\vec{P}$ + 0.2716	$\vec{T}$
IV	$\kappa =$		τ
	$\lambda =$	π + 0.2716	τ
V	$\pi =$		T
	$\tau =$	- P	
VI	$\kappa =$	- L	
	$\lambda =$		K

Vectors, points ■	Homog. linear forms, straight lines
$\vec{C_1} = 0.2\,\vec{P} + 0.8\,\vec{T}$	$\Gamma_1: 0.8\ P - 0.2\ T = 0$
$\vec{C_2} = 0.6\,\vec{P} + 0.4\,\vec{T}$	$\Gamma_2: 0.4\ P - 0.6\ T = 0$
Sum $\vec{C_S} = 0.8\,\vec{P} + 1.2\,\vec{T}$	Sum $\Gamma_S: 1.2\ P - 0.8\ T = 0$
Sum normalized $\vec{C_{SN}} = 0.4\,\vec{P} + 0.6\,\vec{T}$	Sum normalized $\Gamma_{SN}: 0.6\ P - 0.4\ T = 0$

Figure 9.7.7. Fundamental colour triangle **P, D, T** assumed to be rectangular. Various types of transformations between the fundamental and the opponent colour system are given and expressed in distimulus values (point co-ordinates) and chrominance/luminance co-efficients (line co-ordinates). Addition of two colours is expressed in vectors as well as linear forms. The results of addition are renormalised so that the numbers add up to 1.

The linear forms are written beside their straight lines. Besides the deuteranopic fundamental reference system (P, T), Figure 9.7.7 shows also the deuteranopic opponent reference system (K, L), where K = T. In this opponent-colour system, the addition could also be done. The mapping from (P, T) to (K, L) is given by equation I in Figure 9.7.7. Equation II is the inverse of equation I. Equation III shows the change from the fundamental primaries to the opponent primaries. Their matrix is contragredient to that of equation I, i.e. derived from I by transposing and inverting the matrix of I. (In our special case, the matrix is symmetric, therefore, the transposition does not become effective.) It is well known in linear algebra (e.g. Kostrikin and Manin, 1989; Scheibner, 1993) that the dual components (π, τ) are also transformed contragrediently to the initial distimulus values (P, T). Therefore equation IV follows the same scheme as equation III. Finally, equation V show the connection between the distimulus values (P, T) and the coefficients (π, τ) and equation VI shows the connection between the distimulus values (K, L) and the coefficients (κ, λ). Transformations V and VI are of the type of duality (Coxeter, 1974).

9.7.6   CONCLUSIONS

For a more complete description of dichromacy, we recommend: (1) to include the alychne trace as a special imaginary confusion line; and (2) to make use of homogeneous linear forms in order to make dual symmetries evident.

9.7.7   REFERENCES

BECK, J. & RICHTER, M. (1958) Neukonstruktion des Dreifarbenmessgerätes nach Guild-Bechstein, *Die Farbe*, **7**, 141–152.

COXETER, H.S.M. (1974) *Projective Geometry*, Toronto and Buffalo: University of Toronto Press.

KNOTTENBERG, TH. & SCHEIBNER, H. (1993) Berücksichtigung des Abney-Effekts im Rahmen der linearen Gegenfarbentheorieh, *Ophthalmologe*, **90**, 155–160.

KÖNIG, A. (1897) Über Blaublindheit, *Sitzungsberichte der Akademie der Wissenschaften Berlin*, 718–731.

KOSTRIKIN, A.I. & MANIN, YU. I. (1989) *Linear Algebra and Geometry*, New York: Gordon and Breach.

KRÖGER, A. & SCHEIBNER H. (1977) Reduktion der Deuteranopie aus der Trichromasie, *Ber. Dtsch. Ophthalm. Gesellsch.*, **75**, 515–517.

KRÖGER-PAULUS, A. (1980) Reduktion der Deuteranopie aus der normalen Trichromasie, *Die Farbe*, **19**, 77–116.

LOCHNER, D. & SCHEIBNER, H. (1991) Gründung einer linearen trichromatischen Übertragungstheorie auf Buntheitsurteile über ungesättigte Farben, *Fortschritte der Ophthalmologie*, **88**, 68–72.

NUBERG, N.D. & YUSTOVA, E.N. (1958) Researches on dichromatic vision and the spectral sensitivity of the receptors of trichromats. In: National Physical Laboratory, *Visual Problems of Colour*, vol. 2, London: Her Majesty's Stationery Office, pp. 477–486.

ORAZEM, A. & SCHEIBNER, H. (1992) Opponent-colour vision of a deuteranope, *Pflügers Archiv, European Journal of Physiology*, **420**, suppl. R 48.

POKORNY, J. & SMITH, V.C. (1986) Colorimetry and color discrimination. In: Boff, K. R., Kaufman, L. & Thomas, J.P. (Eds) *Handbook of Perception and Human Performance*, vol. 1, New York: John Wiley, pp. 8-1–8-51.

REES, E.G. (1983) *Notes on Geometry*, Berlin: Springer-Verlag.

RUSHTON, W.A.H. (1965) A foveal pigment in the deuteranope, *Journal of Physiology*, **176**, 24–37.

SCHEIBNER, H. (1968) Dichromasie als Homomorphismus der Trichromasie, *Optica Acta*, **15**, 339–349.

SCHEIBNER, H. (1976) Missing colours (Fehlfarben) of Deuteranopes and extreme deuteranomalous observers. In: Verriest, G. (Ed.) *Colour Vision Deficiencies III*, Basel: Karger, pp. 21–26.

SCHEIBNER, H. (1993) Transformation of luminance coefficients, *Journal of the Optical Society of America*, **A10**, 1392–1395.

SCHEIBNER, H. & BRUCKWILDER, R. (1989) Protanopic opponent colour vision. In: Drum, B. & Verriest, G. (Eds) *Colour Vision Deficiencies IX*, Dordrecht, The Netherlands: Kluwer, pp. 125–130.

SCHEIBNER, H. & PAULUS W. (1978) An analysis of protanopic colour vision. In: Verriest, G. (Ed.) *Colour Vision Deficiencies IV*, Basel: Karger, pp. 206–211.

SCHRÖDINGER, E. (1925) Über das Verhältnis der Vierfarben zur Dreifarbentheorie, *Sitzungsberichte der Akademie der Wissenschaften Wien* (IIa), **134**, 471–490.

WRIGHT, W.D. (1946) *Researches on Normal and Defective Colour Vision*, London: Kimpton.

The Two Axes of the Human Eye and Inversion of the Retinal Layers: the Basis for the Interpretation of the Retina as a Phase Grating Optical, Cellular 3D Chip

N. Lauinger

9.8.1 FROM PRENATAL DEVELOPMENT OF THE HUMAN EYE TO THE FORMATION OF TWO EYE AXES

How does the biaxial structure of the adult eye shown in Figure 9.8.1 come about? With an angle α between the photopic visual axis (VA) and the mechanical or optical ocular axis (OA)? The only place to find the answer is in the prenatal development of the eye.

After the formation of the optic cup and stalk by the neural ectoderm (Figure 9.8.2), the latter comes into contact with the body surface epithelium. This is followed by *invagination* of the retina (Figure 9.8.3), where the anterior hemisphere of the optic cup comes into contact with the pigment epithelium hemisphere. It would be possible, even expected from an understanding of optical equipment, for the photoreceptors to grow forward out of the retina, toward the light, and for the ganglion cell axons to grow out rearward, toward the brain (Figure 9.8.4, top). A uniaxial design with a fovea in the center of the axis would be possible. However, development does *not* continue in this way. *Inversion* of the retinal layers takes place specifically (Figure 9.8.4, bottom). In chronological sequence, first a blood vessel forces its way into the interior of the eye at a very early stage, thus cutting open the entire cup in the ocular fissure, until it has captured a central position at the zenith of the primary ocular axis (Figure 9.8.5, left and right), which becomes the papilla. The ocular fissure then immediately closes again. The optic nerve axons of the ganglion cells grow radially toward the papilla and pass through them toward the brain. Finally, the receptors grow out of the retina into the space next to the pigment epithelium.

But what use is an eye with a blind spot at the zenith of the only axis? In any case, the inversion of the retinal layers proves to have top priority during development. It is not a 'regrettable accident'. The consequences are clear: the biaxial and bipolar structure of the central area at the back of the eye is formed. As the human face develops, the angle between the optic stalks becomes smaller (Figure 9.8.6).

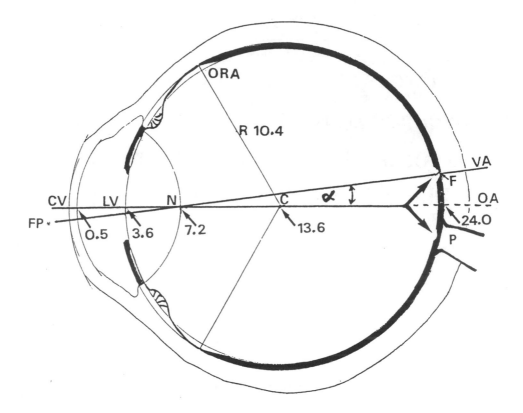

Figure 9.8.1.   Horizontal cross section through the right human eye with ocular axis (OA) and visual axis (VA), α = angle between the two axes. F = fovea, P = papilla, C = centre, N = nodal point, LV = lens vertex, CV = cornea vertex, FP = fixation point, R = radius. The distances from CV or C are given in mm.

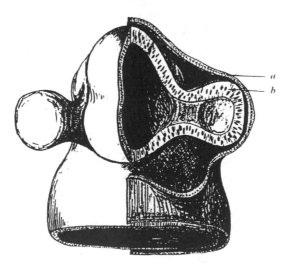

Figure 9.8.2.   Forebrain with optic vesicles (embryo with an overall length of 4 mm, 3rd week, frontal view). a = body surface ectoderm, b = neural ectoderm (Mann, 1949, p. 20).

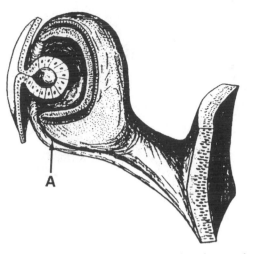

Figure 9.8.3. Optic cup with invagination of the lens and retina. A = ocular fissure in the optic cup, resulting from the entry of the arteria hyaloidea (Mann, 1949, p.26)

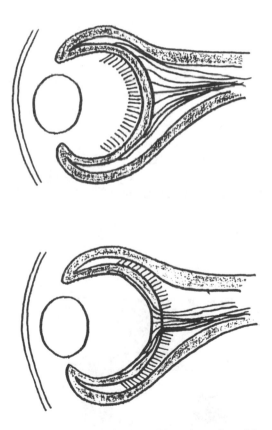

Figure 9.8.4. (Top) Model of an invaginated retina without inversion of the retinal layers; the photoreceptors grow out of the retina toward the light, the optic nerves toward the brain. (Bottom) The situation in the actual invaginated retina with inversion of the retinal layers and opposite growth directions of photoreceptors and optic nerves.

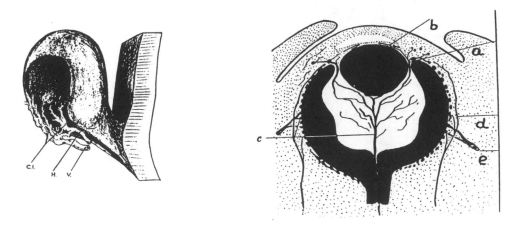

Figure 9.8.5. (Left) Arteria hyaloidea (H) entering the interior of the eye through the ocular fissure (embryo length 5 mm) (Mann, 1949, p. 35) (Right) The papilla is initially at the zenith of the interior of the eye, i.e. at the point of penetration of the eye axis through the retina. The intraocular and part of the extraocular embryonal vessel system of the eye develops via the Arteria hyaloidea; just before birth, it degenerates or is replaced by a new vessel system (a different one in the blueprint). Embryo length 25 mm, 7th week (Mann, 1949, p. 36).

This causes the papilla in both eyes to move toward the nose, leaving space temporally of the primary zenith of the ocular axis into which the retina grows and in which the photopic central region containing the fovea develops. Figure 9.8.7 shows the late insertion of the papillomacular optic nerve bundle into the initially radial path of the optic nerves.

Figure 9.8.8 shows the isopter lines, the retinal zones of the same visual acuity. It can

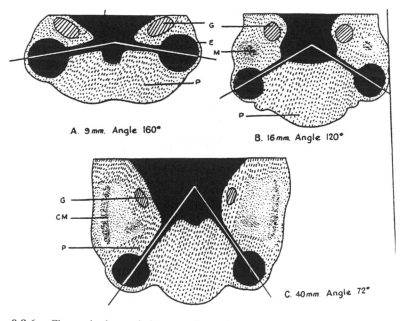

Figure 9.8.6. Change in the angle between the ocular axes and stalks as a consequence of the formation of the face (Mann, 1949, p. 270).

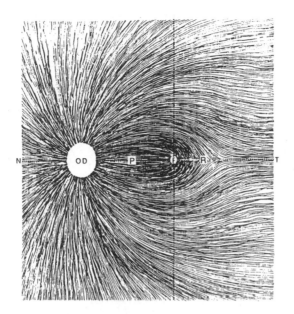

Figure 9.8.7. Path of the optic nerve bundles in the region of the papilla and in the central area of the retina. The papillomacular optic nerve bundle P represents a later inclusion into the optic nerve tracks, which extend basically radially to the papilla. N = nasal, T = temporal, F = fovea, OD = papilla, R = Raphe dividing line (Hogan *et al.*, 1971, p. 536).

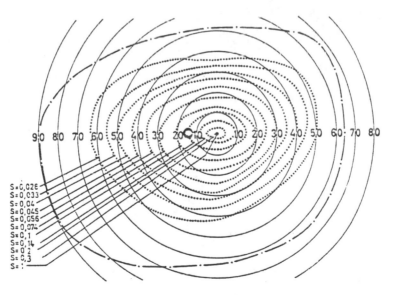

Figure 9.8.8. Isopter lines in the right eye (division of the retinal zones into degrees, S = visual acuity values). The larger isopter ellipses are centred on the primary ocular axis, whose zenith is between the papilla and fovea.

also be seen from them that the peripheral retina (ganglion cell distribution) was centered on the primary ocular axis (zenith between papilla and fovea).

Overall, the sites of the ganglion cells as elements of the retinal (inverted) spatial frequency filter, which is responsible for the visual acuity data in photopic and scotopic vision in this interpretation, are defined by intersections of circles, ellipses and sets of hyperbolas around the two poles (papilla and fovea) (Figure 9.8.10), comparable to the holodiagram reference system known from holography (Figure 9.8.11).

9.8.2   THE 3D PHASE GRATING OPTICAL INTERPRETATION OF THE INVERTED RETINA AND ITS FUNCTIONAL IMPORTANCE

The three cellular layers in the inverted retina (Figure 9.8.12, INL, MNL and ONL) are totally transparent, but have slight refractive index differences between cell nuclei and cell bodies, i.e. are multilayer phase gratings.

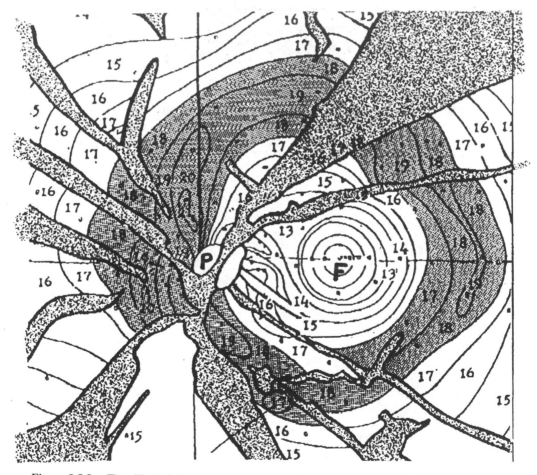

Figure 9.8.9. The elliptical ring zone of greatest rod density (zones 18–20, grey marking by the author, rod density in 10 thousand per mm²) defines the ring zone of sharpest scotopic vision. It encircles papilla (P) and fovea (F) as a dipole (Østerberg, 1935).

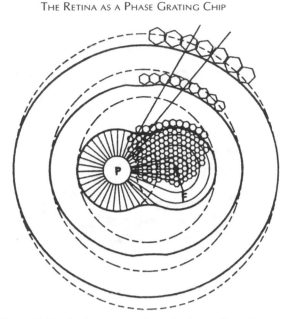

Figure 9.8.10. Ganglion cell distribution concentric to the fovea (F) in the central retinal region and concentric to the papilla (P) and fovea in the peripheral retinal region, as spatial frequency filter in the retinal 3D chip.

The cells themselves can be interpreted as coupled oscillators. Their crystal-optical interpretation may provide an explanation of, inter alia, the following phenomena known from human vision:

- the sites of the four λ_{max} in the visible spectrum, i.e. the spectral points of maximum spectral sensitivity of the cones (447/537/559 nm) and rods (521 nm) as determined by interference-optical laws;
- the Purkinje shift from photopic to scotopic vision and vice versa as an intensity-adaptive 3D grating process;
- the aperture effects in human vision, ie. the Stiles-Crawford effects I (drop in brightness

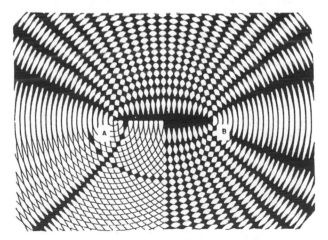

Figure 9.8.11. Abramson holodiagram (Abramson, 1993) for interference optical analysis of holograms.

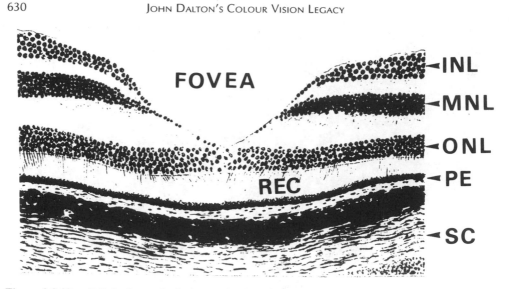

Figure 9.8.12. Cellular layers in the inverted retina (fovea region). INL = inner nuclear layer, MNL = middle nuclear layer, ONL = outer nuclear layer, REC = receptor plane, PE = pigment epithelium layer, SC = sclera (Bargmann, 1967).

for rays incident obliquely on the pupil and retina) and II (hue shift of these rays) as two aspects of a single retinal 3D grating optical effect;

- the transformation of two physical parameters (intensity and wavelength) into three psychological parameters (brightness, hue and saturation);
- the construction of the opponent colour settlement in the crystal-optical trichromatic light processing phase;
- the retinal zone-specific spatial frequency filtering (visual acuity data) based on the grating-optical interpretation of the locations of the ganglion cell bodies;
- in all probability also adaptation mechanisms, as are possible for explaining colour constancy;
- in all probability the time pulse triggering (coherent over an object area of uniform colour) in the chromatic frequency bands whose frequency ratio (447:537:559 = 1:1.2:1.25) is predestined for the occurrence of vibrations in the interference field.

9.8.4 REFERENCES

ABRAMSON, N.H. (1993), Holography as a teaching tool, *Optical Engineering*, **32**(3), 508–513.

BARGMANN, W. (1967) *Histologie und mikroskopische Anatomie des Menschen*, Stuttgart.

HOGAN, M.J., ALVARADO, J.A. & WEDDELL, J.E. (1971) *Histology of the Human Eye*, Philadelphia-London-Toronto: CV Mosby.

MANN, I. (1949) *The Development of the Human Eye*, London: Cambridge University Press.

ÖSTERBERG, G. (1935) Topography of the layer of rods and cones in the human retina, *Acta Ophthalmologica*, Suppl. VI, **13**, 3–4.

Brightness, Hue and Saturation in Photopic Vision: A Diffraction-optical Result of Luminance and Wavelength in the Cellular Phase Grating 3D Chip of the Inverted Human Retina

N. Lauinger

9.9.1   INTRODUCTION

In photopic vision, two physical variables (luminance and wavelength) are transformed into three psychological variables (brightness, hue and saturation). Following on from 3D grating optical explanations of aperture effects (Stiles-Crawford effects SCE I and II; Lauinger, 1992), all three variables can be explained via a single 3D chip effect. The 3D grating optical calculations are carried out using the classical von Laue equation and demonstrated using the example of two experimentally confirmed observations in human vision: saturation effects for monochromatic test lights between 485 and 510 nm in the SCE II and the fact that many test lights reverse their hue shift in the SCE II when changing from moderate to high luminances compared with that on changing from low to medium luminances. At the same time, information is obtained on the transition from the trichromatic colour system in the retina to the opponent colour system.

The inverted retina, with its cells and cell nuclei in hexagonal closest packing, is interpreted as a 3D phase grating with low refractive index differences. Since the formulation of the van Cittert/Zernike theorem in optics, it is thought that incoherent light is converted into partially coherent light on the image-side aperture of the eye, i.e. the amplitude and phase calculation is always required there. The diffraction-optical transformation of white light in photopic vision into three chromatic channels or $h_1h_2h_3$ diffraction orders with λ_{max} ($h_1h_2h_3 = 111$) = 559 nm (RED, L), λ_{max} ($h_1h_2h_3 = 123$) = 537 nm (GREEN, M) and $\lambda_{max}(h_1h_2h_3 = 122)$ = 447 nm (BLUE, S) is described via the direction cosine $\Sigma \cos^2 = \lambda/\lambda = 1$ of the von Laue equation. The explanation of the Purkinje shift from scotopic to photopic vision and of the aperture effects (SCE I/II, Bezold-Brücke phenomenon) themselves had the same basis in an article (Lauinger, 1992).

If, in the von Laue equation, the cosine terms ($h_1\lambda/b_1$, $h_2\lambda/b_2$ and $h_3\lambda/d$) of the direction cosine of the $\alpha_0\beta_0\gamma_0$ angle of incidence and of the $\alpha\beta\gamma$ diffraction angle in the grating and of its interference term are formulated via the same grating spacings (transformed to the local frequency λ in the 111 diffraction order) and wavelengths λ in the $h_1h_2h_3$ triplet, we obtain:

$\Sigma\cos^2\alpha\beta\gamma$	Interference term	$\Sigma\cos^2\alpha_0\beta_0\gamma_0$		$\Sigma\cos^2$
$\cos^2\alpha$	$-\ 2\cos\alpha\cos\alpha_0$	$+\ \cos^2\alpha_0$	$+$	
$\cos^2\beta$	$-\ 2\cos\beta\cos\beta_0$	$+\ \cos^2\beta_0$	$+$	
$\cos^2\gamma$	$-\ 2\cos\gamma\cos\gamma_0$	$+\ \cos^2\gamma_0$	$=$	$\lambda/\lambda = 1$

With the grating spacings for hexagonal geometry in Cartesian co-ordinates ($b_1 = 2\lambda_{max}111$, $b_2 = 4\lambda_{max}111\sqrt{3}$, $d = 4\lambda_{max}111$, $\lambda_{max}111 = 559$ nm), the value for the λ/λ coefficient is always 1 in each of the three diffraction orders (with the respective $\lambda_{max}h_1h_2h_3$ in the numerator). It becomes relevant here, i.e. when considering the aperture effects, in its variation with $\alpha_0\beta_0\gamma_0$, which affects only the interference term. To simplify matters, we will assume that we are dealing with self-luminating visual objects, otherwise the product of illuminant and reflectance of the object would have to be included in the calculation.

9.9.2   THE CALCULATIONS

We will start from monochromatic lights incident perpendicularly or obliquely on the pupil and retina against a white background, which is set up as an equi-energy spectrum giving a 33 per cent equilibrium of the brightness values in the three chromatic diffraction orders (Table 9.9.1, values for $\gamma_0 = 0°$; the base values for the white background have been set arbitrarily at 1060 units each). With reference to experimental data and observations regarding the aperture effects SCE I/II, we will show in detail that

- The three psychological variables, brightness, hue and saturation, are obtained through 3D interference optics from the two physical quantities intensity and wavelength. In the SCE II in particular, desaturation effects occur for chromatic, obliquely incident lights between 480 and 510 nm.
- The reversal of the hue shift in the SCE II – as shown by Valberg and Seim (1991) – on changing from moderate to high luminances has already taken place in the 3D chip of the inverted retina, well before the retinal neurones or the CGL.
- The transition from the trichromatic colour system to the opponent colour system has its origins in diffraction grating optics as early as the inverted retina.

The mathematical calculation is shown in the work by Lauinger (1994), so we will merely give the tabulated and graphic results here.

9.9.3   BRIGHTNESS, HUE AND SATURATION IN PHOTOPIC VISION; THREE COUPLED ASPECTS IN THE 3D INTERFERENCE OPTICAL TRANSFORMATION OF INTENSITY AND WAVELENGTH; SUPERSATURATION AT 480–510 NM IN THE SCE II

Brightness is defined in 3D grating optical terms via the SCE I, hue via the SCE II, and saturation via the relationship between the SCE I and II:

Table 9.9.1. 3D grating optical calculation data for the brightness, hue and saturation values for monochromatic light rays incident obliquely on the pupil and retina against a white background, with standard aperture $\gamma_0 = 0''$ as the reference parameter for all other γ_0 values (2.4''–9.6''). Coefficient $= \lambda/\lambda = \Sigma\cos^2$ in the von Laue equation.

1	2	3	4	5	6	7	8	9	10	11	12	13	14	15	16	17	18	19	20	21	22	23	24	25	26	27	28	29	30
		norm	aperture	0°		0.96		2.4°			0.92		4.6°			0.88			111	7.2°					0.84		9.6°		
coeff. rec.		122	123	111													122	123	111										
h1h2h3	wavel.	blue	green	red	sum	wavel.	SCE I	SCE II	SAT	SAT-II	wavel.	SCE I	SCE II	SAT	SAT-II	wavel.	blue	green	red	sum	SCE I	SCE II	SAT	SAT-II	wavel.	SCE I	SCE II	SAT	SAT-II
	400	1324	1061	1060	3446	383	94	4	10	6	367	92	5	12	8	351	1061	1060	1060	3181	92	5	13	8	336	92	5	13	8
	410	1608	1064	1061	3731	393	89	7	18	11	376	86	9	23	14	360	1063	1060	1060	3183	85	10	24	15	344	85	10	24	15
	420	2010	1069	1062	4141	403	85	9	24	15	386	78	14	35	22	369	1069	1060	1060	3189	77	15	38	23	353	77	15	38	23
	430	2451	1079	1064	4594	412	83	9	26	17	395	73	17	44	27	378	1088	1060	1060	3209	70	20	51	30	361	69	20	51	31
	440	2772	1100	1070	4942	422	85	7	21	15	404	72	16	44	28	387	1136	1060	1060	3256	66	23	55	34	370	65	23	58	35
	450	2832	1137	1081	5050	431	92	2	10	8	413	76	11	35	24	395	1238	1081	1060	3359	67	19	53	33	378	64	22	59	36
	460	2603	1198	1103	4903	441	101	-3	-4	-1	422	67	11	17	13	404	1425	1062	1060	3548	72	13	41	28	387	68	18	52	34
	470	2190	1290	1139	4619	451	109	-9	-18	-9	431	101	-6	-7	-1	413	1715	1065	1061	3841	83	3	20	17	395	73	11	38	27
	480	1756	1417	1198	4372	460	112	-13	-25	-12	441	118	-16	-28	-13	422	2088	1070	1062	4220	97	-9	-8	-8	403	81	0	20	19
	490	1421	1578	1285	4284	470	108	-14	-22	-8	450	118	-23	-41	-18	431	2472	1080	1065	4616	108	-20	-28	-8	412	89	-11	1	11
	500	1217	1758	1404	4379	479	100	-13	-13	-7	459	112	-26	-38	-12	439	2757	1098	1070	4924	112	-28	-41	-12	420	95	-21	-15	5
	510	1118	1937	1551	4606	489	93	-10	-3	7	468	110	-24	-42	-10	448	2844	1128	1079	5051	110	-32	-42	-10	429	98	-28	-27	2
	520	1078	2085	1717	4880	498	89	-6	4	11	477	101	-20	-11	9	457	2701	1176	1095	4971	102	-32	-34	-2	437	99	-33	-33	1
	530	1055	2177	1883	5124	508	89	-4	7	11	487	91	-15	2	16	466	2381	1246	1121	4748	93	-29	-22	7	445	98	-36	-34	2
	540	1061	2193	2025	5278	518	91	-1	6	9	496	82	-10	8	18	474	1991	1342	1162	4495	85	-24	-9	7	454	95	-35	-30	5
	550	1060	2130	2118	5308	527	95	-1	4	5	505	84	-6	10	16	483	1634	1466	1213	4323	81	-18	1	19	462	91	-35	-23	9
	560	1060	2001	2147	5208	537	101	0	-1	-6	514	91	-3	7	9	492	1389	1613	1307	4309	82	-12	6	18	471	88	-32	-15	12
	570	1060	1831	2104	4998	546	106	1	-5	-12	523	99	0	0	1	501	1226	1773	1415	4394	88	-6	6	12	479	88	-27	-8	9
	580	1060	1848	2000	4708	556	112	2	-9	-15	532	110	2	-8	-10	510	1120	1930	1545	4595	98	-2	-8	-2	487	91	-20	-3	2
	590	1060	1478	1851	4389	566	116	4	-13	-19	542	121	6	-16	-21	518	1032	2064	1690	4836	110	2	-19	-24	496	98	-6	-4	-9
	600	1060	1337	1684	4080	575	119	4	-15	-19	551	130	6	-24	-30	527	1037	2158	1838	5062	124	5	-19	-24	504	109	-9	-10	-9
	610	1060	1230	1520	3810	585	120	5	-15	-20	560	137	7	-29	-37	536	1082	2196	1972	5230	137	8	-30	-37	513	123	4	-18	-23
	620	1060	1158	1378	3596	594	118	4	-14	-18	569	139	9	-31	-39	545	1128	2172	2076	5309	148	10	-36	-46	529	136	8	-29	-36
	630	1060	1112	1265	3438	604	115	4	-11	-15	578	138	8	-30	-38	554	1060	2091	2136	5287	154	11	-43	-54	529	149	10	-39	-49
	640	1060	1086	1184	3330	613	112	3	-9	-12	588	134	7	-28	-34	562	1060	1985	2143	5168	155	11	-44	-55	538	158	12	-46	-58
	650	1060	1072	1130	3350	623	109	3	-8	-12	597	123	6	-21	-28	571	1060	1811	2090	4967	152	11	-41	-52	546	163	13	-50	-63
	660	1060	1065	1097	3223	633	106	2	-4	-6	606	121	6	-16	-21	580	1060	1650	2001	4712	146	10	-36	-46	555	164	13	-51	-64
	670	1060	1062	1079	3201	642	103	1	-2	-3	615	115	3	-11	-15	589	1060	1499	1872	4432	130	8	-29	-38	563	161	13	-49	-61
	680	1060	1061	1069	3189	652	101	0	-1	-1	624	110	3	-7	-10	597	1060	1369	1727	4156	130	8	-23	-30	571	156	12	-44	-58
	690	1060	1061	1064	3184	661	101	0	-1	-1	633	107	1	-5	-7	606	1060	1288	1580	3906	123	6	-17	-23	580	148	11	-37	-48
	700	1060	1060	1062	3182	671	101	0	-1	-1	643	104	1	-3	-4	615	1060	1190	1445	3695	116	5	-12	-16	588	140	9	-30	-40
	710	1060	1060	1061	3181	681	100	0	0	0	652	102	0	-2	-2	624	1060	1138	1331	3529	111	3	-8	-11	597	132	8	-24	-32
	720	1060	1060	1060	3180	690	100	0	-1	-1	661	101	0	-1	-1	633	1060	1104	1241	3405	107	2	-5	-7	605	124	6	-17	-24
	730	1060	1060	1060	3180	700	100	0	0	0	670	101	0	-1	-1	641	1060	1083	1175	3319	104	1	-3	-4	613	117	5	-12	-17
	740	1060	1060	1060	3180	709	100	0	0	0	679	101	0	-1	-1	650	1060	1072	1130	3262	103	1	-2	-3	622	112	4	-8	-12
	750	1060	1060	1060	3180	719	100	0	0	0	689	100	0	0	0	659	1060	1066	1100	3226	101	0	-1	-1	630	108	2	-6	-8
	760	1060	1060	1060	3180	729	100	0	0	0	698	100	0	0	0	668	1060	1063	1082	3204	101	0	-1	-1	639	105	2	-3	-5
	770	1060	1060	1060	3180	738	100	0	0	0	707	100	0	0	0	677	1060	1061	1071	3192	100	0	0	0	647	103	1	-2	-3
	780	1060	1060	1060	3180	748	100	0	0	0	716	100	0	0	0	685	1060	1060	1066	3186	100	0	0	0	655	102	1	-1	-2
	790	1060	1060	1060	3180	757	100	0	0	0	725	100	0	0	0	694	1060	1060	1063	3183	100	0	0	0	664	101	0	-1	-1
	800	1060	1060	1060	3180	767	100	0	0	0	734	100	0	0	0	703	1060	1060	1061	3181	100	0	0	0	672	101	0	0	0

$$\text{Brightness} = \text{SCE I }(\gamma_0) = 100 \cdot \frac{(R + G + B)_{\gamma_0}}{(R + G + B)_{\gamma_N}}$$

$$\text{Hue} = \text{SCE II }(\gamma_0) = 100 \cdot \left[\left(\frac{R + G}{R + G + B}\right)_{\gamma_0} - \left(\frac{R + G}{R + G + B}\right)_{\gamma_N}\right]$$

$$\text{Saturation} = \text{SCE II} - \text{SCE I} + 100$$

where R, G and B are red (L), green (M) and blue (S) colour values, γ_0 is the value of the γ angle in the aperture angle triplet ($\alpha_0\beta_0\gamma_0$ of the incident light cone, and γ_N is the γ_0 angle chosen as the reference standard).

The *brightness*, therefore, is a value arising from the ratio between the sum of the brightness values (Σy) in all three diffraction orders of the 3D chip at a certain aperture γ_0 and the corresponding sum at an aperture γ_N chosen as the reference standard.

The *hue* results from the difference between the ratio of the brightness values in the red/green diffraction orders and the sum of the Σy values of all three diffraction orders at a certain aperture and the ratio at a defined γ_N aperture.

The *saturation* results from the difference between the two effects or the ratio of the SCE I and II to one another entering this difference.

Let us first consider the results obtained from the above definitions, shown in Table 9.9.1 for the reference standard $\gamma_N = 0°$. This gives the SCE I/II/SAT values for monochromatic test lights incident obliquely on a white background with $\gamma_0 = 2.4°$, $4.8°$, $7.2°$ and $9.6°$, compared with those for perpendicular incidence of light ($\gamma_0 = 0°$). The brightness values themselves are shown in columns 18–21 for $7.2°$, otherwise only values relative to $\gamma_N = 0°$.

In grating-optical terms, the following takes place: the increasingly oblique incidence of light means that ever shorter wavelengths reach the optically 'effective' grating spacings (transformed to λ) and it is consequently possible for ever longer wavelengths in the visible spectrum to set the λ_{max} transferred with maximum transmission into the three chromatic diffraction orders in a certain spatial direction. This shift to shorter wavelengths in the grating spacings or to a longer wavelength λ_{max} is evident from the γ_0-specific λ/λ coefficient of the direction cosine (line 3), which is always 1 for $\gamma_0 = 0°$. The tabulation of the effects of the coefficient is achieved on the one hand – as shown in the columns headed 'wavel.' – by shortening the wavelengths at $0°$ (column 1) by the particular amount of the λ/λ co-efficient while keeping the $h_1h_2h_3$ λ_{max} triplet constant at 447/537/559 nm in the 3D grating, or, on the other hand, by shifting the three λ_{max} values to longer wavelengths by the amount of the coefficient (red shift of the three λ_{max} from 447/537/559 nm at $0°$ to 508/610/635 nm at $7.2°$). By relating the brightness values in the three colour channels for $7.2°$ to λ in column 1, these new λ_{max} positions in the visible spectrum can be read. The effect corresponds to the fact that, for oblique incidence of light on a grating, the optically 'effective' grating spacing shortens, approximately by the amount of the cosine of the angle of incidence. An ever shorter wavelength thus enters the 'effective' grating spacings transformed to λ. The λ/λ coefficient, which is dependent on the angle of incidence, is therefore obtained in the same way if the three grating spacings in the von Laue equation are always multiplied by $\cos\gamma_0$.

We also obtain the γ_0- and λ-specific SCE I values (curves with the typical three intersections of the 100 per cent base line for $0°$ in column 6 (sum) and with two asymptotic ends at the limits of the visible spectrum), the SCE II values (curves with the typical two intersections of the 0 per cent base line for $0°$, in which R + G is added and offset relative to B on the blue-yellow opponent colour axis, because – as shown in Lauinger (1991) – the R + G diffraction orders differentiate from the yellow diffraction order (λ_{max} = 521 nm) in scotopic vision with increasing intensity in the illumination spectrum. As the brightness values in the B channel tend toward zero in scotopic vision (λ_{max} = 422 nm) and R + G (both λ_{max} = 521 nm) are not yet differentiated from one another, the values can only be offset there as brightnesses), and the SAT values, which are particularly striking in

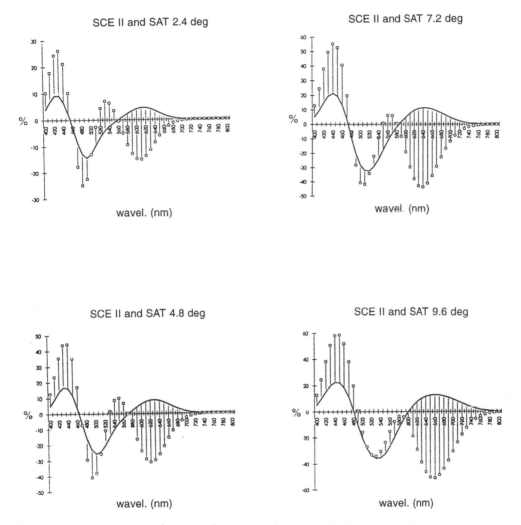

Figure 9.9.1. SCE II curve for monochromatic lights on a white background for various γ_0 angles of incidence from Table 9.9.1 (above 0 line = hue shift toward RED; below 0 line = hue shift toward BLUE) and the corresponding SAT-II values, which illustrate the saturation (negative values) or desaturation effects (positive values) in various wavelength regions, in particular between 485 and 510 nm, as a function of the SCE II. If all the γ_0 values are compared with the standard aperture γ_N = 0° for monochromatic lights from all wavelength regions, hue shifts in one and the same direction and saturation/desaturation effects in the SCE II are obtained. On transition from small to large γ_0 angles (which correspond to large pupillary diameters, i.e. lower luminance in the visual field), the SCE II and SAT effects become stronger. Hue reversals do not occur in the SCE II.

experimental work on the SCE II. For this reason, the (SAT-SCE II) values relevant to Figure 9.9.1 are shown in an additional column. Figure 9.9.1 shows the γ_0- and λ-specific SCE II curves, with a SAT value labelling (corresponding to the SCE I curve, i.e. the relative brightness values) that shifts the saturation toward + for desaturation (relative increase in brightness) and toward - for (super)saturation. As virtually all experimental work on aperture effects has been carried out at between 460 and 600 nm, it must have been evident to sensitive test persons that a supersaturation effect can be detected between 480 and 510 nm:

> The results show hue shifts of the expected kind and a small but significant supersaturation of the apparent colour of an obliquely, compared with a normally incident stimulus, in the wavelength range 485 to 510 nm (Enoch and Stiles, 1961, p. 330)

> Qualitative changes of saturation, particularly an increased saturation of the obliquely incident ray for wavelengths near 500 nm, have been reported by W.S. Stiles (1937) and Walraven and Bouman (1960) quoted in Enoch and Stiles (1961)

9.9.4   THE REVERSAL OF THE HUE SHIFT IN THE SCE II ON TRANSITION FROM MODERATE TO HIGHER LUMINANCES

It seems justified to ask whether the human eye must always use perpendicular incidence of light ($\gamma_N = 0°$) through the centre of the pupil as reference standard, as in the experimental set-ups for measurement of the Stiles-Crawford effects. On adaptation to various luminances, the pupillary diameter varies, and the proportion of the rays incident obliquely on the retinal 3D chip therefore increases with increasing diameter and decreases with decreasing diameter. Let us assume, for example, that the eye selects an annular aperture zone that in each case divides the effective pupillary area in two as a reference standard and let us recalculate the earlier angle values, but with respect to $\gamma_N = 4.8°$. Figure 9.9.2 shows, by comparison with Figure 9.9.1, that the saturation effects always remain the same between 480 and 510 nm. However, the hue shift of most (not all) monochromatic test lights on a white background now reverses on this side of the 4.8° reference zone. Valberg reports the following:

> When the luminance ratio increases from the minimum value ... several test lights display hue shifts first in one direction and then back again (Valberg and Seim, 1991, p. 430).

It thus appears entirely possible to ensure such a law in the inverted retina merely through grating optics. The standardisation of the values in the pupil function, which are nevertheless always only relative ones, in any case requires experimental clarification.

9.9.5   THE 3D GRATING OPTICAL CONNECTION BETWEEN THE TRICHROMATIC AND OPPONENT COLOUR SYSTEMS

The connection between the trichromatic and opponent colour systems has already been mentioned above. It arises from interference-optical laws, because the third grating spacing in the 3D chip ensures adaptation to the energy level by changing the distance between the cellular layers (while the three grating spacings (b_1, b_2 and d) together ensure chromatic adaptation (so-called λ-transformation) by defining the grey/white axis in the colour space by forming a 33 per cent equilibrium as standard for the white point under a certain illuminant). With increasing energy level (reduction in distance between the layers), the red and green diffraction orders in photopic vision differentiate out of the yellow diffraction order of scotopic vision. As the third independent diffraction order, the blue diffraction order becomes relevant at the same time. In scotopic vision (greatest distance between the layers in the 3D chip), the red and green diffraction orders, which are equally tuned 3D grating optically (λ_{max} = 521 nm in each case), in the absence of chromatic differentiation

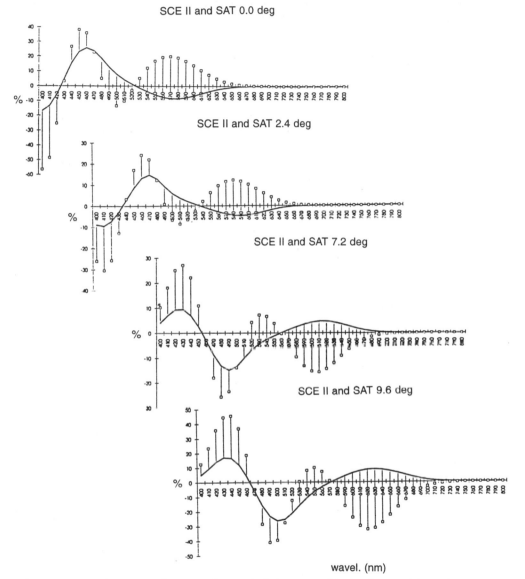

Figure 9.9.2. SCE II curve for monochromatic lights on a white background for various γ_0 angles of incidence with reference aperture at γ_0 = 4.8° (above 0 line = hue shift toward RED; below 0 line = hue shift toward BLUE) and the corresponding SAT-II values, which illustrate the saturation (negative values) or desaturation effects (positive values) in particular between 485 and 510 nm, as a function of the SCE II. If all the γ_0 values are compared with the standard aperture 4.8°, the saturation effects between 485 and 510 nm remain the same as in Figure 9.9.1, but hue reversals occur in the SCE II.

as the yellow diffraction order, are virtually alone in determining brightness vision, for the blue diffraction order is still irrelevant. The blue diffraction order only becomes optically effective (λ_{max} = 447 nm) via the intensity-driven Purkinje shift, and the yellow diffraction order becomes differentiated into the red and green diffraction orders (λ_{max} = 537 and 559 nm respectively). As both medium and long colour channels originate in grating optical terms from the same source (yellow diffraction order), they remain additively linked to one another even later. Red and blue shifts in the aperture effects (SCE I/II) and in the Bezold-Brücke phenomenon (hue shift via intensity variation) can be explained in this way.

9.9.6   CONCLUSIONS

The above results give further evidence for the fact that diffraction gratings at interfaces in human vision (see also Maurice (1957) on the corneal transparency determined by diffraction grating optics) and in particular coupled cellular oscillators in the inverted retina have functional importance for the adaptive preprocessing of visual stimuli. However, all cortical layers exhibit equally the same cellular layer structure as in the retina. It only needs something other than Golgi staining of microscopic specimens to render this clearly visible. However, these cellular layers – as shown by the crystal-optical phase calculation for the retina – act at above cell level or cell-interactively and holographically. Consequently, they can only be analysed in full via amplitude and phase calculations.

9.9.7   REFERENCES

Enoch, J.M., & Stiles, W.S. (1961) The colour change of monochromatic light with retinal angle of incidence, *Optica Acta*, **8**, 329–358.

Lauinger, N. (1991) 3D grating optics of human vision, *Acta Ophthalmologica*, **69** (Suppl. 199), 1991.

Lauinger, N. (1992) 3D grating optical retinal chip and stimulus-adaptive robotic vision, *SPIE*, **1825**, 78.

Lauinger, N. (1994) Brightness, hue and saturation in photopic vision, *SPIE Proceedings International Symposium on Photonics for Industrial Applications*, 31 October to 4 November, Boston, MA.

Maurice, D.M. (1957) The structure and transparency of the cornea, *Journal of Physiology*, **136**, 263.

Stiles, W.S. (1937) *Procedings of the Royal Society*, **B123**, 90.

Valberg, A. & Seim, T. (1991) On the physiological basis of higher colour metrics. In: Valberg, A. & Lee, B.B. (Eds) *From Pigments to Perception*, New York: Plenum Press, p. 425.

Walraven, P.L. & Bouman, M.A. (1960) *Journal of the Optical Society of America*, **50**, 780.

3D Grating Model of Colour Perception

Margarita A. Carbon

9.10.1 INTRODUCTION

In the present chapter, we study a 3D-grating layer model of colour perception based on the diffraction theory of human vision by Lauinger (1991, 1992). According to that theory, visual information processed in the human eye involves trichromatic diffractive Fourier images of a 3D grating formed by the cell layer in the retina of the eye (Figure 9.10.1). The theory presents the eye as a trichromatic modulator, which codes the optical information in a hologram-like manner creating an interference pattern in the Fresnel diffraction zone.

In Section 9.10.2, we solve the wave equation for a light field propagating in an isotropic

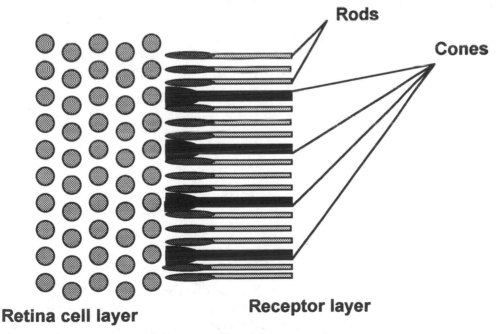

Figure 9.10.1. 3D grating of the retina cells and the receptor layer.

homogeneous dielectric medium with a small 3D grating perturbation in the refractive index, using the 4D spectral method (Carbon and Parygin, 1992). In Section 9.10.3, we derive analytical expressions for the amplitude and intensity of light diffracted by a 3D grating layer for the incident plane wave light. In the near zone of diffraction, the diffracted light forms an interference pattern. In the far diffraction zone, the bandwidth of the diffracted intensity curves is defined by the width of the grating layer, the grating periods, and the ordinal numbers of the diffraction maximum.

In Section 9.10.4, for white collimated light, we compute the wavelength dependence of the diffracted light intensity for various geometries of the grating layer and the incident light. Within the visible spectrum range 0.4–0.7 μm, we obtain the intensity curves of the diffracted light versus wavelength for three basic diffracted maxima with central wavelengths corresponding to blue, green, and red light. Finally, intensity curves are computed for the three diffracted light maxima corresponding to oblique incidence of light on the grating. The blue shifts for the curves agree with the Stiles-Crawford effects (Stiles and Crawford, 1933).

9.10.2   4D SPECTRAL METHOD

Let us introduce the 4D coordinate and 4D frequency vectors:

$$\mathbf{r} = (r_1, r_2, r_3, r_4) \qquad \mathbf{v} = (v_1, v_2, v_3, v_4)$$

and their scalar product:

$$\mathbf{v} \cdot \mathbf{r} = v_1 r_1 + v_2 r_2 + v_3 r_3 - v_4 r_4.$$

In our notation, the 4D Fourier transformations take the forms:

$$\hat{f}(\mathbf{v}) = \int_{-\infty}^{\infty} f(\mathbf{r})\exp\,(i2\pi\mathbf{v}\cdot\mathbf{r})d^4\mathbf{r}, \quad f(\mathbf{r}) = \int_{-\infty}^{\infty} \hat{f}(\mathbf{v})\exp\,(-i2\pi\mathbf{v}\cdot\mathbf{r})d^4\mathbf{v}, \tag{1}$$

where $\hat{f}(\mathbf{v})$ is the 4D Fourier spectrum of the function $f(\mathbf{r})$.

The propagation of the light field $E(\mathbf{r})$ in an isotropic homogeneous dielectric medium is described by the light wave equation (Born and Wolf, 1965) that can be written in the form:

$$\square E(\mathbf{r}) = 0, \tag{2}$$

where:

$$\square \equiv \frac{\partial^2}{\partial r_1^2} + \frac{\partial^2}{\partial r_2^2} + \frac{\partial^2}{\partial r_3^2} - \frac{1}{c^2}\frac{\partial^2}{\partial r_4^2}\varepsilon,$$

and ε is the dielectric permeability of the medium. Let us assume that the dielectric permeability changes through some perturbation in the refractive index of the medium. For the perturbed medium, we have (Balakshii et al., 1985):

$$\tilde{\varepsilon} = \varepsilon + \Delta\varepsilon = [n + \Delta n f(\mathbf{r})]^2 \cong n^2 + 2n\Delta n f(\mathbf{r}) \tag{3}$$

where $\Delta n << n$ is the amplitude of the refractive index perturbation, and $f(\mathbf{r})$ is its spatial distribution. The function $f(\mathbf{r})$ satisfies the existence conditions of the Fourier transform where $|f(\mathbf{r})| \leqslant 1$. Substituting equation (3) into equation (2), we obtain the wave equation for light propagation in the disturbed medium:

$$\Box E(\mathbf{r}) = \frac{2n\Delta n}{c^2} \frac{\partial^2}{\partial r_4^2} E(\mathbf{r}) f(\mathbf{r}). \tag{4}$$

We will solve equation (4) by representing the light field and the perturbation function as 4D Fourier integral expansions into plane wave spectra, i.e.,

$$E(\mathbf{r}) = \int\limits_{-\infty}^{\infty} \hat{E}(\mathbf{v}) \exp(-i2\pi\mathbf{v} \cdot \mathbf{r}) d^4\mathbf{v}, \quad f(\mathbf{r}) = \int\limits_{-\infty}^{\infty} \hat{f}(\mathbf{v}') \exp(-i2\pi\mathbf{v}' \cdot \mathbf{r}) d^4\mathbf{v}'. \tag{5}$$

Substituting equation (5) into equation (4) and carrying out the differentiation gives us:

$$\int\limits_{-\infty}^{\infty} G(\mathbf{v})\hat{E}(\mathbf{v}) \exp(-i2\pi\mathbf{v} \cdot \mathbf{r}) d^4\mathbf{v} = \frac{2n\Delta n}{c^2} \int \int\limits_{-\infty}^{\infty} (v_4 + v_4')^2 \hat{f}(\mathbf{v}') \hat{E}(\mathbf{v}) \exp[-i2\pi(\mathbf{v}' + \mathbf{v}) \cdot \mathbf{r}] d^4\mathbf{v} \tag{6}$$

where

$$G(\mathbf{v}) = v_1^2 + v_2^2 + v_3^2 - \frac{v_4^2 n^2}{c^2}. \tag{7}$$

Shifting the variable $\mathbf{v} \to \mathbf{v} - \mathbf{v}'$ on the left-hand side of equation (6), we obtain:

$$\int\limits_{-\infty}^{\infty} G(\mathbf{v})\hat{E}(\mathbf{v}) \exp(-i2\pi\mathbf{v} \cdot \mathbf{r}) d^4\mathbf{v} = \frac{2n\Delta n}{c^2} \int \int\limits_{-\infty}^{\infty} (v_4^2 \hat{f}(\mathbf{v}') \hat{E}(\mathbf{v} - \mathbf{v}')) \exp[-i2\pi\mathbf{v} \cdot \mathbf{r}] d^4\mathbf{v}' d^4\mathbf{v}. \tag{8}$$

Now we can rewrite equation (8) in the form:

$$\int\limits_{-\infty}^{\infty} [G(\mathbf{v})\hat{E}(\mathbf{v}) - \frac{2n\Delta n v_4^2}{c^2} \int\limits_{-\infty}^{\infty} \hat{f}(\mathbf{v}') \hat{E}(\mathbf{v} - \mathbf{v}') d^4\mathbf{v}'] \exp(-i2\pi\mathbf{v} \cdot \mathbf{r}) d^4\mathbf{v}. \tag{9}$$

From equation (9), we derive the integral equation:

$$G(\mathbf{v})\hat{E}(\mathbf{v}) = 2\frac{\Delta n}{n\lambda^2} \hat{f} * \hat{E}(\mathbf{v}), \tag{10}$$

where $\lambda = c/(nv_4)$ is the wavelength and $*$ denotes the 4D convolution. To solve this integral equation, we will apply the perturbation expansion:

$$\hat{E}(\mathbf{v}) = \sum_{m=0}^{\infty} \hat{E}^{(m)}(\mathbf{v}) \left(\frac{\Delta n}{n}\right)^m, \tag{11}$$

for the diffracted light spectrum, where the zeroth-order approximation:

$$\hat{E}^{(0)}(\mathbf{v}) = \hat{E}_{inc}(\mathbf{v}) \tag{12}$$

is the 4D spectrum of the incident light. Substituting equation (11) into equation (10), and equating terms in the same order of the small parameter $\Delta n/n$, we have the following relation between two successive transitions:

$$\hat{E}^{(m)}(\mathbf{v}) = \frac{2}{\lambda^2 G(\mathbf{v})} \hat{f} * \hat{E}^{(m-1)}(\mathbf{v}).$$

(13)

Using equation (13) with the initial condition (12), we can calculate the diffracted light spectrum (11) for any desired accuracy. Each subsequent approximation for the diffracted light spectrum is defined by the convolution of the previous approximation with the spectrum of the perturbation. The term $G(\mathbf{v})$ (7) introduces some singular points that correspond to the plane-vector eigenmodes of the medium. Substituting the spectrum (11) into the Fourier integral (5), we obtain the diffracted light field:

$$E(r) = \sum_{m=0}^{\infty} \left(\frac{\Delta n}{n}\right)^m \int_{-\infty}^{\infty} \hat{E}^{(m)}(\mathbf{v}) \exp(-i2\pi\mathbf{v}\cdot\mathbf{r}) d^4\mathbf{v}.$$

(14)

The integral in equation (14) must be understood in the sense of the principal value.

9.10.3　DIFFRACTION OF LIGHT BY A 3D-GRATING LAYER

Let us consider the medium with the perturbed refractive index:

$$\tilde{n} = n + \Delta n f_{gr}(\mathbf{r}) = n + \Delta n g(\mathbf{r}) * \text{comb}^3(\mathbf{r}),$$

where $f_{gr}(\mathbf{r})$ is the spatial distribution of a 3D grating that could be presented (Goodman, 1968) as the convolution of the aperture function $g(\mathbf{r})$ with the 3D comb-function:

$$\text{comb}^3(\mathbf{r}) \equiv \sum_{h_i=-\infty}^{\infty} \prod_{i=1}^{3} \delta(r_i - h_i b_i),$$

and b_1, b_2, and b_3 are spatial periods of the grating. From equation (1), we obtain the 4D spectrum of the grating:

$$\hat{f}_{gr}(\mathbf{v}) = \hat{g}(\mathbf{v})\text{comb}^3(\mathbf{v}) = \hat{g}(\mathbf{v}) \sum_{h_i=-\infty}^{\infty} \prod_{i=1}^{3} \delta(b_i v_i - h_i).$$

Suppose now that the grating perturbation is located in the layer with boundaries $z = [-L/2, L/2]$ (see Figure 9.10.2). Here, for the spatial distribution of the perturbation, we will use the function:

$$f(\mathbf{r}) = \text{rect}\frac{r_3}{L} f_{gr}(\mathbf{r}), \quad \text{where } \text{rect}(x) = \begin{cases} 1 & (|x| \le 0.5) \\ 0 & (|x| > 0.5) \end{cases}$$

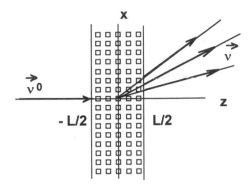

Figure 9.10.2. Diffraction of light by a 3D grating layer with boundaries $z_1 = -L/2$ and $z_2 = L/2$.

According to the properties of Fourier transformations, the 4D spectrum of the grating layer is:

$$\hat{f}(\mathbf{v}) = L\text{sinc}(v_3 L) * [\hat{g}(\mathbf{v})\text{comb}^3(b_i v_i)]$$

$$= \sum_{h_1 h_2 h_3} L \text{ sinc }[(v_3 - \frac{h_3}{b_3})L] \hat{g}(v_1, v_2, \frac{h_3}{b_3})\delta(v_1 - \frac{h_1}{b_1})\delta(v_2 - \frac{h_2}{b_2})\delta(v_4). \tag{15}$$

Here $\text{sinc}(x) = \sin(\pi x)/(\pi x)$.

Consider incident light with a 4D spectrum of monochromatic plane wave with 4D frequency $\mathbf{v}^{(0)}$:

$$\hat{E}_{inc}(\mathbf{v}) = \delta(\mathbf{v} - \mathbf{v}^{(0)}). \tag{16}$$

For weak interaction, using equations (13), (15), and (16), we obtain the 4D spectrum of the diffracted light:

$$\hat{E}_{dif}(\mathbf{v}) = \frac{2L}{\lambda^{(0)^2} G(\mathbf{v})} \sum_{h_1 h_2 h_3} \text{sinc}[(\eta_3 - \frac{h_3}{b_3})L]\hat{g}(\eta_1, \eta_2, \frac{h_3}{b_3})\delta(\eta_1 - \frac{h_1}{b_1})\delta(\eta_2 - \frac{h_2}{b_2})\delta(\eta_4),$$

where $\mathbf{\eta} = \mathbf{v} - \mathbf{v}^{(0)}$. For the diffracted light field, we have:

$$E_{dif}(\mathbf{v}) = \frac{2\Delta n L}{\lambda^{(0)^2}} \sum_{n \, h_1 h_2 h_3} \hat{g}(\frac{h_1}{b_1}, \frac{h_2}{b_2}, \frac{h_3}{b_3}) \tag{17}$$

$$\times \exp[-i2\pi(v_1^{(h_1)}r_1 + v_2^{(h_2)}r_2 - v_4^{(0)}r_4)]\int_{-\infty}^{\infty} \frac{\text{sinc }[(\eta_3 - \eta_3^{(h_3)})L]}{v_3^2 - v_3^{(h_1 h_2)^2}} \exp(-i2\pi v_3 r_3)dv_3,$$

where

$$v_i^{(h_i)} = v_i^{(0)} + \frac{h_i}{b_i}, \quad v_3^{(h_1 h_2)} = \sqrt{\lambda^{(0)^{-2}} - v_1^{(h_1)^2} - v_2^{(h_2)^2}}.$$

The integral in (17) is taken using the theory of residues. For $r_3 > L/2$, we obtain:

$$E_{dif}(\mathbf{v}) = \sum_{h_1 h_2 h_3} A^{(h_1 h_2 h_3)} \exp(-i2\pi \mathbf{v}^{(h_1 h_2)} \cdot \mathbf{r}), \tag{18}$$

where

$$A^{(h_1h_2h_3)} = \frac{i2\pi\Delta nL}{\lambda^{(0)2}\, n\, v_3^{(h_1h_2)}} \hat{g}(\frac{h_1}{b_1},\, \frac{h_2}{b_2},\, \frac{h_3}{b_3})\sin c(\Delta\eta_3 L),$$

$$v^{(h_1h_2)} = (v_1^{(h_1)},\, v_2^{(h_2)},\, v_3^{(h_1h_2)},\, v_4^{(0)}),\quad \Delta\eta_3 = v_3^{(h_1h_2)} - v_3^{(h_3)}. \tag{19}$$

Intensity of light diffracted in maximum $h_1h_2h_3$ in the far field is:

$$I^{(h_1h_2h_3)} = E^{(h_1h_2h_3)}[E^{(h_1h_2h_3)}]^* = |A^{(h_1h_2h_3)}|^2. \tag{20}$$

According to the energy conservation law, the sum of the intensities of all diffracted maxima equals the intensity of the incident light. From that condition, we find the amplitude of the non-diffracted light to be:

$$A^{(000)} = \sqrt{1 - \sum_{h_1h_2h_3} |A^{(h_1h_2h_3)}|^2}.$$

Notice, that the amplitudes of diffracted light are imaginary, i.e., shifted by $\pi/2$ compared to non-diffracted light.

In the near diffraction region, the intensity of the diffracted field creates an interference pattern. Neglecting terms of order $\sim (\Delta n/n)^2$, we can write:

$$I_{dif}(\mathbf{r}) = E_{dif}(\mathbf{r})E_{dif}(\mathbf{r})^* \cong A^{(000)}\{A^{(000)} + 2\sum_{h_1h_2h_3} |A^{(h_1h_2h_3)}|\sin[2\pi(\mathbf{\eta}^{(h_1h_2h_3)}\cdot\mathbf{r})]\},$$

where

$$\mathbf{\eta}^{(h_1h_2h_3)} = \left(\frac{h_1}{b_1},\, \frac{h_2}{b_2},\, \frac{h_3}{b_3} + \Delta\eta_3,\, 0\right).$$

If the incident light is collimated white light, then there is a wavelength dependence for the diffracted light intensity. Using the geometry of coordinate angles presented in Figure 9.10.3, we can express the 4D frequencies of the incident and diffracted light through direction cosines as:

$$v^{(0)} = (\frac{1}{\lambda^{(0)}}\cos\alpha^{(0)},\, \frac{1}{\lambda^{(0)}}\cos\beta^{(0)},\, \frac{1}{\lambda^{(0)}}\cos\gamma^{(0)},\, v_4^{(0)}),$$

$$v^{(h_1h_2)} = (\frac{1}{\lambda^{(0)}}\cos\alpha^{(h_1)},\, \frac{1}{\lambda^{(0)}}\cos\beta^{(h_2)},\, \frac{1}{\lambda^{(0)}}\cos\gamma^{(h_1h_2)},\, v_4^{(0)}), \tag{21}$$

where $\alpha^{(0)}$, $\beta^{(0)}$, and $\gamma^{(0)}$ are co-ordinate angles for the direction of incident light, and for the diffracted light:

$$\cos\alpha^{(h_1)} = \cos\alpha^{(0)} + \lambda^{(0)}\frac{h_1}{b_1},\quad \cos\beta^{(h_2)} = \cos\beta^{(0)} + \lambda^{(0)}\frac{h_2}{b_2},$$

$$\cos\gamma^{(h_1h_2)} = \sqrt{1 - \cos^2\alpha^{(h_1)} - \cos^2\beta^{(h_2)}}. \tag{22}$$

Substituting equations (22) and (21) into equation (19) and calculating equation (20), we obtain for the intensity of the maximum $h_1h_2h_3$ in the far field:

$$I^{(h_1 h_2 h_3)} = \left(\frac{2\pi \Delta n L}{\lambda^{(0)} n \cos \gamma^{(h_1 h_2)}} \right)^2 \hat{g}^2 (\frac{h_1}{b_1}, \frac{h_2}{b_2}, \frac{h_3}{b_3}) \ \text{sinc}^{\ 2} (\Delta \eta_3 L), \tag{23}$$

The function sinc(x) in equation (23) defines the shape of the diffracted light maxima. The condition $\Delta \eta_3 = 0$ gives, for the central wavelengths of the diffracted maxima,

$$\cos \gamma^{(h_1 h_2)} - \cos \gamma^{(0)} - \frac{\lambda h_3}{b_3} = 0. \tag{24}$$

From equations (24) and (22), we derive the von Laue equation:

$$\lambda^{(h_1 h_2 h_3)} = -2 \frac{(h_1 / b_1) \cos \alpha^{(0)} + (h_2 / b_2) \cos \beta^{(0)} + (h_3 / b_3) \cos \gamma^{(0)}}{(h_1 / b_1)^2 + (h_2 / b_2)^2 + (h_3 / b_3)^2}$$

Note that h_3 is negative for the diffracted light that passed through the layer.

For normal incidence ($\cos \gamma^{(0)} = 1$, $\cos \alpha^{(0)} = \cos \beta^{(0)} = 0$) and small diffraction angles ($\lambda h_i / b_i << 1$), equation (23) can be used to estimate the half-bandwidth of the diffracted light intensity maxima in the far field. It appears that the half-bandwidth of the diffracted intensity light depends on the grating layer width, the sizes of the grating cells, and the diffractional numbers as follows:

$$\frac{\Delta \lambda}{\lambda} \cong \frac{0.8 b_1^2}{\lambda L [h_1^2 + (h_2 h_1 / b_2)^2]}.$$

Let us consider the spatial distribution of the diffracted light maxima. For the case of normal incidence, the directional cosines of the diffracted light wave vector are:

$$\cos \alpha^{(h_1)} = \frac{h_1 / b_1}{\sqrt{(h_1 / b_1)^2 + (h_2 / b_2)^2 + (1 / \lambda + h_3 / b_3)^2}},$$

$$\cos \beta^{(h_1)} = \frac{h_2 / b_2}{\sqrt{(h_1 / b_1)^2 + (h_2 / b_2)^2 + (1 / \lambda + h_3 / b_3)^2}}, \tag{25}$$

$$\cos \gamma^{(h_1)} = \frac{h_3 / b_3}{\sqrt{(h_1 / b_1)^2 + (h_2 / b_2)^2 + (1 / \lambda + h_3 / b_3)^2}},$$

while for the directional cosines of the corresponding 3D-grating maxima, we have:

$$\cos \alpha_{gr}^{(h_1)} = \frac{h_1 b_1}{\sqrt{(h_1 b_1)^2 + (h_2 b_2)^2 + (h_3 b_3)^2}},$$

$$\cos \beta_{gr}^{(h_2)} = \frac{h_2 b_2}{\sqrt{(h_1 b_1)^2 + (h_2 b_2)^2 + (h_3 b_3)^2}}, \tag{26}$$

$$\cos \gamma_{gr}^{(h_1)} = \frac{h_3 b_3}{\sqrt{(h_1 b_1)^2 + (h_2 b_2)^2 + (h_3 b_3)^2}}.$$

Equations (25) and (26) describe the reciprocal geometry of the diffracted light mentioned by Lauinger (1991, 1992). For the polar angle ϕ (see Figure 9.10.3) that characterises the position of the maxima in the plane of constant r_3, we have:

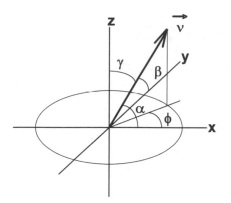

Figure 9.10.3. Geometry of co-ordinate angles.

$$\cos \phi = \frac{h_1 / b_1}{\sqrt{(h_1 / b_1)^2 + (h_2 / b_2)^2}}, \quad \cos \phi_{gr} = \frac{h_1 b_1}{\sqrt{(h_1 b_1)^2 + (h_2 b_2)^2}}.$$

Thus, it follows that the 3D grating with the grating space ratio b_1: b_2 will create, for normal light incidence, a 3D grating image in the plane parallel to the layer boundaries with the grating space ratio $(1/b_1)$: $(1/b_2)$.

9.10.4 ANALYSIS OF THE RESULTS

Using equation (23), we numerically computed the wavelength dependence of the diffracted light intensity for various geometries of the grating layer and the incident light. We assumed that the incident light is collimated white light with uniform wavelength distribution within the visible spectrum range 0.4–0.7μm. We considered the cubic grating layer model with the grating space ratio b_1: b_2: b_3 = 1: $\sqrt{3}$: $\sqrt{3}$ and the cubic cell size a = 0.5 μm. For the cubic cells, the spectrum grating aperture function is:

$$\hat{g}(\frac{h_1}{b_1}, \frac{h_2}{b_2}, \frac{h_3}{b_3}) = \frac{a^3}{b_1 b_2 b_3} \text{sinc}\ (\frac{ah_1}{b_1})\text{sinc}\ (\frac{ah_2}{b_2})\text{sinc}\ (\frac{ah_3}{b_3}).$$

The closest distance between the nodes of the grating d = b_1 was varied within the range 1–5μm. We assumed the thickness of the layer L to be linearly dependent on the grating parameter L = $6b_3$, i.e. six grating distances in the layer along the z-axis. Further, the diffraction numbers h_1, h_2 and h_3 were varied from 0 to 7. For the purpose of the analysis and comparison, we chose those diffracted light intensity curves that corresponded to reasonable geometry of diffracted light and were numerically comparable in value. We also considered as important criteria for colour discrimination the presence of three main diffracted maxima corresponding to red, green, and blue wavelengths.

The most interesting results were obtained at d = 2.2 μm. In Figure 9.10.4(a), we show the wavelength dependence of the diffracted light intensities (in conventional units) for three main diffracted maxima for normal light incidence ($\gamma^{(0)}$ = 0). The shape of these three curves agrees with the curves for tristimulus values of spectrum stimuli of unit irradiance according to Ladd-Franklin and Young theories (Judd, 1962). They also agree with the fundamental sensitivity curves (Lauinger, 1992) of the human eye. This suggests a diffractive origin for the fundamental sensitivity curves.

Figures 9.10.4 (b,c,d) show how the deviation from normal incidence changes the position and shape of the diffracted light intensity curves for the same diffraction maxima. Each of the three curves shows a blue shift for $\gamma = 1°$ (b). As the angle of incidence increases (c and d), the blue shift causes a complete disappearance of the 'blue' maximum from the visible range. Thus, the total information about colour of the incident light, contained in the two remaining visible maxima, will be red-shifted. These facts agree with the Stiles-Crawford effects (Stiles and Crawford, 1933) I and II and could be considered as an affirmation to the diffraction theory of human vision.

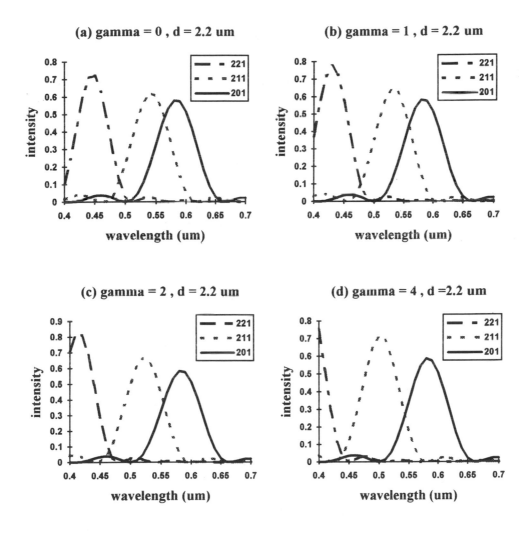

Figure 9.10.4.   Wavelength dependence of diffracted light intensity for normal incidence (a) and deviation from normal incidence (b–d).

9.10.5　SUMMARY AND CONCLUSIONS

We have studied the problem of light diffraction by a 3D grating using the model of a plane grating layer. To solve the problem we used the method of 4D plane wave spectra. We found that the spectrum of light diffracted by a 3D grating layer is defined by the convolution of the incident light spectrum with the spectrum of the layer. For weak interaction, we obtained the analytical expressions for the amplitude and intensity of the diffracted light field for the incident plane-wave light. According to these expressions, the bandwidth of the diffracted intensity curves is defined by the width of the grating layer and the grating periods. In the far field, we found that the geometry of the diffracted light is reciprocal with respect to the geometry of the 3D grating. We derived the von Laue equation from our intensity expression as the condition for the central wavelengths of the diffracted light maxima.

We computed the wavelength dependence of the diffracted light intensity for incident collimated white light. Analysing some interesting triplets of the diffracted light maxima, we concluded that the fundamental sensitivity curves for red, green, and blue colours in human vision could be explained as effects of diffraction of light by 3D grating layer of the retina cells. The physical blue shift of the diffracted light maxima for non-zero incident angle agrees with the shift in hue in human vision (the Stiles-Crawford effects I and II).

The results justify the validity of the diffraction theory of human vision. The presented model could be used in the design of the retinal 3D chip (Lauinger, 1994), and applied to the theory of colour vision devices for robots and computers.

9.10.6　ACKNOWLEDGEMENTS

The author thanks Dr N. Lauinger for his great ideas and discussions on the problems of human vision, and the Institute of Optosensory Systems, Wetzlar, Germany, for sponsoring the presentation of the results.

9.10.7　REFERENCES

BALAKSHII, V. I., PARYGIN, V. N. AND CHIRKOV, L. E. (1985) *Physical Principles of Acoustooptics* [in Russian], Moscow: Radio I Svyaz'.
BORN, M. & WOLF, E. (1965) *Principles of Optics*, New York: Pergamon Press.
CARBON, M. A. & PARYGIN, V. N. (1992) Diffraction of light by a three-dimensional acoustic column, *Optical Engineering*, **31**, 2103–9.
GOODMAN, J. W. (1968) *Introduction to Fourier Optics*, New York: McGraw-Hill.
JUDD, D. B. (1962) Basic correlates of the visual stimulus. In: Stevens, S. S. (Ed.) *Handbook of Experimental Psychology*, New York: John Wiley & Sons, p. 840.
LAUINGER, N. (1991) 3D grating optics of human vision, *Acta Ophthalmologica*, **69**, suppl. 199.
LAUINGER, N. (1992) 3D grating optical retinal chip and stimulus-adaptive robotic vision, *SPIE Vol. 1825 Intelligent Robots and Computer Vision*, **XI**, 78–103.
LAUINGER, N. (1994) Physical optics and human vision, *OE Reports*, No. 123, p. 7.
STILES, W. S. & CRAWFORD, B. H. (1933) The luminous efficiency of rays entering the eye pupil at different points, *Proceedings of the Royal Society (London)*, **B112**, 428–450.

A Zone Model for Colour Vision Based on Discriminability Optimisation

H. Vaitkevičius, Z. Stankevičius and V. Petrauskas

9.11.1 INTRODUCTION

The multiple-stage colour model is rather widely accepted (Svaetichin et al., 1965; Ingling and Tsou, 1977; Formin et al., 1979; Guth, 1991; Ismailov and Sakolov, 1991). But it is not clear what could be a functional meaning of transformation of unipolar R, G, B cone signals into signals of opponent cells. We know only a few papers dealing with this problem (Buchsbaum and Gottshalk, 1983; Vaitkevičius et al., 1984, Vaitkevičius et al., 1993).

Buchsbaum and Gottshalk (1983) supposed that a transformation of the R, G, B cone signals into the signals of three opponent cells (Wh-Bl; R-G; Y-B) both decorrelates signals that are transmitted through the three channels and increases reliability of transmitted information. But in this case it is not clear how this transformation changes a signal/noise ratio when the noise is generated both by single cones and by opponent cells. Any transformation can impair this signal/noise ratio and hence impair the colour discriminability (see Vaitkevičius et al., 1993).

The second group of papers deals with the problem of how the opposition changes colour discriminability. But in this case the authors took into account the noise generated either only by the opponent cells (this noise does not depend upon the transformation sought) or only by the cones.

This paper deals with the problem of the increasing colour discriminability, keeping in mind the noise generated both by the cones and by opponent cells.

9.11.2 THE PRESENTATION OF THE PROBLEM

9.11.2.1 A formal model

Here is the three-stage colour model:

$$S = \{s(\lambda)\} \xrightarrow{\Omega_i} R = \{y_i\} \xrightarrow{\Omega_i} O = \{x_i\} \to D$$

At the first stage energy of light is transformed into signals of three cones (R, G, B or L, M, S). At the second stage the three cone signals are transformed into the signals of three opponent cell signals. For simplicity, let us assume that this transformation is linear. If we take into consideration a noise generated both by cones and by opponent cells then we must modify the earlier described scheme in the following manner:

$$S = s(\lambda) \rightarrow R = \{y_i\} \overset{\varepsilon_i}{\underset{\downarrow}{\rightarrow}} \oplus \rightarrow O = \{x_i\} \overset{\eta_i}{\underset{\downarrow}{\rightarrow}} \oplus \rightarrow D$$

where ε_i ($i = 1, 2, 3$) is the noise generated by a cone; η_i is noise generated by an opponent cell. We incorporate only additive noise. In this case an output signal of the ith opponent cell could be calculated from the following expression:

$$x_i' = \sum_j^3 \alpha_{ij}(y_j + \varepsilon_j) = x_i + \varepsilon_i', \quad \text{where } \varepsilon_i' = \sum_j^3 \alpha_{ij}\varepsilon_j + \eta_i \tag{1}$$

9.11.2.2 The criteria of the colour discriminability

Let the noise generated by cones and opponent cells be uncorrelated, and have Gaussian distribution $N(0, \sigma_j')$. It is obvious that the combined noise ε_i' influences the colour discriminability. An absolute value of a random vector E, i.e. a random quantity $((\varepsilon_1')^2 + (\varepsilon_2')^2 + (\varepsilon_3')^2)^{1/2}$, determines the radius (r) of a region about the point $\{x_i\}$ ($i = 1, 2, 3$), where the stimulus $s(\lambda)$ is mapped. The size of the this radius (r) depends on the probability with which the stimulus is being mapped within this region. To calculate this radius we could use the well-known Tchebyshev inequality

$$p(|E| \geq r) \leq 1 - p_0 = M(\sum_i^3 (\varepsilon_i')^2)/r^2$$

This expression we can rewrite as

$$p(|E| \leq r) \geq p_0 = 1 - \sum_i^3 M((\varepsilon_i')^2)$$

and keeping in mind equation (1) we can calculate a value of r

$$r^2 = \sum_i^3 M((\varepsilon_i')^2)/(1 - p_0) = \sum_i^3 \sum_j^3 \alpha_{ij}^2 \sigma_j^2 + 3\sigma_4^2 \tag{2}$$

where σ_4 is the dispersion of a random quantity η_i, dispersion of which does not depend on i. In this case we have some sphere with a radius of r determined by equation (2) and a volume of $V = 4\pi r^3/3$.

Thus we can determine a volume of a colour body in which all the stimuli are mapped. Let us have an unclosed 3D curve $\{x_i(\lambda)\}$, $i = 1, 2, 3$ and $\lambda \in (\lambda_{380}, \lambda_{720})$. It is natural to satisfy some restrictions $|\alpha_{ij}y_j| \leq a_0$. Let the ends of this unclosed curve be connected by a straight line. Thus we have some closed curve L. Each point of L is connected both with point $\{0, 0, 0\}$ (the origin) and point $\{a_0, a_0, a_0\}$. In other words we have a shape that we call the colour body. It is easy to calculate the volume ($V(\alpha_{ij})$) of this colour body. Now, let us determine the ratio

$$\delta = V(\alpha_{ij})/V(\varepsilon_j') = cV(\alpha_{ij})/\sigma_1^3[\sum_{ij}^3 \alpha_{ij}^2 + 3(\sigma_4/\sigma_1)^2]^{3/2} \tag{3}$$

where c is some coefficient.

It is natural to suggest that this ratio determines the colour discriminability of our system. The greater δ the greater the discriminability. Now we are able to formulate the problem: *we must find a value of the coefficients* α_{ij} *(i.e. an operator* Ω_2*) such that for the three orthogonal functions* $\{x_i(\lambda)\}$*, i = 1, 2, 3, ratio* $\delta = V(\alpha_{ij})/V(\varepsilon'_j)$ *(see equation (1)) is maximal subject to the restriction* $|\alpha_{ij}y_j| \leq a_0$.

But it should be noted that the determined operator $\Omega_2 = \|\alpha_{ij}\|$ is not uniquely specified: the ratio δ is unchanged by rotation.

Let us rotate the co-ordinate system of the determined axis of colour space in such a way that the white colour vector $\mathbf{E}(w)$ will coincide with vector $\{x_1, 0, 0\}$, and vectors $\{0, x_2, 0\}$ and $\{0, 0, x_3\}$ will coincide with the so-called constant hue colour vectors, i.e. vectors conforming to monochromatic light stimuli with wavelength $\lambda = 475, 500$ and 580 nm respectively (see Purdy, 1931).

Thus, it is clear that the sought opponent functions depend on the specification of the concept of white colour. For calculations of the operator Ω_2 we used Smith–Pokorny primaries (Smith and Pokorny, 1972). The operator Ω_2 had been determined for D_{65} and A white light source. It takes the forms

$$\begin{Vmatrix} 0.7 & 0.58 & 0.38 \\ 0.44 & 0.08 & -0.9 \\ 0.55 & -0.8 & 0.24 \end{Vmatrix} \text{ and } \begin{Vmatrix} 0.81 & 0.56 & 0.11 \\ 0.19 & -0.04 & -0.98 \\ 0.54 & -0.83 & 0.17 \end{Vmatrix}$$

respectively: These opponent functions are shown on Figures 9.11.1 and 9.11.2.

9.11.3   THE BASIC PROPERTIES OF THE MODEL

While calculating the properties of the model we shall use the following well-known suggestion:

- the brightness of a stimulus is specified by an absolute value of an associated colour vector (Ingling and Tsou, 1977; Guth *et al.*, 1969; Vaitkevičius *et al.*, 1985, Ismailov and Sokolov, 1991);
- hue is specified by an angle of vector $\{0, x_2, x_3\}$ (i.e. the projection of the colour vector in the plane (x_2, x_3) with axis either x_2 or x_3 (Ismailov and Sokolov, 1991). But in the literature hue is generally specified by the so-called hue coefficients (Hurvich and Jameson, 1955), which could be calculated from this expression $|x_3|/(|x_2| + |x_3|)$ or $|x_2|/(|x_2| + |x_3|)$.
- saturation is determined by an angle between the colour vector and the plane (x_2, x_3) (Ismailov and Sokolov, 1991).

It is suggested that threshold changes in the hue and saturation are specified by just noticeable changes in the above-mentioned angles. This angle was calculated in the following way. We used the just noticeable changes ($\Delta\lambda$) of the wavelength of the monochromatic light (see Wright and Pitt, 1934). Knowing $\Delta\lambda$ and the opponent functions $\{x_i\}$ ($i = 1, 2, 3$), we can calculate just-noticeable changes in a colour vector orientation $\Delta\Psi(\lambda)$. It is assmed that this quantity is constant and it is equal to $\Delta\Psi(\lambda) = [\Delta\Psi(\lambda = 490) + \Delta\Psi(\lambda = 530) + \Delta\Psi(\lambda = 590)\}/3$.

As mentioned above the brightness is determined by the absolute value of a colour vector $\mathbf{E}$: $|\mathbf{E}| = M(\lambda) = [x_1^2(\lambda) + x_2^2(\lambda) + x_3^2(\lambda)]^{1/2}$. This function is shown in Figure 9.11.3 (solid line) together with the experimentally found function (dashed line, see Kulikowski and Walsh (1991)).

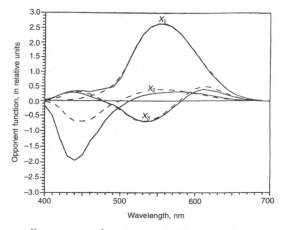

Figure 9.11.1. Spectrally opponent functions. Solid lines are theoretically calculated functions for (A) white light, the dashed lines, redrawn from Ingling and Tsou (1977).

The hue coefficients are shown in Figure 9.11.4 against λ. Hue discrimination as a function of λ is shown in Figure 9.11.5. The saturation as function of λ is shown in Figure 9.11.6.

9.11.4 DISCUSSION

As we can see from the above mentioned figures there are also some discrepancies between calculated and perceptual properties of the visual system of a human being.

The first discrepancy lies in the shapes of the opponent functions, especially for short wavelengths. As may be seen from Figure 9.11.1 and 9.11.2 there are rather large deviations of calculated opponent functions from the perceptual ones in the short wave interval. It is conceivable that there are a few reasons for that discrepancy.

1. It is known that experimentally obtained data for short wavelengths are rather crudely specified – for example, data obtained by Ingling *et al.* (1978) differ by a factor of ten from those obtained by Hurvich and Jameson, (1955).

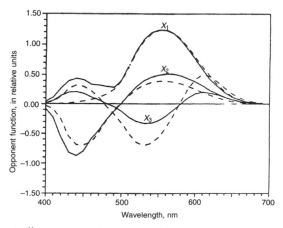

Figure 9.11.2. Spectrally opponent functions. The same as in Figure 9.11.1, but for (D_{65}) white.

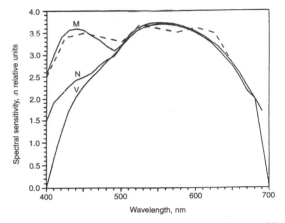

Figure 9.11.3.   The luminosity curves. Dashed line, redrawn from Kulikowski and Walsh (1991). The curve labelled (M) is the relationship between the absolute value of the colour vector and wavelength. The (N) curve is the same function but without 'blue'cones. The curve labelled by (V) is the CIE (1924) curve.

2. It is necessary to take into consideration that the noise generated by blue (S) cones is smaller than that generated by red (L) and green (G) cones. This can influence the shape of the 'optimal' opponent functions used in our model.

The second discrepancy touches on the luminosity curve. Three types of curves are shown in Figure 9.11.3: M (solid line) is the calculated curve, the dashed line is the perceptual spectral sensitivity curve for detection of a test flash (1 hz) taken from the paper of Kulikowski and Walsh (1991). $V(\lambda)$ is the well-known luminosity curve and N is again the calculated curve when (S) cones are switched off.

As may be seen from Figures 9.11.1 and 9.11.2, function $x_1(\lambda)$ is very similar to the luminosity curve $V(\lambda)$. On the basis of this similarity it is suggested that the achromatic first channel is related to our determination of the brightness. But in this case it is not clear how to explain non-additivity of brightness. Therefore we proposed (see also Ingling and Tsou, 1977; Guth *et al.*, 1969) that brightness is specified by the absolute value of the colour

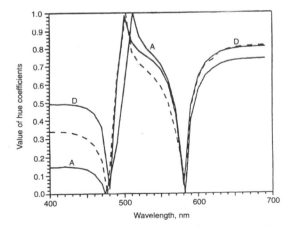

Figure 9.11.4.   Hue coefficient. The dashed line is the relationship redrawn from Hurvich and Jameson, (1955), the solid line is the calculated relationship: (A), (D) – for (A) and (D$_{65}$) white, respectively.

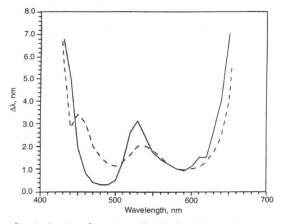

Figure 9.11.5. Hue discrimination function. The dashed line is the relationship redrawn from Wright and Pitt (1934), the solid one is the calculated relationship.

vector (only for white colour, when the output signals of two other opponent signals are equal to zero, $x_2(\lambda) = x_3(\lambda) = 0$, does the achromatic channel specify a brightness). We think that the spectral sensitivity curve (M) reduces to the luminosity curve $V(\lambda)$ when signals of S cones are small (compare the N curve with $V(\lambda)$ curve). The truth of this assumption may be seen from the data described by Kulikowski and Walsh (1991): when stimuli are small and they are presented in the fovea, where there are no S cones the spectral sensitivity curve is similar to the luminosity curve ($V(\lambda)$).

The third discrepancy touches on the brightness additivity curve. This curve as a function of λ is shown in Figure 9.11.7. The constant stimulus has wavelength $\lambda = 525$ nm (see Guth *et al.*, 1969). The dashed line represents the experimental data (taken from Guth *et al.*, 1969). The solid lines A and B represent calculated curves with a ratio noise $(\sigma_4/\sigma_1) = 1$ and $(\sigma_4/\sigma_1) = 8$, respectively. The solid line with filled circles represents the case when S cones are switched off. We are not able to find in the literature any data that could help either to accept or to reject this hypothesis. We think that in this case it is necessary also to take into consideration that the ratio of the signal/noise is smaller for S cones than for R and G cones.

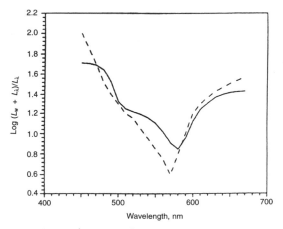

Figure 9.11.6. The saturation as function of wavelength. The dashed line is the relationship redrawn from Wright (1946), the solid one is the calculated relationship.

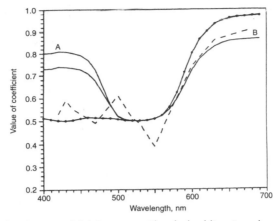

Figure 9.11.7. The brightness additivity curve. The dashed line is redrawn from Guth *et al.* (1969). The solid lines (A) and (B) represent calculated curves with a ratio of noise (σ_4/σ_1) equal to 1 and 8, respectively. The line labelled by solid circles represents the relation without 'blue' cones.

9.11.5   SUMMARY

1. Colour discriminability depends on additive noise generated both by cones and other elements of a neural net. The discriminability is determined by the ratio of the volume of the whole colour body and that of the averaged sphere in which a stable stimulus is mapped with the given probability P_0.
2. It is suggested that three cone signals are transformed in signals of the opponent cells in such a way that the colour discriminability of the whole system would be optimal (the above-mentioned ratio (see equation (3)) would be maximal). The view of the opponent functions depends upon the ratio of the dispersion of the above-mentioned noise generated by cones and other elements of a neural net. The lower the cone noise the greater volume of colour body that is designed for green–red colours (in other words non-additivity of the brightness under the sum of brightness of the green and red stimuli increases).
3. In order to make a more detailed calculation of opponent functions it is necessary to take into consideration that the noise generated by different cones could also be different. Furthermore it is necessary to allow that an efficiency of cones in transformation of light energy of an output signal could be different (Gribakin, 1994).

9.11.6   REFERENCES

Buchsbaum G. & Gottshalk A. (1983) Trichromacy opponent colours coding and optimum colour information transmission in the retina, *Proceedings of the Royal Society, London*, **220**, 1221–1223.

De Valois R.L. & De Valois K.K. (1993) A multi-stage color model, *Vision Research*, **33** (8), 1053–1065.

Fomin, S.V., Sokolov, E.N. & Vaitkevičius, H.H. (1979) *Artificial Sense Organs*. Moscow, Navka, 179p.

Gribakin F. (1994) Personal communication.

Guth S.L. (1991) Model for colour vision and light adaptation, *Journal of Optical Society of America* **A, 8** (6), 976–993.

GUTH S.L., DONKEY N.J. & MARROCO R.T. (1969) On luminance additivity and related topics, *Vision Research* **9**, 537–575.

HURVICH L.M. & JAMESON D. (1955) Some quantitative aspects of an opponent-color theory: brightness, saturation and hue in normal and dichromatic vision, *Journal of Optical Society of America*, **45**, 602–616.

INGLING C.R. & TSOU B.M. (1977) Orthogonal combinations of three visual channels, *Vision Research*, **17**, 1075–1082.

INGLING C.R., RUSSELL P.W. & TSOU B.M. (1978) Red–green opponent spectral sensitivity: disparity between cancellation and direct matching methods, *Science*, **201**, 1221–1223.

ISMAILOV CH.A. & SOKOLOV E.N. (1991) Spherical model of color and brightness discrimination, *Psychological Science*, June, 249–259.

KULIKOWSKI J.J. & WALSH V. (1991) *On the Limits of Color Detection and Discrimination, Vision and Visual Dysfunction*, Vol. 5: *Limits of Vision*. London, Macmillan Press.

PARAMEJ G.V., ISMAILOV CH.A. & SOKOLOV E.N. (1991) Multidimensional scaling of large chromatic differences by normal and color-deficient subjects, *Psychological Science*, **4**, 244–248.

PURDY D.M. (1931) Spectral hue as function of intensity, *American Journal of Psychology*, **43**, 541–559.

SMITH V.C. & POKORNY J. (1972) Spectral sensitivity of color-blind observers and the cone photo pigments, *Vision Research*, **12**, 2059–2071.

SOKOLOV E.N. & VAITKEVIČIUS H.H. (1989) *Neurointellect* (From neurones to neurocomputers), Moscow Nauka, 219 pp.

SVAETICHIN G., NEGISHI K. & FATERCHAND R. (1965) *Cellular Mechanism of Young–Hering Theory*, CIBA Found. Symp. Color Vision, Boston, Little, Brown & Co, pp. 178–202.

VAITKEVIČIUS H.H., DAILYDAITE R., MEŠKAUSKAS A. & SINIUS J. (1984) Opponent processing in the colour analyser and its connection with differential sensitivity, *Symposium on Computational Models of Hearing and Vision*, Summaries, Tallinn.

VAITKEVIČIUS H.H., STANKEVIČIUS Ž. & SOKOLOV E.N. (1993) Opponent color functions and color discriminability, *Sensory System*, **7** (4), 58–66.

WRIGHT, W.D. (1946) *Researches on Normal and Defective Colour Vision*. Hevy Kimpton, London.

WRIGHT W.D. & PITT F.M.S. (1934) Hue discrimination in normal color vision, *Proceedings of the Physical Society*, London, **46**, 459.

Section 10 – Colour Applications

Hyperchromatic Lenses as Potential Aids for the Presbyope

W.N.Charman and H.D.Whitefoot

10.1.1 INTRODUCTION

It has been known since the time of Newton (Shapiro, 1984) that the eye suffers from substantial longitudinal chromatic aberration (LCA). This amounts to about two dioptres across the visible spectrum, with the eye being more myopic for blue light (see, e.g. Charman, 1991, for review). In view of the blur that would be expected to result from this aberration, many authors have sought to demonstrate that visual acuity (VA) in monochromatic light is superior to that in white light. This turns out to be surprisingly difficult, largely because the eye's lower spectral sensitivity at the extremes of the spectrum reduces the effect of the out-of-focus blur associated with the chromatic aberration (Campbell and Gubisch, 1967). It does appear, however, that depth-of-focus (DOF) in white light is slightly greater than that in monochromatic light (Campbell, 1957).

These characteristics of the normal eye led Öhmann (1949) to suggest that there might be advantages in providing the presbyope with a hyperchromatic corrective lens that deliberately enhanced the LCA of the eye. As presbyopes have lost the ability to increase the power of their crystalline lenses to view near objects, Öhmann hypothesised that a lens with enhanced LCA would increase the lens-eye DOF, allowing a clear red image of distant objects and a clear blue image of near objects to be formed on the presbyope's retina. Obviously the concept could only work with polychromatic 'white' light containing a broad spectrum of wavelengths. Öhmann's ideas were elaborated on by Freeman (1984), who pointed out that high levels of LCA could be produced much more easily by a diffractive lens of negative power. The power of a diffractive lens is directly proportional to the wavelength, so that it effectively has much greater dispersion than a refractive lens.

Clearly, the problem with using any hyperchromatic lens is that when the blue image is in focus the red image is substantially blurred, and vice versa. Will the visual system then simply sum the retinal irradiances due to the various wavelengths with weighting according to the CIE V_λ photopic visual efficiency curve (Bradley, 1992), or will it be able to use colour information to 'select' the in-focus quasi-monochromatic image and hence attain better acuity? There is, of course, no doubt that resolution is possible on the basis of colour information, even in the absence of luminance contrast, although limiting grating acuities based on red-green or blue-yellow discrimination are only about one-third of those found for gratings showing luminance contrast (Mullen, 1985). Therefore, we carried out a study to determine whether enhancing the ocular LCA in this way does usefully increase the DOF without the penalty of reduced visual acuity.

10.1.2   METHODS

10.1.2.1 Control of effective ocular LCA

LCA was manipulated with the aid of an achromatising lens consisting of a doublet and triplet separated by air (Powell, 1981). By using the doublet and triplet separately and in combination, the lens-eye LCA could be approximately reversed (triplet), doubled (doublet) or neutralised (complete lens). Figure 10.1.1 shows the measured values of lens-eye LCA for one subject, as obtained using an interference-filter monochromator in conjunction with a Badal optometer (see also Bobier *et al.*, 1992).

10.1.2.2 Visual acuity and depth-of-focus

Monocular depth-of-focus was assessed using a Snellen letter acuity task. Single Snellen letters, produced on a tri-phosphor Super-VGA monitor, were viewed from a distance of 6 m. Each of the 10 characters of the Sloan letter set (Sloan, 1951) appeared dark on a white background. The background luminance was approximately 1000 cdm^{-2} and the room was illuminated to about 600 lux. Ocular focus in the viewing eye was changed at 0.25 D intervals by inserting spectacle trial lenses just behind the components of the Powell lens, care being taken to maintain lens centration and vertex distance. The non-viewing eye was occluded. For each level of focus, the control programme (French, 1993) determined the VA by a staircase procedure, successive steps of the staircase being at intervals of 0.1 logMAR (log$_{10}$ minimum angle of resolution in minutes of arc). With single letters being counted, the threshold criterion used was essentially that employed in clinical practice, that the probability of letter recognition should approach 100 per cent.

Complete through-focus series with high-contrast letters (90 per cent Michelson contrast) were carried out with two subjects. A 56-year-old presbyope (subjective amplitude of accommodation about 1.5 D, objective amplitude about 0.5 D) was tested both under cycloplegia (1 per cent cyclopentolate) with a 4 mm artificial pupil, and with free accommodation and a natural pupil (about 3.5 mm diameter). A second, younger, subject repeated the cycloplegic measurements with the artificial pupil. Further cycloplegic measurements were made with both subjects viewing low-contrast (10 per cent Michelson contrast) letters produced with the same display.

10.1.3   RESULTS

Results for the presbyope under cycloplegia for three of the four LCA conditions are shown in Figure 10.1.2. It is clear that under all conditions the subject achieved a best logMAR of about −0.2 (Snellen 6/4). Little, if any, reduction in high-contrast VA was caused by the enhanced LCA introduced by the doublet. Results with the other subject were very similar.

In general terms, Figure 10.1.2 suggests that DOF tends to increase in the order: corrected LCA (full Powell lens); normal LCA (naked eye); doubled LCA (doublet lens). As is well known, given results of the type shown in Figure 10.1.2, numerical values of DOF depend upon the criterion used to obtain them (e.g. Tucker and Charman, 1974). For the present purposes, it seems reasonable to take the total DOF as the range of dioptric focus over which the acuity exceeds a chosen value. Table 10.1.1 shows values of DOF determined in this way, measured at logMAR values of 0.00 and +0.20, corresponding to Snellen acuities 6/6 and 6/9.5 respectively. With free accommodation the presbyope's through-focus curves were a little broader, due both to the small amount of residual accommodation and to the slightly smaller natural pupil, and the corresponding DOFs were therefore slightly larger (Table 10.1.1). The hyperchromatic doublet lens always gives the largest DOFs and hence appears to be potentially useful to the presbyope, although the increase in DOF over that of the naked eye is quite modest (around 0.5 D).

With the low-contrast letters, however, a somewhat different picture emerges (Figure 10.1.3). Increasing the LCA over the natural level leads to a marked reduction in peak acuity (by about 0.1 logMAR), although the through-focus curves are, perhaps, slightly broader at lower levels of acuity.

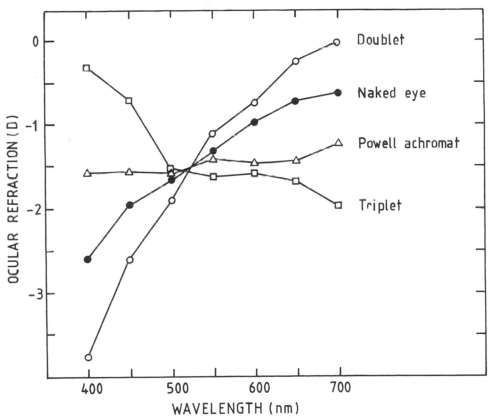

Figure 10.1.1. Effective ocular LCA as measured with and without the various components of the Powell lens (WNC, left eye). ● Naked eye ('normal' LCA); △ complete Powell lens ('zero' LCA); ○ doublet lens ('doubled' LCA); □ triplet lens ('reversed' LCA). The data have not been corrected for the low myopia of the observer or for the small back vertex power of the lenses.

10.1.4   DISCUSSION

These results confirm that a hyperchromatic correction may usefully enhance DOF in high-contrast tasks. This enhancement is, however, achieved at the expense of a loss in retinal image contrast, so that when low-contrast detail is observed the performance is markedly impaired with the hyperchromatic correction. Contrast sensitivity measurements (not given here) confirm the loss in retinal image contrast with the hyperchromatic lens. This poor performance with low-contrast detail obviously limits the possible value of hyperchromatic corrections to presbyopes, although the same criticism could be levelled at many of today's designs of contact lens for the presbyope (Bullimore and Jacobs, 1993). It would obviously be desirable to explore a wider range of values of lens-eye LCA to determine the best compromise level.

Subjectively, the hyperchromatic doublet did not give the impression that the distance image was markedly red or the near image markedly blue. It should be noted, however, that hyperchromatic spectacle lenses would be of limited utility due to their high levels of transverse chromatic aberration when the eye is rotated behind the lens to view objects through the lens periphery. Well-centred hyperchromatic contact or intraocular lenses do not suffer from this problem, because they move with the eye.

It is interesting to note that white-light DOF with the full Powell achromatising lens is consistently less (by about 0.3 D) than that of the naked eye. This difference is rather

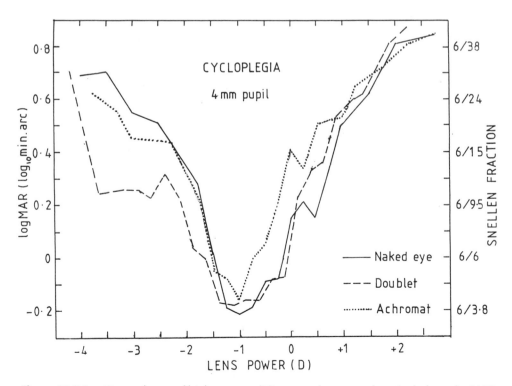

Figure 10.2.2. Dependence of high-contrast (90 per cent), monocular, single-letter logMAR acuity on focus for different conditions of lens-eye LCA: for clarity only three conditions are shown. Subject WNC (56 years, left eye) with cycloplegia and a 4 mm diameter artificial pupil. ——— Naked eye; _ _ _ doublet lens (doubled LCA); ..... full Powell lens (zero LCA).

Table 10.1.1. Full monocular depths-of-focus over which high-contrast, single-letter logMAR acuity levels 0.0 (6/6 Snellen) and +0.2 (6/9.5 Snellen) were achieved for WNC (left eye). The optimal logMAR (Snellen) acuities at best focus are also shown.

Condition	Peak logMAR acuity (Snellen)	DOF (D) at 0.00 logMAR	DOF (D) at +0.20 logMAR
Cycloplegia (4 mm pupil)			
Naked eye (normal LCA)	−0.21 (6/3.7)	1.20	1.81
Powell			
(zero LCA)	−0.18 (6/4.0)	0.84	1.48
Doublet (doubled LCA)	−0.19 (6/3.9)	1.59	2.40
Triplet (reversed LCA)	−0.20 (6/3.8)	0.96	1.60
No cycloplegia (natural pupil)			
Naked eye (normal LCA)	−0.21 (6/3.7)	1.88	2.67
Powell			
(zero LCA)	−0.20 (6/3.8)	1.42	2.30
Doublet (doubled LCA)	−0.22 (6/3.6)	2.25	3.25
Triplet (reversed LCA)	−0.22 (6/3.6)	1.80	2.67

greater than the value of about 0.1 D for four subjects found by Campbell using a 'just perceptible blur' criterion and a 3 mm pupil. The apparent discrepancy can reasonably be accounted for by the better correction for transverse chromatic aberration achieved with the Powell lens used in the present study (Powell, 1981) and to the different tasks, pupil sizes

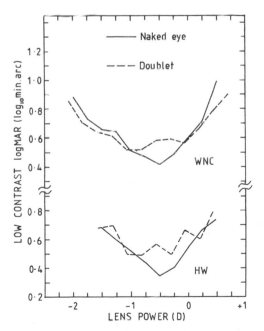

Figure 10.1.3. Dependence of low-contrast (10 per cent), monocular, single-letter logMAR acuity on focus for two subjects under cycloplegia with a 4 mm artificial pupil. ⎯⎯ Naked eye (normal LCA); _ _ _ doublet lens (doubled LCA).

and criteria involved in the estimation of the DOF. There seems little doubt, however, that the natural LCA of the eye does modestly enhance ocular DOF in white light.

10.1.5 REFERENCES

BOBIER, W.R., CAMPBELL, M.C.W. & HINCH, M. (1992) The influence of chromatic aberration on the static accommodation response, *Vision Research*, **32**, 823–832.

BRADLEY, A. (1992) Perceptual manifestations of imperfect optics in the human eye: attempts to correct for ocular chromatic aberration, *Optometry and Vision Science*, **69**, 515–521.

BULLIMORE, M.A. & JACOBS, R.J. (1993) Subjective and objective assessment of soft bifocal contact lens performance, *Optometry and Vision Science*, **79**, 469–475.

CAMPBELL, F.W. (1957) The depth-of-field of the human eye, *Optica Acta*, **4**, 157–164.

CAMPBELL, F.W. & GUBISCH, R.W. (1967) The effect of chromatic aberration on visual acuity, *Journal of Physiology*, **192**, 345–358.

CHARMAN, W.N. (1991) Optics of the human eye. In: Charman, W.N. (Ed.) *Vision and Visual Dysfunction, Vol 1: Visual Optics and Instrumentation*, London: Macmillan, pp. 1–26.

FREEMAN, M.H. (1984) Ophthalmic lenses having negative diffractive power, UK Patent application GB 2 127 988 A, 18th April 1984.

FRENCH, C.N. (1993) PC practice in theory, *Optician*, **205** (5391) March 5, 18–20.

MULLEN, K. (1985) The contrast sensitivity of the human colour vision to red-green and blue-yellow chromatic gratings, *Journal of Physiology*, **359**, 381–400.

ÖHMANN, Y. (1949) Sur l'emploi de lentilles hypochromatiques, pour agrandir la profondeur de champ, dans un état accommodation donné, *Revue d'Optique*, **28**, 105–106.

POWELL, I. (1981) Lenses for correcting the chromatic aberration of the eye, *Applied Optics*, **20**, 4152–4155.

SHAPIRO, A.E. (Ed.) (1984) *The Optical Papers of Isaac Newton, Vol.1, The Optical Lectures 1670–1672*, Cambridge: Cambridge University Press, pp. 579–583.

SLOAN, L.L. (1951) Measurement of visual acuity, *AMA Archives of Ophthalmology*, **45**, 704–725.

TUCKER, J. & CHARMAN, W.N. (1974) The depth-of-focus of the human eye for Snellen letters, *American Journal of Optometry and Physiological Optics*, **52**, 3–21.

Revision of the CIE Recommendations for the Colours of Signal Lights

Barry L. Cole and Jennifer D. Maddocks

10.2.1 INTRODUCTION

The International Commission on Illumination (CIE) first adopted recommendations for the colours of signal lights in 1959. The most recent revision of the recommendations was in 1975 (CIE, 1975). The recommendations have been widely adopted in international and national standards that specify the colours of signals and, as a consequence, have brought about substantial international consistency in colours used in signal systems.

The original recommendations were based largely on experiments on the recognition of signal colours reported by McNicholas (1936), Holmes (1941) and Hill (1947), together with the advice based on the practical experience of the expert members of the CIE. The 1975 revision took account of some new work (Blaise, 1960, 1965) as well as experience in the application of the recommendations, but the changes were not substantial. There were some changes to the restricted boundaries and the blue boundary of white was extended to include the chromaticity for xenon sources. A violet signal colour was introduced because this colour had found some useful application for harbour signals.

At the 21st quadrennial session of the CIE in Venice in 1987, Division 4 of the CIE, which is concerned with lighting and signals for transport, decided that there should be a critical review of the recommendations based on an analysis of experimental reports on the recognition of signal colours as the original recommendations had been adopted. This task fell to a committee of expert members appointed by Division 4.

10.2.2 METHOD

The committee assembled a bibliography of published and unpublished reports on the recognition of signal colours and identified 25 references that reported experimental data (see Appendix). The experimental conditions used in these investigations varied considerably presenting the committee with the challenging task of finding a means to amalgamate the data in a form that would enable the CIE recommendations to be tested against the data.

The data was categorised according to adaptation conditions (night, day) and the illuminances of the signals.[1] The categorisation of illuminances was:

- very dim signals having an illuminance of less than 1 μlux, typical of long distance martime signal lights;
- dim signals between 1 and 10 μlux, typical of distant aviation signal lights;
- moderately bright signals of between 10 and 100 μlux, typical of railroad signals;
- bright signals of between 100 and 1000 μlux, typical of motor vehicle signals and traffic lights and some aviation signals;
- very bright signals of more than 1000 μlux.

The available experimental data were tabulated by the colours used in the experiments, stimulus size and duration and the number of observers and their means of selection. Some reports included colour vision defective observers.

The probability of correct recognition of each colour was extracted from the data and plotted on large scale 1931 CIE chromaticity diagrams. Data for colours that gave a low probability of recognition were discarded because the CIE recommendations for signal colours should define those colours that provide a high degree of certainty of correct recognition. Where there was sufficient data within the report of a particular investigation, the contours for 90 per cent correct recognition were estimated and plotted. Any individual colours that had a probability of correct recognition greater than 0.9 were also plotted as individual points.

These 90 per cent contours and individual colours with a probability of correct recognition greater than 0.90 were then compared with the chromaticity boundaries that defined the colour domains recommended by the CIE for red, yellow, green, white and blue signals.

10.2.3   RESULTS

Figures 10.2.1 and 10.2.2 (in the colour section) show the 90 per cent recognition contours for very dim signals and very bright signals plotted on the 1931 CIE diagram. The figures also show the boundaries of the colour domains defined by the CIE in its 1975 recommendations.

The full set of plots and the tabulated summaries of the experimental data are given in the report of the CIE technical committee (CIE, 1994).

10.2.3.1 Red signal colours

The committee judged that the yellow boundary of the colour domain for red signals extended too far toward yellow so that it included orangish-reds that were not reliably identified as red. It has recommended that the yellow boundary be shifted from $y = 0.335$ to $y = 0.320$. This has the effect of reducing the maximum possible transmission of red signal glasses by 17 per cent and thereby reducing the intensity of red signals. However, it was agreed that the loss of transmission would not seriously limit the range of red signal lights in practice because of the increased efficiency of modern light sources.

The present CIE recommendations have a restricted purple boundary to be used when more certain recognition of red was required. The experimental data did not support the need for this restricted boundary: slight desaturation of red does not appear to decrease the probability of correct recognition and as a consequence the purple boundary is to be abandoned.

There is a second restricted boundary to ensure high probability of correct recognition. This is located at $y = 0.300$ and excludes short wavelength reds. The experimental data support the retention of this restricted boundary.

10.2.3.2 Red signals and colour vision defective users

Persons with a protan colour vision defect have difficulty seeing red signals and the longer the dominant wavelength of the red the greater is their difficulty. This has been one reason why the yellow boundary has in the past been set to include orangish-reds. Moving the yellow boundary to $y = 0.320$ will disadvantage this group of users. However, the experimental data obtained with colour vision defective observers shows that they recognise long wavelength red signals better than orangish-reds. The orangish-red may be better seen by protan observers but is more likely to be wrongly identified by both normal and colour abnormal observers.

The loss of visual range for protan observers arising from a shift of the yellow boundary of red to $y = 0.320$ is marginal and can be compensated by the use of more efficient light sources and optical systems to provide a compensatory increase of signal intensity.

However, it is still desirable that the red colour of signal systems that are used by colour vision defective observers should exclude deep reds that the protan observer may be unable to see even with increases in intensity. This is achieved by defining a further restricted boundary at $y = 0.290$, so that reds for signals used by colour vision defective observers should lie between this boundary and $y = 0.320$. This restricted boundary is unchanged from the 1975 CIE recommendations.

10.2.3.3 Yellow signal colours

The present CIE recommended yellow seems to extend too far toward red, probably because of the desire to encompass 'amber' signals that have been used in road traffic signals in some countries and there is a clear need to draw this boundary back.

Of particular interest was that the experimental data suggest that at higher illuminances 'yellow' shifts to shorter wavelengths. At low illuminances, these shorter wavelengths are not reliably recognised as yellow but longer wavelengths are.

The committee has substantially re-drawn the boundaries of yellow to define a recommended signal colour that lies parallel to the spectral locus between dominant wavelengths 585 nm and 593 nm with an extension to 595 nm wavelengths for low illuminance signals. For high illuminance signals, it is recommended that yellow be constrained to between 585 nm and 590 nm and between 590 nm and 595 nm for low illuminance signals.

10.2.3.4 Green signal colours

The present green signal colour domain extends over a wide area and within it is a restricted domain to be used when certain recognition of green is important. The experimental data show that the broader domain generally lies outside the $p = 0.90$ contours and a revised domain for green is recommended that follows the old restricted boundaries.

There is a further restricted boundary to exclude yellowish-greens which has the purpose of defining greens that may be better recognised by colour vision defective observers. This boundary forms part of the 1975 CIE recommendations and is to be retained. The argument is that colour vision defective observers are better able to recognise bluish-greens as green. This concept was first proposed by Judd (1952) as part of a red, green, blue signal system for panel lights that Judd believed might be reliably recognised by colour vision defective observers. However, while bluish-greens are better recognised by colour vision defectives, the gains are marginal (CIE, 1994).

10.2.3.5 Blue signal colours

At low illuminances only saturated blues with a dominant wavelength between 455 nm and 470 nm are reliably recognised. At very low illuminances, threshold tritanopia makes blue an unreliable signal colour. As a result of reviewing the experimental data, the committee recommends a much more constrained domain for blue than is defined in the 1975 Recommendations. In addition, a very circumscribed area at short wavelengths is defined for very low illuminance blue signals.

Blue signal glasses have a very low transmittance and for this reason an extension of blue toward white is to be permitted when a high intensity signal is required and when confusion with white is not important.

The committee could find no information on the current use of the violet colour domain defined in the 1975 Recommendations, nor is there any support for such a colour from the experimental data. Accordingly, it is recommended that the violet colour be abandoned.

10.2.3.6 White signal colours

The 1975 CIE Recommendations define a complex domain for white that generally follows the line of the Planckian locus. There are three domains, one intended to embrace very low colour temperature sources such as oil lamps, one for incandescent lamps and the third for higher colour temperature sources. White is not reliably recognised in the two low colour temperature domains where it tends to be confused with yellow.

The committee has recommended that the very low colour temperature domain be abandoned and that the domain for incandescent sources be restricted on its yellow boundary at $x = 0.420$.

The committee also considered that the blue boundary of white extended too far toward blue and should be located at $x = 0.300$ instead of $x = 0.285$.

10.2.4   CONCLUSION

The committee has presented its data, reasoning and recommendations in a technical report (CIE, 1994) and has drafted a CIE/ISO Standard for Signal Colours to replace the 1975 CIE recommendations. The draft is under consideration by the National Committees of the CIE and ISO.

10.2.5   NOTE

1 Illuminance (E) is used in this context to specify the amount of light from a signal that reaches the observers' eyes. Illuminance is the amount of light per unit area in the plane of the observer's eye.

It is defined as $E = F/A$, where F is the luminous flux in lumens and A the area in metres. The unit of E is the lux. Illuminance is dependent on the intensity of the signal (I in candelas) and the inverse of the square of the observation distance d, such that $E = I/d^2$.

10.2.6   REFERENCES

BLAISE, P. (1960) Sur la vision colorée en signalisation maritime, *Conférence Internationale des Services de Signalisation Maritime*, Washington DC, Rapport 5.4.1.

BLAISE, P. (1965) Vision des feux violets et leur utilisation en signalisation maritime, *Conférence Internationale des Services de Signalisation Maritime*, Rome, Rapport 5.1.5.

CIE (1975) *Colors of Light Signals*, CIE Publication No 2.2, Paris: CIE.

CIE (1994) *Review of Official Recommendations of the CIE for the Colours of Signal Lights*, CIE Publication 107-1994, Vienna: CIE.

HILL, N. E. G. (1947) The recognition of coloured signal lights which are near the limit of visibility, *Proceedings of the Physical Society*, **59**, 560–574.

HOLMES, J. G. (1941) The recognition of coloured signal lights, *Transactions Illumination of Engineering Society*, **6**, 71–97.

JUDD, D. B. (1952) *Standard Filters for Electronic Equipment*, Michigan: Armed Forces Nat Res Council Vision Committee, University of Michigan.

McNICHOLAS, H. J. (1936) Selection of colours for signal lights, *Journal for Research at the National Bureau of Standards*, **17**, 955–980.

10.2.7   APPENDIX: KEY REFERENCES

BLAISE, P. (1960) Sur la vision colorée en signalisation maritime, *Conference Internationale des Services de Signalisation Maritime*, Washington, DC September – October 1960: Rapport 5.4.1.

BLAISE, P. (1965) Vision des feux violets et leur utilisation en signalisation maritime. *Conférence internationale des Services de Signalisation Maritime*, Rome, May: Rapport 5.1.5.

BLAISE, P. (1985) Influence de la diffusion de Rayleigh sur les couleurs en signalisation maritime, *XI Conférence de l'Association Internationale de Signalisation Maritime*, Brighton.

CIE Publication No 2 (1959) *Colors of Light Signals*, Paris: Commission Internationale l'Eclairage.

CIE Publication No 2.2 (1975) *Colors of Light Signals*, Paris: Commission Internationale l'Eclairage.

COLE, B.L. & BROWN, B. (1966) Optimum intensity of red road-traffic signal lights for normal and protanopic observers, *Journal of the Optical Society of America*, **56**, 516–522.

COLE, B.L. & VINGRYS, A.J. (1983). Do protanomals have difficulty seeing red lights? *Proceedings of CIE 20th Session*, Amsterdam, CIE Publication 56, EO4, Paris: Commission Internationale l'Eclairage, pp. 1–3.

DAS, S.R. (1966) Recognition of signal colors by a different set of color names, *Journal of the Optical Society of America*, **56**, 789–794.

FARNSWORTH, D. (1946) Confusions of colored lights at small subtense by protans and deutans, NSMRL, Report Number 108, US Naval Submarine Medical Research Laboratory, Groton, CT.

FREEDMAN, M., DAVIT, P.S., STAPLIN, L.K. & BRETON, M.E. (1985) Traffic signal brightness: An examination of nighttime dimming, Final report, Report Number FHWA/RD-85-005, National Technical Information Service, Springfield, Virginia.

HALSEY, R.M. (1959) Identification of signal lights. I. Blue, green, white and purple, *Journal of the Optical Society of America*, **49**, 45–55.

HALSEY, R.M. (1959) Identification of signal lights. II. Elimination of the purple category, *Journal of the Optical Society of America*, **49**, 167–169.

HALSEY R.M. & CHAPANIS, A. (1951) On the number of absolutely identifiable spectral hues, *Journal of the Optical Society of America*, **41**, 1057–1058.

HALSEY, R.M. & CHAPANIS, A. (1954) Chromaticity-confusion contours in a complex viewing situation, *Journal of the Optical Society of America*, **44**, 442–454.

HEATH, G.G. & SCHMIDT, I. (1959) Signal color recognition by color defective observers, *American Journal of Optometry and Archives of the American Academy of Optometry*, **36**, 421–437.

HILL, N.E.G. (1947) The recognition of coloured signal lights which are near the limit of visibility. *Proceedings of the Physical Society*, **59**, 560–574.

HOFMANN, H. (1975) Recognition of colours of light signals in photopic and scotopic vision. *Proceedings of 18th CIE Session, London*, CIE Publication No. 36, P-75-04, Paris: Commission Internationale l'Eclairage, pp. 63–69.

HOFMANN, H. (1975) Uber das Bemessen der Leuchtdichte, Farbart und Darbietungszeit von Signallichtern unter verschiedenen Beobachtungsbedingungen, Dr Ing Dissertation, Darmstart.

HOLMES, J.G. (1941) The recognition of coloured signal lights, *Transactions Illumination of Engineering Society*, **6**, 71–97.

HONJYO, K. & NONAKA, M. (1970) Perception of white in a 10 degree field. *Journal of the Optical Society of America*, **60**, 1690–1694.

INGLING, C.R., SCHEIBNER, H.M.O. & BOYNTON, R.M. (1970) Color naming of small foveal fields. *Vision Research*, **10**, 501–511.

IKEDA, M. & UEHIRA, I. (1989) Unique hue loci and implications, *Colour Research and Application*, **14**, 318–324.

JUDD, D.B. (1952) *Standard Filters for Electronic Equipment*, Michigan: Armed Forces Nat Res Council Vision Committee, University of Michigan.

KAISER, P.K. (1968) Colour names of very small fields varying in duration and luminance, *Journal of the Optical Society of America*, **59**, 640–643.

KINNEY, J.A.S., PAULSON, H.M. & BEARE, A.N. (1979) Color defectives' judgments of signal lights at sea: A Replication, NSMRL Report Number 897, US Naval Submarine Medical Research Laboratory, Groton, CT.

KINNEY, J.A.S., PAULSON, H.M. & BEARE, A.N. (1979) The ability of color defectives to judge signal lights at sea, *Journal of the Society of America*, **69**, 106–113.

LEWIS, M.F. & STEEN, J.A. (1971) Color defective vision and the recognition of aviation color signal light flashes, Report Number FAA-AM-71-27, Federal Aviation Administration, Washington, DC.

LURIA, S.M. (1967) Color-name as a function of stimulus-intensity and duration, *American Journal of Psychology*, **80**, 14–27.

MCNICHOLAS, H.J. (1936) Selection of colours for signal lights, *Journal for Research at the National Bureau of Standards*, **17**, 955–980.

NATHAN, J., HENRY, G.H. & COLE, B.L. (1964) Recognition of colored road traffic light signals by normal and color-vision-defective observers. *Journal of the Optical Society of America*, **54**, 1041–1045.

SLOAN, L.L. & HABEL, A. (1955) Color signal systems for the red-green color blind. An experimental test of the three-color signal system proposed by Judd, *Journal of the Optical Society of America*, **45**, 592–598.

SLOAN, L.L. & HABEL, A. (1955) Recognition of red and green point sources by color-deficient observers, *Journal of the Optical Society of America*, **45**, 599–601.

SMITH, A.J. (1990) Colour measurements at the interface of two colours in a high intensity projector, personal communication.

STEEN, J.A. & LEWIS, M.F. (1971) Color defective vision and day and night recognition of aviation color signal light flashes, Report Number FAA-AM-71-32, Federal Aviation Administration, Washington, DC. [Also in: *Aerospace Medicine*, **43**, 34–36 (1972).]

VERRIEST, G., NEUBAUER, O., MARRÉ, M. & UVIJLS, A. (1980) New investigations concerning the relationships between congenital colour vision defects and road traffic security, *International Ophthalmology*, **2**, 87–99.

VINGRYS, A.J. (1984) An analysis of colour vision standards in the transport industry, PhD thesis, Melbourne University.

VINGRYS, A.J. & COLE, B.L. (1988) Are colour vision standards justified for the transport industry? *Ophthalmic and Physiological Optics*, **8**, 257–274.

VINGRYS, A.J. & COLE, B.L. (1993) The ability of colour vision defective observers to recognise an optimised set of red, green and white signal lights. In: Drum, B. (Ed.) *Colour Vision Deficiencies XI*, Dordrecht: Kluwer, pp. 87–95.

WEITZMAN, D.O. & KINNEY, J.A.S. (1967) Appearance of color for small, brief, spectral stimuli, in the central fovea, *Journal of the Optical Society of America*, **57**, 665–670.

A Methodology for Producing Maximally Discriminable, Nameable Colours in Control Room Displays

Darren Van Laar, Richard Flavell, Ian Umbers and Jonathan Smalley

10.3.1 INTRODUCTION

Over the years, Nuclear Electric (NE) and its predecessor the Central Electricity Generating Board (CEGB) have developed colour conventions for use in its power stations (Umbers and Collier, 1990). Colours for use with VDUs in power stations have often been restricted either by the small number of colours available or through a combination of past practice and subjective judgements. This has not always proved to be satisfactory, for example:

- the precise reproduction of the selected colours even on similar hardware is not always possible;
- certain important/useful colours, e.g. red and blue, are insufficiently bright;
- conspicuity of certain colours is not consistent with the importance of the information they convey;
- colours change as a result of display hardware degradation.

In the mid-1980s, an attempt was made to overcome some of these difficulties. A set of 13 nameable, discriminable colours was derived from Kelly (1966). This set of colours was implemented on a VDU by translating the Munsell references through CIE co-ordinates into RGB values for a calibrated monitor. The overall perceptual differences within this colour set in terms of both the minimum and maximum colour difference (ΔE^*) between any pair of colours and the average ΔE^* were:

Minimum ΔE^*: 14.2;   Average ΔE^*: 63.4;   Maximum ΔE^*: 127.1

10.3.2 PRACTICAL PRODUCTION OF A SET OF NAMEABLE DISCRIMINABLE COLOURS

In operational terms, to create a set of maximally discriminable colours, it is necessary to make the ΔE^* distance between all pairs of colours as large as possible while ensuring that all the colours lie within the monitor gamut. This may be turned into a structured problem by trying to maximise the distance between the pair of colours that are minimally separated. Additional constraints on the colour set, such as requirements for the colours to be 'recognisable' and 'nameable', cannot be mathematically defined, and yet are extremely important properties for the final set of colours. Therefore, instead of a purely mathematical procedure to derive a good set of colours, the following method was adopted.

1. The number of colours required in the set, and the names of the colours within the set was specified.
2. For each colour in turn, a colour was selected in xyY co-ordinates that matched to the desired name.
3. Calculate ΔE^* for each pair of colours.
4. Identify the pair of colours that was responsible for the overall minimum ΔE^*.
5. If possible the separation between this pair should be increased. This may be achieved by changing the hue and saturation, or by changing the luminance difference, i.e.
   a. if the colours were intrinsically close in terms of hue because of their colour names, such as red and orange, then increase the separation of their luminances by changing the Y values;
   b. if the colours were intrinsically different in hue, then increase the differences between the xy co-ordinates of the two colours.

If the separation between the pair of colours of minimum ΔE^* in the set had been successfully increased so that this pair was no longer responsible for the minimum separation, then this procedure was repeated from step 4.

6. If the separation between this pair of colours cannot be successfully increased, this may be because there are a number of pairs of colours that have approximately the same minimal ΔE^* separation. In this case go back to step 1 and reconsider the number and names of the colours.

The resulting set of primary colours, starting from a set of nameable colours and repeating the method described above a number of times, is shown below. Notice that the minimum ΔE^* has nearly trebled and that the average ΔE^* has nearly doubled compared with the original Kelly set:

$$\text{Minimum } \Delta E^*: 38.9; \quad \text{Average } \Delta E^*: 113.3; \quad \text{Maximum } \Delta E^*: 238.2$$

10.3.3   AN ALTERNATIVE ALGORITHM FOR GENERATING A COLOUR SET

It was suggested above that the mathematical algorithms constructed to identify sets of maximally discriminable colours (cf. De Corte, 1988) were inappropriate in this case, because of the nameability requirement, but also because of the very local nature of the algorithms. However a simple mathematical algorithm is proposed below that starts from step 2 above, i.e. a good first set of colours, and tries to increase the separation between the colours in a systematic fashion. The algorithm is based on the idea that the naming constraints, whilst in reality unquantifiable, essentially restrict the colour to a small area of Luv space. Thus, if step 2 can initially locate a colour within Luv space, constraints can then be constructed to limit the subsequent movement of the colour to a small cuboid centred on this original point. Furthermore, because subsequent movement is small, little error is introduced by locally linearising the problem.

Let L_i, u_i, v_i be the original location of the ith colour in Luv; ΔL_i, Δu_i, Δv_i be the unknown subsequent movement; ΔL_{ij}, Δu_{ij}, Δv_{ij}, ΔE_{ij} be the current known separation between colours i,j.

Hence,

$$(\Delta E_{ij})^2_{new} = [L_i + \Delta L_i - L_j - \Delta L_j]^2 + [u_i + \Delta u_i - u_j - \Delta u_j]^2 + [v_i + \Delta v_i - v_j - \Delta v_j]^2 \ \forall i,j$$

Expanding and ignoring second-order terms, we get:

$$(\Delta E_{ij})^2_{new} \approx (\Delta E_{ij})^2 + 2\Delta L_{ij}(\Delta L_i - \Delta L_j) + 2\Delta u_{ij}(\Delta u_i - \Delta u_j) + 2\Delta v_{ij}(\Delta v_i - \Delta v_j) \ \forall i,j$$

Thus, to maximise the minimum separation, we can write:

Max λ st.

$$\lambda - 2\Delta L_{ij}(\Delta L_i - \Delta L_j) + 2\Delta u_{ij}(\Delta u_i - \Delta u_j) + 2\Delta v_{ij}(\Delta v_i - \Delta v_j) \leq (\Delta E_{ij})^2 \ \forall i > j$$

In order to limit the movement around the Luv space, let d_L, u_L be the downwards (negative) and upwards (positive) percentage movements in L, etc., i.e. $d_L L_i \leq \Delta L_i \leq u_L L_i \ \forall i$ with similar constraints on Δu_i, Δv_i.

As an example of this approach, we have taken the new colour set and permitted a 2 per cent variation around each colour in u'v'L* space. Table 10.3.1 shows the result of a sequence of such optimisations, each result produced by permitting a 2 per cent variation around the previous optimal set. This set was found experimentally to still be nameable. The perceived advantages of the linear optimisation over the more complex algorithms published (such as De Corte, 1990) is that it is very simple to implement (indeed the results were obtained using a spreadsheet), that it is extremely quick, and that it would appear to provide considerable pragmatic improvement.

10.3.4   CONCLUSIONS

This paper has presented a practical methodology for the specification of colour sets of high discriminability. The approach first used a somewhat subjective step to increase the separation of colour pairs. Subsequently an optimisation technique was adopted to reduce the dependency on skilled subjective judgements. Throughout the process, attention was paid to important aspects such as nameability. The methodology also paves the way for improved control in the specification of colour requirements in other applications. Expected future developments include the procedures for gamma correction and monitor calibration, and a further specification of colour usage.

Table 10.3.1. Increasing the minimum ΔE^* through a sequence of optimisations, with discriminations for optimisation number 9

Optimisation number	Minimum ΔE^*
1	41.5
5	45.2
9	49.0
Minimum ΔE^*: 49.0; Average ΔE^*: 111.7; Maximum ΔE^*: 240.6	

10.3.5   REFERENCES

De Corte, W. (1988) Ergonomically optimal CRT colours for nonfixed ambient illumination conditions, *Colour Research & Applications*, **13**(5), 327-331.

De Corte, W. (1990) Recent developments in the computation of ergonomically optimal sets of CRT colours, *Displays Technology Applications*, **11**, 123–128.

Kelly, K.L. (1966) Twenty-two colours of maximum contrast, *Colour Engineering*, **3**, 26–27.

Umbers, I. G. & Collier, G.D. (1990) Coding techniques for process plant VDU formats, *Applied Ergonomics*, **21**(3), 187–198.

Qualitative Assessment of Compatibility of a Mixture of Disperse Dyes Using Colour Coordinates

S. R. Shukla, S. S. Dhuri and V. C. Gupte

10.4.1 INTRODUCTION

Textile colourists are required to produce a given shade, many times by using a mixture of dyes selected on the basis of their similar dyeing properties. In practice, however, the dyer frequently has to use dyes from several sources, or from dyes with different dyeing characteristics for reasons such as economy, non-availability of a specific dye or the need to produce a non-standard shade. The dyer has to know the mixing behaviour of the dyes for which data are often not available. Dyes dyed in admixture are termed compatible in that particular colour used if, during dyeing, the colour builds up in such a manner that the ratio of the component dyes on the fibre remains the same throughout the dyeing process giving an ontone build up of the colour without any change in the hue. Such an ideal dyeing depends on many different factors (Beckmann and Hoffmann, 1983).

Predictive tests for assessing compatibility enable formulation of possible recipes for ideal dyeing that can be checked, if necessary, by laboratory tests. The traditional and most common method of assessing the results of compatibility tests is to observe visually the degree of ontone build up during dyeing. Half-dyeing-time values and the diffusion number (Blackburn and Gallagher, 1980) have been used for predicting compatibility. Beckmann (1970) established a dye classification according to the dyeing rates under the standardised conditions. All these techniques of assessing the compatibility are tedious, although useful, because in each case the concentration dependence of exhaustion has to be taken into account.

Special compatible mixtures of dyes have also been used. Mitsubishi (1983) recommended trichromatic colour combinations of dyes having similar dyeing rates with reduced concentration dependence. According to Beckman *et al.* (1972), it is worth using several dyes of similar colour in a combination, instead of a large quantity of a single dye as dyes tend to exhaust independently. Schlaeppi *et al.* (1982) and Richter (1983) gave particular emphasis to the use of specifically developed auxiliary products.

677

Table 10.4.1. Disperse dyes used in the present work

Mixture	CI generic name	Manufacturer's name	λ max (nm)	Molecular weight
M₁	CI Disperse Orange 30	Sandoz (India) Ltd	430	450.29
	CI Disperse Orange 25	Sandoz (India) Ltd	470	323.36
	CI Disperse Brown 1	Atul Products Ltd	460	433.69
M₂	CI Disperse Yellow 23	Sandoz (India) Ltd	400	302.34
	CI Disperse Red 11	Atic Industries Ltd	530	268.27
	CI Disperse Blue 56	Atic Industries Ltd	630	305.70
M₃	CI Disperse Yellow 23	Sandoz (India) Ltd	400	302.34
	CI Disperse Red 1	Atul Products Ltd	490	314.35
	CI Disperse Violet 4	Chemiequip Ltd	560	252.27

Colour measurement systems help the textile colourist to analyse the colour. Hue of any colour and its development throughout the dyeing cycle is of great importance to a practical dyer, in addition to the depth of a shade. He judges the development of hue expressed by different colour coordinates through the use of colour measurement systems such as the CIELab system.

The technique of qualitative assessment of compatibility of three different tertiary mixtures of disperse dyes, dyed on polyester fabric, is reported in this paper with the help of various plots drawn using the CIELab colour coordinates and the K/S values.

10.4.2 METHODS

10.4.2.1 Materials

Heat-set and texturised 100 per cent polyester fabric was used for dyeing with the mixtures of disperse dyes described in Table 10.4.1. Lyogen DFTI liquid, supplied by Sandoz (India) Limited, was used as a non-ionic levelling agent. The other reagents used were of 'Chemically Pure' grade.

10.4.2.2 Dyeing Method

The polyester fabric pieces were dyed with the tertiary mixtures of disperse dyes containing dyes in equal proportions at a total applied depth of 4.5 per cent by the usual high temperature dyeing technique using a liquor ratio of 50:1. The dyeing was started at 40°C and the temperature was raised to 130°C at a rate of 1°C min⁻¹. The dyeing was continued further for 60 min at 130°C, the total dyeing time being 150 min.

In each set 12 samples were withdrawn from the dyebath at intervals of 10 min from 70°C onwards. The penultimate sample was taken after 40 min at 130°C, and the last one at the end of the dyeing process. Of the 10 samples in each set 2 were dyed at increments of 10 percentage points up to 100 per cent of the total applied depth of the dye mixture at 130°C for 60 min. After dyeing, all the samples were given a reduction – clearing treatment followed by soaping, washing and final air-drying.

10.4.2.3 Colour measurement

The colour of the dyed samples under illuminant D_{65} was measured for the 10° standard observer on a Match Scan II spectrophotometer attached to an IBM personal computer, over the range of 400–700 nm. The results were recorded in terms of the CIELab colour coordinates L*, b* and a*, and C*. The computer calculated colour differences from the standard (undyed) fabric, and also the DL*, Db*, Da* and DC* values, with the indications of lighter/darker, redder/greener, yellower/bluer and the difference in saturation. The K/S values of the dyed samples were also obtained from the computer through the strength evaluation program.

10.4.3   RESULTS AND DISCUSSION

For uniform dyeing of polyester, the dyes should be compatible with each other even after complete development of hue, especially during the latter stages of dyeing. In case of a mixture containing dyes having different hues such as, red, yellow and blue, the measurement of the amounts of individual dyes in the fibre at the respective absorption maxima (λ_{max}) is simple and quick, giving an idea about their compatibility. This technique fails when the dyestuffs have either close hues wherein enough separation of the individual λ_{max} is not possible or when the dyes interact with each other and do not indicate their individual λ_{max} peaks. In practice, many such dye combinations are required to be used and the above technique cannot predict their compatibility.

Figure 10.4.1 gives the plot of K/S versus wavelength for the three selective disperse dye mixtures M_1, M_2 and M_3, described in Table 10.4.1. The mixture M_1 contained the dyes having similar hues, all lying in the red-yellow sector of the colour space, and gave only a single broad peak. The mixtures M_2 and M_3 contained the dyes with widely different hues.

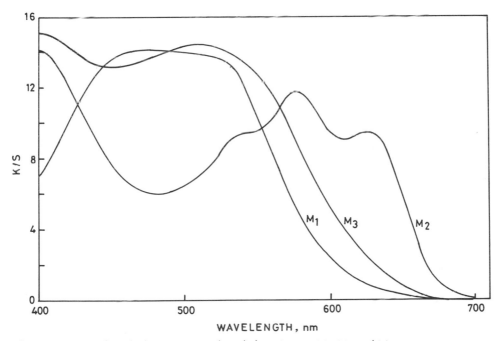

Figure 10.4.1.   Plot of K/S versus wavelength for mixtures M_1, M_2 and M_3.

However, mixture M_2 showed distinct peaks, making it feasible to use the simpler technique of estimation of the amount of individual dyes on the fibre for predicting the compatibility of these dyes in the mixture. Mixture M_3, on the other hand, although containing dyes with widely different hues, showed only two peaks indicating possible interaction between the red and violet dyes.

It was suggested by Datye and Mishra (1984), while dyeing various disperse dye mixtures of different hues on different fibres, that during the dyeing of an ideally compatible dye mixture, the depth of shade of the samples after absorption of each successive 10 per cent dye portion (set 2) should almost match with the corresponding shade of the samples of set 1 taken out at each successive 10 min interval at a constant rate of heating of 1°C min^{-1}. The degree of compatibility of a given mixture can then be demonstrated qualitatively by the closeness of approach or complete overlap between the two curves for these two sets.

When this technique was applied to mixture M_1 containing dyes with very close hues and from different molecular weight groups, it was found that, at lower total applied depths only, the mixture behaved compatibly as indicated by the complete overlap between the two curves drawn for the two sets in the plots of DL* versus DC* and Db* versus Da* (Shukla and Dhuri, 1992a). At the higher total applied depth of 4.5 per cent, however, the two curves showed significant separation from each other, meaning, thereby, that the mixture M_1 behaved incompatibly (Figure 10.4.2).

A dyer judges the development of hue by comparison with a standard in the form of hue terms, namely a* (redder/greener), b* (yellower/bluer) and the lightness L* (lighter/darker). The plot of DL* versus DC* indicates the effect of the build up of colour on the lighter/darker appearance of the sample whereas the plot of Db* versus Da* indicates the change in tone of the shade as the dyeing proceeds. That is, it indicates the build up of the hue of a colour describing the position of the colour developed on the dyed fibre in the colour space.

The changes in the hue of any colour on the dyed substrate may arise out of a number of factors of which the differences in the build up of the individual dyes from a mixture are

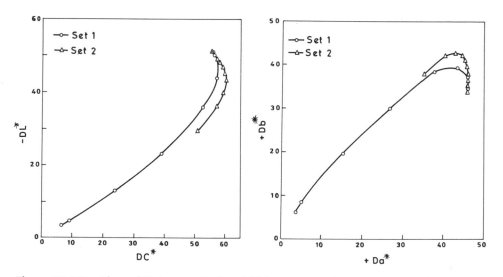

Figure 10.4.2. Plots of DL* versus DC* and Db* versus Da* for mixture M_1 in the absence of Lyogen DFTI.

mainly responsible. It is, therefore, necessary to take into account the changes in the hue of a final shade arising out of the increase in the amount of dye on the fibre. As the Kubelka-Munk (K/S) function is the only parameter proportional to the amount of dye on the fibre, the changes in the colour coordinates, namely DL*, Da* and Db*, were plotted against the K/S values of the dyed samples to study the build up of hue during dyeing. Although these plots are not shown in the present paper, their nature as regards the degree of overlap between the two curves for the two sets was similar to those plots for DL* versus DC* and Db* versus Da*. With increase in the K/S, as shown in Figure 10.4.2, DL*, Db*, Da* all showed an increase, with only Db* decreasing slightly towards the end of dyeing, which may be due to the preferential removal of the dye CI, Disperse Orange 25, having lower molecular weight and higher colour strength as compared with the other two dyes, during the reduction-clearing treatment of the dyed samples thereby decreases its contribution towards the yellowness of the final shade on the fabric.

The plots of DL* versus DC* and Db* versus Da* for mixture M₂, given in Figure 10.4.3, indicate that for both the sets, there was no systematic build up of the colour on the fabric as the dyeing proceeded. Even towards the end of the dyeing, the two curves did not overlap indicating the totally incompatible behaviour of the mixture M₂. Similar were the observations for the plots of these different colour co-ordinates against K/S values.

From Figure 10.4.4, giving such plots for mixture M₃, it can be seen that a very slight overlap of the two curves for the two sets was obtained only towards the extreme end of the dyeing process. Although darkness increased with the dyeing, the chroma initially increased and then decreased as the dyeing proceeded at the high temperature. In the plot of Db* versus Da*, both the parameters increased initially, followed by a sharp decrease and showed only a slight portion of overlap between the two curves for the two sets towards the extreme end of the dyeing process.

It may be noted that although it is said that the dyes from similar molecular weight groups should behave compatibly by exhausting the substrate at similar rates, the dyes in mixtures M₂ and M₃, which are all in the low molecular weight category, showed no

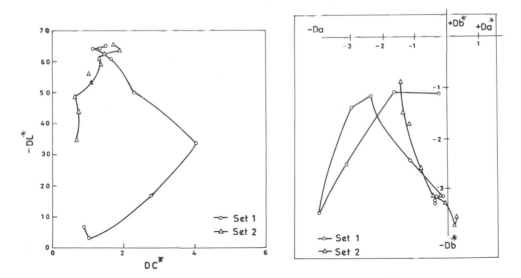

Figure 10.4.3.   Plots of DL* versus DC* and Db* versus Da* for mixture M₂ in the absence of Lyogen DFTI.

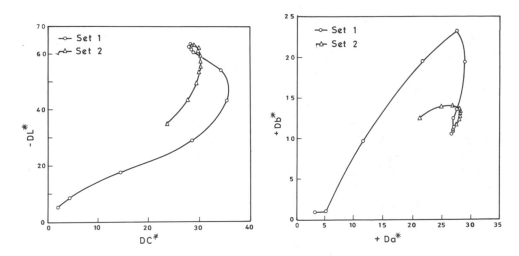

Figure 10.4.4.   Plots of DL* versus DC* and Db* versus Da* for mixture M₃ in the absence of Lyogen DFTI.

compatibility as indicated by the various plots drawn by making use of the colour coordinates as well as the K/S values.

All the CIELab colour coordinates and the K/S values can, thus, be made use of in the qualitative assessment of the compatibility of different disperse dye mixtures. The parameter K/S of the total shade is more appropriately related to the dye absorption making the technique more useful for a practical dyer.

The levelness of a dyeing on polyester depends on the rate at which a dye exhausts onto the fibre and on the extent of its migration at the top dyeing temperature. Ideally, the exhaustion phase itself should be controlled so as to minimize the migration phase. This is particularly relevant for the dyes which do not tend to behave compatibly. For this purpose, in addition to the various dyeing systems and efficient dyeing machinery, non-ionic dyeing assistants have been employed (Schlaeppi *et al*, 1982).

All the three mixtures did not show compatibility at the higher total applied depth. Hence, it was decided to see whether the compatibility can be improved by addition of a non-ionic levelling agent into the dyebath. Figure 10.4.5 gives the plots of DL* versus DC* and Db* versus Da* for mixture M₁ dyed in the presence of Lyogen DFTI (Shukla and Dhuri, 1992b). The changes in the behaviour of various colour coordinates were found to be similar to those observed in the absence of Lyogen DFTI. However, the two curves for the two sets showed complete overlap right from the beginning of the dyeing process in all the plots, including those drawn using K/S values (not shown). This means that the mixture M₁ behaved as an ideally compatible one, even at higher depths, in the presence of the non-ionic levelling agent. As the dyeing proceeded, the DC* values reached a maximum at the top temperature of 130°C and then decreased with further increase in the time of dyeing at 130°C.

Almost complete coincidence of the two curves in the plots of DL* versus DC* (Figure 10.4.5) and Db* versus Da* (Figure 10.4.6) as well as DL* versus K/S, Db* versus K/S and Da* versus K/S for the two sets in the presence of Lyogen DFTI indicates that although the use of a non-ionic levelling agent in the dyeing of polyester with disperse dyes helps in ensuring uniform dye transfer in the critical temperature range, it lowers the final

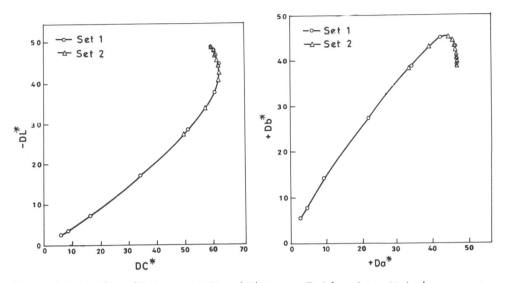

Figure 10.4.5. Plots of DL* versus DC* and Db* versus Da* for mixture M₁ in the presence of Lyogen DFTI.

exhaustion of the dyebath leading to variations in hue which, although slight, may be of concern to a practical dyer.

It is likely that during the initial stages of dyeing, the dye exhausts slowly onto the fibre in the presence of this levelling agent, which releases the dyes from the aqueous phase in a controlled manner from the beginning of the dyeing process itself, thereby improving the compatibility of these disperse dyes (mixture M_1) applied in admixture at any depth. It results in a uniform build up, both in terms of the amount of dye on the fibre as well as the hue.

The K/S values of the dyes, when dyed individually and in mixture M_2, were nearly the same at the respective maximum, indicating their almost similar exhaustion behaviour due

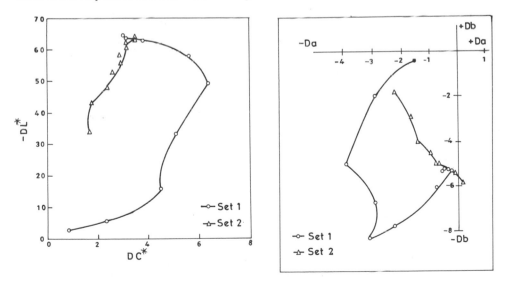

Figure 10.4.6. Plots of DL* versus DC* and Db* versus Da* for mixture M_2 in the presence of Lyogen DFTI.

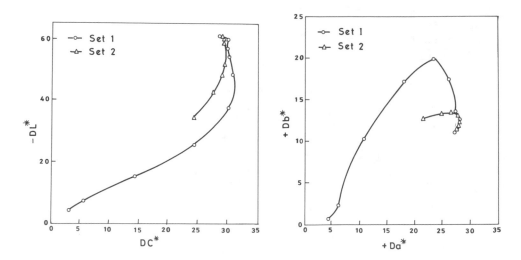

Figure 10.4.7. Plots of DL* versus DC* and Db* versus Da* for mixture M₃ in the presence of Lyogen DFTI

to their close molecular weights. The plots DL* versus DC* and Db* versus Da* for both the sets of samples dyed in the presence of Lyogen DFTI, are shown in Figure 10.4.6. It may be observed that, even in the presence of Lyogen DFTI, the nature of plots remained the same and no overlap between the two curves for the two sets was observed.

Similar plots for the two sets of mixture M₃ dyed in the presence of Lyogen DFTI are given in Figure 10.4.7. Some overlap can be observed during dyeing at the top temperature of 130ºC indicating slight improvement in the build up of the hue of the mixture M₃. Lyogen DFTI, thus, seems to have improved the compatibility of the dyes in the tertiary mixture M₃ to some extent.

It may be concluded that when the compatibility of such mixtures using simple analytical techniques fails, the overlap method based on the plots of colour co-ordinates can be used. However, this allows only qualitative evaluation of compatibility. Moreover, when a tertiary mixture contains two dyes having significant differences in individual λ_{max} values, but showing a single peak in their binary mixture, the method based on K/S function of the total shade, as has been proposed to evaluate compatibility of dyes having close hues can be used.

10.4.4　REFERENCES

BECKMANN, W. (1970) Recent development in dyeing texturised polyester, *Textile Chemists and Colourists*, **2**,(20), 350–357.

BECKMANN, W. & HOFFMANN, F. (1983) Connections between compatibility of dyes and levelness – A constantly recurring problem, *Melliand Textilberishte*, **64**, 828–833.

BECKMANN, W., HOFFMANN, F. & OTTEN, H. G. (1972) Practical significance, theory and determination of compatibility of dyes on synthetic – polymer fibres, *Journal of Society of Dyers and Colourists*, **88**, 354–360.

BLACKBURN, D. & GALLAGHER, V. C. (1980) Disperse dyes for polyester – A new approach to compatibility, *Journal of Society of Dyers and Colourists*, **96**, 237–245.

DATYE, K.V. & MISHRA, S. (1984) Compatibility of dye mixtures, *Journal of Society of Dyers and Colourists*, **100**, 334–337.

MITSUBISHI CHEMICAL INDUSTRIES LTD (1983) Disperse azo dye mixtures, *Chemical Abstract*, **98**, 79.

RICHTER, P. (1983) Synchronously dyeing disperse dyes for high temperature dyeing of polyester fibres and polyester – cellulosic fibre blends, *Melliand Textilberishte*, **64**, 347–353.

SCHLAEPPI, F., WAGNER, R.D. & McNEILL, J.L. (1982) High temperature dyeing of polyester and polyester/cotton, *Textile Chemists and Colourists*, **14**(12), 257–268.

SHUKLA, S.R. & DHURI, S.S. (1992a) Assessing the compatibility of disperse dye mixtures by the use of colour coordinates, *Journal of Society of Dyers and Colourists*, **108**, 139–144.

SHUKLA, S.R. & DHURI, S.S. (1992b) Improving the compatibility of disperse dye mixtures using levelling agent – assessment through colour coordinates, *Journal of Society of Dyers and Colourists*, **108**, 395–399.

Real-time Colour Recognition for Machine Vision Systems

Bruce G. Batchelor and Paul F. Whelan

10.5.1 INTRODUCTION

Consider the task of designing a machine to inspect printed cardboard and plastic cartons, such as those used for food products, household goods, toiletries, etc. These are often printed in several colours. Inspecting such items could be achieved by first isolating the different colours and then applying conventional (i.e. monochrome) image analysis procedures to each of the colour separations. In this chapter, we shall discuss electronic filters that are capable of performing such a separation of colours (Intelligent Camera, 1990; Plummer, 1991). A Programmable Colour Filter (PCF) might, for example, isolate the yellow streak on a margarine tub, so that it can be examined in detail. Once a yellow streak has been inspected, other coloured features can be treated in the same way. Of course, such a filter should be able to tolerate wide variations in the brightness of the scene being examined; it should be sensitive to colour, not intensity. Other possible applications include: reading resistor colour codes, identifying coloured wires, inspecting iconic displays on car dashboards, etc.

Previous work by the authors has shown that colour recognition can be used to good effect in a symbolic programming environment (Prolog has been used for several years as a medium for programming vision systems. See Batchelor, 1991, 1992; Batchelor and Whelan, 1993, 1995). This approach to colour recognition requires machines that can quickly learn to recognise colours such as 'margarine-tub yellow', 'margarine-tub red', given a few examples of each. The samples on which such an inspection machine is to be designed would most conveniently be obtained by examining a small number of margarine tubs on a production line.

10.5.1.1 The naming of colours

The axiom on which this article is based is that the names of colours cannot be defined mathematically. The standard CIE (1931) Chromaticity Diagram should be regarded as a conceptual aid, because it cannot form a precise basis for discriminating between colours. The position of the boundary between any two named colours in the Chromaticity Diagram is plotted for an hypothetical *standard observer*, working in carefully controlled lighting conditions. In a practical situation, however, an industrial machine vision system is likely to be taught by a person untrained in colour science, working in a factory environment, where the lighting is highly variable. Schettini (1993) points out that camera, lighting and filter combinations affect the RGB values measured by a video camera.

Several authors have represented the colours of ordinary everyday objects as points plotted on the Chromaticity Diagram (Chamberlain and Chamberlain, 1980). However, it should be noted that each point represents just one instance of a broad class of objects. The set of all ripe tomatoes, for example, is represented more accurately by a cluster of points, while ripening tomatoes generate a broad serpentine curve in the Chromaticity Diagram. The Chromaticity Diagram does not include definitions for the range of such colours as 'margarine-tub yellow' or even 'sky blue'. The fact that people recognise colours by some mental process that is not fully understood simply has to be accepted (Optical Society of America, 1953; Chamberlain and Chamberlain, 1980). The authors suggest that a colour recognition filter, used when inspecting artefacts such as food packaging, household goods and pharmaceutical cartons, could be designed using the principle of teaching-by-showing.

10.5.1.2 Notation

The set notation introduced in this section allows us to define colour generalisation process in formal mathematical terms. Generalisation is seen as being an essential function in any learning system. Let $<X>$ denote the set of colours of objects in that class defined by human beings and which is called X. A machine that is designed for colour recognition, might well use the conventional RGB colour separations. To take account of this fact, we shall therefore take $\{X\}$ as being the set of all of those (R,G,B)-vectors that can be associated with the label X. Notice that in this notation, $<X>$ is defined by a person, while $\{X\}$ is a set of 3-element (R,G,B)-vectors, derived by a machine.

10.5.1.3 Recognition and generalisation of colours

Implicit in our approach to colour recognition is the concept of teaching by showing. It is important, of course, to make the maximum use of each colour sample, since they may be difficult and/or expensive to collect. It is impossible, in practice, to obtain more than a very small proportion of all the colours of a class such as $<yellow>$, so we must teach our machine using a few well chosen samples and leave it to generalise. Generalisation is universally accepted as being essential in *all* pattern recognition machines, of which the PCF is an example.

Given that $<daffodil> \cup <canary> \cup <banana> \cup <lemon> \subseteq <yellow>$, it is reasonable to expect that $\{daffodil\} \cup \{canary\} \cup \{banana\} \cup \{lemon\} \subseteq \{yellow\}$. Now, we want to find some operation upon the set $\{daffodil\} \cup \{canary\} \cup \{banana\} \cup \{lemon\}$ that will generate an enlarged set E, such that $E \supseteq \{daffodil\} \cup \{canary\} \cup \{banana\} \cup \{lemon\}$ and $\forall X:X \in E \rightarrow X \in \{yellow\}$. An important but ill-defined condition is that the set E should be as small as possible, thereby avoiding over-generalisation.

This is one of the two types of colour generalisation we discuss in this chapter. It is appropriate for those situations in which we are interested in *colour recognition* (single colour class), as distinct from *colour discrimination* (more than one colour class). We shall present one procedure for generalisation in colour recognition (*Procedure 4*, defined below). A different type of colour generalisation is needed when we have to discriminate between colours. For reasons of economy, we might, for example, need to use a small data set to learn to distinguish between {apple} and {tomato} and wish to make the discrimination more reliable, so that colours in these sets that were not represented in the training data are classified appropriately.

10.5.2 COLOUR RECOGNITION

The inspection of coloured objects and surfaces by machine has, of course, been studied by numerous researchers over many years. Particular attention has been paid to the characterisation and matching of subtle colouring of fabrics, paint, paper, printing and automobiles. As very precise colour measurement is needed in these areas, non-imaging techniques have been widely used. It should be understood that the approach that we have taken is quite different, for we are concerned with relatively coarse, high-speed recognition and discrimination processes. A typical application for the techniques we shall discuss is the inspection of packages and containers for food, domestic goods and pharmaceutical products on a factory production line. A review of previous work in this area can be found in Batchelor and Whelan (1995).

10.5.2.1 Real-time recognition of colours in electronic hardware

Figure 10.5.1 shows the block diagram of a colour recognition system designed by Plummer (1991). This is built into a small self-contained commercially available image processing unit, called the Intelligent Camera (1990). The authors used the Intelligent Camera, in conjunction with control software written in Prolog (Batchelor, 1991, 1992) in the experiments reported below. Another implementation using a real-time RGB/HSI converter chip (Umbaugh et al., 1992) is suggested in Figure 10.5.2. A third implementation relies upon the use of the x,y parameters used to define the standard Chromaticity Diagram, see Figure 10.5.3. These last two configurations have not yet been implemented.

Notice that in Figures 10.5.1–3, the output from the Look-Up Table (LUT) is a stream of 8-bit values, which may be regarded as forming intensities in a monochrome image. This image can be analysed in a conventional monochrome image processing sub-system. All of these hardware systems can be fully simulated in a software environment, but not necessarily in real-time. While it is the accepted wisdom that the HSI representation is better able than RGB to discriminate colours as we perceive them, this hardware arrangement is, in fact, quite general, in that the LUT in Figure 10.5.1 can be programmed to generate H, S and I, given R, G and B. Hence, Figure 10.5.1 is able to implement any functions that Figures 10.5.2 and 10.5.3 can. A further advantage of Figure 10.5.1 is that it relies upon cheap standard memory devices, rather than custom ICs or real-time divider circuits. Our discussion hereafter is based upon the system using a LUT with RGB inputs, as illustrated in Figure 10.5.1.

The LUT forms the heart of the *Programmable Colour Filter*. The use of high-speed random access memory (RAM) to form a look-up table, together with 'flash' analogue-to-digital converters, makes the PCF very fast indeed. It is well able to perform transformations upon a digitised video signal, in real time. Training the PCF consists of calculating appropriate values for each of the LUT's 2^{18} storage cells. (See Batchelor (1992) and Batchelor and Whelan (1993, 1994) for details on the programming of the PCF). Once the

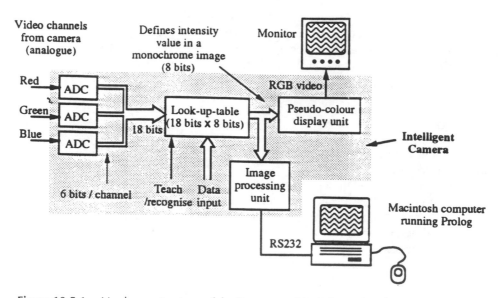

Figure 10.5.1. Hardware structure of the Programmable Colour Filter, based upon RGB inputs to the LUT. This is the block diagram of the implementation of this technique in the Intelligent Camera (1990: Plummer 1991) and was used by the authors in the experiments reported here.

PCF has been programmed, the colour recognition process takes place in real-time and does not increase the computational load needed for image analysis in any way.

10.5.3   PROCEDURES FOR COLOUR GENERALISATION

The colour scattergram (generated by projecting all RGB vectors onto the colour triangle, this is a convenient representation of the distribution of colours within the input (Batchelor and Whelan, 1993, 1994)), may be displayed as a grey-scale image, in which intensity indicates the number of pixels with the same values of hue and saturation. (See Figure

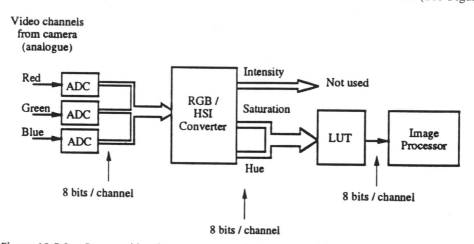

Figure 10.5.2. Proposed hardware structure of a Programmable Colour Filter, based upon HSI inputs to the LUT, using a real-time RGB/HIS converter chip (Umbaugh et al., 1992).

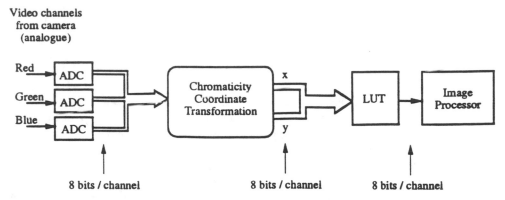

Video channels
from camera
(analogue)

Figure 10.5.3. Proposed hardware structure of a Programmable Colour Filter, based on the *xy* parameters used in defining the standard Chromaticity Diagram.

10.5.4 for some results.) The colour scattergram must be simplified before any further processing takes place. An obvious step is to threshold it. This process will generate a compact blob for each region of similar colours.

Our approach to colour generalisation consists of adjusting the sizes of the blobs created by thresholding the colour scattergram. It will be necessary to do this in such a way that blobs, which were distinct when the (multi-cluster) scattergram was first thresholded, remain separate. In a typical application, a number of coloured scenes are used to design the PCF. As each scene is being viewed, a scattergram is generated in the colour triangle. Noise is then removed from the scattergram, using common image processing operations, such as low-pass filtering. This is followed by thresholding. If the input scene consists of a single colour, such as <margarine-tub yellow>, thresholding the scattergram, after clean-up, creates a single blob, B_i. This process is repeated for each colour we wish to use to design the PCF. As each new blob ($B_i, i = 1, \ldots, n$) is generated, it is superimposed on the colour triangle. Therefore, prior to generalisation, the colour triangle consists of a number of blob regions, each of which corresponds to one of the trained colours. The aim of the generalisation procedures is to expand these regions, forming the regions $C_i, i = 1, \ldots, n$. By projecting the C_i back onto the colour cube, we generate the contents of the PCF look-up table. If the C_i have been generated appropriately, the resulting colour recognition process is more reliable than it would have been if the smaller blobs B_i had been used instead (Batchelor and Whelan, 1993, 1994). The definitions of four suggested procedures for colour generalisation are as follows:

- Procedure 1 – Simple Dilation: Each blob, B_i, in the colour triangle is dilated (expanded) by a single pixel for a fixed number of iterations. The number of iterations is denoted by the variable N. The resultant blob is C_i.
- Procedure 2 – Dilation with Preservation of Connectivity: A single layer of background pixels is stripped from the (binary) image in the colour triangle. Unlike the previous approach, pixels critical for connectivity are retained. The number of iterations in this 'onion peeling' operation is denoted by the variable N.
- Procedure 3 – Watershed: This approach involves finding the watershed for each of the blobs B_i. The watershed is generated by finding the medial axis transformation of the image background.
- Procedure 4 – Convex Hull Generalisation: The convex hull is drawn around the set of blobs B_i ($i = 1, \ldots, n$) in the colour triangle. It is reasonable to expect that points within

this convex hull will correspond to a generalisation of the observed colours, $\{A_i\}, i = 1,$ ... ,n.

10.5.4   DEMONSTRATION OF COLOUR RECOGNITION

We have devised a demonstration of colour recognition, using a multi-colour pattern, similar to those found on a number of product logos. Figure 10.5.4(a) (for Figures 10.5.4(a) to (i) see the colour section) shows the original artwork of the multi-colour pattern used in our experiments. (This was produced using the Photoshop image processing software, running on a Macintosh computer, and a Kodak ColorEase laser printer.) When this image was used in the experiments, a narrow white border was included within the camera's field of view. Figure 10.5.4(b) shows the RGB colour separations. (The top-left image contains the red component, the top-right, green and the bottom-left, blue.) Figure 10.5.4(c) contains the resulting colour scattergram. Notice that there are seven blobs, corresponding to the six colour bands in Figure 10.5.4(a), plus the central spot, which represents the narrow white border mentioned in relation to Figure 10.5.4(a). Figure 10.5.4(d) is a pseudo-colour display of the colour scattergram. Notice that the dark regions in the colour scattergram are more clearly visible when the pseudo-colour display is switched on. (Evident as purple cloud-like structures in Figure 10.5.4(d).) The colour scattergram was thresholded, and all minor blobs removed (Figure 10.5.4.(e)). The remaining major blobs were assigned colours (by the program) in an arbitrary manner.

Figure 10.5.4(f) is the output of the programmable colour filter, obtained by training on the blobs of Figure 10.5.4(e). (To obtain Figure 10.5.4(f), the camera was focused again on the image in Figure 10.5.4(a).) Notice that the colour bands in Figure 10.5.4(f) contain dark spots and are separated by dark streaks. Both of these effects are caused by the blobs in Figure 10.5.4(e) being too small. The white border of Figure 10.5.4(a) is visible here as a yellow edge. (It should be clearly understood that no attempt should be made to associate the natural and pseudo-colours in Figures 10.5.4(a) and 10.5.4(f).).

Figure 10.5.4(g) illustrates the result of applying colour generalisation (Procedure 3) on Figure 10.5.4(c). When the PCF is trained on the new image, containing the enlarged blobs, the performance is greatly improved (see Figure 10.5.4(h)). Notice the absence of dark spots and streaks, compared to Figure 10.5.4(f). Hence, the new PCF is robust and is able to distinguish the colours in the simulated logo, reliably and accurately.

Recognising a colour logo, such as that in Figure 10.5.4(a), as the anticipated logo can be performed quite easily, simply by measuring the proportions of each of the component colours and noting their position and shape. Thus, colour pattern recognition can be reduced to combining the results of a series of very simple binary image analysis operations.

10.5.5   DISCUSSION AND CONCLUSIONS

The idea of using a look-up table to perform colour recognition is not new but has considerable appeal for such tasks as recognising (ripe) fruit on a tree, recognising resistor colour codes, tracing wiring, inspecting food products, cartons and pharmaceutical packaging. It lends itself to implementation in fast electronic hardware. Commercial equipment has been available for colour recognition for some years. The colour scattergram is a useful tool which allows the user to associate areas of the colour triangle with colours that he or she can recognise and name. Once a colour scattergram has been generated, the user can think about colour in convenient terms, using the concepts of blob position, shape and size. He or she can also apply a wide range of image processing operators to the colour triangle. This is possible because the colour triangle is an image, like any other. Colour recognition is achieved in real time, although the subsequent procedures for image analysis may not be. Four techniques for colour generalisation have been described and have been studied extensively by ourselves, using an interactive image processing system. As a result of their experience, the authors are convinced that the techniques described above provide a useful addition to the range of facilities available for recognising colours. It is possible to extend the range of colours recognised by the PCF to any extent desired. In Procedure 2, for example, the parameter N can be adjusted at will; if N is increased, the degree of generalisation will become higher. It is possible for a person, working with an interactive system, to experiment with the colour generalisation parameter to obtain the best results for a given application. On the other hand, a program can be written which chooses a suitable value for N, according to some pre-defined criterion.

10.5.6 REFERENCES

BATCHELOR, B.G. (1991) *Image Processing in Prolog*, Berlin & New York: Springer Verlag.

BATCHELOR, B.G. (1992) Colour Recognition in Prolog, *Proceedings of the SPIE Conference on Machine Vision Applications, Architectures and Systems Integration*, SPIE **1823**, 294–305.

BATCHELOR, B.G. & WHELAN, P.F. (1993) Generalisation Procedures for Colour Recognition, *Proceedings of the SPIE Conference on Machine Vision Applications, Architectures and Systems Integration II*, SPIE **2064**, 36–46.

BATCHELOR, B.G. & WHELAN, P.F. (1995) Real-time Colour Recognition in Symbolic Programming for Machine Vision Systems, *Machine Vision and Applications*, **8**, 385–398.

CHAMBERLAIN, G.J. & CHAMBERLAIN, D.G. (1980) *Colour: Its Measurement, Computation and Application*, London: Heyden & Son, pp. 18–45.

INTELLIGENT CAMERA (1990) Image Inspection Ltd, Unit 7, First Quarter, Blenheim Road, Kingston, Surrey.

OPTICAL SOCIETY OF AMERICA (1953) *The Science of Colour*. Optical Society of America Committee on Colorimetry: 99–144.

PLUMMER, A.P. (1991) Inspecting Coloured Objects Using Grey Scale Vision Systems, *Proceedings of the SPIE Conference on Machine Vision Applications, Architectures and Systems Integration*, SPIE **CR36**, 78–92.

SCHETTINI, R. (1993) A segmentation algorithm for color images, *Pattern Recognition Letters*, **14**, 499–506.

UMBAUGH, S.E., MOSS, R.H. & STOECKER, W.V. (1992) Automatic color segmentation algorithm with application to identification of skin tumor borders, *Computerized Medical Imaging and Graphics*, **16**(3), 227–235. [Refers to Part no. DT 2871, Data Translation Ltd.]

A System for Precision Ophthalmic Tinting and Its Role in the Treatment of Visual Stress

Arnold Wilkins

10.6.1 INTRODUCTION

Tinted glasses have a long history of use in optometric practice, not only as protective filters, but also in the treatment of eye-strain (Giles, 1965; pp. 263–281). It is only recently, however, that the advent of 'plastic' (resin) spectacle lenses has made it possible to obtain almost any desired spectral transmission cheaply and quickly. The technology has been used for cosmetic dyeing for more than a decade, but only in the last few years has the breadth of its therapeutic potential been realised. The purpose of this chapter is to describe a new system for precision ophthalmic tinting and the clinical results obtained using the system.

When resin lenses are tinted, the lenses are simply dipped for a few minutes into hot organic dyes. Molecules of dye penetrate the surface, and are held beneath the surface when the lens cools, and so the dye deposition is independent of the lens thickness. Because the dyes do not interact chemically with one another, it is possible to deposit successive layers and, by combining the spectral absorbance of several dyes, to obtain any desired tint.

Helen Irlen (Irlen, 1983; Irlen and Lass, 1989; Irlen, 1991) developed a system for dyeing lenses, available at the Irlen Institutes she founded. She described a 'scotopic sensitivity syndrome' which included many non-specific symptoms of visual fatigue (e.g. blurring, headache). Wilkins and Neary (1991) examined 20 patients described as suffering this syndrome. A variety of optometric and psychophysical tests were undertaken with and without Irlen's lenses. The glasses improved the speed of visual search and reduced the anomalous perceptual effects seen in epileptogenic gratings. The perceptual effects seen in such gratings are known to be associated with headache and eye-strain (Wilkins *et al.*, 1984) and are symptoms of what has been termed *pattern glare* (Wilkins and Nimmo-Smith, 1984). An 'intuitive colorimeter' was designed to facilitate further investigation of the effects of coloured light on perception (Wilkins *et al.*, 1992a). The instrument turned out to be valuable in the clinical investigation of patients, and this discovery led to the development of a system for precision ophthalmic tinting (Wilkins *et al.*, 1992b). Open trials using the system (Maclachlan *et al.*, 1993) motivated a double-masked study (Wilkins *et al.*, 1994), which indicated that the benefits from lenses tinted using the system are more than can reasonably be attributed simply to placebo effects.

10.6.2   A SYSTEM FOR PRECISION OPHTHALMIC TINTING

The system for precision ophthalmic tinting has been in use in optometric practice in the UK since 1992. It enables an ophthalmic tint to be chosen according to a patient's subjective assessment of its effects on perception and visual comfort. A precise tint can be selected rapidly and efficiently. The system uses the Intuitive Colorimeter and associated tinted trial lenses (see below). The Colorimeter is used to assist the patient in obtaining a suitable colour. This colour is then matched with a combination of tinted trial lenses, which are given to the patient to try out, and alter, if necessary. After the combination has been selected, the chosen lenses are used to guide the dyeing of spectacle lenses. Each aspect of this system will now be described in turn.

10.6.3   INTUITIVE COLORIMETER

The Intuitive Colorimeter is a simple apparatus for mixing coloured light that enables the three subjective dimensions of colour (hue, saturation and brightness) to be varied separately. Figure 10.6.1 shows the instrument in profile. The main viewing window on the front of the instrument has a sliding cover which can be raised to reveal an inner surface on which visual material can be placed. The material is illuminated by coloured light and separate controls on the side of the instrument allow the hue, saturation and brightness to be controlled. The instrument is designed to be placed on a table with the examiner sitting on the patient's right. The controls on the right side of the instrument can then be operated by either the examiner or the patient. One control changes the hue, another changes the saturation, and two alter the luminance without altering the colour. One attenuator reduces the luminance by half (■), and one reduces the luminance by three-quarters (■), i.e. to one-quarter of the unattenuated value. Operating the two attenuators together reduces the luminance to one eighth the unattenuated value.

Figure 10.6.2 shows a simplified cross section of the instrument. A collimated cylindrical beam of white light from a tungsten-halogen lamp (L) is reflected from a cold-light mirror (M) and passes through a wheel (W) and into a box with matt white inner surfaces (S). The wheel is divided into three sectors, each covered with a different filter so as to transmit light of a different colour. One sector transmits long-wavelength light (and is red in colour), one intermediate wavelengths (appearing green) and one short wavelengths (blue). The coloured light is mixed as it is reflected and scattered from the inner surfaces of the box. Text (T) is mounted on one surface of this box and viewed through a window in the front.

When the wheel is concentric with the beam, the three filters each pass a similar proportion of the light, and white light results when the beam is mixed. However, the wheel is free to slide downwards so that the beam can pass eccentrically through it. The area of the filters through which the light passes is then no longer the same. The colour of the mixed light becomes progressively deeper and deeper (increasingly saturated) as eccentricity increases. The wheel is also free to rotate. This changes the colour (hue). Figure 10.6.3 gives a demonstration of the principle of the Colorimeter, which is an extension of the colorimeters described by Burnham (1952) and Gunkel and Cogan (1978). The Intuitive Colorimeter has several advantages for assessing the subjective effects of coloured light: (1) It provides a standard source of illumination of appropriate[1] and constant luminance that allows colour (CIE UCS 1976 hue angle, h_{uv}) and depth of colour (CIE UCS 1976 saturation, s_{uv}) to be varied separately and therefore intuitively; (2) the variation is continuous rather than discrete; (3) a large range of colours (gamut) is available (colours that are outside the gamut are very strongly saturated, and could be reproduced only with inappropriately dark lenses); (4) no coloured surfaces are visible within the Colorimeter, so it is possible to study chromaticity independent of the particular spectral power distribution of the illuminating light, and related colour constancy mechanisms; (5) the perceptual effects of colour can be studied while the patient's eyes are colour-adapted; and (6) the assessment is quick and efficient.

10.6.4 TRIAL LENSES

The Intuitive Colorimeter is designed to be used to provide a chromaticity that is optimum for visual perception and visual comfort. This chromaticity is then matched using trial lenses. The trial lenses serve six purposes: (1) they provide a calibrated colour standard; (2) they enable a patient to try out a tint under different lighting conditions before it is made up; (3) they allow the adjustment of the tint; (4) they indicate the amount of each dye necessary to achieve the required spectral transmission thereby enabling practitioners to issue an

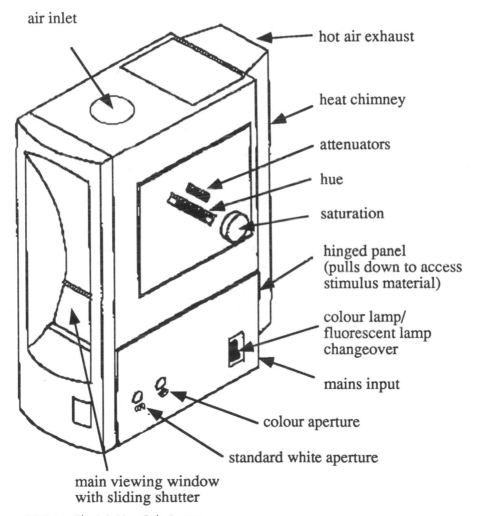

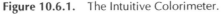

Figure 10.6.1. The Intuitive Colorimeter.

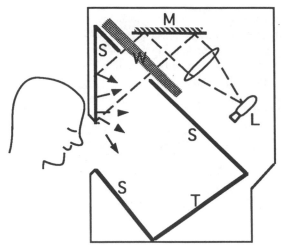

Figure 10.6.2. Cross section of Intuitive Colorimeter.

accurate prescription; (5) they govern the dyeing of spectacle lenses; and (6) they allow practitioners to check the accuracy of the dyeing.

The dyes for the trial lenses have been selected on the basis of six principles: (1) the dyes are stable; (2) the spectral transmission curves of lenses tinted with the dyes are as smooth as possible so as to reduce metamerism when lenses are combined; (3) the dyes are suitable for rapid tinting; (4) the hue angles of the dye colours are chosen so as to sample colour space evenly; (5) a large number of dyes (seven) has been chosen so there is one colour from the selection that will closely match any Colorimeter chromaticity; and (6) it is simple to superimpose trial lenses of similar colour to obtain a desired shade, and the choice of trial lenses necessary is intuitively obvious. When absorbed by a lens, the dyes have the following colour appearances: rose, orange, yellow, green, turquoise, blue and purple.

The trial lenses have different degrees of deposition of each of the above dyes so as to vary the saturation of colour. The lenses are arranged in pairs: two with identical transmission (one lens for each eye). Five pairs with increasing saturation are provided for five of the seven dyes (but with six pairs for rose and purple). In Figure 10.6.4 the peripheral

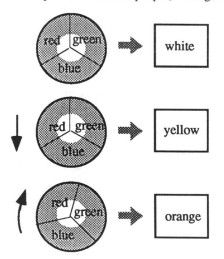

Figure 10.6.3. Principle of Intuitive Colorimeter.

panels show the transmissions of the lenses. Each curve represents the transmission of a trial lens (0–100 per cent, y-axis) as a function of wavelength (400–700 nm, x-axis). The chromaticity co-ordinates of the lenses of each dye are shown in the UCS diagram in the central panel of Figure 10.6.4 (large points).

The deposition of dye increases geometrically from one pair of lenses to the next. Thirty-one levels of deposition can be obtained by superimposing the trial lenses, adding them in all possible combinations.

The trial lenses for two dyes can be combined so that $31 \times 31 = 961$ tints are obtainable having colours (chromaticity co-ordinates) in between those of the two dyes. Figure 10.6.4 (central panel) shows the chromaticity co-ordinates of the 961 combinations of orange and rose, the 961 combinations of rose and purple, purple and blue, blue and turquoise, etc. As can be seen, a large area of the UCS diagram can be evenly and densely sampled (6727 points in all) using only two dyes at a time, both with similar hue angle. The sixth rose and purple lenses can be used to increase the gamut still further.

The spectral transmission of each lens is measured and used by a computer program that computes ultra-violet absorption, blue light transmission and Q-values for signal lights. The program issues guidelines for the optometrist and also (in non-technical form) for the patient. The guidelines are based on British Standard 2724 for sunglasses and concern ultra-violet protection, and the extent to which the tint is likely to interfere with the perception of traffic signals. The Precision Tinting System is patented by the Medical Research Council

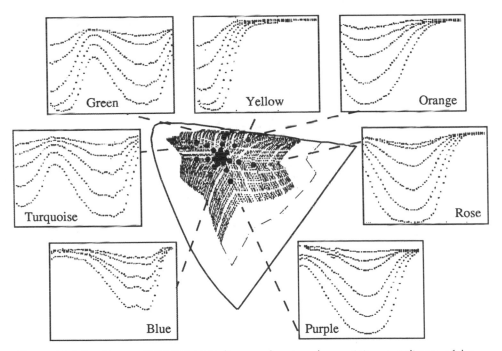

Figure 10.6.4. Centre: CIE 1976 UCS diagram showing chromaticity co-ordinates of the trial lenses (large points) and combinations of these lenses, when the dyes with neighbouring hue were combined two at a time (small points). For example, the small points with hue angles between purple and rose were obtained with combinations of purple and rose trial lenses. Periphery: transmissions of the trial lenses (0–100%, y-axis) as a function of wavelength (400–700 nm, x-axis). The dashed line shows the limits of the chromaticities available when the sixth rose and purple dyes are used.

and manufactured by Cerium Visual Technologies (Tenterden, Kent, England), who offer a commercial tinting service, now available internationally.

Over the first year that the tinting system was introduced into clinical practice in the UK, more than 1000 tints were prescribed. Figure 10.6.5 shows the chromaticities of these tints and confirms the preponderance of blue and green tints noted in open trials (Maclachlan *et al.*, 1993). Most prescriptions were based on a combination of two trial lenses, and such a combination is sufficient for a large range of chromaticities. The greater frequency of green and blue tints cannot be attributed to an artefact of the number of lenses used for the prescription. Figure 10.6.6 provides a histogram of the photopic transmission of the tints.

10.6.5 EXAMINATION PROCEDURE

For some patients, there are circumscribed regions of colour space within which perceptual distortions abate, and visual discomfort is reduced (Maclachlan *et al.*, 1993; Wilkins *et al.*, 1992a,b). The examination procedure is aimed at locating these regions without inducing discomfort, and then refining the measurements under conditions of colour adaptation. In a darkened room, the patient looks through the observation window of the Colorimeter and observes an array of random letters. The letters are arranged in strings to resemble words in a paragraph of text. The assessment is carried out under binocular viewing conditions unless there are indications that the optimal tint may differ in the two eyes and the patient is prepared to countenance wearing spectacles with differently coloured lenses.

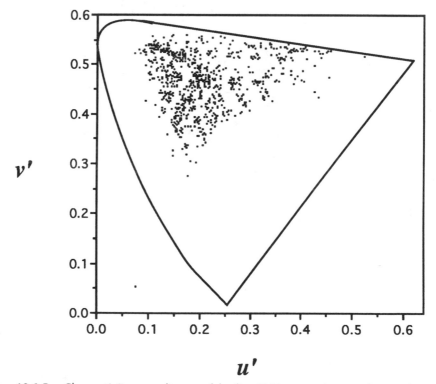

Figure 10.6.5. Chromaticity co-ordinates of the first 1000 spectacles tinted using the MRC system for Precision Ophthalmic Tinting.

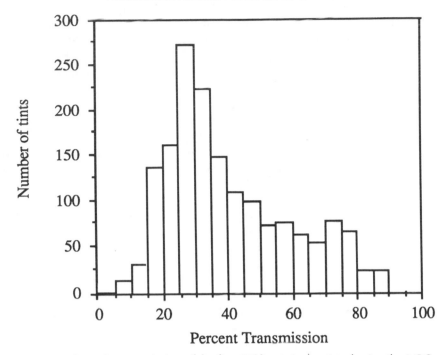

Figure 10.6.6. Photopic transmission of the first 1000 spectacles tinted using the MRC system for Precision Ophthalmic Tinting.

The test procedure recommended in the Intuitive Colorimeter Manual (Wilkins, 1993) can be summarised as follows. An initial screening procedure is undertaken at constant luminance (~ 20 cdm^{-2}) with the eyes adapted to white light. Beginning with a hue angle (h_{uv}) close to 0 degrees (a rose hue), saturation (s_{uv}) is slowly increased from white ($u' = 0.23$, $v' = 0.44$) to a moderately saturated rose ($s_{uv} \sim 0.8$) and then decreased until the light is again white. The observer is required to report any effects of the colour and compare them with white. The hue angle is then increased by 30 degrees and the procedure is repeated. Twelve hue angles (orange, yellow, green, etc.) are examined in this way. The purpose of the initial screening is to determine the range of hue angles that are beneficial and identify any that are aversive.

Following the screening, a second detailed examination takes place. The best hue angle is selected from the alternatives identified in the initial screening, if necessary by forced choice between the alternatives, presented in succession. Saturation is then optimised at this best hue angle, usually by a method of adjustment. Hue angle is optimised at the chosen saturation, usually by forced choice between two similar hue angles. At the revised hue angle thus obtained saturation is again adjusted. This procedure is repeated as necessary and will often, but not always, result in a stable choice of colour, particularly if the subject reports benefit. The procedure is based on the assumption that there are stable regions of colour space within which perception is improved. Note that during the detailed examination the eyes remain exposed to light of a particular colour, and the assessment is conducted while the eyes are colour adapted. The above adjustments are initially made at a constant photopic luminance similar to that which a person might experience under conditions of normal office lighting when wearing tinted glasses that absorb about half the light (Mills and Borg, 1993). The measurements are then checked at lower luminance levels.

The chosen colour is visible through the circular aperture in the side of the Colorimeter. Another circular aperture reveals a surface lit with a standard white light (CIE type F3) that is switched on when the sliding cover on the main viewing window is closed, preventing the entry of ambient light. In a darkened room both apertures appear as light sources rather than as surfaces. The combination of trial lenses likely to match the Colorimeter setting is obtained from tables. The combination of lenses is placed in front of the Standard aperture and the match is verified by the patient, adjusting the combination if necessary. A 'white' fluorescent lamp (CIE type F3) was chosen for the standard because: (1) it is a type of lamp that is commonly used for lighting offices and schools; (2) its spectral power distribution is easily controlled; (3) it has a chromaticity midway between that of daylight and incandescent light.[2] Because the apertures have the appearance of light sources, the matching of their colour is straightforward.

The stack of trial lenses that matches the Colorimeter setting is selected by combining lenses from one main colour and one subsidiary colour. The main colour is the one that predominates and gives most of the colour appearance. The subsidiary colour is added to it to fine-tune the colour. The dye colours have been chosen so that the colour of the combination of two dyes is intuitively obvious, for example, a combination of blue and purple gives a purpley blue. As Figure 10.6.4 shows, the colour appearance of the two apertures can always be matched very closely by superimposing over the Standard aperture lenses from a main colour and just one colour with neighbouring hue, that is by combining lenses of just two colours and hence of just two dyes.

Once selected, the combination of trial lenses is worn by the patient under a variety of typical viewing conditions and lighting so that any adjustments to the combination of trial lenses can be made. Some patients prefer a lower saturation than that selected in the Colorimeter, presumably to reduce the darkness of the lenses and their effect on the appearance of surface colours.

10.6.6 RELIABILITY OF THE PROCEDURE

The reliability of the Colorimeter examination procedure has been assessed in three independent trials. In the first of these trials, 15 normal adults from the MRC Applied Psychology Unit subject panel aged 30–61 years (mean 50 years) were examined. They were assessed initially and then 24–26 months later by a different examiner who had no knowledge of the subjects' previous performance. The observers did not receive any treatment or other intervention in the two-year interval between examinations. Five subjects were emmetropic and ten wore their usual near correction. None was receiving orthoptic treatment. The optimal hue angle was assessed at each examination and the minimum absolute angular difference between the hue angles (h_{uv}) was calculated. For example, if a hue angle of 285° had been chosen on the first occasion and 205° on the second, the angular difference would have been 80°; if the first hue angle had been 305° and the second 10°, then the angular difference would have been 65°. The mean angular difference for the 15 subjects was 63.1°. If the hue angles had been chosen randomly and all hue angles had been equally likely, the expected angular difference would have been 90°. However, the chosen hue angles tend to cluster between 90 and 270°, as can be seen from Figure 10.6.5. Therefore the expected value is difficult to obtain from distribution theory, and a randomisation technique was used to calculate the expected value. A given subject's initial hue was randomly paired with another subject's second hue and the angular difference obtained. Random permutations were undertaken, re-pairing all subjects, and the mean angular difference calculated. The process was repeated 10 000 times by computer and only on 114 occasions was the value lower than 63.1º. The p-value for the chance occurrence is therefore 0.0114. The 99 per cent confidence limits for the p-value were 0.0084 and 0.0140.

Data from two other trials have been treated in a similar way. The first was from a double-masked study by Wilkins *et al.* (1994) who examined children aged 9–14 years, offering them spectacles with lenses that matched an optimal Colorimeter setting or a suboptimal setting, comparing the incidence of headaches and eye-strain (Evans *et al.*, this volume, pp. 709–715). The children were examined for a second time at the end of the study, approximately one year after the first examination. During the interval most of the children wore coloured glasses. The mean angular difference between the optimal hue angle on the first and second assessments was 62.9º ($p = 0.0035$). The second trial was undertaken by Jenny Brown, who, working in optometric practice, assessed patients every six months on average. As in the above trial most were wearing coloured glasses. In 30 consecutive cases, the mean angular difference was 49.7º ($p < 0.0001$).

10.6.7 A REBUTTAL OF RECENT CRITICISM

In a recent abstract, Mason *et al.* (1994) criticised the Colorimeter on three counts.

1. *The assessment was 'unreliable'.* The subjects examined by Mason *et al.*, 'reported distortions whatever the colour'. If their subjects were unable to find a colour that could alleviate symptoms it is perhaps unsurprising that their settings were 'unreliable', although no statistics are quoted. It is clear from the previous section that normal observers generate reliable data when examined using the recommended techniques.
2. *Two or more colours cannot be presented in immediate succession.* Although this was not possible on the prototype Colorimeter used by Mason *et al.* because the hue wheel had a low gear ratio, the gearing has been changed on the production model and it is now simple to change colours rapidly. It is not, however, recommended that two colours are presented in immediate succession unless they have similar hue angle because the changing state of adaptation of the eyes may complicate any comparison.
3. *Colours cannot be presented simultaneously for comparison.* The Colorimeter does not permit the simultaneous presentation of different colours for a *fundamental* but subtle reason. As outlined above, the Colorimeter was designed to assess the effects of coloured light and to do so under conditions in which the eyes are adapted to that illuminant colour. Changing the colour of a light source is similar to wearing a coloured lens. It is for this reason that the Colorimeter provides a good guide to the colour appropriate for tinted spectacles.

As Mason *et al.* point out, young children often find the effects of colour easier to assess when two colours are presented simultaneously. However, the state of adaptation of the eye then depends upon many factors, and the colour selection would not be appropriate for lenses. Simultaneous comparison of two colours is best achieved when the eyes are adapted to a conventional (white) light source and the colours are perceived as surfaces rather than as lighting. This can readily be achieved using overlays (e.g. Irlen, 1991; Wilkins, 1994). These are sheets of coloured plastic that can be placed side by side over a page of text that is illuminated conventionally. The British College of Optometry has issued guidelines suggesting that children should use overlays for a trial period before being assessed for tinted glasses.

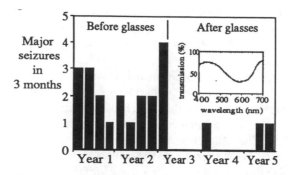

Figure 10.6.7. Incidence of major tonic clonic seizures before and after the provision of coloured spectacles.

As might be expected, the choice of colour for spectacles is predictable from the choice of colour in the Colorimeter and not from the choice of coloured overlays (Wilkins *et al.*, 1992a).

10.6.8 CLINICAL USE OF PRECISION TINTS

10.6.8.1 Reading

Children with reading difficulty can benefit from a reduction of eye-strain and headaches, as detailed in the chapter by Evans *et al.* (this volume, pp. 709–715).

10.6.8.2 Photosensitive epilepsy

Patients with photosensitive epilepsy are liable to seizures induced by light, particularly when it flickers. An electroencephalographic response to flickering light is usually obtained in these patients. The colour of the flickering light can affect the electroencephalographic response, although with differences between individual patients as to which colour is the most epileptogenic (Harding and Jeavons, 1994). It has long been reported that photo-sensitive patients may benefit from wearing coloured spectacles (Newmark and Penry, 1979), although most reports preceded the development of an effective anticonvulsant therapy (sodium valproate). Benefit is typically reported with spectacles that absorb red light. The author has examined several patients with photosensitive epilepsy using the Colorimeter (usually with concurrent EEG recording to reduce the risk of seizures). Spectacles tinted using the subjective methods described above appear to have successfully reduced seizures. In most cases to date, the interpretation is complicated by concurrent changes in medication, but in a girl with intractable major seizures the seizure reduction was immediate, sustained and, since there were no concurrent changes in medication, unequivocal. Her mother kept a seizure diary summarised in Figure 10.6.7. The patient wore the spectacles on a cord around her neck and put them on whenever she felt the need.

10.6.8.3 Migraine

Many adults with migraine and a sensitivity to light appear to benefit from precision tints (Maclachlan *et al.*, 1993; Wilkins *et al.*, 1992a), although double-masked studies remain to be conducted.

10.6.8.4 Colour vision deficiency

Fletcher and Voke (1985) and Birch (1993) have reviewed the literature on the use of coloured filters to ameliorate the effects of Daltonism in everyday life. They discuss the advantages and disadvantages of monocular and binocular filters, different filters in the two eyes, and filters that partially cover the field of view. They also present several case histories of patients who appeared to benefit from wearing binocularly tinted spectacles covering the entire field of view, some of whom preferred to wear their spectacles continuously. The author has also seen two patients who appeared to benefit from binocular tints, reporting that colours appeared less glaring. Both cases had an acquired colour vision deficiency. They reported that coloured surfaces appeared more normal with their chosen filter (selected from the range of trial tints) and, in one case, errors of colour naming were reduced considerably. These preliminary observations deserve further exploration.

10.6.9 WHY PRECISION TINTING WORKS

The following is one possible explanation as to why precision tints have their beneficial effects. It is only one among many, but has the merit of parsimony.

1. In patients with photosensitive epilepsy there is considerable convergent evidence that seizures can be triggered in the visual cortex (Darby *et al.*, 1986; Wilkins, *et al.*, 1980, 1981).
2. The seizures can sometimes be provoked by patterns of stripes, and sometimes only by stripes in a limited range of orientations (Chatrian *et al.*, 1970; Soso *et al.*, 1980; Wilkins, *et al.*, 1979).
   Inference: The trigger can be quite focal in the visual cortex, involving a small hyperexcitable area with columns of cells having the appropriate orientation specificity.
3. The visual stimuli that trigger seizures in patients with photosensitive epilepsy provoke in others feelings of discomfort and anomalous perceptual distortions (Marcus and Soso, 1989; Wilkins *et al.*, 1984).
   Inference: Some of the perceptual effects are due to a spread of excitation in the visual cortex sufficient to excite neurones inappropriately, but not sufficient to provoke a seizure.
4. People with migraine or with migraine in the family are particularly susceptible to the perceptual distortions seen in epileptogenic visual stimuli (Marcus and Soso, 1989; Wilkins *et al.*, 1984). In those with consistently lateralised visual aura the distortions are similarly lateralised (Khalil, 1991).
   Inference: In these individuals the visual cortex of one or both hemispheres may be unusually excitable.
5. Text has spatial characteristics that resemble those of stressful patterns (Watt *et al.*, 1990; Wilkins, 1991; Wilkins and Nimmo-Smith, 1987).

6. Reading can provoke anomalous visual effects (Wilkins, 1991), headaches (Wilkins and Nimmo-Smith, 1984) and photosensitive epilepsy (Wilkins and Lindsay, 1985).

7. Covering the lines that are not being read, leaving only three visible lines, reduces these adverse effects (Wilkins and Lindsay, 1985; Wilkins and Nimmo-Smith, 1984).

Inference: Certain spatial characteristics of text induce 'pattern glare' and make it stressful, particularly for individuals with cortical hyperexcitability.

8. Some cortical neurones are tuned for wavelength or for colour appearance. None can be indifferent to the spectral power distribution of the stimulating light (Lennie and D'Zmura, 1988).

Inference: The colour of the illuminating light changes the pattern of excitation in the cortical network.

9. People with migraine show a consistency not shown by age and sex matched controls regarding their choice of coloured light for reading, avoiding red illumination (Chronicle and Wilkins, 1991).

10. Certain children report a reduction in distortion with light of a certain colour, different for each individual, but usually complementary to red (Maclachlan *et al.*, 1993; Wilkins *et al.*, 1992a).

11. These children usually have migraine in the family and suffer frequent headaches (Maclachlan *et al.*, 1993).

12. There are several early reports (Newmark and Penry, 1979) and one recent report (Takahashi and Tsukahara, 1992) emphasising the effectiveness of glasses that absorb red light in the treatment of photosensitive epilepsy.

13. Precision Tints (both blue and other colours, selected according to routine subjective methods) reduce the photoconvulsive EEG response to flickering light and patterns whereas neutral tints of similar photopic transmission are less effective (recent unpublished observations).

14. Precision Tints reduce seizures in some patients (see above).

Inference: The colour that is therapeutic changes the pattern of excitation in the cortical network so as to avoid local areas of hyperexcitability.

15. The patterns that provoke seizures have characteristics that are reminiscent of the properties of magnocellular cells (Wilkins, 1995): patterns of stripes are not epileptogenic if the stripes differ in colour but not in brightness; the effects of pattern motion suggest that directionally sensitive neurones are involved in seizure induction; the effects of binocular fusion would be consistent with the action of disparity-tuned neurones; the low spatial resolution of cells in the magnocellular system would be consistent with the spatial frequencies at which aversive effects occur; the high temporal resolution would be consistent with the effects of flicker; epileptiform EEG activity in response to patterns is usually maximal over electrodes which record from parieto-occipital cortex.

16. Children with reading difficulty have a deficit in transient system function (Lovegrove *et al.*, 1986) implicating magnocellular dysfunction (Livingstone *et al.*, 1991).

17. They often have poor sensitivity at mid-range spatial frequencies but good sensitivity at high spatial frequencies (Lovegrove *et al.*, 1986).

18. They often complain of glare from the page (Wilkins *et al.*, 1992a).

Inference: There may be a link between pattern glare and magnocellular function.

Drawing together the above inferences, it is proposed that when observers who report perceptual distortion choose a coloured light that improves clarity and comfort of text, they may be selecting a distribution of excitation in the visual cortex that reduces the excitation in hyperexcitable regions. It is unclear why the magnocellular system appears to be preferentially involved.

10.6.10   NOTES

1. A luminance of 20 cdm^{-2} is used for this examination initially because this is the luminance expected under conventional office lighting (Mills and Borg, 1993) when wearing a lens that absorbs about half the light.
2. Note that when the saturation control is at its minimum the colorimeter has a chromaticity similar to that of daylight (D65).

10.6.11   REFERENCES

BIRCH, J. (1993) *Diagnosis of Defective Colour Vision*, Oxford: Oxford University Press.
BURNHAM, R.W. (1952) A colorimeter for research in colour perception, *American Journal of Psychology*, **65**, 603–608.
CHATRIAN, G.E., LETTICH, E., MILLER, L.H. & GREEN, J.R. (1970) Pattern-sensitive epilepsy. Part 1: An electroencephalographic study of its mechanisms, *Epilepsia*, **15**, 125–149.
CHRONICLE, E. & WILKINS, A.J. (1991) Colour and visual discomfort in migraineurs, *Lancet*, **338**, 890.
DARBY, C.E. PARK, D.M., & WILKINS, A.J. (1986) EEG characteristics of epileptic pattern sensitivity and their relation to the nature of pattern stimulation and the effects of sodium valproate, *Electroencephalography and Clinical Neurophysiology*, **63**, 517–525.
FLETCHER, R.J. & VOKE, J. (1985) *Defective Colour Vision: Fundamentals, Diagnosis and Management*, Bristol: Adam Hilger.
GILES, G.H. (1965) *The Principles and Practice of Refraction and its Allied Subjects*, 2nd edn, London: Hammond Hammond.
GUNKEL, R. & COGAN, D. (1978) Colorimetry by a new principle, *Archives of Ophthalmology*, **96**, 331–334.
HARDING, G.F.A. & JEAVONS, P.M. (1994) *Photosensitive Epilepsy* (new edn), London: MacKeith Press.
IRLEN, H. (1983) Successful treatment of learning difficulties. Paper presented at the First Annual Convention of the American Psychological Association. Anaheim, California, USA.
IRLEN, H. (1991) *Reading by the Colors: Overcoming Dyslexia and Other Reading Disabilities through the Irlen Method*, New York: Avery Publishing Group
IRLEN, H. & LASS, M.N. (1989) Improving reading problems due to symptoms of scotopic sensitivity syndrome using Irlen lenses and overlays, *Education*, **109**(4), 413–417.
KHALIL, N. (1991) Investigations of visual function in migraine by visual evoked potentials and visual psychophysical tests, PhD Thesis, University of London.
LENNIE, P. & D'ZMURA, M. (1988) Mechanisms of colour vision, *CRC Critical Reviews in Neurobiology*, **3**(4), 333–399.
LIVINGSTONE, M.S., ROSEN, G.D., DRISLANE, F.W. & GALABURDA, A.M. (1991) Physiological and anatomical evidence for a magnocellular defect in developmental dyslexia, *Proceedings of the National Academy of Science*, **88**, 7943–7947.
LOVEGROVE, W., MARTIN, F., & SLAGHUIS, W. (1986) A theoretical and experimental case for a residual deficit in specific reading disability, *Cognitive Neuropsychology*, **3**, 225–267.
MACLACHLAN, A., YALE, S. & WILKINS, A.J. (1993) Open trial of subjective precision tinting: follow-up of 55 patients, *Ophthalmic and Physiological Optics*, **13**, 175–178.
MARCUS, D.A. & SOSO, M.J. (1989) Migraine and stripe-induced discomfort, *Archives of Neurology*, **46**, 1129–1132.

MASON, A.J.S., FOWLER, M.S. & STEIN, J.F. (1994) Evaluation of the Intuititive Colorimeter, *Investigative Ophthalmology and Visual Science*, **35**(4), 1754.

MILLS, E. & BORG, N. (1993) Trends in recommended lighting levels: an international comparison. In: *Proceedings of the 2nd European Conference on Energy-Efficient Lighting*, Arnhem, The Netherlands, September 26–29.

NEWMARK, M.E. & PENRY, J.K. (1979) *Photosensitivity and Epilepsy: A Review*, New York: Raven Press.

SOSO, M.J. LETTICH, E. & BELGUM, J.H. (1980) Pattern-sensitive epilepsy II: Effects of pattern orientation and hemifield stimulation, *Epilepsia*, **21**, 313–323.

TAKAHASHI, T. & TSUKAHARA, Y. (1992) Usefulness of blue sunglasses in photosensitive epilepsy, *Epilepsia*, **33**(3), 517–521.

WATT, R.J., BOCK, J. THIMBLEBY, H. & WILKINS, A.J. (1990) Visible aspects of text. In: *Applying Visual Psychophysics to User Interface Design*, British Telecom, pp 309–325.

WILKINS, A.J. (1991) Visual discomfort and reading. In: Stein, J.F. (Ed.) *Vision and Visual Dyslexia*, Basingstoke: Macmillan, pp. 155–170.

WILKINS, A.J. (1993) *A System for Precision Ophthalmic Tinting: Manual for the Intuitive Colorimeter*, Cerium Visual Technologies, 27pp.

WILKINS, A.J. (1994) Overlays for classroom and optometric use, *Ophthalmic and Physiological Optics*, **14**, 97–99.

WILKINS, A.J. (1995) *Visual Stress*, Oxford: Oxford University Press.

WILKINS, A.J. & LINDSAY, J. (1985) Common forms of reflex epilepsy: physiological mechanisms and techniques for treatment. In: Pedley, T.A. & Meldrum, B.S. (Eds.) *Recent Advances in Epilepsy II*, Edinburgh: Churchill Livingstone, pp. 239–271.

WILKINS, A.J. & NEARY, C. (1991) Some visual, optometric and perceptual effects of coloured glasses, *Ophthalmic and Physiological Optics*, **11**, 163–171.

WILKINS, A.J. & NIMMO-SMITH, M.I. (1984) On the reduction of eye-strain when reading, *Ophthalmic and Physiological Optics*, **4**, 53–59.

WILKINS, A.J. & NIMMO-SMITH, M.I. (1987) The clarity and comfort of printed text, *Ergonomics*, **30**(12), 1705–1720.

WILKINS, A.J., DARBY, C.E. & BINNIE, C.D. (1979) Neurophysiological aspects of pattern-sensitive epilepsy, *Brain*, **102**, 1–25.

WILKINS, A.J., BINNIE, C.D. & DARBY, C.E. (1980) Visually-induced seizures, *Progress in Neurobiology*, **15**, 85–117.

WILKINS, A.J., BINNIE, C.D. & DARBY, C.E. (1981) Interhemispheric differences in photosensitivity: I. Pattern sensitivity thresholds, *Electroencephalography and Clinical Neurophysiology*, **5**, 461–468.

WILKINS, A.J., NIMMO-SMITH, I., TAIT, A., McMANUS, C., DELLA SALA, S., TILLEY, A., ARNOLD, K., BARRIE, M. & SCOTT, S. (1984) A neurological basis for visual discomfort, *Brain*, **107**, 989–1017.

WILKINS, A.J., MILROY, R., NIMMO-SMITH, I., WRIGHT, A., TYRRELL, R., HOLLAND, K., MARTIN, J., BALD, J., YALE, S., MILES, T., & NOAKES, T. (1992a) Preliminary observations concerning treatment of visual discomfort and associated perceptual distortion, *Ophthalmic and Physiological Optics*, **12**, 257–263.

WILKINS, A.J., NIMMO-SMITH, I. & JANSONS, J. (1992b) A colorimeter for the intuitive manipulation of hue and saturation and its role in the study of perceptual distortion, *Ophthalmic and Physiological Optics*, **12**, 381–385.

WILKINS, A.J., EVANS, B.J.W., BROWN, J.A., BUSBY, A.E., WINGFIELD, A.E., JEANES, R.J. & BALD, J. (1994) Double-masked placebo-controlled trial of precision spectral filters in children who use coloured overlays, *Ophthalmic and Physiological Optics*, **14**(4), 365–370.

Optometric Characteristics of Children with Reading Difficulties who Report a Benefit from Coloured Filters

Bruce J.W. Evans, Arnold J. Wilkins, Ann Busby and Rebecca Jeanes

10.7.1   INTRODUCTION

In 1983 Irlen described 'scotopic sensitivity syndrome', a condition that she said is characterised by the presence of certain symptoms which are alleviated by tinted lenses. The symptoms, which principally occur when reading, can be described as eyestrain, headache, and anomalous visual effects and the benefit from tinted lenses is claimed to be idiosyncratic and very specific (Irlen, 1991). A review of the literature noted that the putative condition and associated therapy lacked both a sound theoretical basis and rigorous placebo-controlled trials (Evans and Drasdo, 1991). The condition, in fact, was first described in detail by Meares (1980) and the term 'Meares-Irlen Syndrome' may be most appropriate.

Recently, Wilkins et al. (1994) have carried out the first double-masked placebo-controlled trial of a tinted lens therapy for children who report these symptoms. The results of this study will be briefly summarised. New research will also be presented in which some of the subjects in the original trial are compared with a control group to investigate the optometric correlates of the syndrome. The aim of this research is to further understanding of the aetiology of Meares-Irlen Syndrome.

10.7.2   RESUMÉ OF DOUBLE-MASKED TRIAL

The aims of the previous study were to determine whether the 'tinted lens treatment' represents anything more than a placebo. To concentrate our sample, we studied children aged 9–14 years who had eyestrain or headaches, and who had been voluntarily using and claiming to benefit from a coloured overlay for at least three weeks. The children were all well-adapted to any necessary refractive corrections (which were worn for all testing at the relevant viewing distance) and subjects with binocular vision anomalies that required treatment (according to conventional criteria; Pickwell, 1991) were excluded.

A new instrument, the Intuitive Colorimeter (Wilkins *et al.*, 1992), was used to find an optimal chromaticity for each subject, which was reported to improve their perception of printed text. The colorimeter was then used to identify a second chromaticity, of very similar colour to the first, which was described by the subject as having a less beneficial effect on the text. Two pairs of tinted CR39 spectacles were made for each subject; one of which matched the optimal chromaticity ('experimental tint'): the other matched the sub-optimal chromaticity ('control tint'). There was no systematic variation in the saturation or transmission of the experimental and control lenses and the mean chromaticity difference between them was equivalent to six just-noticeable-differences (Wilkins *et al.*, 1994).

The subjects wore each pair of tinted spectacles, in random order, for a period of four weeks, with an interval of at least four weeks between each pair. Because of colour adaptation, children were unaware of the precise colour of their colorimetry settings. Several other measures were taken to ensure that the study was double-masked (Wilkins *et al.*, 1994) and when the subjects were questioned at the end of the study it was confirmed that they were unaware of which pair of tints matched their preferred colorimeter setting. Throughout the study the children completed daily symptom diaries, detailing occurrences of eyestrain and headache. Sixty-seven children entered the study and 36 completed the symptom diaries.

The experimental tint reduced symptoms of eyestrain and headache significantly more than the control tint. Thus, the study showed that coloured filters can help to reduce eyestrain and headaches for reasons that cannot be solely attributed to a placebo effect. The prevalence of colour vision defects in the study population, as detected by Ishihara and 100-hue testing, was similar to that expected in a normal population (Wilkins *et al.*, 1994).

10.7.3   MATCHED CONTROL GROUP STUDY

To discover more about why some children are helped by tinted lenses, we decided to compare the optometric characteristics of a sample of the children from the tinted lens trial with a matched control group.

10.7.3.1 Subject selection and matching

Sixteen of the children in the original trial came from Upbury Manor School in Kent and these were defined as the tinted lens group for the matched group study. We screened a further 92 children from the same school to select controls. Forty-five children were excluded because they had symptoms and/or demonstrated a positive response to testing with coloured overlays and four because they gave unreliable results during testing with coloured overlays. A further 12 children were excluded because they had been prescribed glasses but were not wearing them, and two were excluded for medical reasons. The remaining 29 were tested with a group IQ test and with the Suffolk reading test. Twenty-five of these were selected on the basis of these test results so as to match the tinted lens group in chronological age, IQ (Raven *et al.*, 1988a,b), and reading performance (Suffolk Reading Test).

10.7.3.2 Methods

The children were investigated (without using any coloured filters) with the following optometric tests: near visual acuity with a logMAR chart, objective refraction by distance fixation retinoscopy (Evans et al., 1994a); distance and near cover test, near dissociated heterophoria, near associated heterophoria, stereo-acuity (Randot Test, contoured circles), AC/A ratio, near vergence reserves, near point of convergence, and amplitude of accommodation (Evans et al., 1994b). The spatial contrast sensitivity of the tinted lens group was assessed with the Vistech near contrast sensitivity charts (taking the median result for each spatial frequency from all three charts) and the temporal contrast sensitivity (at 10 Hz) of both groups was assessed by varying the modulation contrast of a sinusoidally flickering low spatial frequency target (Evans et al., 1995).

Some people experience eyestrain, headaches, and anomalous visual effects when viewing certain types of striped patterns and this 'pattern glare' has been extensively studied by Wilkins et al. (1984). Wilkins and Neary (1991) suggested that pattern glare might account for a benefit from tinted lenses in Meares-Irlen Syndrome. We tested for pattern glare using two high contrast square wave gratings, one with spatial properties that should cause pattern glare (pattern glare grating) and the other of low spatial frequency, which should not cause pattern glare (control grating). Subjects were asked scripted questions to detect if they perceived any of the following perceptual distortions when they viewed the gratings: colours, bending, blurring, flicker, shimmering, disappearing and re-appearing. The total number of distortions that a subject reported with a given grating was taken as their pattern glare score for that grating. This procedure is the usual method of quantifying pattern glare and has been described in more detail by Evans et al. (1995, 1996).

10.7.3.3 Results

No extra-ocular muscle palsies or strabismus were detected in either group. The groups did not significantly differ in terms of visual acuity, refractive error, cover test results, near dissociated or associated heterophoria, or AC/A ratio. The median near point of convergence was slightly ($p = 0.085$) more remote in the tinted lens group (5.25 cm) than in the control group (4.5 cm) and the mean amplitude of accommodation was lower in the tinted lens group (14 D cf 17 D; $p = 0.014$). The convergent and divergent vergence reserves were reduced in the tinted lens group (see Figure 10.7.1), who also had significantly worse near stereo-acuity (medians: tinted lens group, 35"; control group, 20"; Mann-Whitney U Test, $p = 0.0022$). The tinted lens group reported significantly more pattern glare than the control group in the grating that was designed to cause pattern glare (medians: tinted lens group, 4; control group, 2; Mann-Whitney U Test, $p = 0.025$), but not in the control grating (medians: tinted lens group, 0; control group, 0; Mann-Whitney U Test, $p = 0.90$).

The temporal contrast sensitivity (at 20 Hz) was not significantly different in the two groups. The spatial contrast sensitivity data were compared with the results obtained in a previous study of dyslexic and control children. We compared data from 50 of the children in the tinted lens trial (not just those from Upbury Manor School) with the data from 37 dyslexic and 42 control children (Evans et al., 1995). The tinted lens ('Meares-Irlen

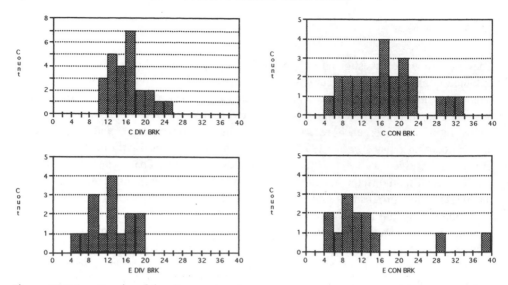

Figure 10.7.1. Graphs of the divergent and convergent vergence reserves ('DIV BRK' and 'CON BRK', respectively) in the control ('C') and tinted lens ('E') groups. The units for the abscissa are prism diopters.

Syndrome') group did not differ significantly from the controls at any of the spatial frequencies tested (1, 2, 4, 8, 12 cpd).

10.7.4   DISCUSSION

The present study investigated the optometric correlates of Meares-Irlen Syndrome, which is claimed to occur more commonly in dyslexic (50 per cent) than in good readers (10 per cent) (Irlen, 1991). A previous study used similar methods to investigate the optometric correlates of dyslexia (Evans *et al.*, 1994a,b), and it is interesting to compare the results of these two studies (see Table 10.7.1). Dyslexic children are believed, on average, to show reduced spatial contrast sensitivity to low spatial frequencies and impaired temporal contrast sensitivity (Lovegrove *et al.*, 1986). These anomalies have been described as a deficit of the transient visual system. Dyslexic children also frequently show signs of binocular instability (Evans *et al.*, 1994b), which has been characterised as reduced vergence amplitude and stability (Giles, 1960). Evans *et al.* (1993) linked the dyslexic's binocular instability, a motor deficit, with the impaired flicker perception, a sensory deficit. The present study suggests that children with Meares-Irlen Syndrome share the motor visual correlates of dyslexia, but do not demonstrate the sensory visual correlates. More research is needed to study these sensory factors using larger groups and more sensitive psychophysical techniques.

The symptoms of Meares-Irlen Syndrome are non-specific and the increased prevalence of subtle ocular motor anomalies in the tinted lens group raises the question of whether ocular motor factors might somehow be the mechanism for a benefit from coloured filters. This hypothesis is related to claims that children with the symptoms of Meares-Irlen Syndrome can be treated as effectively with optometric vision therapy as with coloured filters (Blaskey *et al.*, 1990). However, we think that this hypothesis is unlikely for the following reasons (Evans *et al.*, 1996). In the matched group research we questioned the children and their parents about whether the subjects had been observed to cover one eye

Table 10.7.1. Comparing the optometric correlates of Meares-Irlen Syndrome with the optometric correlates of dyslexia

Variable	Meares-Irlen Syndrome	Dyslexia
refractive error	normal	normal
heterophobia	normal	normal
vergence amplitude	reduced	reduced
accommodation	reduced	reduced
stereo-acuity	reduced	normal
spatial CSF	normal	reduced at low SFs
temporal CSF (20 Hz)	normal	reduced

when reading. Clinically, this symptom is taken to be a sign of binocular anomalies (Pickwell, 1991, p. 31), yet we found it to be no more common in the tinted lens than in the control group. Further, although the vergence reserves, amplitude of accommodation, and stereo-acuity were statistically significantly worse in the tinted lens group, the differences between the groups were slight and unlikely to be clinically significant. These observations suggest that our selection criteria to exclude subjects with clinically significant ocular motor anomalies were sufficiently rigorous to allow the conclusion that the benefit from colour in our tinted lens group was not the result of ocular motor anomalies.

Nevertheless, we investigated the possibility that there was a tendency for our subjects to prefer a chromaticity that would modify their accommodation in such a way as to reduce any heterophoria. Analyses showed that there was not a statistically significant effect of this type. Finally it should be noted that the double-masked placebo-controlled trial supports Irlen's claim that the chromaticity of the optimal coloured glasses can be highly specific. We know of no other ocular motor mechanism which shows this high chromatic specificity.

10.7.5   CONCLUSIONS

The double-masked placebo-controlled trial suggests that people who experience eyestrain, headaches, and anomalous visual effects whilst reading sometimes report a reduction in their symptoms when they use individually and precisely prescribed coloured filters. This benefit is not solely attributable to a placebo effect (Wilkins et al., 1994), although a placebo effect is doubtless a factor in at least some cases. One method of reducing the number of 'placebo cases' when prescribing precision tinted lenses is to screen initially with coloured overlays and to only carry out intuitive colorimetry once a person has shown a sustained benefit from an overlay. This method is used routinely with children (Irlen, 1991; Wilkins, 1994), although it should be noted that our study confirmed theoretical predictions that the colour of a person's optimal tinted spectacles cannot be predicted from the colour of their preferred overlay.

Our group of subjects who, on average, showed a benefit from coloured filters were compared with an asymptomatic control group who did not report a benefit from colour but who were matched for age, IQ, and reading performance. Optometric testing showed that the tinted lens group did not differ significantly from the control group in their visual acuity, refractive error, and heterophoria. However, the tinted lens group had a reduced vergence and accommodative amplitude and poorer stereo-acuity than the control group. This suggests that the tinted lens group demonstrated the motor optometric correlates of dyslexia (Evans et al., 1994b). Our finding that they did not manifest the sensory optometric correlates of dyslexia (Evans *et al.*, 1994a) requires replication with more sensitive psychophysical tests than the clinical nature of our study permitted. The tinted lens group did demonstrate more pattern glare than the controls, and we feel that this is likely to be an important part of the explanation for the efficacy of coloured filters.

Our results suggest that the benefit from coloured filters is not simply derived from a correction of ocular motor anomalies. However, since we excluded subjects with clinically significant orthoptic problems and still found an increased prevalence of subtle ocular motor anomalies in our tinted lens group it seems likely that there is an increased risk of people with Meares-Irlen Syndrome suffering from ocular motor anomalies that might require treatment. This is in agreement with the literature (Blaskey *et al.*, 1990) and, therefore, we think it important that before trying coloured filters people should have a thorough optometric examination and any clinically significant conventional visual anomalies should be corrected.

10.7.6   ACKNOWLEDGEMENT

We are grateful to the pupils and their parents, and to the staff of Upbury Manor School for their cooperation. We are also grateful for financial support from: the Medical Research Council, Cerium Visual Technologies, the Paul Hamlyn Trust, and Dollond and Aitchison. Finally, we thank Clement Clarke International, Vistech Inc, and Cibavision for donating equipment.

10.7.7   REFERENCES

BLASKEY, P., SCHEIMAN, M., PARISI, M., CINER, E.B., GALLAWAY, M., & SELZNICK, R. (1990) The effectiveness of Irlen filters for improving reading performance: a pilot study, *Journal of Learning Disabilities*, **23**, 604–612.

EVANS, B.J.W. & DRASDO, N. (1991) Tinted lenses and related therapies for learning disabilities – a review, *Ophthalmic and Physiological Optics*, **11**, 206–217.

EVANS, B.J.W., DRASDO, N. & RICHARDS, I.L. (1993) Linking the sensory and motor visual correlates of dyslexia. In: Wright, S.F. & Groner, R. (Eds) *Facets of Dyslexia and its Remediation*, Amsterdam: Elsevier Science, pp. 179–191.

EVANS, B.J.W., DRASDO, N. & RICHARDS, I.L. (1994a) An investigation of some sensory and refractive visual factors in dyslexia, *Vision Research*, **34**, 1913–1926.

EVANS, B.J.W., DRASDO, N. & RICHARDS, I.L. (1994b) Investigation of binocular and accommodative function in dyslexia, *Ophthalmic and Physiological Optics*, **14**, 5–19.

EVANS, B.J.W., BUSBY, A., JEANES, R. & WILKINS, A.J. (1995) Optometric correlates of Meares–Irlen Syndrome: a matched group study, *Ophthalmic and Physiological Optics*, **15**, 481–487.

EVANS, B.J.W., WILKINS, A.J., BROWN, J., BUSBY, A., WINGFIELD, A., JEANES, R. & BALD, J. (1996) A preliminary investigation into the aetiology of Meares–Irlen Syndrome, *Ophthalmic and Physiological Optics*, in press.

GILES, G.H. (1960) *The Principles and Practice of Refraction*, London: Hammond, Hammond and Company.

IRLEN, H. (1991) *Reading by the Colors: Overcoming Dyslexia and Other Reading Disabilities through the Irlen Method*, New York: Avery.

IRLEN, H. (1983) 'Successful treatment of learning difficulties', presentation at The Annual Convention of the American Psychological Association, Anaheim, California.

LOVEGROVE, W., MARTIN, F., & SLAGHUIS, W. (1986) A theoretical and experimental case for a visual deficit in specific reading disability, *Cognitive Neuropsychology*, **3**, 225–267.

Meares, O. (1980) Figure/ground, brightness contrast, and reading disabilities, *Visible Language*, **14**, 13–29.

Pickwell, D. (1991) *Binocular Vision Anomalies: Investigation and Treatment*, London: Butterworths.

Raven, J.C., Court, J.H. & Raven, J. (1988a) *Manual For Raven's Progressive Matrices and Vocabulary Scales: Section 3*, London: Lewis.

Raven, J.C., Court, J.H. & Raven, J. (1988b) *Manual For Raven's Progressive Matrices and Vocabulary Scales: Section 5a*, London: Lewis.

Wilkins, A.J. (1994) Overlays for classroom and optometric use, *Ophthalmic and Physiological Optics*, **14**, 97–99.

Wilkins, A.J. & Neary, C. (1991) Some visual, optometric and perceptual effects of coloured glasses, *Ophthalmic and Physiological Optics*, **11**, 163–171.

Wilkins, A.J. & Nimmo-Smith, I. & Jansons, J.E. (1992) Colorimeter for the intuitive manipulation of hue and saturation and its role in the study of perceptual distortion, *Ophthalmic and Physiological Optics*, **12**, 381–385.

Wilkins, A.J., Evans, B.J.W., Brown, J., Busby, A., Wingfield, A., Jeanes, R. & Bald, J. (1994) Double-masked placebo-controlled trial of precision spectral filters in children who use coloured overlays, *Ophthalmic and Physiological Optics*, **14**, 365–370.

Wilkins, A.J., Nimmo-Smith, I., Tait, A., McManus, C., Della Sala, S., Tilley, A., Arnold, K., Barrie, M. & Scott, S. (1984) A neurobiological basis for visual discomfort, *Brain*, **107**, 989–1017.

The Magnocellular Defect of Dyslexics

J.F. Stein

Between 5 and 10 per cent of 7–10-year-old children experience severe difficulty learning to read (Rutter and Yule, 1975). Developmental dyslexia is diagnosed if the child's reading is more than two standard deviations behind what would be expected from his intelligence in other areas, usually as measured by Performance IQ. This problem is much commoner in boys than girls, and it seems to run in families. It is often associated with minor language problems, such as lisping and stammering, mixed handedness, inability to tell left from right, missequencing of the days of the week and months of the year and a tendency to allergies such as asthma and hay fever. In short it is probably a syndrome that has a neurological basis.

This idea was very unpopular until recently, both because it seemed to offer dyslexics very little hope of improvement and also because many denied that dyslexia existed at all. It was strongly argued that dyslexia was a term embraced by the middle classes to conceal their children's backwardness! But the neurological basis of dyslexia has recently received much greater support from the finding that dyslexics often lack the normal anatomical asymmetry of the language areas in the temporal lobe. In non-dyslexics, the planum temporale on the left is on average three times greater than that on the right, whereas in dyslexics the two sides are equal or that on the right is larger (Galaburda et al., 1985). Furthermore, Galaburda and colleagues found in post-mortem brains of dyslexics that neuropathological abnormalities such as ectopias and microgyrias are common, particularly in the language areas on the left as well as in their homologues in the right hemisphere.

Quite commonly dyslexics complain that letters and words appear to move around when they look at small print. Hence, they are never quite sure how the words they are trying to read should appear; and so they tend to missequence and misspell words. As a result they make characteristic errors when trying to read. Because their mind's eye presents them with a confused jumble of letters, if they pronounce what they see, they tend to produce nonsense rather than real words (Cornelissen et al., 1991). We believe that this perceptual instability, which amounts to mild oscillopsia, probably results from their having unstable binocular eye movement control (Fowler, 1991); this is analogous to the more severe degree of oscillopsia that often accompanies breakdown of ocular motor control in conditions such as nystagmus. When these children attempt to fixate a small target, such as a letter, their eyes tend to move around more than those of non-dyslexic subjects (Eden *et al.*, 1994). This instability is also apparent when the children attempt to pursue a moving target with their eyes. Instead of being able to follow it smoothly, their eyes tend to lag behind; so they need to make many catch-up saccades (saccadic intrusions) to keep it on the fovea (Adler-Grinberg and Stark, 1978). Nobody's eyes are entirely stationary during fixation; but the binocular control of these dyslexics is very much worse than normal, and also, unlike non-dyslexics, they do not seem to be able to learn to compensate for these eye movements.

For the last 15 years Bill Lovegrove and his colleagues in Australia have been collecting evidence that the 'transient' component of visual processing is impaired in dyslexics (Lovegrove *et al.*, 1982). This system is responsible for tracking rapid temporal changes. It is most sensitive to low contrast and low spatial and high temporal frequencies; hence, it responds well to visual motion. In dyslexics, both static and flicker contrast sensitivity measurements, together with visible persistence and masking studies, point to the same conclusion, that their transient system is compromised. We have been able to confirm that English dyslexics have the same problems. They, too, exhibit impaired transient system function in static and flicker contrast sensitivity tests (Mason *et al.*, 1993). We have also shown that they have an elevated threshold for detecting motion in random dot displays (Cornelissen *et al.*, 1995); this is known to be a sensitive test of transient function.

Another way of measuring transient system function in humans is to measure the visual evoked potentials in response to flickering low contrast stimuli. We, and others, have shown that in dyslexics these are reduced and delayed (Livingstone *et al.*, 1991; Maddock *et al.*, 1992). This delay implies that the neuronal systems responsible for transient processing are in some way impaired, which Livingstone and colleagues (1991) were able to show is indeed the case. The magnocellular layers of the LGN in five dyslexic brains were found to be disorganised and the number and size of the magnocells reduced compared with non-dyslexics. As the magnocellular system is thought to underpin transient processing this result is not unexpected.

Thus, dyslexics appear to have impaired development of the magnocellular processing of their visual system and also impaired ocularmotor control. What is the connection between the two? The magnocellular system is known to be responsible for timing events in the visual world, and therefore for signalling the motion of visual targets. It is not surprising, therefore, to find that the magnocellular system dominates ocularmotor control. The superior colliculus, which is responsible for reflex control of eye movements, receives its main input from the magnocellular system. The main output of the cortical visual system involved with controlling eye movements is the dorsomedial 'where' stream that culminates in the PPC. It, too, is dominated by the magnocellular system. Therefore, if the magnocellular layers of the LGN are inactivated in monkeys, ocularmotor control is most severely affected (Merigan and Maunsell, 1993). In particular, smooth pursuit is impaired and fixation becomes less stable. It will not have escaped the reader's attention that these are precisely the problems that we have found to afflict dyslexics.

Magnocells are not confined to the visual system; they are found in all the sensory and motor systems. The neurological abnormality that causes dyslexia can express itself in many other ways besides visuomotor problems. Most dyslexics also have auditory processing defects. An important skill for learning to read and for practised readers to read unfamiliar words, is the ability to segment the sounds of words. These must be broken down to their constituent phonemes in order to match with the graphemes that represent them. Dyslexics are extremely bad at such phonemic segmentation; they fail in rhyming, alliteration, pig latin and many other tests that require phonological analysis (Bradley and Bryant, 1983; Liberman *et al.*, 1974; Snowling, 1987).

Recent evidence suggests that, like their visuomotor impairment, the phonological problems of dyslexics are probably also caused by a more fundamental processing defect. They require a longer than normal processing time to distinguish consonants reliably (phonemic categorisation – Tallal and Schwartz, 1980). Likewise they confuse consonant vowel pairs, particularly sybillants, more easily than normals do (Cornelissen *et al.*, 1996). This is probably because their ability to analyse sounds that are changing rapidly in time (sound transients) is slightly impaired. We have recently shown that many basic sound processing operations that depend upon detecting temporal transients as opposed to identifying spectral cues, may be compromised in dyslexics. Thus, their pitch discrimination is significantly worse than non-dyslexics, as is their ability to detect small frequency or amplitude modulations. Likewise, their ability to detect temporal differences between the two ears, as measured by the binaural masking level difference is significantly worse than non-dyslexics (McAnally, 1994). All these problems may result from impaired magnocellular transient function in the auditory domain. Recently, Rosen and colleagues (1996) have shown that the magnocellular division of the auditory medial geniculate nucleus is disorganised and that the neurons are smaller, as was found to be the case for the LGN. What was particularly interesting was that, whereas in normal subjects the magnocellular nucleus on the left is larger, this difference was not found in dyslexics. The lack of hemispheric asymmetry favouring the left in dyslexics may well correlate with this.

In summary, it seems that dyslexics have impaired development of magnocellular neurons in the brain. This may explain both their phonological and visuomotor problems. In the case of the visual system, impaired magnocellular development seems to lead to lowered contrast sensitivity at low spatial frequencies, reduced flicker contrast sensitivity, impaired motion detection, delayed flicker evoked potentials, and unstable ocularmotor control. Unstable ocularmotor control at a crucial stage in development leads to unstable visual perceptions, hence visual confusions and the visual non-word errors that dyslexics characteristically make.

How does any of this relate to colour vision, the subject of this volume? Empirically it has been discovered that many children with reading problems benefit from viewing print through coloured filters. In fact, some people are making fortunes out of this unproven treatment. We routinely test all the children with visual problems who we see with a selection of coloured overlays (neutral density, red, blue, green, yellow) through which to look at print. Usually the children see no differently through them; and the child expresses no preference for a particular colour.

Occasionally, however, a child presents with low vision in both eyes for which we can find no retinal or refractive cause, and finds that the yellow filters help them to see much more clearly. Typically, these children have low Snellen acuity, reduced accommodation and vergence, reduced stereoacuity and lowered contrast sensitivity, particularly at low spatial frequencies. In this small group (about one per cent of all our referrals) the yellow spectacles reverse these impairments; and if the children are less than 8 years old, a few months of wearing the yellow spectacles may correct their vision permanently (Fowler *et al.*, 1992). Unfortunately, however, whatever the cause of the problem, it seems to be irreversible in older children.

The effect of yellow filters cannot be explained by placebo or psychological effects. We have also ruled out chromatic aberration as the cause. Moreover, the children are not colour blind; we have not found any of the classical cone defects in any of them. Our current hypothesis is that yellow filters help them, because, for some reason, they have an abnormal sensitivity to blue. In non-dyslexics, blue probably makes a small inhibitory input to the achromatic luminance system. Possibly in these children this inhibitory input is much greater than usual; hence the use of yellow filters helps them by their 'negative blue' effect.

A rather larger number of children, perhaps 7.5 per cent of those referred to us, complain of photophobia, and that print and text seem to move around and shimmer. Many are helped by blue filters. These children may have a higher than normal contrast sensitivity at high spatial frequencies; but we have not confirmed these clinical results yet using more accurate psychophysical tests. We have shown, however, that they have a higher threshold than normals for detecting motion in random dot displays. One possibility is that these children have overactive transient systems; the 'negative yellow' effect of blue filters would limit this. Another possibility is that the transient, luminance channel inhibits the sustained chromatic channels more in these children for some reason. Blue filters might alleviate this by cutting transient activity; but we do not know yet whether this is the right explanation.

In summary, we have found two groups of patients with visual symptoms who are helped by coloured filters. Our hypothesis is that these filters change the balance between the magnocellular, transient, achromatic or luminance channel compared with the parvocellular, sustained, or chromatic channel; and that this is the way coloured filters improve their visual processing.

10.8.1   REFERENCES

ADLER-GRINBERG, D. & STARK, L. (1978) Eye movements, scan paths and dyslexia, *American Journal of Optometry and Physiological Optics*, **55**, 557–570.

BRADLEY, L. & BRYANT, P. (1983) Categorising sounds and learning to read – a causal connection, *Nature*, **301**, 419–421.

CORNELISSEN, P., BRADLEY, L., FOWLER, M.S. & STEIN, J.F. (1991) What children see affects how they read, *Developmental Medicine & Child Neurology*, **33**, 755–762.

CORNELISSEN P.L., RICHARDSON, A.R., MASON, A, FOWLER, M.S. & STEIN, J.F. (1995) Contrast sensitivity and coherent motion detection measured at photopic luminance levels in dyslexics & controls, *Vision Research*, **35**, 1483–1494.

CORNELISSEN, P.L., HANSEN, P.C., BRADLEY, L. & STEIN, J.F. (1996) Analysis of perceptual confusions between 9 sets of consonant-vowel sounds in normal and dyslexic adults, *Cognition* (in press).

EDEN, G.F., STEIN, J.F., WOOD, H.M. & WOOD, F.B. (1994) Differences in eye movements and reading problems in dyslexic and normal children, *Vision Research*, **34**, 1345–1358.

FOWLER, M.S. (1991) Binocular instability in dyslexics. In: Stein, J.F. (Ed.) *Vision and Visual Dysfunction, Vol 13*, London: Macmillan Press.

FOWLER, M.S., MASON, A.J.S., RICHARDSON, A.J. & STEIN, J.F. (1992) Yellow glasses improve the vision of children with binocular amblyopia, *Lancet*, **340**, 724.

GALABURDA, A., ROSEN, G. & SHERMAN, G.P. (1985) Developmental dyslexia: four consecutive cases with cortical anomalies, *Annals of Neurology*, **18**, 222–233.

LIBERMAN, I.Y., SHANKWEILER, D., FISCHER, F.W. & CARTER, B. (1974) Explicit syllable and phoneme segmentation in the young child, *Journal of Experimental Child Psychology*, **18**, 201–212.

LIVINGSTONE, M.S., ROSEN, G.D., DRISLANE, F.W. & GALABURDA, A.M. (1991) Physiological and anatomical evidence for a magnocellular defect in developmental dyslexia, *Proceedings of the National Academy of Science*, **88**, 7943–7947.

LOVEGROVE, W.J., MARTIN, F., BOWLING, A., BLACKWOOD, M., BADCOCK D. & PAXTON, S. (1982) Contrast sensitivity functions and specific reading disability, *Neuropsychologia*, **20**(3), 309–315.

McANALLY, K. (1994) Reduced auditory temporal resolution in dyslexic subjects? *Poster presentation at the 23rd Rodin Academy International Conference*, Malta.

MADDOCK, H., RICHARDSON, A. & STEIN, J.F. (1992) Reduced and delayed visual evoked potentials in dyslexics, *Journal of Physiology*, **459**, 130P.

MASON, A., CORNELISSEN, P., FOWLER, M.S. & STEIN, J.F. (1993) Contrast sensitivity, ocular dominance and reading disability, *Clinical Visual Science*, **8**, 345–353.

MERIGAN, W.H. & MAUNSELL, J.R. (1993) How parallel are the primate visual pathways? *Annual Review of Neuroscience*, **16**, 369–402.

ROSEN, G., GALABURDA, A. & SHERMAN, G. (1996) Impaired magnocellular organisation in the medial geniculate nucleus of dyslexics, *Annals of the New York Academy of Science*, (in press)

RUTTER, M. & YULE, W. (1975) Specific reading retardation, *Journal of Child Psychiatry*, **16**, 181–197.

SNOWLING, M (1987) *Dyslexia*, London: Blackwells.

TALLAL, P & SCHWARTZ, J. (1980) Temporal processing, speech perception and hemispheric asymmetry, *Trends in Neurosciences*, **3**, 309–311.

Visual Defence or Facilitation Processes Favoured by Alarming or Playful Colours

Paolo Bonaiuto, Anna Maria Giannini, Valeria Biasi,
Margherita Miceu Romano and Marino Bonaiuto

10.9.1 INTRODUCTION

The colour perception can be itself an occasion in which anomalies take place: from dischromatopsias described by John Dalton, to certain colour incongruities and related illusions (Bonaiuto et al., 1990b; Bruner and Postman, 1949; Bruner et al., 1951). However, do colours, even when exactly perceived, influence the perception of other anomalies, for example, object, shape, size, or position incongruities? Based on our work, the answer is positive. This article summarises some experiments showing that colours, because of their meanings and physiognomic properties, can contribute toward mobilising defence or facilitation processes in incongruity perception.[1]

We show how emotional properties, also mediated by colours, can influence structural qualities of objects leading to surprising underevaluation or overevaluation effects. These effects can be understood only by referring to the general dynamic of perception processes, including interest in avoiding or preventing 'negative' emotions and facilitating pleasant ones.

10.9.2 PERCEPTUAL DEFENCE OR FACILITATION TOWARD AN INCONGRUENT BUILDING SHAPE

Experimental subjects were volunteer university students or graduates, equally divided for sex, between 19 and 39 years of age. All participants were examined separately.

The first investigation was carried out in the 1980s by Bonaiuto, Giannini and Bonaiuto (1992). A tridimensional model of a modern building, with a square base, six storeys and an attic, was used in two versions. The model is 40 cm high and observed from a distance of 2 m. There is a horizontal fracture line halfway up the building, with partial sliding of the upper part forward, over the lower part. Therefore, the building has a *bayonet shape*; the slipping is 27 per cent of the lateral width of the facade. This model was shown to the subject in two different positions: from the front, so that the sliding appears anterior-posterior, tending to flatten out – this situation can be defined as perceptually *ambiguous* – or in profile, with lateral sliding (toward the right) in full view – perceptually *unequivocal* situation. Each subject saw two versions of the building in each position (from the front or in profile). The two versions present contrasting emotional qualities because of their colour and several symbolic details, in which colour again plays an important role.

1. Building with *alarming* and *threatening* decoration, also sad and serious. The plaster is primarily grey-violet; the door and window frames are yellow; red and black curtains can be glimpsed through the windows. Details include: vases with dried flowers, lighted candles, a black, yellow and red lantern, black, grey or yellowish cloth, the symbol of the skull, a sculpture of a long grey amphora surmounted by a sort of black vulture; a dried-up plant, chains, coats of arms, scythes, halberds.
2. Building with *playful* and *reassuring* decoration, also happy and protective. The walls are mostly bright pink; the door and window frames are emerald green; beyond the windows – with white and blue reflections – orange curtains with red polka dots can be glimpsed. Details include: flower pots with many small green leaves and multi-coloured flowers, multi-coloured Chinese lanterns, lamps, small flags and balloons, a kite, some toys and an abstract sculpture with bright colours.

The apparent building shapes were evaluated by 24 subjects. Comparison scales containing seven shapes derived from a rectangle were used, to present the sliding of the upper part with respect to the lower part, with values increasing from 0 per cent to 54 per cent of the width of the rectangle (Figure 10.9.1). Both 'ascending' and 'descending' scales were used for each position of the building and for each 'emotional' version of the model (random sequence).

The attribution of the 'negative' or 'positive' appearance in terms of *emotional qualities* was checked by using other groups of subjects; they completed several 7-point evaluation scales with pairs of contrasting adjectives, providing strongly divergent semantic profiles (alarming, threatening, serious, sad, etc., first building, versus reassuring, protective, playful, happy, etc., second building).

A further check consisted in the construction and use of two 'non-buildings', i.e. of control objects with the same shapes and dimensions as the two described models, but without architectural details. They were homogeneous for colour, one bright pink and the other grey-violet, with the same basic colours used in the above-described architectural models. Using the same procedure as the one adopted for building models, these were shown to a new group of 24 persons.

Overall, in terms of evaluation of shape, the effects obtained with these four objects are significant. With building models, a striking underevaluation effect linked to the ambiguous perceptual conditions was found, as well as an overevaluation effect in the unequivocal ones. On the whole, the anomaly is underestimated in the model with the

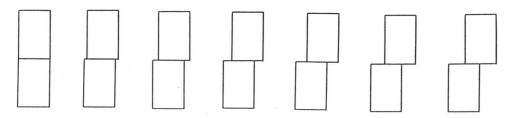

Figure 10.9.1. The apparent building shapes presented to the subjects.

alarming and threatening appearance; and is overestimated in the other model (Figure 10.9.2).

Interesting findings also emerge with the control objects. Examined using the scale of adjectives, the 'non buildings' show slight differences similar to those for the buildings, i.e. the pink object appears a little more playful and a little less alarming than the grey-violet one. The same objects, examined using the comparison scale for visual shape, show a weak structural effect similar to that observed much more strikingly with the architectural models (Figure 10.9.3). The shape irregularity is slightly, but significantly, more appreciated in the bright pink object. However, with respect to the architectural models, the differences between the two objects are significantly reduced, and there is no real overestimation of the shape anomaly in the unequivocal perceptual conditions.

10.9.3 PERCEPTUAL DEFENCE OR FACILITATION TOWARD SCENES OF CONGESTED URBAN TRAFFIC

In a more recent investigation, another environmental anomaly was proposed as an experimental situation: a scene of *very congested urban traffic* (Bonaiuto *et al.*, 1993b,

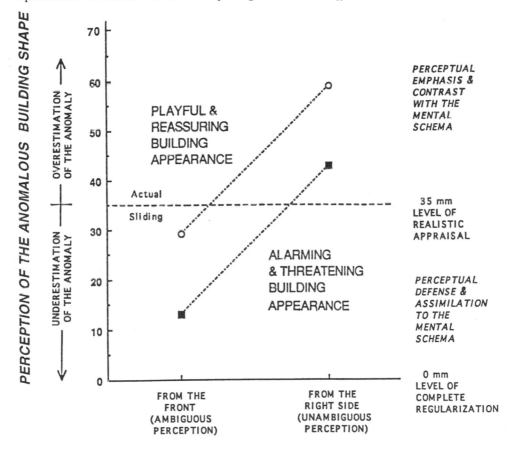

OBSERVATION CONDITIONS

Figure 10.9.2. The perception of the building models by the subjects.

1993c). Here, the *apparent number of cars* constitutes the dependent variable, for psychological measurement. Preference was given to the most crucial observation conditions, i.e. the unequivocal ones.

A very detailed illustration of 27 cars, crowding an intersection, was prepared; they appear between high buildings and other urban elements (the edge of a public park, a pavement corner with a news-stand). The scene, on vertical rectangular pasteboard, measures 25 x 32 cm.

Two contrasting versions of the same scene were prepared in colour, using water colour on collages made with photographs of real cars; colour photocopies of the originals were then made.

1. The first congested urban traffic scene has an overall *alarming* and *threatening* colour decoration and appears sad and serious. The facades of the buildings are characterised by predominantly grey-violet colours; tones, decorations and details are the same as those in the previous experiment. The 27 cars are consistent with this environment: the dominant colours and shades are violet, grey, black, olive green, with touches of yellow and dark red; there are also worrisome symbols.

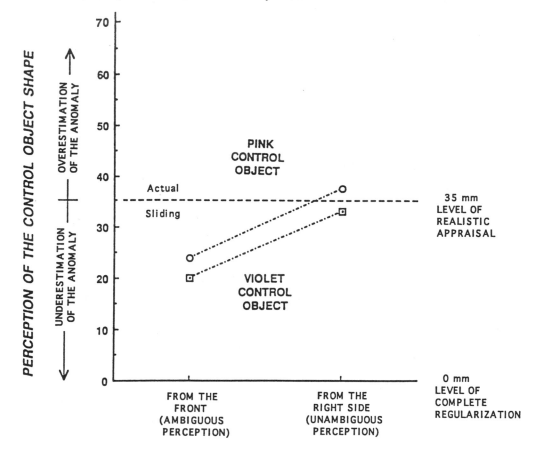

Figure 10.9.3. The perception of the control objects by the subjects.

2. In the contrasting experimental table, colour decoration of the congested urban traffic scene can be defined as *playful* and *reassuring*, as well as happy and protective. Again, taking indications from our previous experiment, the facades of the buildings are primarily pink, with touches of blue, white and light green. The 27 cars are in harmony with the surrounding scene; their colours and shades include bright pink, orange, light blue and light green, with touches of bright red and yellow, with a smooth look; the symbols are joyful.

The experimental material also includes three training scenes, with 9, 17 and 27 cars outlined simply in black and white (Figure 10.9.4). The subject, seated at a table, must immediately – at first glance and without counting – tell how many cars he/she sees in each scene.

To avoid the interference of systematic individual differences in the tendency to over- or underestimate the number, we regulated access to one or the other test scene in order to balance the mean values of the cars seen in the training tables by the two opposing experimental groups. Each group included 32 participants (*between subjects* design).

Another important control condition was created by preparing two additional coloured tables in which the dominating colours cited above, i.e. the violet-grey, olive green 'alarming' series, or the pink-orange, light blue, light green 'playful' series, are applied to a group of 27 simple squares, similar to those in Figure 10.9.5. We assumed that there are no particular mental schemata and expectations, concerning these geometrical figures, comparable to those which can be reasonably hypothesised for urban traffic. Again, two groups of 32 subjects were examined with a procedure similar to the previous one.[2]

At this point, our hypotheses can be better outlined in these terms: overall, it is expected that in these unequivocal perceptual conditions there will be a general overestimation of the number of cars, because of the pro-active contrast between the congested urban traffic

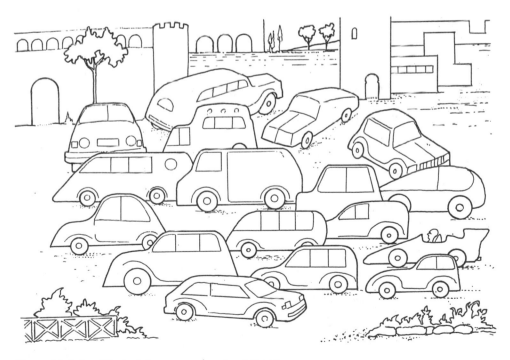

Figure 10.9.4. The training scene showing 17 cars.

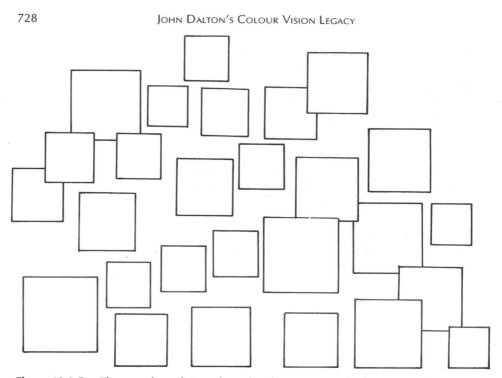

Figure 10.9.5.   The contol condition where the objects are simple squares.

scene and the mental schema of normal traffic. But it is also expected that the scene of congested traffic in the 'playful and reassuring' version will allow for greater perceptual acceptance and, therefore, a relative overestimation of the environmental anomaly, expressed by the number of cars indicated by the subjects at first glance. The contrasting scene, i.e. 'alarming and threatening', should lead to perceptual defence and thus, to an estimation of a significantly lower number, at least with respect to the other scene; with the possibility of an interesting conflict with the contrast factor due to mental schema, in any case, favouring overestimation. With regard to the two control tables (coloured squares), there should be neither overestimations nor significant differences in the perception of numbers.

The results of the experiment, expressed in Table 10.9.1, seem to confirm the hypotheses.[3]

10.9.4   DISCUSSION

Three different types of psychological processes must be considered to understand the observed phenomena.

First, underevaluation of incongruities in the ambiguous perceptual conditions is a process of confirmation of expectations and coincides with a pro-active assimilation effect of the actual perceptual image to the corresponding mental schema (for example, the general schema of a building, is a very regular shape).

In the unambiguous perceptual conditions, the opposite effect occurs (a contrast effect) and shape anomalies, or anomalous numerosity, are emphasised. Consideration of these processes follows a remarkable phenomenological and psychodynamic tradition (Bonaiuto, 1965, 1967, 1970, 1978; Bonaiuto et al., 1986; Bonaiuto et al., 1987, 1990a, 1992; Bonaiuto et al., 1993a; Musatti, 1931). References and comparisons are also proposed with works by Usnadze (1939), Volkmann (1951), Natadze (1960), Sherif and Hovland (1961), Bevan and Turner (1964).

Second, consideration of the connections between a specific structural and/or chromatic order and several emotionally relevant tones, which are summarised in the qualifications of 'alarming', 'playful', etc., derives directly from both pictorial practice and tradition and from previous studies on expressiveness related to shapes and colours (Arnheim, 1949; Bonaiuto, 1967, 1978; Canestrari, 1961; Lersch, 1932; Metzger, 1954, 1963; Werner, 1940).

Third, consideration of defence or facilitation processes in perception is dictated by the reality of the observations made (without recourse to these processes the observations would be incomprehensible) and is connected historically with classical works by Bruner and Postman (1947), Postman, Bruner and McGinnies (1948), McGinnies (1949), Dixon (1981) and others.

10.9.4.1 Further comments on the traffic experiment.

With the second traffic scene (playful and reassuring) and with respect to a realistic appraisal (27 cars), the increase given by perceptual facilitation is favoured in the results; this process goes in the same direction as contrast with the mental schema and, therefore, increases the overestimation, which could have been expected also in the absence of the special role of the emotional qualities.

Table 10.9.1 Average estimation of the number of cars in the training or test tables regarding the traffic scene, and average apparent number of squares in the corresponding control tables

Experimental or control situations		Average apparent number of objects		Comparison by rows with analysis of variance
		Subjects presented with the emotionally alarming and threatening test table (or control table)	Subjects presented with the emotionally playful and reassuring test table (or control table)	
Training tables (T) before coloured scenes of congested traffic	T_1 9 cars	8.69	8.83	$F_{1,62} = 0.00$; ns
	T_2 17 cars	16.05	16.00	$F_{1,62} = 0.00$; ns
	T_3 27 cars	25.84	26.98	$F_{1,62} = 1.84$; ns
Test tables: coloured scenes of congested traffic with 27 cars		26.58	31.38	$F_{1,62} = 12.95$ $p < 0.001$
Corresponding control tables: assemblages of 27 coloured squares		25.18	25.22	$F_{1,62} = 0.00$; ns

In the opposite case, the decrease in the number because of perceptual defence conflicts with the contrast direction with respect to the mental schema; this contrast always favours an overestimation of the number of cars in the scene, which is always one of congested traffic. Therefore, in the latter situation (i.e. with the 'alarming and threatening' traffic table) these two components tend to balance each other and the appraisal becomes close to the realistic one.

Other factors agreeing or conflicting with the emotional message given by colours can be added and experimentally tested; it is also possible to carry out experiments with only colours, without the presence of other symbols or messages. Our research group is conducting investigations in both of those directions.

10.9.5   NOTES

1   The experiments have been partially described and discussed elsewhere (Bonaiuto et al., 1992; Bonaiuto et al., 1993b). A paper recently published in Italy contains four colour plates that reproduce the coloured configurations exactly: building models and traffic scenes with playful or alarming colours (Bonaiuto et al., 1993c; see for an eventual replication of the experiments and an examination of the colour figures, described here). Both the investigations and the authors' participation in related national or international conferences, were supported by: C. N. R. (Committees 08, 10 and 13), Ministero della Pubblica Instruzione, Ministero dell'Università e della Ricerca Scientifica e Tecnologica, Università di Roma 'La Sapienza', and ISAPS (1983–1993).

2   The emotional qualities in the coloured experimental tables (cars) or control tables (squares) were measured – similar to the experiment with the models of fractured buildings – using groups of subjects that were not part of the main experiment; they used evaluation scales with contrasting pairs of adjectives. Also, in this new investigation (and particularly in the case of 'traffic'), the semantic profiles are strongly divergent, in agreement with the experimental assumptions.

3   According to the methodological cautions expressed, the means of the perceived numerosity for the training tables in the two experimental groups dealing with the traffic scenes were equivalent, i.e. they showed no significant differences. Also, overall they appear rather realistic. Due to their simplified drawing style, the three training tables, which hint at a very broad urban environment, do not necessarily favour the experience of congested traffic; further, one of these tables presents only nine outlines of cars and, thus, is easy to estimate exactly.

10.9.6   REFERENCES

ARNHEIM, R. (1949) The Gestalt theory of expression, *Psychological Review*, **56**, 156–171.

BEVAN, W. & TURNER, E.D. (1964) Assimilation and contrast in the estimation of numbers, *Journal of Experimental Psychology*, **67**, 458–462.

BONAIUTO, P. (1965) Tavola d'inquadramento e di previsione degli 'effetti di campo' e dinamica delle qualità fenomeniche, *Giorn. Psich. Neuropat.*, **93** (4 suppl.), 1443–1685 (reprint, Rome: Kappa).

BONAIUTO, P. (1967) *Le motivazioni dell'attività nell'età evolutiva. Analisi fenomenologica, riferimenti e indicazioni per la sperimentazione*, Milan: CMSR (reprint, Rome: Kappa).

BONAIUTO, P. (1970) Sulle ricerche psicologiche europee in tema di monotonia percettiva e motoria ('Sensory Deprivation' e simili). Il processo della saturazione di qualità fenomeniche, *Rassegna Neuropsich.*, **24** (3-4), 1–114 (reprint, Rome: Kappa).

BONAIUTO, P. (1978) *Forme lineari e bande colorate. Un reattivo per la valutazione delle capacità di percepire l'espressività visuale*, Rome: Università di Roma 'La Sapienza'.

BONAIUTO, P., MICEU ROMANO, M. & BONAIUTO F. (1986) Phenomena of reduction or increase in perceptual irregularity of architectural structures and environments. In: Krampen, M. (Ed.), Environment and Human Action, Berlin: Hochschule der Kunste, pp. 18–22.

BONAIUTO, P., GIANNINI, A.M. & BONAIUTO, M. (1987) Elaborazione de conflitto cognitivo nella percezione di architetture. In: Bianchi, E., Perussia, F. & Rossi, M. (Eds), Immagine soggettiva e ambiente. Problemi, applicazioni e strategie della ricerca, Milan: Unicopli, pp. 99–116.

BONAIUTO, P., GIANNINI, A.M. & BONAIUTO, M. (1990a) Piloting mental schemata on building images. In: Fusco, A., Battisti, F. & Tomassoni, R. (Eds), Recent Experiences in General and Social Psychology in Italy and Poland, Milan: Angeli, pp. 85–130.

BONAIUTO, P., MICEU ROMANO, M. & BONAIUTO, M. (1990b) 'Colour modification effects in the perception of colour incongruities', presentation at the 13th European Conference on Visual Perception, Paris.

BONAIUTO, P., GIANNINI, A.M. & BONAIUTO, M. (1992) Metamorphoses of building perception: Experimental observations. In: Mazis, A. & Karaletsou, C. (Eds), Socio-Environmental Metamorphoses: Builtscape, Landscape, Ethnoscape, Euroscape. Vol II, Thessaoloniki: Aristotle University Thessaloniki Publications Office, pp. 294–301.

BONAIUTO, P., GIANNINI, A.M. & BARTOLI, G. (1993a) Incongruity perceptions, personality features and attitudes towards transgressive behavior descriptions. In: Van Heck, G.L., Bonaiuto, P., Dreary, I.J. & Nowack, W. (Eds), Personality Psychology in Europe. Vol 4, Tilburg: Tilburg University Press, pp. 85–104.

BONAIUTO, P., GIANNINI, A.M. BIASI, V., MICEU ROMANO, M. & BONAIUTO M. (1993b) Contrasting meaningful influences of environmental physiognomic properties on perceptual paradoxes, presentation at the 3rd Hungarian-Italian Psychology Conference.

BONAIUTO, P., GIANNINI, A.M. BIASI, V., MICEU ROMANO, M. & BONAIUTO, M. (1993c) Qualità emotive, emozioni reali e percezione ambientale, presentation at the Convegno Annuale di Studi sulle Emozioni, Lecce, Attualità in Psicologia, 9 (1), 129–157.

BRUNER, J.S. & POSTMAN, L. (1947) Emotional selectivity in perception and reaction, Journal of Personality, 16, 69–77.

BRUNER, J.S. & POSTMAN, L. (1949) On the perception of incongruity: A paradigm, Journal of Personality, 18, 206–223.

BRUNER, J.S., POSTMAN, L. & RODRIGUEZ, J. (1951) Expectation and the perception of color, American Journal of Psychology, 64, 216–227.

CANESTRARI, R. (1961) Espressione ed espressività, presentation at the 2° Colloquio Internaz. Espressione Plastica, Bologna.

DIXON, N.F. (1981) Preconscious Processing, New York: Wiley.

LERSCH, P. (1932) Gesicht und Seele, Leipzig: Reinhardt.

METZGER, W. (1954) Psychologie, Darmstadt: Steinkopf.

METZGER, W. (1963) I fondamenti dell'esperienza estetica, presentation at the 2° Colloquio Internaz. Espressione Plastica, Bologna.

McGINNIES, E. (1949) Emotionality and perceptual defense, Psychological Review, 56, 244–251.

MUSATTI, C.L. (1931) Forma e assimilazione, Archivio Italiano di Psicologia, 9, 61–156.

NATADZE, R. (1960) Emergence of set on the basis of imaginal situations, British Journal of Psychology, 51, 237–245.

POSTMAN, L., BRUNER, J.S. & McGINNIES, E. (1948) Personal values as selective factors in perception, Journal of Abnormal Social Psychology, 43, 142–154.

SHERIF, M. & HOVLAND, C.I. (1961) Social Judgement. Assimilation and Contrast Effects in Communication and Attitude Change, New Haven: Yale University Press.

USNADZE, D. (1939) Untersuchungen zur Psychologie der Einstellung, Acta Psychologica, 4, 323–360.

VOLKMANN, J. (1951) Scales of judgement and their implications for social psychology. In: Rohrer, J.H. & Sherif, M. (Eds), Social Psychology at the Crossroads, New York: Harper.

WERNER, H. (1940) Comparative Psychology of Mental Development, New York: Harper.

Index